Handbook of Evidence-Based Critical Care

D1088655

Handbook of Evidence-Based Critical Care

2nd Edition

Paul Ellis Marik
MBBCh, FCP(SA), FRCP(C), FCCP, FCCM, FACP

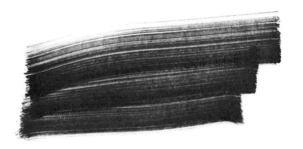

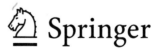 Springer

Paul Ellis Marik, MD
Division of Pulmonary and Critical
  Care Medicine
Eastern Virginia Medical School
Norfolk, VA, USA
marikpe@evms.edu

ISBN 978-1-4419-5922-5   e-ISBN 978-1-4419-5923-2
DOI 10.1007/978-1-4419-5923-2
Springer New York Dordrecht Heidelberg London

Library of Congress Control Number: 2010921986

Printed on acid-free paper

Springer is part of Springer Science+Business Media (www.springer.com)

To Susan, Ernie and Molly,
who have enriched my life.

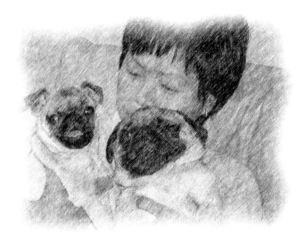

Acknowledgments

This book is dedicated to my mentors and students who have taught me everything I know and inspired me to learn even more.

Preface

Learning without thinking is useless. Thinking without learning is dangerous

– Confucius

Since the publication of the first edition of *The Handbook of Evidence-Based Critical Care* in 2001, the landscape of critical care medicine has changed enormously. Numerous randomized controlled studies (RCTs) that have changed the daily practice of critical care medicine have been published. Furthermore, our understanding of the complex pathophysiology of the critically ill and injured has advanced, new therapies have emerged (and some have fallen by the wayside), and we have refined how we monitor and manage our patients. We have also recognized our limitations and improved end-of-life care. In all, we are *wiser* and more attuned to the challenges of providing care to the sickest of the sick. However, the basic guiding principles of critical care medicine have not changed; compassionate, dedicated and thoughtful clinicians, who evaluate the functioning of the "whole" patient, ponder their disease processes and pathophysiology and provide the highest level of *evidence-based* interventions with the goal of restoring the patient to a quality of life which he/she values. The second edition of *The Handbook of Evidence-Based Critical Care* chronicles the remarkable progress made in the last decade and sets the stage for what is yet to come!

The focus of this handbook is on issues that pertain specifically to the ICU. As such the reader is referred to standard medical and surgical texts as well as online resources for more complete information on the wide spectrum of conditions and diseases from which ICU patients may suffer.

Paul Ellis Marik
Norfolk, Virginia

Contents

Part I

Introduction to Critical Care Medicine

As critical care medicine has evolved into a discreet specialty that crosses anatomical and other artificial boundaries and deals with an enormous array of human conditions, it has become evident that to achieve the best outcomes for our very complex patients, all our clinical decisions should be based on the *best available evidence*. The complexity of the critically ill patient together with the vast armamentarium of therapeutic options available makes it essential that we critically evaluate established and emerging clinical practices. Bone throwing, bloodletting, witchcraft, and other forms of hocus-pocus have no role in modern critical care. However, it is important to realize that critical care medicine can be practiced only by close observation of the patient (at the bedside), by contemplation, and by the integration of a large data base of evidence-based medicine together with a good deal of humility.

The *Handbook of Evidence-Based Critical Care* is not a reference text but presents a practical *evidence-based approach* to the management of critically ill ICU patients. Due to the vast number of therapeutic interventions that ICU physicians make daily, the topics are presented as narrative summaries of the *best available evidence* rather than as systematic reviews of each and every intervention. While all attempts have been made to be current, due to the exponential growth of medical knowledge, some of the information presented may already be outdated when this book comes to print. The reader therefore should keep up-to-date with the current medical literature. In keeping with the goal of providing an evidence-based approach to critical care, references are provided to support the evidence presented.

ALERT

The guidelines presented in the book are not meant to replace clinical judgment but rather to provide a framework to patient management. Individual clinical situations can be highly complex and the judgment and wisdom of an experienced and knowledgeable intensivist with all available information about a specific patient is essential for optimal clinical management.

■ REFERENCES

1. Osler W. Preface. The Principles and Practice of Medicine. 8th ed. New York: D. Appleton & Co.; 1918.
2. Sackett DL, Richardson WS, Rosenberg W, Haynes RB. Evidence-Based Medicine. How to Practice and Teach EBM. New York: Churchill Livingstone; 1997.

3. Science. http://en.wikipedia.org/wiki/Science. Wikipedia. Accessed December 3, 2009.
4. Rissmiller R. Patients are not airplanes and doctors are not pilots [Letter]. *Crit Care Med.* 2006;34:2869.
5. Laurance J. Peter Pronovost: champion of checklists in critical care. *Lancet.* 2009;374:443.

2

Classic Critical Care Papers

A limited number of publications have had a dramatic impact on the practice of critical care medicine. These publications are regarded as "compulsory" reading for residents, fellows, and other practitioners of critical care medicine. Surprisingly, although not unexpectedly, those publications with the potential to have the most dramatic positive impact on patient care have been slow to be adopted, while publications of questionable scientific rigor are frequently adopted with an unexplained religious fervor. This chapter reviews those papers which have dramatically altered the practice of critical care medicine (for good or bad) as well as those "classic" papers that have shaped the history of critical care medicine.

Perhaps the most important publication in the history of critical care medicine is that of the ARDSNet low vs. standard tidal volume study.[1] This study demonstrated a significant reduction in 28-day mortality in patients randomized to the low tidal volume group (6 ml/kg PBW) as compared to the traditional tidal volume (12 ml/kg PBW) group. The results of this study are supported by extensive experimental and clinical studies. Furthermore, high tidal volumes are associated with progressive lung injury in patients who initially do not have acute lung injury. A tidal volume of 6–8 ml/kg is therefore considered the standard of care for *all* ICU patients. A follow-up study by the ARDSNet group suggested that a fluid management strategy that aims to keep patients "dry" improves patient outcome (significant increase in ventilator-free days).

Kress and colleagues[2] demonstrated that in patients who are receiving mechanical ventilation, daily interruption of sedative drug infusions decreases the duration of mechanical ventilation and the length of stay

P.E. Marik, *Handbook of Evidence-Based Critical Care*,
DOI 10.1007/978-1-4419-5923-2_2,
© Springer Science+Business Media, LLC 2010

in the intensive care. Ely and colleagues[3,4] have demonstrated that a non-physician-directed protocol of spontaneous breathing trials expedites weaning and shortens the duration of mechanical ventilation. Recently, Girard and colleagues[5] demonstrated that a wake up and breathe protocol that pairs daily spontaneous awakening trials (i.e., interruption of sedatives) with daily spontaneous breathing trials results in better outcomes for mechanically ventilated patients than do the "standard approaches." This approach should be considered the standard of care in all ICU patients.

Blood transfusions and the choice of resuscitation fluid have until recently been a controversial issue. In a landmark study, Hebert and colleagues[6] compared a conservative (transfusion for Hb <7 g/dl) vs. liberal (transfusion for Hb <10 g/dl) blood transfusion protocol. In this study the complication rate and 28-day mortality tended to be lower in the conservative group. These results of this study are supported by a meta-analysis of cohort studies, which clearly establishes the benefits of a restrictive blood transfusion strategy.[7] The SAFE study demonstrated the safety of albumin in critically ill patients,[8] while the VISEP study demonstrated an increased risk of renal failure and death in critically ill patients resuscitated with a hydroxyethyl starch solution.[9]

Beginning in the 1960s, Dr. Max Harry Weil[10,11] (the father of critical care medicine) demonstrated the relationship between lactate and the reversibility of shock. Furthermore, in what is now a landmark study, Dr. Weil and colleagues[12] demonstrated a marked difference in arterial and mixed venous acid–base status in patients undergoing CPR. These studies ushered in our current approach to the monitoring of tissue oxygenation in the critically ill patients.

In 1982, Shoemaker and colleagues[13] published a study suggesting that achieving "supranormal" levels of oxygen delivery improved the outcome of critically ill patients. This approach became very fashionable in the late 1980s and the early 1990s and became part of the ICU culture encouraging the (excessive) use of the pulmonary artery catheter (PAC). Subsequent, RCTs were unable to demonstrate the benefit of this approach with the suggestion that driving up oxygen delivery to the "magical" end points proposed by Shoemaker and colleagues may be harmful (this became a popular theme!).[14,15]

The "classic" study by Connors et al.[16] in 1996 raised the possibility that the PAC may be harmful in critically ill patients. Subsequent studies have been unable to demonstrate any benefit associated with the use of the PAC.[17] While the use of the PCWP (pulmonary capillary wedge pressure) as measured using the PAC has fallen into disfavor, the central venous pressure (CVP) continues to be used universally to guide fluid management despite convincing evidence that this measurement is as useful as flipping a coin.[18]

The diagnosis and treatment of ventilator-associated pneumonia (VAP) is an important issue in the ICU. Fagon and colleagues[19] compared a diagnostic approach based on lower respiratory tract sampling and quantitative culture with that of the "standard approach." Compared with the non-invasive strategy, the invasive strategy was associated with fewer deaths at 14 days, earlier resolution of organ dysfunction or less antibiotic use in patients suspected of having VAP. Chastre and colleagues[20] compared 8 vs. 15 days of antibiotic therapy in patients with VAP. There was no difference in outcome between the two groups (with the possible exception of those with pseudomonas pneumonia).

Until recently, the optimal dosing of intermittent hemodialysis (IHD) and continuous renal replacement therapy in the ICU was unclear with data suggesting that more aggressive renal replacement therapy (RRT) was associated with improved renal recovery. The VA/NIH Acute Renal Failure Trial Network randomized 1,124 patients with ARF to receive intensive or less intensive RRT.[21] Hemodynamically stable patients underwent IHD (6 vs. 3 times per week) and hemodynamically unstable patients underwent CVVHD (35 vs. 20 ml/kg/h). There was no difference in clinical outcomes between the two groups of patients.

November the 8th was a dark day in the history of critical care. On that day two "studies" were published in the *New England Journal of Medicine* which changed (overnight) the way critical care was practiced around the world.[22,23] Rivers and colleagues[23] randomized 288 patients with severe sepsis and septic shock to "early goal-directed therapy (EGDT)" or standard care. EGDT was reported to be associated with a 16% absolute reduction of hospital death (35% relative reduction in death). Based on this single study, EGDT became adopted as the "standard of care" around the world and has become the cornerstone of the recommendations of the *Surviving Sepsis Campaign*.[24,25] It is however important to recognize that this was an unblinded, small, single-center study with investigators who were highly "invested" in the outcome of the study. By any stretch of the imagination the results of this study were "too good to be true." Recent evidence questions the validity of the findings of the study (see *Wall Street Journal*, lead report, August 14th 2008).[26] While the concept of EGDT intuitively makes sense, the role of the "central venous oxygen saturation" and a CVP >8 cm H_2O as the end points of resuscitation in septic patients is questionable (and not validated) as is the liberal use of blood and other interventions called for by the EGDT protocol (see Chapters 8, 10, and 51). Stay tuned to this interesting saga; a sequel is in the works! [Protocolized Care for Early Septic Shock (ProCESS); NCT00510835]

On the same day that the EGDT study was published, the *Leuven Intensive Insulin Therapy Trial #1* appeared in the *NEJM*.[22] This study compared the outcome of patients randomized to an insulin infusion protocol that achieved "tight glycemic control" (blood glucose 70–110 mg/dl) as compared to "standard glycemic control" (blood glucose 180–200 mg/dl). This study demonstrated a significant reduction in morbidity and mortality in the patients randomized to the "tight glycemic group." Similar to EGDT, based on this single-center, unblinded study performed by highly "invested" investigators, "tight glycemic control" became adopted overnight as the standard of care throughout the world.[27] Subsequent studies have failed to reproduce the findings of van den Berghe et al. and "tight glycemic control" should now be abandoned.

The role of corticosteroids in patients with sepsis and ARDS is controversial. Landmark studies by Annane et al. and Meduri et al. suggested that corticosteroids reduced 28-day mortality in ICU patients with septic shock and ARDS (late), respectively.[28,29] The results of more recent studies have further fueled this controversy.[30–32]

■ REFERENCES

1. Ventilation with lower tidal volumes as compared with traditional tidal volumes for acute lung injury and the acute respiratory distress syndrome. *N Engl J Med*. 2000;342:1301–1308.
2. Kress JP, Pohlman AS, O'Connor MF, et al. Daily interruption of sedative infusions in critically ill patients undergoing mechanical ventilation. *N Engl J Med*. 2000;342:1471–1477.
3. Ely EW, Baker AM, Dunagan DP, et al. Effect on the duration of mechanical ventilation of identifying patients capable of breathing spontaneously. *N Engl J Med*. 1996;335:1864–1869.
4. Ely EW, Bennett PA, Bowton DL, et al. Large scale implementation of a respiratory therapist-driven protocol for ventilator weaning. *Am J Respir Crit Care Med*. 1999;159:439–446.
5. Girard TD, Kress JP, Fuchs BD, et al. Efficacy and safety of a paired sedation and ventilator weaning protocol for mechanically ventilated patients in intensive care (Awakening and Breathing Controlled trial): a randomised controlled trial. *Lancet*. 2008;371:126–134.
6. Hebert PC, Wells G, Blajchman MA, et al. A multicenter, randomized, controlled clinical trial of transfusion requirements in critical care. Transfusion Requirements in Critical Care Investigators, Canadian Critical Care Trials Group. *N Engl J Med*. 1999;340:409–417.
7. Marik PE, Corwin HL. Efficacy of RBC transfusion in the critically ill: a systematic review of the literature. *Crit Care Med*. 2008;36: 2667–2674.
8. Finfer S, Bellomo R, Boyce N, et al. A comparison of albumin and saline for fluid resuscitation in the intensive care unit. *N Engl J Med*. 2004;350:2247–2256.

9. Brunkhorst FM, Engel C, Bloos F, et al. Intensive insulin therapy and pentastarch resuscitation in severe sepsis. *N Engl J Med.* 2008;358: 125–139.
10. Broder G, Weil MH. Excess lactate: an index of reversibility of shock in human patients. *Science.* 1964;143:1457–1459.
11. Weil MH, Afifi AA. Experimental and clinical studies on lactate and pyruvate as indicators of the severity of acute circulatory failure (shock). *Circulation.* 1970;41:989–1001.
12. Weil MH, Rackow E, Trevino R. Difference in acid–base state between venous and arterial blood during cardiopulmonary resuscitation. *N Engl J Med.* 1986;315:153–156.
13. Shoemaker WC, Appel PL, Waxman K, et al. Clinical trial of survivors cardiorespiratory patterns as therapeutic goals in critically ill postoperative patients. *Crit Care Med.* 1982;10:398–403.
14. Gattinoni L, Brazzi L, Pelosi P, et al. A trial of goal-oriented hemodynamic therapy in critically ill patients. *N Engl J Med.* 1995;333: 1025–1032.
15. Hayes MA, Timmins AC, Yau E, et al. Elevation of systemic oxygen delivery in the treatment of critically ill patients. *N Engl J Med.* 1994;330:1717–1722.
16. Connors AF, Speroff T, Dawson NV, et al. The effectiveness of right heart catheterization in the initial care of critically ill patients. *JAMA.* 1996;276:889–897.
17. Harvey S, Harrison DA, Singer M, et al. Assessment of the clinical effectiveness of pulmonary artery catheters in management of patients in intensive care (PAC-Man): a randomised controlled trial. *Lancet.* 2005;366:472–477.
18. Marik PE, Baram M, Vahid B. Does the central venous pressure predict fluid responsiveness? A systematic review of the literature and the tale of seven mares. *Chest.* 2008;134:172–178.
19. Fagon JY, Chastre J, Wolff M, et al. Invasive and non-invasive strategies for management of suspected ventilator-associated pneumonia. *Ann Intern Med.* 2000;132:621–630.
20. Chastre J, Wolff M, Fagon JY, et al. Comparison of 8 vs. 15 days of antibiotic therapy for ventilator-associated pneumonia in adults: a randomized trial. *JAMA.* 2003;290:2588–2598.
21. Palevsky PP, Zhang JH, O'Connor TZ, et al. Intensity of renal support in critically ill patients with acute kidney injury. *N Engl J Med.* 2008;359: 7–20.
22. van den Berghe G, Wouters P, Weekers F, et al. Intensive insulin therapy in critically ill patients. *N Engl J Med.* 2001;345:1359–1367.
23. Rivers E, Nguyen B, Havstad S, et al. Early goal-directed therapy in the treatment of severe sepsis and septic shock. *N Engl J Med.* 2001;345:1368–1377.

24. Dellinger RP, Carlet JM, Masur H, et al. Surviving Sepsis Campaign guidelines for management of severe sepsis and septic shock. *Crit Care Med*. 2004;32:858–873.

25. Dellinger RP, Levy MM, Carlet JM, et al. Surviving sepsis Campaign: international guidelines for management of severe sepsis and septic shock: 2008. *Crit Care Med*. 2008;36:296–327.

26. Burton TM. New therapy for sepsis infection raises hope but many questions (lead article). *Wall St J*. 2008;A1.

27. Marik PE, Varon J. Intensive insulin therapy in the ICU: is it now time to jump off the bandwagon? *Resuscitation*. 2007;2007:191–193.

28. Annane D, Sebille V, Charpentier C, et al. Effect of treatment with low doses of hydrocortisone and fludrocortisone on mortality in patients with septic shock. *JAMA*. 2002;288:862–871.

29. Meduri GU, Headley S, Golden E, et al. Effect of prolonged methylprednisolone therapy in unresolving acute respiratory distress syndrome. A randomized controlled trial. *JAMA*. 1998;280:159–165.

30. Sprung CL, Annane D, Keh D, et al. Hydrocortisone therapy for patients with septic shock. *N Engl J Med*. 2008;358:111–124.

31. The Acute Respiratory Distress Syndrome Network. Efficacy and safety of corticosteroids for persistent acute respiratory distress syndrome. *N Engl J Med*. 2006;354:1671–1684.

32. Marik PE. Critical illness related corticosteroid insufficiency. *Chest*. 2009;135:181–193.

3

Critical Care Medicine 101

Patients in the ICU need to be managed by doctors who can see the "big picture," be able to integrate and understand the patients' complex multi-system disease, and formulate an integrative plan that is evidence based, systematic, and is in keeping with the patients' treatment goals and values while being consistent with reality. Intensivists are realists who provide physiologically based interventions with the goal of limiting disease and improving outcomes; voodoo and other fantasy-based treatments have no role in the ICU. This chapter reviews the concepts and basic interventions which should be addressed when admitting a "generic patient" to the ICU. A number of issues need to be addressed regardless of the type of ICU to which the patient is being admitted and the patient's diagnosis.

It is important to note that no two patients are ever the same and that patients do not read medical textbooks or "policies and procedures." Furthermore, patients respond differently to the same intervention. Each patient's care must therefore be individualized based on the patient's unique demographics, comorbidities, acute disease processes, response to physiologically based interventions, and their values and goals. "Policies and procedures" and "bundles of care" have a limited place in the ICU. Parallels are often drawn between the airline industry and the practice of medicine. In general, this is a dangerous position to take. As Southwest Airlines understands, all 737-300s are build exactly the same and respond exactly in the same way when the same set of knobs and levers are pulled; patients, however, are not 737s (they are infinitely more complex and much more unpredictable).

P.E. Marik, *Handbook of Evidence-Based Critical Care*, **13**
DOI 10.1007/978-1-4419-5923-2_3,
© Springer Science+Business Media, LLC 2010

■ HOW AN ICU DIFFERS FROM OTHER AREAS OF THE HOSPITAL

An ICU is a place where patients undergo intensive and continuous physiological monitoring, where the critical care team applies physiologically based interventions and monitors the response to these interventions, which then serves as the basis for further interventions. It is therefore clear that critical care medicine can be practiced only at the bedside; office-based "intensivists" have no place in the ICU.

■ FACTORS TO CONSIDER WHEN A PATIENT IS ADMITTED TO THE ICU

- The patient's age (chronological not physiological)[1] (see Chapter 55).
- Comorbidities, particularly the following:
    - Cardiac disease and ventricular function.
    - Underlying lung disease.
    - Baseline renal function (the baseline and current estimated GFR should be calculated on admission in *all* patients).[*]
    - Use of immunosuppressive drugs.
- The diagnoses and differential diagnoses.
- Is this patient septic?
- Does this patient have SIRS (leaky capillaries)?
- Does this patient have acute lung injury (ALI)?
- What is the status of this patient's intravascular volume? (see Chapter 8)?
    - Normal.
    - Increased.
    - Decreased.
- Does this patient have evidence of impaired tissue/organ perfusion (see Chapter 8)?
    - Decreased urine output.
    - Cold/clammy skin.
    - Mottled peripheries.
    - Increased lactate concentration.
    - Hypotension.

---

[*]Estimated GFR (Cockcroft–Gault equation) $= (140\text{–age}) \times (\text{weight in kg}) \times (0.85 \text{ if female})/(\text{creatinine} \times 72)$

- The patients' code status, preferences for life-supportive therapy, and goals/expectations of treatment *must* be determined when the patients are admitted to the ICU.
- Determine the adequacy of venous access.
- Communicate with the patients' nurse and respiratory therapist.
- Keep the family informed.
- Measure the patients' height and weight on admission (see Chapters 14 and 19).

■ INITIAL "GENERIC" TREATMENT ORDERS

- Fluids:
  - State the type of fluid and the infusion rate.
- Oxygenation
  - Nasal cannula/Venturi mask.
- Initial ventilator settings:
  - AC rate 6–8 ml/kg Ideal Body weight (IBW).
  - Flow rate 60 l/min.
  - FiO$_2$ 100%.
  - PEEP 5–10 cm H$_2$O.
- ICU patients are at a high risk for deep venous thrombosis (DVT) and therefore *all* ICU patients require DVT prophylaxis. This should be individualized based on the patient's risk of DVT, risk of bleeding, risk of HIT, and renal function (see Chapter 21):
  - Subcutaneous heparin (5,000 U BID, TID).
  - Subcutaneous low molecular weight heparin.
  - Subcutaneous fondaparinux (2.5 mg q day).
  - Sequential compression devices.
  - Combination of SCD and anti-coagulant.
- Routine stress ulcer prophylaxis is not required in patients who are receiving enteral nutrition (see Chapter 32):
  - PPI or H2RB in those who require stress ulcer prophylaxis.
- Nutrition (see Chapter 31):
  - Unless specifically contraindicated or the patient's length of stay in the ICU is expected to be less than 24 h, all patients should be fed enterally once they have been resuscitated.
- All patients require chlorhexidine (or equivalent) mouth wash and regular oral hygiene.[2,3]
- All patients should be nursed head up 30° unless contraindicated for some reason (reduces risk of VAP).[4]
- Ocular lubricant to prevent exposure keratopathy.[5]
- Sedation should be titrated to the RASS score (see Chapter 9).

- All ICU patients should be regularly screened (at least daily) for the presence of delirium using a validated delirium assessment tool (see Chapter 47).
- Sedation with benzodiazepines should be avoided (see Chapters 9 and 47).

■ REFERENCES

1. Marik PE. Management of the Critically Ill Geriatric Patient. *Crit Care Med*. 2006;34(Suppl):S176–S182.
2. Koeman M, van der Ven AJ, Hak E, et al. Oral decontamination with chlorhexidine reduces the incidence of ventilator-associated pneumonia. *Am J Respir Crit Care Med*. 2006;173:1348–1355.
3. Chan EY, Ruest A, O'Meade M, et al. Oral decontamination for prevention of pneumonia in mechanically ventilated adults: systemic review and meta-analysis. *Br Med J*. 2007-doi:10.1136/bmj.39136.528160.BE.
4. Drakulovic MB, Torres A, Bauer TT, et al. Supine body position as a risk factor for nosocomial pneumonia in mechanically ventilated patients: a randomised trial. *Lancet*. 1999;354:1851–1858.
5. Ezra DG, Chan MP, Solebo L, et al. Randomised trial comparing ocular lubricants and polyacrylamide hydrogel dressings in the prevention of exposure keratopathy in the critically ill. *Intensive Care Med*. 2009;35:455–461.

4

House Officers' Guideline 1: Housekeeping

Intensive care units embody the miraculous advances of modern medicine. An ICU provides an environment where high-quality, compassionate, physiologically orientated, and evidence-based medicine can be practiced. The ICU is an exciting and challenging place to work and provides a remarkable learning environment. The keys to a successful rotation in the ICU are (1) teamwork and (2) a systematic, disciplined, and organized approach to patient care.

■ ADMISSION HISTORY AND PHYSICAL EXAMINATION

It is essential that a detailed and systematic history and physical examination be performed on all patients admitted to the ICU. This should include past medical and surgical history, current mediations as well as details of the current illness. The patient's *code status* and the presence of advance directives should be established on admission to the ICU. The initial physical examination frequently serves as the baseline reference, and it should include a basic neurological examination (including reflexes, motor power, evaluation of mental status, and funduscopic examination). Following the history and physical examination, and review of the available laboratory data and chest radiograph, a differential diagnosis and a management plan should be formulated.

The patient's weight and height should be measured directly with a scale and tape measure on admission to the ICU. These values should not

P.E. Marik, *Handbook of Evidence-Based Critical Care*,
DOI 10.1007/978-1-4419-5923-2_4,
© Springer Science+Business Media, LLC 2010

be estimated as they are frequently *wrong*[1]; the height and the weight are used in dosing calculations as well as estimating GFR and predicted body weight (PBW); so the correct data should be used.

■ DAILY EXAMINATION

It is essential that the patient's flow sheet (paper or electronic) over the last day be thoroughly reviewed and the major events of the last 24 h be documented. Most ICUs use a 24-h flow sheet which runs from midnight to midnight. Hence when reviewing and documenting the patient's progress over the "last day," the last 24-h period (midnight–midnight) as well as the progress since midnight should be reviewed. The following serves as a guideline for the daily progress note:

ALERT

It is important to be systematic and develop a template for your daily progress notes.

General

Primary and secondary diagnoses, overall condition of the patient, and events of the last 24 h.

Vital Signs (24-h Min and Max and Current)

- Temperature
- Blood pressure
- Pulse (rate and rhythm)
- Respiratory rate
- Arterial saturations

Fluid balance and urine output are *vitally* important in the daily and ongoing evaluation of the ICU patient. The following should be recorded:

- 24 h in.
- 24 h out.
- 24 h urine.
- Output of each drain should be noted.
- *Cumulative fluid balance.*
- 6 h in.
- 6 h out.
- 6 h urine.

Additional Observations

- The doses of all pressors should be documented.
- The presence of all pulses and the adequacy of peripheral perfusion.
- Limb symmetry and swelling (DVT).
- Presence of rashes and decubitus ulcers.
- The presence of all invasive lines, tubes, and devices should be noted including the duration of each central line.

The Ventilator

The ventilator is an extension of the patient and it is therefore essential that the following features be recorded (see Chapter 14):

- Mode
  - Assist controlled
  - Pressure controlled
  - Pressure support
  - APRV (Airway Pressure Release Ventilation)
  - SIMV (Synchronised Intermittent Mandatory Ventilation)
- Rate (set)
- Tidal volume (V_t)
  - Total
  - Milliliters per PBW(kg)[*] (*This is very NB*)
- Minute ventilation
- FiO_2
- PEEP
- Most recent blood gas analysis (if within past 24 h)

ALERT

Patients require a daily spontaneous breathing trial if criteria met (see Chapter 16).

Heart

Heart sounds and murmurs.

---

[*]Lung volume is indexed to predicted body weight (PBW) which is dependent on sex and height:

Male $= 50 + 0.91$ (height in centimeters $- 152.4$)

Female $= 45.5 + 0.91$ (height in centimeters $- 152.4$)

Chest

Symmetry of air entry (i.e., presence of breath sounds) and presence of rhonchi or crackles.

Abdomen

The presence of distension and tenderness (especially right upper quadrant), the type of enteral feeds, evidence of reflux, gastric residual volumes, and the presence of diarrhea (see Chapters 31 and 38).

CNS

A focused neurological examination is essential, particularly in patients receiving hypnotic/sedative agents, and should include the following:

- Level of consciousness and response to commands
- Pupillary size and response
- Eye movements
- Limb movements: spontaneous and in response to noxious stimuli (pain)
- Presence of deep tendon reflexes

ALERT

Patients require daily awakenings to determine neurological status and allow re-evaluation of sedation (see Chapters 9 and 16).

Importance of the Daily Neurological Examination

Critically ill patients in the ICU are at risk of developing serious neurological complications including ICU psychosis, septic encephalopathy, critical illness polyneuropathy, entrapment neuropathies, compartment syndromes, cerebral edema, intracerebral hemorrhages (related to coagulopathies), cerebral ischemia (related to hemodynamic instability), and cerebral embolism. These conditions can be detected and diagnosed only by physical examination. Furthermore, these conditions may frequently be masked in patients who are sedated. If the patient does not respond to a noxious stimulus, the sedation must immediately be stopped to facilitate further neurological evaluation.

■ LABORATORY TESTS

All ICU patients require the following tests daily (if a patient does not require these tests, he/she probably does not need to be in the ICU!):

- Complete blood count:
  - Hemoglobin.
  - White cell count (differential and band count).
  - Platelet count.
- Urea and electrolytes.
- Oxygenation should be assessed in all patients (usually by pulse oximetry and blood gasses when appropriate).
- Ca^{2+}, Mg, and phosphorus should be measured every 2–3 days or more frequently if clinical circumstances dictate.
- All other laboratory tests should be ordered on merit; standing laboratory tests are not cost effective.
- It is not cost effective to perform a complete blood count and urea and electrolyte tests more frequently than every 24 h unless special circumstances dictate, such as the following:
  - Diabetic ketoacidosis, hypernatremia, hyponatremia, where Na^+ and K^+ should be tested every 2–4 h.
  - In patients who are bleeding, a hematocrit should be followed no more frequently than every 6 h (it takes 72 h for the hematocrit to stabilize following blood loss).

ALERT

- Pay special attention to a falling platelet count (see Chapter 53)
  - HIT
  - Drug-induced thrombocytopenia
- Patients with hypernatremia receiving 3% NaCl should have electrolytes followed every 1–2 h

---

■ IMAGING

- Daily chest X-rays are not cost effective.
- Chest X-rays should be performed only on demand (as clinical circumstances dictate).[2,3]

the hereafter; this implies that not all dying patients need (or will benefit from) admission to an ICU.

Once a patient is admitted to the ICU the appropriateness of continuing care in the ICU should be evaluated in an ongoing fashion; the fact that aggressive life-supportive therapy has been provided to a patient does not imply that it cannot be withdrawn. Patients should only remain in the ICU as long as they continue to derive benefit from the physiological support provided in the ICU. When all the ICU beds are filled, the ICU/Critical Care Director or his designee will have the responsibility to admit/discharge patients from these units. Triage decisions should be made explicitly, fairly, and justly. Ethnic origin, race, sex, social status, sexual preference or financial status should not be considered in triage decisions. Triage decisions may be made without patient, surrogate, or attending physician consent.

In evaluating the appropriateness of an admission to the ICU, the priority of the admission as well as the disease-specific or physiological indications for admission (as outlined below) should be determined.

■ PRIORITIZATION OF POTENTIAL ICU ADMISSIONS

This system defines those patients that will benefit most (priority 1) to those that will not benefit at all (priority 4) from admission to an ICU.

Priority 1

These are critically ill, unstable patients in need of *intensive treatments and monitoring* that cannot usually be provided outside of the ICU. Examples of such treatments include ventilator support, continuous titration of vasoactive drug infusion. These patients have no limits placed on the extent of therapy they are to receive. Illustrative case types include postoperative or acute respiratory failure patients requiring mechanical ventilatory support and shock or hemodynamic instability requiring invasive monitoring and/or titrated vasoactive drugs.

Priority 2

These are patients that require the *intensive monitoring* services of an ICU and are at risk to require immediate intensive treatment. No limits are placed on the extent of therapy these patients are to receive. Examples of these patients include patients with underlying heart, lung, renal, or central nervous system disease who have an acute severe medical illness or have undergone major surgery, and those patients requiring invasive hemodynamic monitoring.

Priority 3

These are critically ill, unstable patients whose previous state of health, underlying disease, or acute illness reduces the likelihood of recovery and therefore benefit from ICU treatment. These patients may receive intensive treatment to relieve acute illness but therapeutic efforts may stop short of measures such as intubation or cardiopulmonary resuscitation. Examples include patients with metastatic malignancy complicated by infection, pericardial tamponade or airway obstruction, or patients with end-stage heart or lung disease complicated by a severe acute illness.

Priority 4

These are patients who are generally not appropriate for ICU admission. Admission of these patients should be on an individual basis, under unusual circumstances and at the discretion of the ICU attending physician/ICU director. These patients can be placed in the following categories:

- Little or no additional benefit from ICU care (compared to non-ICU care) based on low risk of active intervention that could not safely be administered in a non-ICU setting (i.e., too well to benefit from ICU care). These include patients with peripheral vascular surgery, hemodynamically stable diabetic ketoacidosis, conscious drug overdose, mild congestive heart failure.
- Patients with terminal, irreversible illness who face imminent death (i.e., too sick to benefit from ICU care). This includes patients with severe irreversible brain damage, irreversible multi-organ system failure, metastatic cancer unresponsive to chemotherapy and/or radiation therapy (unless the patient is on a specific treatment protocol), brain-dead non-organ donors, patients in a persistent vegetative state, patients who are permanently unconscious.

This group *includes* patients with decision-making capacity who decline intensive care and/or invasive monitoring and who elect to receive comfort care only. This group *excludes* brain-dead patients who are organ donors or potential organ donors (these patients require intensive monitoring and/or treatment in an ICU).

Transfer from Another Hospital: Variable Priority

The priority of transfers from other hospitals should be based on the current ICU census as well as the nature of the patient's acute condition and the risks of interhospital transfer. Consent for transfer must be obtained from the patient or his/her surrogate by the transferring attending physician prior to transfer.

■ DISEASE-SPECIFIC INDICATIONS FOR ICU ADMISSION

Cardiovascular System

- Acute myocardial infarction (AMI) complicated by ongoing pain, arrhythmias, CHF, or hemodynamic instability
- Patients suffering an AMI who are candidates for or have received reperfusion therapy
- Unstable angina
- Cardiogenic shock
- Acute congestive heart failure with respiratory failure and/or requiring hemodynamic support
- Hypertensive emergencies, i.e., accelerated hypertension with encephalopathy, chest pain, pulmonary edema, aortic dissection, or eclampsia

Pulmonary System

- Acute respiratory failure requiring emergent ventilatory support, including non-invasive positive-pressure ventilation
- Severe asthma, with FEV1 or peak flow <40% predicted, pulsus paradoxus >18 mmHg, pneumothorax or pneumomediastinum, $PaCO_2$ >40 mmHg, or an "exhausted" patient
- Hemodynamically unstable patients with pulmonary emboli and/or patients who are candidates for thrombolytic therapy

Neurological Disorders

- Patients suffering a CVA who are candidates for or have received thrombolytic therapy [i.e., within a 3 (4.5 h)-h window following the onset of the CVA] and patients with cerebellar or brain-stem CVAs
- Central nervous system or neuromuscular disorders with deteriorating neurological or ventilatory function
- Patients with subarachnoid hemorrhage (Hunt and Hess grades I–IV)

Drug Ingestion and Drug Overdose

- Hemodynamically unstable drug ingestion
- Drug ingestion with significantly altered mental status with inadequate airway protection
- Seizures following drug ingestion

- Drug ingestion requiring mechanical ventilation
- Drug ingestion requiring acute hemodialysis/hemoperfusion

Gastrointestinal Disorders

- Gastrointestinal bleeding from any source with
  - Hemodynamic instability:
    - Systolic arterial pressure <100 mmHg
    - Pulse rate >120 beats/min
    - Postural hypotension after 1,000 ml of fluid resuscitation (but excluding postural hypotension on presentation alone)
    - Hypotension requiring pressors
  - Ongoing bleeding (bright red blood on NG aspirate; red or maroon blood per rectum)
  - Rebleeding
  - Erratic mental status
  - "Unstable" comorbid disease
  - Coagulopathy (INR >1.6 and/or PTT >40 s)
- Fulminant hepatic failure
- Chronic liver failure with
  - Grade III/IV encephalopathy
  - Oliguria
  - GI bleeding
- Acute hemorrhagic pancreatitis (three or more Ranson criteria)

Endocrine

- Diabetic ketoacidosis with severe acidosis, hemodynamic instability, or altered mental status
- Hyperosmolar state with coma and/or hemodynamic instability
- Thyroid storm or myxedema coma
- Severe hyponatremia, hypernatremia, or hypercalcemia with altered mental status
- Hyperkalemia, severe and acute
- Adrenal crisis

Renal Disorders

- Patients who require acute emergent dialysis
  - Severe hypertension
  - Pulmonary edema
  - Hyperkalemia

Postoperative Care

- Postoperative patients requiring hemodynamic monitoring, ventilatory support, treatment of hemodynamic instability or airway monitoring

- Neurosurgical patients requiring hemodynamic monitoring or aggressive titrated treatment of intracranial hypertension and vasospasm, etc.

Miscellaneous

- Septic shock or sepsis syndrome requiring hemodynamic monitoring or hemodynamic or respiratory support.

■ PHYSIOLOGICAL INDICATION FOR ICU ADMISSION

- Apical pulse <40 or >150 beats/min (>130 beats/min if age >60 years)
- Mean arterial pressure (MAP) <60 mmHg after adequate fluid resuscitation (2,000 ml) or the need for vasoactive agents to maintain a MAP >60 mmHg
- Diastolic blood pressure >110 mmHg *and* one of the following:
  - Pulmonary edema
  - Encephalopathy
  - Myocardial ischemia
  - Dissecting aortic aneurysm
  - Eclampsia or pre-eclampsia (diastolic >100 mmHg)
  - Subarachnoid hemorrhage (diastolic >100 mmHg).
- Respiratory rate >35 breaths/min (sustained) and respiratory distress
- PaO_2 <55 mmHg with $FiO_2 \geq 0.4$ (acute)
- Serum potassium >6.5 mEq/l (acute)
- pH_a <7.2 or >7.6 (diabetic ketoacidosis pH_a <7.0)
- Serum glucose >800 mg/dl
- Serum calcium >15 mg/dl
- Temperature (core) <32°C

■ DISCHARGE CRITERIA

In order to maximize the efficient use of ICU resources, the discharge process should be ongoing and continuous. Once admitted, it may be possible to determine whether a patients is too well to benefit or too sick to benefit from continued intensive care (see Chapter 62). Patients should be discharged from the ICU when it can be determined that the patient is no longer benefitting from being in the ICU. The discharge process should be a collaborative one between the intensivist, the primary care physician or surgeon, and the nursing staff to assure that the needs of the patients can be met by the receiving unit. General criteria for ICU discharge have been met when the need for intensive care is no longer present because of the following:

- The indication for initial or continued treatment has reverted spontaneously or with therapy.
- Therapy provided has not reversed the reason for admission and little benefit will be attained from continued intensive therapy.
- The need for intensive monitoring is no longer present.
- The patient has responded to treatment but the long-term prognosis is such that continuing further care is unacceptable to the patient or his surrogate.

■ REFERENCE

1. Guidelines for intensive care unit admission, discharge, and triage. Task Force of the American College of Critical Care Medicine, Society of Critical Care Medicine. *Crit Care Med*. 1999;27:633–638.

6

House Officers' Guidelines 2: Procedures

ALERT

- The tradition of *See one, Do one, Teach one* can no longer be condoned. The safety and well being of the patient is one's overriding concern.
- If you do not know how to do it, do not do it!
- Before doing a procedure, make sure that you have all the equipments required.
- Make sure you know how to get out of trouble should the procedure "go wrong."
- If you fail after 2–3 attempts at the procedure, *stop*. Ask a more experienced operator for help.
- Check the platelet count, PTT, and INR before any invasive procedure (see Chapters 52 and 53).
  - As a general rule the risk of bleeding is related to the skill of the operator rather than the ability of the blood to clot (however this helps).
  - Patients receiving therapeutic anti-coagulants tend to bleed; stop anti-coagulants prior to the procedure.
- Obtain informed consent from the patient (or surrogate), unless an emergency. Explain the benefits and risks (including death). See Chapter 65.

P.E. Marik, *Handbook of Evidence-Based Critical Care*,
DOI 10.1007/978-1-4419-5923-2_6,
© Springer Science+Business Media, LLC 2010

- Murphy's First Law of Procedures:
  - Nature sides with the hidden flaw.
- Murphy's Second Law of Procedures:
  - If a procedure can go wrong, it will go wrong usually at the most inopportune time.
- Murphy's Third Law of Procedures:
  - If a patient can bleed, he/she will bleed.
- Murphy's Fourth Law of Procedures:
  - Never persuade a patient to agree to a procedure that they have declined or are hesitant about; these are the patients that will suffer a complication.
- Murphy's Fifth Law of Procedures:
  - Never "force" a device into a patient; if it does not "go in easily," it will go into the wrong place.

■ CENTRAL VENOUS ACCESS

Most ICU patients require a central line. Indications include the following[1-9]:

- Use of *any* vasopressor agent. Dopamine, epinephrine, and norepinephrine infusion should *never* run through a peripheral line.
- Multiple mediations, infusions, antibiotics, etc.
- Patient requiring volume/blood resuscitation with inadequate peripheral venous access.
- Placement:
  - A fully stocked procedure cart is highly recommended.
  - ICU nurse should be at bedside to assist (and observe) the operator.
  - Full body drape is recommended.
  - An antibiotic-/anti-microbial-coated catheter is recommended in units which have a high baseline incidence of catheter-related bloodstream infection I (>5/1,000 catheter days).
  - Use a "chuck" (absorptive pad) to prevent covering the bed in blood.
  - Clean up your mess after you are completed; do not leave it up to the nurse.
- Site of placement:
  - First choice should depend on patient's body habitus, existing and previous lines, and your degree of comfort with each site.
  - Ultrasound guidance is highly recommended for placement of internal jugular (IJ) lines and visualization of the inguinal anatomy in obese patients.

- The femoral site is suggested in highly coagulopathic patients, in emergency situations, in patients with severe bullous lung disease, etc.
- The femoral site is compressible should the artery be accidentally stuck (as opposed to the IJ or the subclavian).
- It is nearly impossible to cause a pneumothorax or a hemothorax when placing a femoral line.[7,8] Caution should be used when placing an IJ or a subclavian line in patients with ALI/ARDS or severe COPD; a pneumothorax can be fatal.
- Catheter-related bloodstream infection (see Chapter 11). As a general rule the risk of CRBI is lowest for a subclavian CVC followed by an IJ and then a femoral catheter.
- Femoral catheters have a significantly higher risk of thrombosis (2% vs. 20%).[10,11] "Aggressive" DVT prophylaxis is indicated in these patients (see Chapter 21).
- A CXR is required after an IJ/subclavian to confirm correct placement and to exclude a pneumothorax.
- Document procedure in patient's chart (with date and time).
- As a general rule, if you think a central venous catheter is infected, it is better to remove and place at a new site rather than to "replace" over a guidewire. A guidewire exchange is acceptable in patients with limited venous access; however, the catheter tip *must* be cultured and the line removed if the cultures are positive (>10 cfu).

Subclavian Vein Catheterization

- *Advantages*: Consistent identifiable landmarks, easier long-term catheter maintenance, relatively high patient comfort.
- *Disadvantages*:
    - Pneumothorax (1–2%).
    - Subclavian artery puncture (1%).
    - Difficult to perform under ultrasound guidance.
- *Contraindications*:
    - Subclavian puncture is a relative contraindication in patients with a coagulopathy and/or a pulmonary compromise (dependent on the expertise of the operator).
- *Anatomy*: It is continuation of axillary vein, beginning at the outer border of first rib, extending 3–4 cm along the undersurface of clavicle, and joining ipsilateral internal jugular vein behind the sternoclavicular joint.
- *Position* (most important): The patient is placed supine with arms at the side and head turned to the opposite side. Trendelenburg position (15–30°), with a small bedroll placed between the shoulder blades.

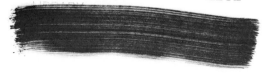

- Infraclavicular approach (blind):
  - Identify the clavicle, the suprasternal notch, and the acromium–clavicular junction.
  - The operator's position is next to patient's ipsilateral shoulder. Feel along the inferior border of the clavicle moving from medial to lateral until you feel a "give" in the tissue resistance. This point is approximately at the junction between the medial and the middle thirds of the clavicle and at the point of the first "S bend" in the clavicle.
  - The skin and the subcutaneous tissue should now be infiltrated with 1% lidocaine. The thumb of the left hand is now placed "in" the suprasternal notch to serve as a landmark.
  - A 2 3/4-in., 14-gauge needle is mounted on a syringe and directed cephalad from the "point" until the tip abuts under the clavicle. With the needle hugging the inferior edge of clavicle the needle is now advanced toward the suprasternal notch (the thumb of your left hand). The needle is advanced until the subclavian vein is entered.

Internal Jugular Vein Catheterization

- *Advantages*: Minimal risk for pneumothorax, preferred in patients with hyperinflation and those receiving mechanical ventilation.
- *Disadvantages*: Carotid artery puncture (2–10%) with blind technique.
- Anatomy: It emerges from the base of the skull through jugular foramen and courses posterolateral to the internal carotid artery in the carotid sheath and runs beneath the sternocleidomastoid muscle.
- *Position* is supine with 15° Trendelenburg and the head turned gently to the opposite side.
- *Central approach* (blind):
  - The skin is punctured at the apex of the triangle formed by the two muscle bellies of sternocleidomastoid muscle and the clavicle, at a 30–45° angle with the frontal plane and directed at the nipple on the same side.
- *Ultrasound approach*:
  - The IJ vein is typically anterior and lateral to the artery.
  - The IJ vein can be distinguished by the fact that the vein is compressible, non-pulsatile, and distensible by the Trendelenburg position.
  - Screening US to assess the degree of overlap of carotid artery by the IJ vein, the compressibility of the vein, and the presence of internal echoes that may signify clot.

– Color Doppler can be used to visualize distinct arterial and venous pulsations (color dependent on direction of the probes in relation to flow and not the "color" of the blood).
– Once the appropriate site is selected, the site is sterilized and draped with full barrier precautions.
– Using US to mark the skin and proceeding without real-time guidance is not recommended.
– The US probe is placed in a sterile sheath; this step requires an assistant. Sterile gel must be placed on the probe and the outside of the sheath.
– As the procedure is performed in real time, a "finder" needle is not required.
– In the "one-handed" method, the operator controls the ultrasound probe with the non-dominant hand and the needle with the dominant hand.
– Passage of the introducer needle into the IJ vein can be performed either with a transverse (short axis) view or a longitudinal (long axis) view.
– The primary advantage of the longitudinal view is that it allows better visualization of the advancing needle tip.
– Once the IJ vein is entered with the introducer, the US probe is placed on the field and the typical Seldinger technique used to place the central venous catheter.

Femoral Vein Catheterization

• *Advantages*: *Safe*, easily accessible, do not need Trendelenburg. Safe to perform in patients with a coagulopathy.
• Disadvantages: Limits flexion of leg at the hip, increased risk of CRBI and thrombosis.
• *Anatomy*: It is the continuation of popliteal vein and becomes external iliac vein at inguinal ligament. It lies medial to the femoral nerve and the femoral artery in the femoral sheath at the inguinal ligament.
• *Technique*:
    – Clean and shave the area. The patient is placed supine with the leg extended and slightly abducted at hip.
    – Palpate for the femoral arterial pulsation; the site of puncture is 1–1.5 cm medial to the femoral arterial pulsation below the inguinal ligament. In a patient with no palpable femoral pulse, it is 1–1.5 cm medial to the junction of medial third and lateral two-thirds of a line joining the anterior superior iliac spine and the pubic tubercle.

- A 14-gauge needle is placed at the site of puncture and advanced at a 45–60° angle to the frontal plane with the tip pointed cephalad.
- After obtaining return of venous blood, the syringe and the needle are depressed to skin level and free aspiration of blood reconfirmed.

ALERT

- *Do not place a femoral line in a kidney transplant patient.*
- *Do not place a central line on the same side as a dialysis fistula* (femoral or subclavian CVC).
- *Do not* remove a CVC (subclavian or IJ) in an upright patient (may cause air embolism).

Complications of Central Venous Access

- Catheter-related bloodstream infection (see Chapter 11).
- Local infection.
- Local bleeding.
- Venous air embolism :
  - Entry of air into the central venous system through the catheter can be fatal.
  - It is best prevented by positioning the patient in 15° Trendelenburg position during catheter insertion.
  - It will manifest as tachypnea, wheezing, hypotension, and "mill wheel" murmur over precordium.
  - The patient should be immediately turned onto his/her left side in the Trendelenburg position and air aspirated after advancing the catheter into the right ventricle.
- Venous thrombosis (see Chapter 21).
- Pneumothorax and/or hemothorax:
  - Occurs due to injury to pleura and underlying lung.
  - Small pneumothorax can be observed, but medium to large pneumothoraces will require chest tube insertion.
  - As a general rule, all intubated patients with a pneumothorax require a chest tube.
- Arterial puncture:
  - If occurs, apply sufficient pressure for at least 10 min.
  - Arterial puncture may be confirmed by pulsatile flow and high hydrostatic pressure.

- Catheter tip migration and perforation of free wall of cardiac chamber.
- Vascular erosions:
  - Uncommon.
  - Typically occur 1–7 days after catheter insertion.
  - Cause sudden dyspnea with new pleural effusion or hydromediastinum on chest radiograph.
  - More common with left-sided catheter placement
- *Occlusion of catheter*: It is common. Best treated by replacement of catheter.
- *Retained catheter fragment*: Catheter tips may get sheared off by traction on beveled tip of inserting needle or by fracture of catheter due to improper fixation and excessive movement.
- *Inadvertent venous catheter placement*: Placement into the internal jugular vein or the opposite subclavian vein from subclavian vein approach is not uncommon.

■ ARTERIAL LINES

- In most patients, blood pressure can be monitored using the traditional time-honored technique used by Florence Nightingale, RN, namely using an adequately sized blood pressure cuff and a mercury or an automated manometer.
- Indications for an arterial line include the following:
  - Ongoing shock and hemodynamic instability.
  - Frequent requirement for arterial blood gas analysis.
  - Patients requiring frequent titration of vasoactive agents.
  - To measure pulse pressure variation and for pulse contour analysis (see Chapter 8).
- Preferred site:
  - My preference is the femoral artery unless the patient has severe peripheral arterial disease. The femoral artery was placed superficially in the groin to make the intensivist's life easier!
  - The radial artery is okay; however, check for the patency of the ulnar artery and monitor perfusion of the thumb.

■ NASO/OROGASTRIC TUBES

- Almost all ICU patients require a naso/orogastric tube or a feeding tube.[12–16]
- As a general rule, an orogastric tube is preferred over a nasogastric tube to limit the risk of sinusitis.

- In patients who require endotracheal intubation, it is preferable to place the ET tube before the NG/OG tube.
- In patients with previous trans-sphenoidal surgery, maxilla-facial and/or facial fracture placement should always be performed under direct vision (not blind) by an operator experienced in this technique (e.g., ENT surgeon).
- All intubated patients require an OG tube:
  - Decompresses the stomach (air and gastric contents).
  - Allows early enteral feeding (see Chapter 31).
  - Allows PO medication.
  - Allows assessment of gastric residuals.
- Placement:
  - Tell the patient what you are doing (if awake).
  - Ask them to swallow as the tube "goes in."
  - Lubricate the end of the tube with "surgilube."
  - Flex the neck.
  - Gently push the tube past the naso/oropharynx and into the esophagus.
  - *Never force* the tube.
  - If the patient coughs, remove and attempt again.
  - If you are having difficulty, it may help to soften the tube with warm water.
  - In those difficult cases, placement may be achieved under direct vision either using a standard or a fiber-optic laryngoscope. An experienced intensivist, a surgeon or an ENT is required for this maneuver.
- Confirming placement in the "stomach":
  - Inject air and auscultate over the epigastrium (Whoosh test).
  - Aspirate; stomach contents or bile confirms placement.
  - An abdominal (or half–half) X-ray is required in all patients to confirm placement.

■ FEEDING TUBES

- Small bore-feeding tubes are "designed" to go into the lung; This is a *bad* thing.[7,18]
- Feeding tubes should *not* be placed by those inexperienced in the technique.
- Devices that allow accurate placement using electromagnetic guidance technology are currently available (GPS for the feeding tube). This method is highly recommended.[18]

- In patients with lesions of the upper airway and those with previous trans-sphenoidal surgery, placement should be performed under direct vision using a portable fiber-optic laryngoscope (by ENT surgeon, general surgeon, or intensivist).
- When placed by under direct vision and when using the GPS device, a confirmatory X-ray may not be required unless uncertain about the position of tube.

■ THORACENTESIS AND PARACENTESIS

- The old dictum that *any body cavity can be needled with a strong arm and a 14-gauge needle* can no longer be supported.
- Ultrasound guidance is recommended for all thoracentesis and paracentesis regardless of the perceived size of the fluid collection; the lung and the bowel have a funny habit of being where they should not be:
    - This is preferably performed by the intensivist/fellow at the bedside using a portable ultrasound device.
    - Alternatively this procedure can be performed by the radiologist; however, the radiologist should not mark the spot with an "X" for needling at a later time (the fluid moves).
- The literature has clearly demonstrated that the complication rate (including *death*) is significantly less when these procedures are done using ultrasound.[19-27]
- A study of 27 patients requiring paracentesis showed that the success of blind paracentesis was directly related to the amount of ascitic fluid present.[28] In six of the eight patients in whom fluid was found in the left or the right flank, air-filled bowel loops were observed by ultrasound between the abdominal wall and the fluid, in the expected path of a blind puncture. The site of accumulation of ascitic fluid depends on the quantity of ascites, its etiology, and the presence of peritoneal adhesions. Therefore, ultrasound not only confirms the presence of ascites but also is used to locate the best site to perform a successful paracentesis, especially when dealing with smaller volumes of fluid.[29]

■ CLINICAL PEARLS

- If you do not know how to do a procedure, do not do it.
- Most ICU patients require a central line and an oro/nasogastric tube.
- Only those with "experience" should place a thin bore-feeding tube.

- When doing a procedure, make sure that you have all the necessary equipments.
- Clean up once you are done.

■ REFERENCES

1. Pronovost PJ, Needham D, Berenholtz S, et al. An intervention to decrease catheter related bloodstream infections in the ICU. *N Engl J Med.* 2006;355:2725–2732.
2. Feller-Kopman D. Ultrasound-guided internal jugular access: a proposed standardized approach and implications for training and practice. *Chest.* 2007;132:302–309.
3. McGee DC, Gould MK. Preventing complications of central venous catheterization. *N Engl J Med.* 2003;348:1123–1133.
4. Cook D, Randolph A, Kernerman P, et al. Central venous catheter replacement strategies: a systemic review of the literature. *Crit Care Med.* 1997;25:1417–1424.
5. Niel-Weise BS, Stijnen T, van den Broek PJ. Anti-infective-treated central venous catheters: a systematic review of randomized controlled trials. *Intensive Care Med.* 2007;33:2058–2068.
6. Galpern D, Guerrero A, Tu A, et al. Effectiveness of a central line bundle campaign on line-associated infections in the intensive care unit. *Surgery.* 2008;144:492–495.
7. Deshpande KS, Hatem C, Ulrich HL, et al. The incidence of infectious complications of central venous catheters at the subclavian, internal jugular, and femoral sites in an intensive care unit population. *Crit Care Med.* 2005;33:13–20.
8. Parienti JJ, Thirion M, Megarbane B, et al. Femoral vs jugular venous catheterization and risk of nosocomial events in adults requiring acute renal replacement: A randomized controlled trial. *JAMA.* 2008;299:2413–2422.
9. Mermel LA, Farr BM, Sherertz RJ, et al. Guidelines for the management of intravascular catheter-related infections. *CID.* 2001;32:1249–1272.
10. Merrer J, De Jonghe B, Golliot F, et al. Complications of femoral and subclavian venous catheterization in critically ill patients: a randomized controlled trial. *JAMA.* 2001;286:700–707.
11. Trottier SJ, Veremakis C, O'Brien J, et al. Femoral deep vein thrombosis associated with central venous catheterization: results from a prospective, randomized trial. *Crit Care Med.* 1995;23:52–59.
12. Deutschman CS, Wilton P, Sinow J, et al. Paranasal sinusitis associated with nasotracheal intubation; a frequently unrecognized and treatable source of sepsis. *Crit Care Med.* 1986;14:111–114.
13. Baskin WN. Acute complications associated with bedside placement of feeding tubes. *Nutr Clin Pract.* 2006;21:40–55.

14. Holzapfel L, Chevret S, Madinier G, et al. Influence of long-term oro- or nasotracheal intubation on nosocomial maxillary sinusitis and pneumonia: results of a prospective, randomized, clinical trial. *Crit Care Med.* 1993;21:1132–1138.

15. Rouby JJ, Laurent P, Gosnach M, et al. Risk factors and clinical relevance of nosocomial maxillary sinusitis in the critically ill. *Am J Respir Crit Care Med.* 1994;150:776–783.

16. Fassoulaki A, Pamouktsoglou P. Prolonged nasotracheal intubation and its association with inflammation of paranasal sinuses. *Anesth Analg.* 1989;69:50–52.

17. Iyer KR, Crawley TC. Complications of enteral access. *Gastrointest Endosc Clin N Am.* 2007;17:717–729.

18. Gray R, Tynan C, Reed L, et al. Bedside electromagnetic-guided feeding tube placement: an improvement over traditional placement technique? *Nutr Clin Pract.* 2007;22:436–444.

19. Beaulieu Y, Marik PE. Bedside ultrasonography in the ICU, Part 2. *Chest.* 2005;128:1766–1781.

20. Feller-Kopman D. Ultrasound-guided thoracentesis. *Chest.* 2006;129: 1709–1714.

21. Diacon AH, Brutsche MH, Soler M. Accuracy of pleural puncture sites: a prospective comparison of clinical examination with ultrasound. *Chest.* 2003;123:436–441.

22. Diacon AH, Theron J, Bolliger CT. Transthoracic ultrasound for the pulmonologist. *Curr Opin Pulm Med.* 2005;11:307–312.

23. Feeney CM, Yoshioka H. A fatal case of pulmonary hemorrhage from thoracentesis. *West J Med.* 1993;158:638–639.

24. Grogan DR, Irwin RS, Channick R, et al. Complications associated with thoracentesis. A prospective, randomized study comparing three different methods. *Arch Intern Med.* 1990;150:873–877.

25. Keske U. Ultrasound-aided thoracentesis in intensive care patients. *Intensive Care Med.* 1999;25:896–897.

26. Mayo PH, Goltz HR, Tafreshi M, et al. Safety of ultrasound-guided thoracentesis in patients receiving mechanical ventilation. *Chest.* 2004;125:1059–1062.

27. Roch A, Bojan M, Michelet P, et al. Usefulness of ultrasonography in predicting pleural effusions >500 ml in patients receiving mechanical ventilation. *Chest.* 2005;127:224–232.

28. Bard C, Lafortune M, Breton G. Ascites: ultrasound guidance or blind paracentesis? *Can Med Assoc J.* 1986;135:209–210.

29. McGibbon A, Chen GI, Peltekian KM, et al. An evidence-based manual for abdominal paracentesis. *Dig Dis Sci.* 2007;52:3307–3315.

7

Chronic Critical Illness

Intensive care unit physicians frequently provide care to patients who survive initial life-threatening events but are unable to recover to the point that they are fully independent of life support. These patients are known as "chronically critically ill." Chronic critical illness (CCI) is usually defined as an ICU patient who requires more than 21 days of assisted ventilation. Although prolonged dependence on mechanical ventilation is a hallmark of CCI, CCI is not simply an extended period of acute critical illness but a discreet syndrome encompassing distinctive derangements of metabolism, organ dysfunction, and endocrine and immunologic function.[1–3]

Depending on the setting, CCI patients account for between 5 and 10% of adult ICU admissions. Mechanically ventilated patients with a history of prior pulmonary disease and who require renal replacement therapy are at the greatest risk of CCI.[1,4–6] These patients are usually elderly with a slight male predominance. Patients suffering postoperative complications make up the majority of the CCI patients. These are usually patients with underlying cardiopulmonary disease who have undergone cardiac or abdominal surgery. Trauma and burn patients as well as those with acute lung injury (ARDS) and patients with chronic respiratory failure (usually COPD) make up the majority of the remaining patients. CCI occurs in the setting of multiple episodes of sepsis with SIRS, multi-organ dysfunction syndrome (MODS), and respiratory failure. The prognosis of these patients is generally poor; however, surprisingly the hospital survival is about 50% with a 1-year survival of approximately 25%.

■ METABOLIC SYNDROME OF CCI

Chronic elevations in cortisol, catecholamines, and cytokines, resulting from recurrent infection and inflammation, act in concert to depress

P.E. Marik, *Handbook of Evidence-Based Critical Care*,
DOI 10.1007/978-1-4419-5923-2_7,
© Springer Science+Business Media, LLC 2010

hypothalamic–pituitary growth hormone, gonadal and thyroid axes, as well as modulate renal, bone, and energy metabolism. These derangements lead to clinical manifestations, such as altered body composition (increased fat and decreased lean mass), hyperglycemia, osteoporosis, and immune dysfunction.[3,7]

Stress Hyperglycemia

Although stress hyperglycemia has not been well studied in CCI, this is likely to be a common problem due to peripheral insulin resistance and increased hepatic gluconeogenesis. While glycemic control appears to have a limited role in the acute phase of critical illness (see Chapter 39), glycemic control may assume a more important role in reducing organ dysfunction in CCI. While the optimal target glucose has yet to be determined, a serum glucose of between 140 and 180 mg/dl would appear to be a reasonable target.

Somatotropic Axis

In health, growth hormone (GH) secretion is pulsatile, with large mainly nocturnal peaks superimposed on a barely detectable baseline level. This pattern of secretion is controlled by the balance between hypothalamic releasing hormone (GHRH) and the inhibitory effects of somatostatin. The actions of GH are mediated directly by way of peripheral GH receptors and indirectly through the enhanced synthesis of insulin-like growth factor (IGF). The pulsatility of GH release is important for its peripheral metabolic functions, particularly the maintenance of IGF-1 levels.

Acute illness is characterized by high peak and interpulse concentrations of GH as well as an increase in GH pulse frequency with reduced levels of insulin-like growth factor-1 (IGF-1) and IGF-binding protein-3. These changes have been interpreted to represent acquired resistance to GH. Increased GH results in lipolytic, insulin-antagonizing, and immunostimulating actions, while the indirect IGF-1-mediated effects of GH are attenuated. These changes prioritize essential substrates such as glucose, fatty acids, and amino acids toward survival rather than anabolism. This pattern contrasts with pattern in CCI in which the pulsatile secretion of GH is suppressed with very low mean nocturnal concentration of GH. These findings are suggestive of relative GH deficiency, which is postulated to play a role in the wasting syndrome of CCI. These changes appear to be more severe in men.

In view of its anabolic properties, GH was considered a potentially beneficial adjuvant therapy in reversing the feeding-resistant catabolism of critical illness. A number of studies in a wide range of catabolic disorders demonstrated an improvement in surrogate end points including improvements in nitrogen balance and improvement in protein synthesis.[8] To investigate the effect of administration of GH (in high doses) in critically ill patients, Takala et al.[9] carried out two parallel randomized controlled trials (RCTs). A total of 532 patients who had been in the ICU for 5–7 days and who were expected to require intensive care for at least 10 days were enrolled. The in-hospital mortality rate was significantly higher in patients who received GH in both studies. Among the survivors, length of ICU stay was prolonged in the GH group. The study has been criticized for the very high dose of GH used, which may have been associated with insulin resistance and hyperglycemia, worsened concealed hypoadrenalism and hypothyroidism, and promoted apoptosis in compromised tissue. The deleterious effects of GH are probably multi-factorial, complex, and related to the timing, dosing, and mode of administration. Furthermore, due to the non-pulsatile mode of administration, the direct effects of GH may have been enhanced (lipolytic, insulin antagonizing) without an enhancement of the indirect effects of the hormone (similar effect to that of acute illness). However, studies that administered IGF-1 alone have also produced disappointing results.[10] A safer and more physiological approach may be to re-establish the pulsatile nature of pituitary secretion of growth hormone and thyroid-stimulating hormone (TSH) by administering a continuous infusion of GHRH and thyrotropin-releasing hormone (TRH).[11] The clinical benefit of such an approach has yet to be determined. These data suggest that at this time, GH or GH analogues should not be given to critically ill patients, as the clinical benefits of such therapy remain unproven.

TSH–Thyroid Axis

The acute phase of critical illness is characterized by low levels of T3 with normal levels of TSH and T4. This syndrome known as the "sick euthyroid syndrome" is caused by decreased peripheral conversion of T4 to T3. This contrasts with the pattern in CCI, in which the TSH is low (or low-normal), with low T4 and T3 levels. The pulsatility in the TSH secretory pattern is dramatically diminished and like the GH axis, the loss of TSH pulse amplitude is related to low levels of thyroid hormone. CCI is associated with decreased thyrotropin-releasing hormone (TRH) gene expression in the hypothalamic paraventricular nuclei. This suggests that the production and/or the release of thyroid hormones is reduced in the chronic phase of critical illness due to reduced hypothalamic stimulation of the thyrotrophs, in turn leading to reduced stimulation of the thyroid gland.

The administration of T4 has failed to demonstrate a benefit in critically ill patients. This is however not surprising in view of the impaired conversion of T4 to T3. In a study of severely burned patents given 200 μg T3 daily, there was no evidence of benefit from thyroid replacement.[12] In patients with the SES, treatment with T4 or T3 alone may not be beneficial. The administration of TSH secretagogues seems to have a more "physiological" effect; however, RCTs are required to determine whether this therapy improves outcome. It is suggested that TSH, T3, and T4 should be measured in CCI patients and those with overt biochemical hypothyroidism together with clinical features compatible with hypothyroidism should be treated with low doses of T3.

Luteinizing Hormone–Testosterone Axis

Similar to that of GHRH and TRH, the pulsatile secretion of LH is decreased. Circulating levels of testosterone become extremely low (often undetectable) in men, whereas estimated free estradiol concentrations remain normal, suggesting increased aromatization of adrenal androgens.

HPA Axis

In CCI, serum ACTH levels are low, while cortisol levels may remain elevated, indicating that cortisol release in this phase may be driven through an alternative pathway. It has been suggested that adrenal steroidogenesis is shifted toward glucocorticoid production and away from mineralocorticoid and androgen production. Some patients however may develop the "adrenal exhaustion syndrome" in which the cortisol levels are low and the adrenal gland becomes unresponsive to ACTH.[13,14] Circulating levels of adrenal androgens such as dehydroepiandrosterone sulfate, which have immunostimulatory properties on Th1 helper cells, are low during CCI.

Changes in dehydroepiandrosterone (DHEA) and dehydroepiandrosterone sulfate (DHEAS) levels during critical illness are complex. DHEAS levels are decreased but DHEA (biologically active form) has been reported to be increased. However, a high cortisol-to-DHEA ratio has been reported to be associated with a poor outcome.[15] This suggests that combined treatment with hydrocortisone and DHEA may be more beneficial than hydrocortisone monotherapy in critically ill patients; however, clinical trials are required to confirm this postulate.

Metabolic Bone Disease

Metabolic bone disease is prevalent in the CCI patient population. Prolonged immobilization and cytokine-mediated events increase the risk of bone hyper-resorption. Vitamin D deficiency is extremely common, resulting from lack of exposure to sun, malnutrition, malabsorption, and impaired renal or hepatic function.[16] Nierman and Mechanick[17] demonstrated that 92% of CCI patients had bone hyper-resorption due to either vitamin D deficiency and/or immobilization. These authors have used the combination of pamidronate and calcitriol [1,25(OH)$_2$ vitamin D] to control bone hyper-resorption.[18]

Energy Metabolism

In contrast to the early phase of severe illness, patients with CCI are no longer able to efficiently use fatty acids as metabolic substrates. They store fat with feeding, both in adipose tissue and as fatty infiltrates in vital organs such as the pancreas and the liver, but they continue to waste large amounts of protein from skeletal muscle and from organs, which causes impairment of vital functions, weakness, and delayed or hampered recovery.

CCI patients are best fed enterally (gastric); TPN should be avoided at all costs. The optimal nutritional formula for these patients has yet to be determined. Immune-enhancing nutritional formulas with added arginine, glutamine, omega-3 FA, and anti-oxidants have been demonstrated to improve the outcome of malnourished patients undergoing elective surgery. While these formulas have not been specifically tested in CCI patients, on theoretical grounds an immune-enhancing diet would have value in these patients. One should avoid overfeeding; a target of 25 kcal/kg/day (non-protein calories) is recommended. Indirect calorimetry may be useful in these patients to determine caloric requirements as well as the preferred source of calories. Additional supplementation of high-quality protein may be required. The role of additional glutamine and selenium requires investigation. A low arginine formula should be used in infected patients.

■ NEUROMUSCULAR ABNORMALITIES

Neuromuscular problems are extremely common in CCI patients. These include critical illness polyneuropathy, delirium, metabolic encephalopathy (with coma), and myopathy. These problems further delay weaning from mechanical ventilation and increase the morbidity and mortality associated with this syndrome.

Critical Illness Polyneuropathy

Critical illness polyneuropathy (CIP), first described by Bolton in 1983, is defined as a predominantly motor, axonal dysfunction of peripheral nerves in the setting of SIRS, MODS, and respiratory insufficiency.[19-21] Postmortem examination of peripheral nerve specimens from patients with CIP has shown primary degeneration of motor and sensory nerves that supply the limbs and the respiratory system. Although this denervation is more widespread and severe in the distal muscle groups, the phrenic nerve, the diaphragm, and intercostal muscles are also involved.

Classically CIP is associated with a symmetric predominantly distal paresis, with legs involved worse than arms, along with impaired sensory testing in the feet and hyporeflexia. CIP is difficult to diagnose clinically and is often suspected when critically ill patients are otherwise improving yet continue to have difficulty in weaning from mechanical ventilation. In most patients the initial neurological symptom of CIP is failure to wean. The definitive diagnosis of CIP is made by EMG and nerve conduction studies. EMG is characterized by the following:

- Widespread fibrillations and positive sharp waves
- Reduced amplitude of compound muscles and sensory nerve action potentials
- Relatively normal conduction studies

There are no proven treatments that will speed the recovery of peripheral nerve function in patients who have developed CIP. CIP is associated with prolonged weaning difficulties, a long convalescence, and a high mortality. Both the time to liberation from mechanical ventilation and the mortality are directly related to the severity of polyneuropathy.

Critical Illness Myopathy

Critical illness myopathy (CIP) is characterized by a diffuse non-necrotizing myopathy accompanied by fiber atrophy, fatty degeneration of muscle fibers, and fibrosis. Clinically, patients with CIM may demonstrate weakness, failure to wean, or paresis. Creatinine phosphokinase (CPK) levels are relatively normal, consistent with a myopathy and not a myositis. CIM remains difficult to distinguish clinically from CIP because they share similar clinical characteristics and may occur in the same patient. Although the presence of normal sensory nerve action potentials with small compound muscle action potentials on electrodiagnostic studies may suggest a component of CIM, muscle biopsy remains the gold standard for diagnosis. However, because there is no effective treatment for CIM, the indications for invasive biopsies are unclear.

Brain Dysfunction

Coma and delirium are reported to occur in up to 65% of CCI patients.[22] Unlike the delirium of acutely ill patients which usually lasts about 48 h, the delirium occurring in CCI patients may persist for a prolonged period of time. Follow-up studies reveal that most of the hospital survivors including those living at home remain profoundly cognitively impaired.[22]

Septic encephalopathy is an acute, reversible, generalized disturbance in cerebral function, initially manifested by alteration in attention and alertness, in the presence of sepsis. It is essentially a diagnosis by exclusion, as many factors such as sedative drugs, encephalitis, liver or renal failure, hypoperfusion, fever, adrenal insufficiency, cerebral vascular accidents, and drug fever either alone or in combination may result in disturbed cerebral function.

■ MANAGEMENT OF CCI

The management of CCI patients is essentially supportive with meticulous attention being paid to prevent infections, to minimize further muscle breakdown, and to promote recovery with successful weaning. The management plan should include the following.

Testing

- T4, T3, and TSH to exclude hypothyroidism
- PTH and vitamin D to evaluate for metabolic bone disease
- ACTH stimulation test if not on steroids
- EMG – to diagnose CIP (important for prognosis)
- EEG if comatose or poorly responsive (important for prognosis)
- Prealbumin and albumin weekly

General Management

- All ventilator-dependent patients should have a tracheotomy performed.
- A small bore feeding tube should be placed in stomach; consider a PEG tube.
- Air mattress or kinetic bed to prevent bed sores.
- VAP precaution measure.
- Immune-enhancing enteral nutrition. *Avoid TPN.*
- *Avoid* blood transfusion at all costs. Blood t/f increases the risk of further organ dysfunction and death.[23]

- Although EPO (erythropoietin) has not been shown to improve the outcome of general ICU patients,[24] high-dose EPO (40,000 U once or twice weekly) should be considered to minimize the requirement for blood transfusion. Check ferritin levels and supplement with iron as required.
- PICC line for venous access.
- Monitor volume status; prevent volume overload.
- Daily physiotherapy; mobilize out of bed if possible and early exercise program (see below).
- DVT prophylaxis.
- Replete magnesium and phosphorus as required.
- Unless contraindicated (drug interactions), consider treatment with a statin. Statins have important immunoregulatory and anti-thrombotic properties which may be beneficial in CCI patients.[25–29]
- Consider supplementation with selenium and zinc.[30–32]
- Limit use of corticosteroids; only for hemodynamic instability and use the lowest dose possible.
- Avoid benzodiazepines.
- Use opiates sparingly for pain.
- Consider daily dosing with olanzapine or with haloperidol PRN.[33,34]
- Consider nighttime dosing with melatonin.[35]
- Maintain day/night sleep cycle with natural light during day.
- Consider music therapy.

Stress Hyperglycemia

- Use intermediate-acting insulin (lente or NPH) every 12 h.
- Rapid-acting insulin sliding scale 4–6 h
- Aim for blood glucose of between 140–180 mg/dl.
- Avoid long-acting insulins and oral hypoglycemic agents.

Metabolic Bone Disease

- Pamidronate 30 mg for 3 days
- Calcitriol 0.25 μg on day 4

Anabolic Steroids

Oxandrolone is an oral anabolic steroid with enhanced anabolic activity and minimal androgenic activity when compared with testosterone. In burn patients, chronically malnourished renal dialysis patients, as well as

malnourished patients with COPD and HIV, anabolic steroids in combination with enhanced calorie and protein diet have been shown to
improve body mass and muscle strength. On the basis of these observations the role of oxandrolone in critically ill patients has been examined
in two RCT.[36,37] Both of these studies failed to demonstrate a benefit,
with the study in CCI patients demonstrating an increase in the duration
of mechanical ventilation as well as ICU length of stay. Based on the
results of these studies, anabolic steroids cannot be recommended in CCI
patients.

Exercise Program

A number of studies have demonstrated that early mobilization and
physical activity are feasible and safe in respiratory failure patients
requiring mechanical ventilation.[38,39] Burtin and colleagues[40] initiated
an individually tailored exercise training protocol during the early ICU
stay of patients requiring mechanical ventilation. The results of this
study suggested that exercise training may enhance recovery of exercise
capacity, self-perceived functional status, and muscle strength. Similarly,
Schweickert and colleagues[41] performed an RCT in which patients who
remained ventilator dependant for more than 3 days were randomized to
early physical and occupational therapy which was coupled with daily
awakenings. Patients in the intervention group had shorter duration of
delirium and more ventilator-free days with significantly more patients
returning to an independent functional status.

■ REFERENCES

1. Carson SS, Bach PB. The epidemiology and costs of chronic critical
   illness. *Crit Care Clin*. 2002;18:461–476.
2. van den Berghe G. Neuroendocrine pathobiology of chronic critical
   illness. *Crit Care Clin*. 2002;18:509–528.
3. Mechanick JI, Brett EM. Endocrine and metabolic issues in the
   management of the chronically critically ill patient. *Crit Care Clin*.
   2002;18:619–641.
4. Venker J, Miedema M, Strack van Schijndel RJ, et al. Long-term
   outcome after 60 days of intensive care. *Anaesthesia*. 2005;60:541–546.
5. Spicher JE, White DP. Outcome and function following prolonged
   mechanical ventilation. *Arch Intern Med*. 1987;147:421–425.
6. Gracey DR, Naessens JM, Viggiano RW, et al. Outcome of patients
   cared for in a ventilator-dependent unit in a general hospital. *Chest*.
   1995;107:494–499.

7. van den Berghe G. Neuroendocrine pathobiology of chronic critical illness. *Crit Care Clin.* 2002;18:509–528.

8. Chung TT, Hinds CJ. Treatment with GH and IGF-1 in critical illness. *Crit Care Clin.* 2006;22:29–40.

9. Takala J, Ruokonen E, Webster NR, et al. Increased mortality associated with growth hormone treatment in critically ill adults. *N Engl J Med.* 1999;341:785–792.

10. Goeters C, Mertes N, Tacke J, et al. Repeated administration of recombinant human insulin-like growth factor-I in patients after gastric surgery. Effect on metabolic and hormonal patterns. *Ann Surg.* 1995;222: 646–653.

11. van den Berghe G, Wouters P, Weekers F, et al. Reactivation of pituitary hormone release and metabolic improvement by infusion of growth hormone-releasing peptide and thyrotropin-releasing hormone in patients with protracted critical illness. *J Clin Endocrinol Metab.* 1999;84:1311–1323.

12. Becker RA, Vaughan GM, Ziegler MG, et al. Hypermetabolic low triiodothyronine syndrome of burn injury. *Crit Care Med.* 1982;10: 870–875.

13. Marik PE, Zaloga GP. Adrenal Insufficiency in the Critically Ill: a new look at an old problem. *Chest.* 2002;122:1784–1796.

14. Guzman JA, Guzman CB. Adrenal exhaustion in septic patients with vasopressor dependency. *J Crit Care.* 2007;22:319–323.

15. Arlt W, Hammer F, Sanning P, et al. Dissociation of serum dehydroepiandrosterone and dehydroepiandrosterone sulfate in septic shock. *J Clin Endocrinol Metab.* 2006;91:2548–2554.

16. Lee P, Eisman JA, Center JR. Vitamin D deficiency in critically ill patients. *N Engl J Med.* 2009;360:1912–1913.

17. Nierman DM, Mechanick JI. Bone hyperresorption is prevalent in chronically critically ill patients. *Chest.* 1998;114:1122–1128.

18. Nierman DM, Mechanick JI. Biochemical response to treatment of bone hyperresorption in chronically critically ill patients. *Chest.* 2000;118:761–766.

19. Bolton CF, Laverty DA, Brown JD, et al. Critically ill polyneuropathy: electrophysiological studies and differentiation from Guillain–Barre syndrome. *J Neurol Neurosurg Psy.* 1986;49:563–573.

20. Bolton CF, Gilbert JJ, Hahn AF, et al. Polyneuropathy in critically ill patients. *J Neurol Neurosurg Psy.* 1984;47:1223–1231.

21. Bolton CF. Sepsis and the systemic inflammatory response syndrome: neuromuscular manifestations. *Crit Care Med.* 1996;24:1408–1416.

22. Nelson JE, Tandon N, Mercado AF, et al. Brain dysfunction: another burden for the chronically critically ill. *Arch Intern Med.* 2006;166: 1993–1999.

23. Marik PE, Corwin HL. Efficacy of RBC transfusion in the critically ill: a systematic review of the literature. *Crit Care Med.* 2008;36:2667–2674.

24. Corwin HL, Gettinger A, Fabian TC, et al. Efficacy and safety of epoetin Alfa in critically ill patients. *N Engl J Med.* 2007;357: 965–976.
25. Almog Y. Statins, inflammation, and sepsis: hypothesis. *Chest.* 2003;124:740–743.
26. Glynn RJ, Danielson E, Fonseca FA, et al. A randomized trial of rosuvastatin in the prevention of venous thromboembolism. *N Engl J Med.* 2009;360:1851–1861.
27. Kruger P, Fitzsimmons K, Cook D, et al. Statin therapy is associated with fewer deaths in patients with bacteraemia. *Intensive Care Med.* 2006;32:75–79.
28. Merx MW, Weber C. Statins in the intensive care unit. *Curr Opin Crit Care.* 2006;12:309–314.
29. Novack V, Terblanche M, Almog Y. Do statins have a role in preventing or treating sepsis? *Crit Care.* 2006;10:113.
30. Geoghegan M, McAuley D, Eaton S, et al. Selenium in critical illness. *Curr Opin Crit Care.* 2006;12:136–141.
31. Angstwurm MW, Engelmann L, Zimmermann T, et al. Selenium in Intensive Care (SIC): results of a prospective randomized, placebo-controlled, multiple-center study in patients with severe systemic inflammatory response syndrome, sepsis, and septic shock. *Crit Care Med.* 2007;35:118–126.
32. Wong HR, Shanley TP, Sakthivel B, et al. Genome-level expression profiles in pediatric septic shock indicate a role for altered zinc homeostasis in poor outcome. *Physiol Genomics.* 2007;30:146–155.
33. Lacasse H, Perreault MM, Williamson DR. Systematic review of antipsychotics for the treatment of hospital-associated delirium in medically or surgically ill patients. *Ann Pharmacother.* 2006;40:1966–1973.
34. Skrobik YK, Bergeron N, Dumont M, et al. Olanzapine vs haloperidol: treating delirium in a critical care setting. *Intensive Care Med.* 2004;30:444–449.
35. Bourne RS, Mills GH, Minelli C. Melatonin therapy to improve nocturnal sleep in critically ill patients: encouraging results from a small randomised controlled trial. *Crit Care.* 2008;12:R52-doi:10.1186/cc6871.
36. Bulger EM, Jurkovich GJ, Farver CL, et al. Oxandrolone does not improve outcome of ventilator dependent surgical patients. *Ann Surg.* 2004;240:472–478.
37. Gervasio JM, Dickerson RN, Swearingen J, et al. Oxandrolone in trauma patients. *Pharmacotherapy.* 2000;20:1328–1334.
38. Bailey P, Thomsen GE, Spuhler VJ, et al. Early activity is feasible and safe in respiratory failure patients. *Crit Care Med.* 2007;35: 139–145.
39. Morris PE, Goad A, Thompson C, et al. Early intensive care unit mobility therapy in the treatment of acute respiratory failure. *Crit Care Med.* 2008;36:2238–2243.

40. Burtin C, Clerckx B, Robbeets C, et al. Early exercise in critically ill patients enhances short-term functional recovery. *Crit Care Med.* 2009;37:2499–2505.
41. Schweickert WD, Pohlman MC, Pohlman AS, et al. Early physical and occupational therapy in mechanically ventilated, critically ill patients: a randomised controlled trial. *Lancet.* 2009;373:1874–1882.

8

Fluid Resuscitation and Volume Assessment

Volume replacement remains the cornerstone of resuscitation in the critically ill and injured patient. The initial therapeutic intervention in hypotensive patients, oliguric patients, and patients with evidence of poor organ/tissue perfusion is volume resuscitation. However, both under-resuscitation and volume overload increase morbidity and mortality in critically ill patients. Uncorrected hypovolemia, leading to inappropriate infusions of vasopressor agents, may increase organ hypoperfusion and ischemia.[1] However, overzealous fluid resuscitation has been associated with increased complications, increased length of ICU and hospital stay, and increased mortality.[2,3] The resuscitation of all critically ill patients therefore requires an accurate assessment of the adequacy of organ/tissue perfusion (and oxygenation), the patients' intravascular volume status, and fluid responsiveness (the hemodynamic response following a fluid challenge). Fluid management is one of the most important (and difficult) issues in the critically ill patient. However, the volume status of each and every ICU patient needs to be assessed on an ongoing basis. The intensivist needs to ask the following questions:

- Does this patient have adequate organ perfusion?
  - Mean arterial pressure (cerebral and abdominal perfusion pressures)
  - Urine output
  - Mentation
  - Capillary refill
  - Skin perfusion/mottling
  - Cold extremities
  - Cold knee's (Marik's sign; temperature gradient between thigh and knee)

P.E. Marik, *Handbook of Evidence-Based Critical Care*,
DOI 10.1007/978-1-4419-5923-2_8,
© Springer Science+Business Media, LLC 2010

- Blood lactate
- Arterial pH, BE, and HCO_3
- Mixed venous oxygen saturation ($SmvO_2$) or central venous oxygen saturation ($ScvO_2$)
- Mixed venous pCO_2
- Tissue pCO_2 (sublingual capnometry or equivalent)
- Gastric impedance spectroscopy
- Skeletal muscle tissue oxygenation StO_2
• What is this patient's intravascular volume?
- See below
• Does this patient have tissue edema?
- Generalized edema
- Pulmonary edema on chest radiograph
- Increased extravascular lung water (PiCCO technology)
- Increased intra-abdominal pressure
• Is this patient volume responsive?
- Pulse pressure variation (PPV) and/or stroke volume variation (SVV)
• Does this patient have preserved LV function?
- ECHO
• If the patient has inadequate organ perfusion and is volume responsive, what volume expander do I use?
- Lactated Ringer's solution (Hartmann's solution)
- 5% albumin
- Normal saline
- 1/2 normal saline
- Blood

■ VOLUME DEPLETION

The intravascular volume of an average 70 kg man is approximately 5 L of which 2 L is red cell volume and 3 L plasma volume. The intravascular, extracellular fluid compartment equilibrates with the extracellular, extravascular fluid compartment (ECF ~ 11 L), with a reduction in one compartment leading to a reduction of the other. However, critically ill patients may have an expanded extracellular, extravascular compartment (tissue edema) with a contracted intravascular compartment. It is important to distinguish between these forms of volume depletion as the management may differ:

Volume Depletion with Depleted Extravascular Compartment

• Acute blood loss
- Trauma
- GI bleed

- Gastrointestinal tract losses (diarrhea, vomiting, fistula)
- Decreased fluid intake due to acute medical conditions
- Diabetic ketoacidosis
- Heat exhaustion
- "Dehydration"

Volume Depletion with Expanded Extravascular Compartment

- Sepsis
- Pancreatitis
- Trauma
- Surgery
- Burns
- Liver failure
- Cardiac failure

A reduction in intravascular volume results in a fall in stroke volume, which is initially compensated for by an increase in heart rate thereby maintaining cardiac output. However, with further volume depletion cardiac output and then blood pressure falls. This is associated with a reduction in organ perfusion. At the organ level, local autoregulatory mechanism comes into play in an attempt to maintain tissue perfusion. A reduction in renal perfusion normally results in dilatation of the glomerular afferent arteriole and constriction of the glomerular efferent arteriole so that glomerular capillary hydrostatic pressure and glomerular filtration rate (GFR) remain constant. However, a decrease in *renal perfusion pressure* below the autoregulatory range (mean arterial pressure < 70 mmHg) leads to an abrupt fall in GFR and urine output (oliguria). In the elderly and in patients with diseases affecting the integrity of the afferent arterioles, lesser degrees of hypotension may cause a decline in renal function and oliguria. While primary renal disease and urinary tract obstruction may lead to oliguria, intravascular volume depletion with renal hypoperfusion is the commonest cause of oliguria in clinical practice. Other features of intravascular volume depletion include the following:

- Concentrated urine
- Postural hypotension
- Tachycardia (and postural tachycardia)
- Pulse pressure variation (PPV) and stroke volume variation (SVV)

■ IS MY PATIENT FLUID RESPONSIVE?

Fundamentally the only reason to give a patient a fluid challenge is to increase stroke volume and cardiac output. This assumes that the patient is on the ascending portion of the Frank–Starling curve and has "recruitable" cardiac output. Once the left ventricle is functioning near the "flat" part of the Frank–Starling curve, fluid loading has little effect on cardiac output and only serves to increase tissue edema and to promote tissue dysoxia. In normal physiologic conditions, both ventricles operate on the ascending portion of the Frank–Starling curve.[4] This mechanism provides a functional reserve to the heart in situations of acute stress.[4] In normal individuals, an increase in preload (with volume challenge) results in a significant increase in stroke volume. In contrast, only about 50% of patients with circulatory failure will respond to a fluid challenge.[5] It is therefore crucial during the resuscitation phase of all critically ill patients to determine whether the patient is fluid responsive or not; this determines the optimal strategy of increasing cardiac output and oxygen delivery.

ALERT

The only reason to give a patient a fluid challenge is to increase stroke volume. The concept of "filling up the tank" is meaningless and reflects a poor understanding of human physiology.

■ "STATIC" MEASURES OF INTRAVASCULAR VOLUME

The Central Venous Pressure (CVP) and Pulmonary Capillary Wedge Pressure (PCWP)

The central venous pressure (CVP) is frequently used to guide fluid management. The basis for using the CVP comes from the dogma that the CVP reflects intravascular volume; specifically it is widely believed that patients' with a low CVP are volume depleted while patients with a high CVP are volume overloaded. Furthermore, the "5-2" rule which was popularized in the 1970s is still widely used today for guiding fluid therapy.[6] According to this rule, the change in CVP following a fluid challenge is used to guide subsequent fluid management decisions.

While the CVP describes the pressure of blood in the thoracic vena cava it is a very poor indicator of both intravascular volume and fluid responsiveness. In a recent report the pooled correlation coefficient between the CVP and the measured blood volume was 0.16 (95% CI 0.03–0.28).[7] The pooled correlation coefficient between the baseline CVP and change in stroke index/cardiac index was 0.18 (95% CI 0.08–0.28). The pooled area under the ROC curve was 0.56 (95% CI 0.51–0.61). The pooled correlation between the delta-CVP and the change in stroke index/cardiac index was 0.11 (95% CI 0.015–0.21).The results of this systematic review clearly demonstrates that there is no association between the CVP and circulating blood volume and that the CVP does not predict fluid responsiveness. It is very important to note that a patient with a CVP of 2 mmHg is as likely to be fluid responsive as a patient with a CVP of 20 mmHg.[8] Based on this data the CVP should no longer (NEVER) be measured in the ICU, operating room, or emergency room.

Since the introduction of the pulmonary artery catheter (PAC) almost 30 years ago, the pulmonary artery wedge pressure (PCWP) was assumed to be a reliable and valid indicator of left ventricular preload. However, it was not long after the introduction of the PAC that studies began to appear demonstrating that the PCWP was a poor reflection of preload. Recent studies have clearly demonstrated that the PCWP is a poor predictor of preload and volume responsiveness.[5,8,9] Indeed, the PCWP suffers many of the limitations of the CVP. The PCWP is an indirect reflection of left ventricular end-diastolic pressure (LVEDP) and not left ventricular end-diastolic volume or LV preload.

ALERT

The CVP is a relic from the past and should never be measured in modern critical care medicine (except in acute cor pulmonale). The CVP and PCWP are no more useful than the "phases of the moon" in evaluating a patient's volume status.

Other Static Indices of Intravascular Volume

The right ventricular end-diastolic volume (RVEDV), left ventricular end-diastolic area (LVEDA), inferior vena-caval diameter, intrathoracic blood volume index (ITBVI), and global end-diastolic volume index (GEDVI) have all been shown to be poor predictors of volume responsiveness and should not be used to guide volume replacement.[10]

■ "DYNAMIC" MEASURES OF INTRAVASCULAR VOLUME

As discussed above, multiple studies have demonstrated that the CVP, PCWP, RVEDVI, and LVEDA do not predict volume responsiveness.[7,11,12] It has therefore become generally accepted that "estimates of intravascular volume based on any given level of filling pressure (or volume) do not reliably predict a patients response to fluid administration."[12] Over the last decade a number of studies have been reported which have used heart–lung interactions during mechanical ventilation to assess fluid responsiveness. Specifically, the pulse pressure variation (PPV) derived from analysis of the arterial waveform and the stroke volume variation (SVV) derived from pulse contour analysis have been shown to be highly predictive of fluid responsiveness.

Stroke Volume Variation (SVV) and Pulse Pressure Variation (PPV)

The principles underling the PPV (and SVV) are based on simple physiology (see Figure 8-1). Intermittent positive pressure ventilation induces cyclic changes in the loading conditions of the left and right ventricles. Mechanical insufflation decreases preload and increases afterload of the right ventricle (RV). The RV preload reduction is due to the decrease in the venous return pressure gradient that is related in the inspiratory increase in pleural pressure.[11] The increase in RV afterload is related to the inspiratory increase in transpulmonary pressure. The reduction in RV preload and increase in RV afterload both lead to a decrease in RV stroke volume, which is at a minimum at the end of the inspiratory period. The inspiratory reduction in RV ejection leads to a decrease in LV filling after a phase lag of two or three heart beats because of the long blood pulmonary transit time. Thus the LV preload reduction may induce a decrease in LV stroke volume, which is at its minimum during the expiratory period. The cyclic changes in RV and LV stroke volume are greater when the ventricles operate on the steep rather than the flat portion of the Frank–Starling curve (see Figure 8-2). Therefore, the magnitude of the respiratory changes in LV stroke volume is an indicator of biventricular preload dependence.[11]

A recent meta-analysis demonstrated that the PPV and SVV measured during volume controlled mechanical ventilation predicted with a high degree of accuracy (ROC of 0.94 and 0.84, respectively) those patients likely to respond to a fluid challenge as well the degree to which the stroke volume is likely to increase.[13] The predictive value was maintained in patients with poor LV function. Furthermore, with remarkable consistency these studies reported a threshold PPV/SVV of 12–13%. In this study the area under the ROC curves was 0.55 for the CVP, 0.56 for the GEDVI, and 0.64 for the LVEDAI. The enormous appeal of using the PPV/SVV as a marker of volume responsiveness is that it dynamically predicts an individual patient's position on his or her Starling curve and this is independent of ventricular function and compliance as well as pulmonary pressures and mechanics (see Figure 8-3).

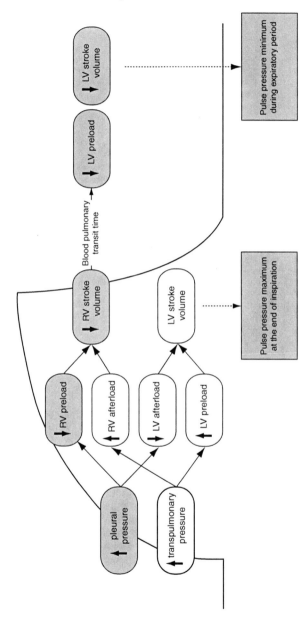

Figure 8-1. Hemodynamic effects of mechanical ventilation. The cyclic changes in LV stroke volume are mainly related to the expiratory decrease in LV preload due to the inspiratory decrease in RV filling. reproduced with permission from Crit Care/Current Science Ltd.

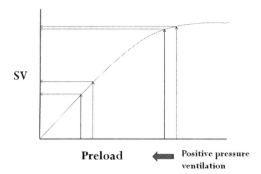

Figure 8-2. The cyclic changes in RV and LV stroke volume are greater when the ventricles operate on the steep rather than the flat portion of the Frank–Starling curve.

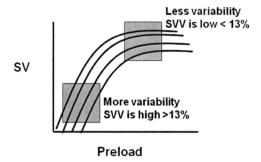

Figure 8-3. Arterial waveform analysis during positive pressure ventilation predicts an individual patients' position on his/her Starling curve and allows optimization of cardiac performance.

While the respiratory variation in vena-caval diameter and stroke volume as measured by echocardiography (see below) has been demonstrated to predict fluid responsiveness, they do not perform as well as the PPV/SVV, require intensivists with a high degree of expertise in echocardiography, and are not conducive to minute-to-minute monitoring. This suggests that currently the PPV/SVV is the most accurate predictor of volume responsiveness in critically ill patients. It should be noted that the PPV was a more accurate predictor of volume responsiveness than the SVV. This may be related to the fact that the PPV is a direct measurement, while the SVV is derived from pulse contour analysis which makes a number of assumptions. Changes in vascular tone alter the contour of the pulse wave which may result in erroneous calculations of stroke volume.[14,15]

It should be appreciated that both arrhythmias and spontaneous breathing activity will lead to misinterpretations of the respiratory variations in pulse pressure/stroke volume. Furthermore, for any specific preload condition the PPV/SVV will vary according to the tidal volume. Reuter and colleagues demonstrated a linear relationship between tidal volume and SVV.[16] De Backer and colleagues evaluated the influence of tidal volume on the ability of the PPV to predict fluid responsiveness.[17] These authors reported that the PPV was a reliable predictor of fluid responsiveness only when the tidal volume was at least 8 mL/kg. For accuracy, reproducibility and consistency we suggest that the tidal volume be increased to 8–10 mL/kg ideal body weight prior to and after a fluid challenge.

Dynamic Changes in Aortic Flow Velocity/Stroke Volume Assessed by Esophageal Doppler

The esophageal Doppler technique measures blood flow velocity in the descending aorta by means of a Doppler transducer. The probe is introduced into the esophagus of sedated, mechanically ventilated patients and then rotated so that the transducer faces the aorta and a characteristic aortic velocity signal is obtained. The cardiac output is calculated based on the diameter of the aorta (measured or estimated), the distribution of the cardiac output to the descending aorta, and the measured flow velocity of blood in the aorta. As esophageal Doppler probes are inserted blindly, the resulting waveform is highly dependent on correct positioning. The clinician must adjust the depth, rotate the probe, and adjust the gain to obtain an optimal signal.[18] Poor positioning of the esophageal probe tends to underestimate the true cardiac output. There is a significant learning curve in obtaining adequate Doppler signals and the correlations are better in studies where the investigator was not blinded to the results of the cardiac output obtained with a PAC.[19]

A meta-analysis by Dark and Singer demonstrated a 86% correlation between cardiac output as determined by esophageal Doppler and PAC.[20] Although the correlation between the two methods was only modest, there was an excellent correlation between the change in cardiac output with therapeutic interventions. Furthermore, the respiratory variation in aortic blood flow velocity with positive pressure ventilation has been demonstrated to be a reliable predictor of fluid responsiveness.[21] While esophageal Doppler has utility in aiding in the assessment of the hemodynamic status of critically ill patients, this technology has been slow to be adopted. This is likely the consequence of a number of factors including the less than ideal accuracy of the cardiac output measurements, the long learning curve, the inability to obtain continuous reliable measurements, and the practical problems related to presence of the probe in the patients' esophagus.

Positive Pressure Ventilation Induced Changes in Vena-Caval Diameter

Cyclic changes in superior and inferior vena-caval diameter as measured by echocardiography have been used to predict fluid responsiveness.[22,23] This technique has a number of limitations, including the fact that sub-costal echocardiography may be difficult in obese patients and those that have undergone laparotomy. Furthermore, changes in IVC diameter are affected by intra-abdominal pressure making this technique unreliable in patients with high intra-abdominal pressure.

Dynamic Changes in Aortic Flow Velocity/Stroke Volume Assessed by Echocardiography

The respiratory changes in aortic flow velocity and stroke volume can be assessed by Doppler echocardiography. Feissel and colleagues demonstrated that the respiratory changes in aortic blood velocity predicted fluid responsiveness in mechanically ventilated patients.[24] In this study the LVEDAI was unable to predict fluid responsiveness.

The dynamic indices of volume responsiveness reviewed above are dependent on the cyclic changes in intrathoracic pressure induced by positive pressure ventilation and are not applicable to spontaneously breathing patients. However, changes in aortic flow velocity and stroke volume induced by passive leg raising in non-ventilated patients have been demonstrated to be predictive of volume responsiveness.[25,26]

Echocardiographic methods of assessing volume status (aortic flow velocity, stroke volume, LVEDA, IVC/SVC diameter) require intensivists with specialized expertise and skill who have undergone rigorous training in these techniques. There is a long learning curve with a lack of reproducibility. Furthermore, the requirement for 24 h availability and the non-continuous nature of the data limit the applicability of these techniques in the ICU environment. However, as more intensivists embrace this technology, in the hands of experienced operators it can be a useful adjunctive tool to determine fluid responsiveness as well as to assess ventricular function.

■ END-POINTS OF VOLUME RESUSCITATION

Not all patients who are volume responsive require additional fluid challenges. The ideal end-point(s) of fluid resuscitation remains the "holy grail" of critical care medicine. This is complicated by the fact that both under- and over-resuscitation are associated with increased morbidity and mortality. Therefore the patient should receive sufficient fluid to restore "adequate organ perfusion and not a drop more." An integration of the following parameters will allow the intensivist to determine the adequacy of volume resuscitation and if/when a vasopressor agent should be initiated:

- Urine output
- Urine sodium and osmolarity
- Mean arterial pressure (cerebral and abdominal perfusion pressure)
- BUN
- PPV (or SVV)
- Heart rate
- Lactate
- Arterial pH, BE, and HCO_3
- Mixed venous oxygen saturation $SmvO_2$ or $ScvO_2$
- Mixed venous pCO_2
- Tissue pCO_2 (sublingual capnometry or equivalent)
- Gastric impedance spectroscopy
- Skeletal muscle tissue oxygenation StO_2 as measured by NIRS
- Extravascular lung water (see below)
- Intra-abdominal pressure (see below)
- Technology yet to be developed

Once resuscitated, it is preferable to keep patients with ARDS and sepsis (and SIRS) on the "dry side of the road"; allow the BUN to creep up to 30–40 mg/dL; however, do not allow acute renal failure to develop.[3] Monitoring of extravascular lung water and intra-abdominal pressure is very useful in this setting (see below).

It is important to note that while "lactic acidosis," $SmvO_2/ScvO_2$, and StO_2 may reflect the adequacy of tissue perfusion and oxygenation in patients with hypovolemic, hemorrhagic, and cardiogenic shock this does NOT apply to patients with severe sepsis/septic shock/SIRS. In patients with sepsis, tissue CO_2 tension (microvascular flow) and gastric impedance spectroscopy (cellular well being) may be better end-points of resuscitation (see Chapter 10).

■ MEASURES OF VOLUME OVERLOAD

While the dynamic changes in pulse pressure and stroke volume together with clinical indices of organ perfusion are useful for detecting intravascular volume depletion we have few reliable measures of volume overload. An elevated CVP and PCWP are measures of RV and LV dysfunction (failure) and not volume status. Some have suggested that patients receive volume resuscitation until they develop pulmonary edema (indicating that the "tank is full"); this is clearly an absurd approach.[27] Radiographic and clinical signs of pulmonary edema and clinical evidence of anasarca are late signs of volume overload and poor end-points for fluid resuscitation. Extravascular lung water as determined by transpulmonary thermodilution and intra-abdominal pressure monitoring are two techniques that "measure" tissue edema and may aid in the assessment of volume overload.

Extravascular Lung Water

Extravascular lung water (EVLW) may be calculated from the descending limb (indicator dissipation) of the transpulmonary thermodilution curve and is a method of quantifying the degree of pulmonary edema (hydrostatic and permeability).[28] This technique has been shown to compare favorably with the double indicator dilution technique and the ex vivo gravimetric method.[29-31] Furthermore, this technique can detect small (10–20%) increases in lung water.[32] The "normal" value for EVLW is reported to be 5–7 mL/kg with values as high as 30 mL/kg during severe pulmonary edema. In an intriguing study, Sakka et al. found that the mortality was about 65% in ICU patients with an EVLW > 15 mL/kg whereas the mortality was 33% in patients with an EVLW < 10 mL/kg.[33] EVLW has been demonstrated to be an accurate indicator of the severity of lung injury and a reliable prognostic indicator in patients with sepsis-induced acute lung injury.[34,35] EVLW should be indexed to IBW rather than actual body weight.[36] It is likely that using EVLW to guide fluid therapy *may* reduce positive fluid balance, duration of mechanical ventilation, and ultimately patient outcome.

Intra-Abdominal Pressure Monitoring

Intra-abdominal pressure (IAP) is the pressure concealed within the abdominal cavity.[37] The World Society of the Abdominal Compartment Syndrome (WSACS, www.wsacs.org) has recently developed consensus definitions outlining standards for IAP measurement as well as diagnostic criteria for intra-abdominal hypertension (IAH). According to the consensus guidelines IAH is defined as an intra-abdominal pressure $\geq$ 12 mmHg and abdominal compartment syndrome (ACS) is defined as an IAP above 20 mmHg with evidence of organ dysfunction/failure.[38] The abdominal perfusion pressure (APP) is a more accurate predictor of visceral perfusion (MAP-IAP) with a target above 60 mmHg correlating with improved survival.[37] Major risk factors for intra-abdominal hypertension (IAH) include the following:

- Abdominal surgery/trauma
- High volume fluid resuscitation (> 3,500 mL/24 h)
- Massive blood transfusion (> 10 units/24 h)
- Large burns
- Ileus
- Damage control laparotomy
- Liver failure with ascites
- Severe pancreatitis
- Liver transplantation

Physical examination is inaccurate in detecting IAH. Currently IAP is best measured using the intravesicular method. Continuous methods for monitoring IAP have been reported.[39] The following key principles must be followed in the measurement of IAP:

- IAP should be expressed in mmHg
- IAP should be measured at end-expiration and in Complete supine position (note: elevated HOB increases IAP)
- Transducer zeroed in midaxillary line at level of iliac crest
- Maximal instillation of 25 mL sterile saline
- IAP should be measured 30–60 s after instillation of fluid

The IAP should be measured in all "at-risk patients" with repeated measures in those with IAH and following clinical deterioration.

Management of IAH

The 24 h fluid balance has been shown to be an independent predictor of IAH.[40] Therefore a restrictive fluid strategy is recommended in patients at risk of IAH and those with IAH (however MAP must be maintained with cautious volume loading and vasopressors if required). Resuscitation with 5% albumin should be considered in these patients (see below); maintain APP > 60 mmHg:

- Improve abdominal wall compliance
  - Sedation and analgesia
  - Avoid HOB > 30°

- Evacuate intra-abdominal contents
  - Orogastric tube decompression
  - Rectal decompression
  - Prokinetic agents
- Evacuate abdominal fluid collections
  - Paracentesis
  - Percutaneous drainage
- Correct positive fluid balance
  - "cautious diuresis"
  - Ultrafiltration
- Optimize ventilation
  - Keep mean airway pressures as low as possible
  - Prevent ventilator dyssynchrony
- Surgical decompression

■ WHAT TYPE OF FLUID?

This age-old debate has become somewhat of a non-issue in recent years and may be best summarized as follows:

- Hydroxyethyl starch (HES) solutions are associated with an increased risk of renal failure (and death) and have a "limited" role in critical care medicine[41]
- Albumin (5% in NaCl) is SAFE[42] and may have a role (together with lactated Ringer's solution) in the resuscitation of patients with
  - Sepsis
  - Cirrhosis
  - Pancreatitis
  - Burns
- Packed –red blood cells AND lactated Ringer's (LR) are the volume expanders of choice in hemorrhagic shock
  - In traumatic blood loss, RBC should be given with FFP and platelets in a ratio of 1:1:1 (see Chapter 51, blood transfusion)
- 0.9% NaCl is better known as "AbNormal Saline," is associated with the following complications, and is best avoided
  - Decreased glomerular filtration rate (GFR)
  - Metabolic acidosis; both hyperchloremic non-AG as well as AG acidosis
  - Coagulopathy with increased bleeding
- Patients with traumatic head injury should be resuscitated with crystalloids (LR); albumin should be avoided[42]
- A glucose (5 or 10%) containing solution should be used in patients with cirrhosis (high risk of hypoglycemia)

ALERT

0.9% NaCl (AbNormal Saline) is a non-physiologic solution (sodium 154 meq/L, Cl 154 meq/L, and pH < 6) with limited indications.

5% Albumin

While the type of fluid used in the resuscitation of patients with sepsis has not been definitively shown to affect outcome, subgroup analysis of the SAFE study suggested a trend toward a favorable outcome in patients who received albumin.[42] This is supported by experimental studies[43] and patients with malaria (similar pathophysiology to gram-negative sepsis).[44] Albumin has a number of features that may be theoretically advantageous in patients with sepsis (and SIRS) including the following:

- Maintains endothelial glycocalyx and "endothelial function"
- Anti-oxidant properties
- Anti-inflammatory properties
- May limit "third" space loss

Our preference is to give a mixture of both albumin and LR ($\pm$ 50–50) in patients with sepsis (and SIRS) in an attempt to maintain intravascular volume and yet limit the total amount of fluid given.

Albumin should be considered the volume expander of choice in patients with underlying liver disease (cirrhosis).[45,46] Albumin is particularly useful in patients with spontaneous bacterial peritonitis, hepatorenal syndrome, and following a paracentesis (see Chapter 33).

Lactated Ringer's (Hartmann's Solution) vs. 0.9% NaCl (AbNormal Saline)

Despite differences in composition, normal saline and lactated Ringer's solution are frequently considered equivalent and lumped under the term "balanced salt solution." For reasons that are unclear, normal saline appears to be the preferred replacement fluid of medical physicians while lactated Ringer's solution is the choice of surgeons. Furthermore, while no body fluid has an electrolyte composition similar to that of normal saline, this fluid is frequently referred to as "physiologic salt solution" (PSS). However, both experimental and clinical data have demonstrated that these fluids are NOT equivalent (see below) and that in most clinical situations LR is the fluid of choice.

Metabolic Acidosis

Numerous studies have demonstrated the development of a hyperchloremic metabolic acidosis in human volunteers and patients resuscitated with normal saline.[47–50] While the clinical implications of these finding are unclear, the additional loss (renal) of HCO_3 in the setting of reduced buffering capacity only adds to the acid–base burden characteristic of hypoperfused states.[48] Furthermore, resuscitation with normal saline may produce a "dilutional acidosis."

In addition it should be noted that the lactate (in LR) is converted to glucose (mainly in the liver); this reaction consumes hydrogen ions, thereby generating HCO_3-[51]:

$$2CH_3CHOHCOO^- + 2H^+ \Rightarrow C_6H_{12}O$$

Lactate   glucose

Many erroneously believe that LR may worsen or cause a "lactic acidosis"; this is impossible as lactate (the base) has already donated H^+ ions; LR generates HCO_3- in the liver and kidney. Although the lactate concentration (base) may increase with LR this increase is associated with an increase in HCO_3- and an increase in pH (even with liver disease). This observation was elegantly demonstrated by Phillips et al., who in a swine hemorrhagic shock model compared the acid–base status of animals resuscitated with LR and NS (see Table 8-1 below).[52]

Table 8-1. Laboratory data at end of study (Phillips et al.).

	Normal Saline	Ringer's Lactate
Lactate	1.3	6.0
HCO_3	16.7	27.8
pH	7.17	7.41

These results are strikingly similar to the work of Healey et al. who compared resuscitation with blood + normal saline vs. blood + lactated Ringer's solution in a murine massive hemorrhage model (see Table 8-2 below).[53] Note the significantly improved survival in the LR group.

Table 8-2. Laboratory data at end of study (Healey et al.).

	NS + Blood	LR + Blood
pH	7.14	7.39
Na	147	135
Cl	130	109
HCO_3	9.4	19.7
Survival	50%	100%

Coagulopathy

Studies in surgical patients have demonstrated that as compared to LR volume replacement with NS results in greater blood loss with a greater need for blood transfusion.[49] The cause of the coagulopathy is unclear and is only partly explained by the difference in Ca^{2+} between the two solutions.

Renal Function

Solutions high in chloride have been shown experimentally to reduce GRF (due to tubulo-glomerulo feedback).[54] Clinical studies have found indices of renal function to be worse in surgical patients randomized to NS as opposed to RL.

D-Lactate

It should be noted that LR solution is a racemic mixture containing both the L- and D-isomers of lactate. Small animal hemorrhagic shock models have suggested that the D-isomer is pro-inflammatory and increases apoptotic cell death.[55–57] The clinical implication of these findings is unclear.

ALERT

As LR has added potassium (K^+ 4–5 mEq/L) this solution should be used with caution in patients with acute renal failure and hyperkalemia.

■ RESUSCITATION IN SPECIFIC DISEASE STATES

Hemorrhage

In patients who have lost blood, fluid moves from the interstitial to the intravascular compartment in an attempt to restore blood volume; the hemoglobin concentration falls by hemodilution (in the absence of volume resuscitation it takes about 72 h for Hct to stabilize). Therefore, both the intravascular and extravascular, extracellular compartments are decreased following blood loss. Experimental hemorrhage models have demonstrated a higher mortality when animals are resuscitated with blood alone, as compared to blood and crystalloids. Patients who have lost blood should therefore be resuscitated with crystalloid (LR), followed by blood. Due to both a consumptive and a dilutional coagulopathy, patients with traumatic hemorrhage should proactively receive platelets and FFP together with packet red blood cells (in a ratio of 1:1:1). In all other patients, platelets and FFP should only be transfused based on coagulation parameters and ongoing bleeding. In both "medical" and surgical bleeding, the goal should be to restore tissue perfusion and oxygenation and not to achieve a "normal" hemoglobin (a hemoglobin above 7–8 g/dL is usually just fine) (see Chapter 51).

Dehydration

Patients who are dehydrated (from diarrhea, vomiting, diabetic osmotic diuresis, etc.) have lost both intravascular and extravascular, extracellular fluid. Volume replacement with crystalloids (LR) will resuscitate both compartments.

Sepsis (and SIRS)

As a consequence of "leaky capillaries" and "third space loss" these patients have a decreased effective intravascular compartment and tissue edema (enlarged interstitial compartment). As less than 20% of infused crystalloid remains intravascular in these patients, the volume of crystalloids should be limited. The combination of albumin and LR is recommended.

Burns

Due to the thermal injury these patients have a massive loss of interstitial fluid as well as a generalized capillary leak. Patients should be resuscitated with crystalloid (LR) during the first 24 h.

■ MANAGEMENT OF OLIGURIA

While primary renal diseases and urinary tract obstruction may lead to oliguria, intravascular volume depletion with renal hypoperfusion is the commonest cause of oliguria in clinical practice (see Chapter 42). The management of oliguria due to intravascular volume depletion is *aggressive fluid resuscitation*. "Lasix is not a volume expander!"

Diuresis with loop diuretics in patients with normal or reduced effective intravascular volume is invariably associated with a fall in intravascular volume, a fall in plasma volume, a fall in GFR, and a rise in blood urea nitrogen (BUN). The fall in GFR has been correlated with the fall in intravascular volume. Contraction of the intravascular volume and fall in GFR may occur in the absence of a fall in cardiac output. Volume depletion is associated with a greater rise in the BUN than in the plasma creatinine due to increased passive reabsorption of urea which follows the hypovolemia-induced increase in sodium and water resorption in the kidney. An increasing BUN/creatinine ratio in a patient receiving a diuretic is a reliable sign of intravascular volume depletion and should prompt the immediate discontinuation of these agents.

ALERT

Lasix® is the "Devil's medicine" and has no role in acute oliguria/acute renal failure.

Contrary to popular belief the GFR falls (rather than rises) with loop diuretics. In the mammalian kidney there is close coordination between the processes of glomerular filtration and tubular reabsorption. Coordination between the glomerulus and tubule is mediated by a system of tubulo-glomerular feedback which operates within the juxtaglomerular apparatus of each nephron. Microperfusion experiments have demonstrated that an increase in flow rate of tubule fluid through the loop of Henle following the use of a loop diuretic is followed by a reduction in single nephron GFR. This has been shown to be mediated via feedback control by the macula densa which is the flow-dependent distal sensing site. When the tubular glomerular feedback pathway is interrupted with a loop diuretic, there is an attenuation of the pressure-induced afferent arteriolar dilatation with impairment in blood flow autoregulation. In patients with extracellular volume depletion this effect is exaggerated with a dramatic fall in GFR.

■ CLINICAL PEARLS

- The initial treatment of hypotension is a fluid challenge (lactated Ringer's solution)
- The initial treatment of oliguria is a fluid challenge (lactated Ringer's solution)
- Lactated Ringer's is the replacement fluid of choice in most clinical scenarios
- Pulse pressure variation (on mechanical ventilation) should be used to determine "fluid responsiveness"
- The measurement of extravascular lung water and intra-abdominal pressure should be used to prevent volume overload during "large volume" resuscitation

■ REFERENCES

1. Murakawa K, Kobayashi A. Effects of vasopressors on renal tissue gas tensions during hemorrhagic shock in dogs. *Crit Care Med.* 1988;16:789–792.
2. Vincent JL, Sakr Y, Sprung CL, et al. Sepsis in European intensive care units: results of the SOAP study. *Crit Care Med.* 2006;34:344–353.
3. The National Heart, Lung, and Blood Institute Acute Respiratory Distress Syndrome (ARDS) Clinical Trials Network. Comparison of two fluid-management strategies in acute lung injury. *N Engl J Med.* 2006;354:2564–2575.
4. Braunwald E, Sonnenblick EH, Ross J. Mechanisms of cardiac contraction and relaxation. In: Braunwald E, ed. *Heart Disease.* Philadelphia, PA: W.B.Saunders Company; 1988:383–425.
5. Michard F, Teboul JL. Predicting fluid responsiveness in ICU patients: a critical analysis of the evidence. *Chest.* 2002;121:2000–2008.
6. Weil MH, Henning RJ. New concepts in the diagnosis and fluid treatment of circulatory shock. Thirteenth annual Becton, Dickinson and Company Oscar Schwidetsky Memorial Lecture. *Anesth Analg.* 1979;58:124–132.
7. Marik PE, Baram M, Vahid B. Does the central venous pressure predict fluid responsiveness? A systematic review of the literature and the tale of seven mares. *Chest.* 2008;134:172–178.
8. Osman D, Ridel C, Ray P, et al. Cardiac filling pressures are not appropriate to predict hemodynamic response to volume challenge. *Crit Care Med.* 2007;35:64–68.
9. Michard F, Boussat S, Chemla D, et al. Relation between respiratory changes in arterial pulse pressure and fluid responsiveness in septic patients with acute circulatory failure. *Am J Respir Crit Care Med.* 2000;162:134–138.
10. Marik PE. Techniques for assessment of intravascular volume in critically ill patients. *J Intensive Care Med.* 2009;24:329–337.
11. Michard F, Teboul JL. Using heart-lung interactions to assess fluid responsiveness during mechanical ventilation. *Crit Care.* 2000;4: 282–289.
12. Vincent JL, Weil MH. Fluid challenge revisited. *Crit Care Med.* 2006;34:1333–1337.
13. Marik PE, Cavallazzi R, Vasu T, et al. Dynamic changes in arterial waveform derived variables and fluid responsiveness in mechanically ventilated patients. A systematic review of the literature. *Crit Care Med.* 2009;37:2642–2647.
14. Opdam HI, Wan L, Bellomo R. A pilot assessment of the FloTrac cardiac output monitoring system. *Intensive Care Med.* 2007;33:344–349.
15. Lorsomradee S, Lorsomradee S, Cromheecke S, et al. Uncalibrated arterial pulse contour analysis versus continuous thermodilution

technique: effects of alterations in arterial waveform. *J Cardiothorac Vasc Anesth*. 2007;21:636–643.

16. Reuter DA, Bayerlein J, Goepfert MS, et al. Influence of tidal volume on left ventricular stroke volume variation measured by pulse contour analysis in mechanically ventilated patients. *Intensive Care Med*. 2003;29:476–480.

17. De Backer D, Heenen S, Piagnerelli M, et al. Pulse pressure variations to predict fluid responsiveness: influence of tidal volume. *Intensive Care Med*. 2005;31:517–523.

18. Lefrant JY, Bruelle P, Aya AG, et al. Training is required to improve the reliability of esophageal Doppler to measure cardiac output in critically ill patients. *Intensive Care Med*. 1998;24:347–352.

19. Valtier B, Cholley BP, Belot JP, et al. Noninvasive monitoring of cardiac output in critically ill patients using transesophageal doppler. *Am J Respir Crit Care Med*. 1998;158:77–83.

20. Dark PM, Singer M. The validity of trans-esophageal Doppler ultrasonography as a measure of cardiac output in critically ill adults. *Intensive Care Med*. 2004;30:2060–2066.

21. Monnet X, Rienzo M, Osman D, et al. Esophageal Doppler monitoring predicts fluid responsiveness in critically ill ventilated patients. *Intensive Care Med*. 2005;31:1195–1201.

22. Barbier C, Loubieres Y, Schmit C, et al. Respiratory changes in inferior vena cava diameter are helpful in predicting fluid responsiveness in ventilated septic patients. *Intensive Care Med*. 2004;30:1740–1746.

23. Feissel M, Michard F, Faller JP, et al. The respiratory variation in inferior vena cava diameter as a guide to fluid therapy. *Intensive Care Med*. 2004;30:1834–1837.

24. Feissel M, Michard F, Mangin I, et al. Respiratory changes in aortic blood velocity as an indicator of fluid responsiveness in ventilated patients with septic shock. *Chest*. 2001;119:867–873.

25. Maizel J, Airapetian N, Lorne E, et al. Diagnosis of central hypovolemia by using passive leg raising. *Intensive Care Med*. 2007;33:1133–1138.

26. Lamia B, Ochagavia A, Monnet X, et al. Echocardiographic prediction of volume responsiveness in critically ill patients with spontaneously breathing activity. *Intensive Care Med*. 2007;33:1125–1132.

27. Hollenberg SM, Ahrens TS, Annane D, et al. Practice parameters for hemodynamic support of sepsis in adult patients: 2004 update. *Crit Care Med*. 2004;32:1928–1948.

28. Isakow W, Schuster DP. Extravascular lung water measurements and hemodynamic monitoring in the critically ill: bedside alternatives to the pulmonary artery catheter. *Am J Physiol Lung Cell Mol Physiol*. 2006;291:1118–1131.

29. Michard F, Schachtrupp A, Toens C. Factors influencing the estimation of extravascular lung water by transpulmonary thermodilution in critically ill patients. *Crit Care Med*. 2005;33:1243–1247.

30. Sakka SG, Ruhl CC, Pfeiffer UJ, et al. Assessment of cardiac preload and extravascular lung water by single transpulmonary thermodilution. *Intensive Care Med.* 2000;26:180–187.
31. Katzenelson R, Perel A, Berkenstadt H, et al. Accuracy of transpulmonary thermodilution versus gravimetric measurement of extravascular lung water. *Crit Care Med.* 2004;32:1550–1554.
32. Fernandez-Mondejar E, Rivera-Fernandez R, Garcia-Delgado M, et al. Small increases in extravascular lung water are accurately detected by transpulmonary thermodilution. *J Trauma.* 2005;59:1420–1423.
33. Sakka SG, Klein M, Reinhart K, et al. Prognostic value of extravascular lung water in critically ill patients. *Chest.* 2002;122:2080–2086.
34. Chung FT, Lin SM, Lin SY, et al. Impact of extravascular lung water index on outcomes of severe sepsis patients in a medical intensive care unit. *Respir Med.* 2008;102:956–961.
35. Kuzkov VV, Kirov MY, Sovershaev MA, et al. Extravascular lung water determined with single transpulmonary thermodilution correlates with the severity of sepsis-induced acute lung injury. *Crit Care Med.* 2006;34:1647–1653.
36. Berkowitz DM, Danai PA, Eaton S, et al. Accurate characterization of extravascular lung water in acute respiratory distress syndrome. *Crit Care Med.* 2008;36:1803–1809.
37. Cheatham ML. Intraabdominal pressure monitoring during fluid resuscitation. *Curr Opin Crit Care.* 2008;14:327–333.
38. Malbrain ML, Cheatham ML, Kirkpatrick A, et al. Results from the International Conference of Experts on Intra-abdominal Hypertension and Abdominal Compartment Syndrome. I. Definitions. *Intensive Care Med.* 2006;32:1722–1732.
39. Balogh Z, De Waele JJ, Malbrain ML. Continuous intra-abdominal pressure monitoring. *Acta Clin Belg Suppl.* 2007;1:26–32.
40. Cheatham ML, Malbrain ML, Kirkpatrick A, et al. Results from the International Conference of Experts on Intra-abdominal Hypertension and Abdominal Compartment Syndrome. II. Recommendations. *Intensive Care Med.* 2007;33:951–962.
41. Brunkhorst FM, Engel C, Bloos F, et al. Intensive insulin therapy and pentastarch resuscitation in severe sepsis. *N Engl J Med.* 2008;358:125–139.
42. Finfer S, Bellomo R, Boyce N, et al. A comparison of albumin and saline for fluid resuscitation in the intensive care unit. *N Engl J Med.* 2004;350:2247–2256.
43. Walley KR, McDonald TE, Wang Y, et al. Albumin resuscitation increases cardiomyocyte contractility and decreases nitric oxide synthase II expression in rat endotoxemia. *Crit Care Med.* 2003;31:187–194.
44. Maitland K, Pamba A, English M, et al. Randomized trial of volume expansion with albumin or saline in children with severe malaria:

preliminary evidence of albumin benefit. *Clin Infect Dis.* 2005;40: 538–545.

45. Fernandez J, Monteagudo J, Bargallo X, et al. A randomized unblinded pilot study comparing albumin versus hydroxyethyl starch in spontaneous bacterial peritonitis. *Hepatology.* 2005;42:627–634.

46. Sort P, Navasa M, Arroyo V, et al. Effect of intravenous albumin on renal impairment and mortality in patients with cirrhosis and spontaneous bacterial peritonitis. *N Engl J Med.* 1999;341:403–409.

47. Scheingraber S, Rehm M, Sehmisch C, et al. Rapid saline infusion produces hyperchloremic acidosis in patients undergoing gynecologic surgery. *Anesthesiology.* 1999;90:1265–1270.

48. Kellum JA, Bellomo R, Kramer DJ, et al. Etiology of metabolic acidosis during saline resuscitation in endotoxemia. *Shock.* 1998;9:364–368.

49. Waters JH, Gottlieb A, Schoenwald P, et al. Normal saline versus lactated Ringer's solution for intraoperative fluid management in patients undergoing abdominal aortic aneurysm repair: an outcome study. *Anesth Analg.* 2001;93:817–822.

50. Reid F, Lobo DN, Williams RN, et al. (Ab)normal saline and physiological Hartmann's solution: a randomized double-blind crossover study. *Clin Sci.* 2003;104:17–24.

51. White SA, Goldhill DR, White SA, et al. Is Hartmann's the solution? *Anaesthesia.* 1997;52:422–427.

52. Phillips CR, Vinecore K, Hagg DS, et al. Resuscitation of hemorrhagic shock with normal saline vs. lactated Ringer's: effects on oxygenation, extravascular lung water and hemodynamics. *Crit Care.* 2009; 13:R30.

53. Healey MA, Davis RE, Liu FC, et al. Lactated ringer's is superior to normal saline in a model of massive hemorrhage and resuscitation. *J Trauma.* 1998;45:894–899.

54. Wilcox CS. Regulation of renal blood flow by plasma chloride. *J Clin Invest.* 1983;71:726–735.

55. Deb S, Martin B, Sun L, et al. Resuscitation with lactated Ringer's solution in rats with hemorrhagic shock induces immediate apoptosis. *J Trauma.* 1999;46:582–588.

56. Ayuste EC, Chen H, Koustova E, et al. Hepatic and pulmonary apoptosis after hemorrhagic shock in swine can be reduced through modifications of conventional Ringer's solution. *J Trauma.* 2006;60:52–63.

57. Alam HB, Rhee P. New developments in fluid resuscitation. *Surg Clin North Am.* 2007;87:55–72.

9

Sedation and Analgesia

Today we will be mixing ... the Draught of Peace, a potion to calm anxiety and soothe agitation. Be Warned: if you are too heavy-handed with the ingredients you will put the drinker into a heavy and sometimes irreversible sleep, so you will need to pay attention to what you are doing.

– Potions teacher Severus Snape addressing Harry Potter and his classmates at Hogwarts School of Witchcraft and Wizardry

Anxiety is an almost universal feature of ICU patients. Clinically significant anxiety has been reported in up to 70% of ICU patients. Severe anxiety is not limited to mechanically ventilated patients; indeed Treggiari-Venzi and colleagues demonstrated that up to 30% of non-intubated SICU patients had severe anxiety.[1] Consequently, sedation is an integral component of the management of the ICU patient. The primary objective of sedation is to allay anxiety, enhance patient comfort, promote sleep, and facilitate mechanical ventilation. The desirable level of sedation/hypnosis will depend in large part upon the patient's acute disease process as well as the need for mechanical ventilation. However, the ideal level of sedation is one from which the patient can be easily aroused with maintenance of the normal sleep–wake cycle.

Assessing the degree of sedation and titrating the drug regimen to predetermined end points is essential as both oversedation and inadequate sedation are associated with significant complications. Complications of under-sedation include severe anxiety with delusional behavior, interference with medical and nursing care, sympathetic overactivity with increased myocardial oxygen consumption, self-injury, and self-extubation. Severe anxiety with inadequate sedation has been reported to be the most important factor leading to unplanned extubations. Oversedation is associated with significant morbidity including

P.E. Marik, *Handbook of Evidence-Based Critical Care*,
DOI 10.1007/978-1-4419-5923-2_9,
© Springer Science+Business Media, LLC 2010

prolonged intubation with an increased risk of pulmonary complications and disorientation and delirium (ICU psychosis) following emergence (see Chapter 47). In addition, oversedation may mask significant neurological and neuromuscular complications.

In anxious patients it is important to exclude treatable causes of anxiety and not just increase the amount of sedative drugs being used. Treatable causes of anxiety include the following:

- Uncontrolled pain (NB)
- Ventilator settings inappropriate (esp. inadequate flow rate) – respiratory incoordination
- Drug or alcohol withdrawal syndrome
- Increased work breathing, e.g., pneumothorax, kinked/blocked tube
- Pulmonary edema
- Loud ventilator alarms and monitors
- Poor communication with patient as regards diagnosis, therapy, etc.

ALERT

"Doctor, doctor, my patient is very agitated!"
What is your next step?

a. Give 2 mg Ativan to the nurse.
b. Give 10 mg Haldol to the patient.
c. Take 5 mg morphine for yourself.
d. Look at your patient.

■ ASSESSING THE LEVEL OF SEDATION

Ongoing clinical evaluation is the most effective method of assessing sedation. In order to provide a more consistent and objective means of assessing the degree of sedation, a number of sedation scales have been developed. Reliable sedation scales can enhance communication among caregivers, improve consistency in drug administration, be used in sedation protocols, and improve precision of medication titration as patient needs change over time. The routine use of a sedation scale, including frequent adjustments of the sedation target as needed, is strongly endorsed by evidence-based guidelines.[2]

The Glasgow Coma Scale (GCS) was developed to assess the level of consciousness of trauma patients. This scale is commonly used in neurosurgical ICUs. The GCS is however essentially a measure of pathological obtundation and cannot be recommended for monitoring the level of sedation in ICU patients.

The Ramsay Sedation Scale and variations of this scale are a frequently used method of assessing and documenting sedation in the ICU. The Ramsay scale was reported by Ramsey and colleagues in 1974 in a study which assessed the use of alphaxalone–alphadolone (Althesin) in 30 ICU patients.[3]

   I. Anxious and agitated
   II. Cooperative, orientated, and tranquil
   III. Drowsy, responds to verbal commands
   IV. Asleep, responds briskly to light stimulation
   V. Asleep, sluggish response to stimulation
   VI. Asleep, no response to stimulation

The Ramsey scale, however, has a number of significant limitations when used to assess the level of sedation in ICU patients, namely the following:

- The six levels of the scale are not mutually exclusive; for example, a patient may be agitated (Level 1) yet poorly responsive (Level 5).
- The levels are not clearly defined nor are they fully inclusive.
- The scale cannot accurately document various degrees of agitation.
- It is difficult to link the scale to protocolized sedation orders.

The Ramsay Sedation Scale is essentially a measure of the level of consciousness rather than reflecting the degree of agitation or hypnosis of ICU patients.

Over 25 instruments have been developed to measure consciousness in the ICU.[3,4] The Richmond Agitation–Sedation Scale (RASS), which was specifically designed to assess sedation in the ICU, is a scale which has been most extensively tested for reliability and validity in adult ICU patients and is currently recommended as the sedation scale of choice.[5,6] RASS is a 10-point scale, with four levels of anxiety or agitation [+1 to +4 (combative)], one level to denote a calm and alert state (0), and 5 levels of sedation (−1 to −5) culminating in unarousable (−5).

The Richmond Agitation–Sedation Scale (RASS)

+4	Combative
+3	Very agitated
+2	Agitated
+1	Restless
0	Alert and calm
−1	Drowsy
−2	Light sedation
−3	Moderate sedation
−4	Deep sedation
−5	Unarousable

■ SEDATIVE AND ANALGESICS

Lorazepam

- *Kinetics.* Half-life of 10–20 h; less lipid soluble than diazepam; slower onset of action (2–5 min) with peak effect at 30 min; metabolized in liver to inactive metabolites by glucuronide conjugation; least affected by liver and renal disease; longer duration of action due to smaller volume of distribution (10–20 h).
- *Dose.* 1–2 mg q 4–6 h IV. If poor response, change to an IV infusion of lorazepam at 2 mg/h and then titrate to effect, increasing by 1–2 mg/h not more frequently than every 15 min:
  - In patients with severe alcohol withdrawal syndrome, the starting dose of lorazepam may be increased to 10 mg/h depending on the degree of agitation.

Midazolam

- *Kinetics.* Half-life of 4–6 h (shortest); hepatic transformation to active metabolite which is renally cleared; rapid onset (1–3 min), peak 5 min, duration 1–2.5 h. Accumulates with prolonged infusion. Half-life prolonged in
  - elderly
  - CHF
  - liver disease
  - renal disease
  - MOF
- *Dose.* Boluses of 1–5 mg every 5 min until desired effect achieved. May be used in patients who are extremely restless and thrashing about in the bed and at risk of injuring/extubating themselves:
  - Patients with alcohol withdrawal syndrome may require increased dosages with boluses of 2–5 mg every 5 min until desired effect is achieved.

Midazolam is not recommended for sustained sedation because prolonged administration results in extended pharmacological activity, caused by accumulation of parent drug, especially in patients who are obese, have low serum albumin, or have renal impairment. Prolonged sedative activity from midazolam may also be related to accumulation of its active metabolite, α-hydroxymidazolam, especially in patients with renal insufficiency. In addition, because it is metabolized by cytochrome P450 3A4, this drug is subject to significant interactions with several inhibitors and substrates of this enzyme system, including fluconazole, fentanyl, and propofol.

Benzodiazepines should be avoided in

- patients with liver failure
- non-intubated COPD patients

Propofol

- *Kinetics*. Half-life of 30–60 min. Onset 30 s; offset few minutes (does not accumulate). Even when the drug is used for several days, the return to a conscious state occurs within 10–15 min. Propofol is metabolized by glucuronide and sulfate conjugation. Dose reduction is not required in patients with hepatic or renal disease.
- *Dose*. Produces stable and predictable levels of sedation. The starting dose of propofol is 5 μg/kg/min. The dose should be increased by 5 μg/kg/min every 15 min until the desired effect is achieved (RASS level). Normal dose range is between 15 and 100 μg/kg/min (depends on the desired effect and co-administered drugs).
- Propofol has no analgesic properties and therefore analgesics may be required.
- The emulsion in which propofol is contained represents approximately 0.1 g of fat (1.1 kcal) for every milliliter. This high lipid load may result in excessive CO_2 production, as well as hyperlipidemia when used for prolonged periods of time in the ICU. Significant elevation of serum triglyceride levels has been reported with prolonged infusions of propofol. It is currently recommended that the lipid profile be monitored closely if patients receive the drug for more than 72 h and that appropriate adjustments be made to the enteral/parenteral nutritional formulations (see Chapter 31).
- Propofol should not be used in non-intubated patients as the patient may rapidly lose control of their airway (VERY NB).

Dexmedetomidine

- Dexmedetomidine is a selective α2-adrenergic receptor agonist with anxiolytic, analgesic, sedative, and sympatholytic properties.
- Dexmedetomidine results in a state of "cooperative sedation" and is associated with EEG changes commensurate with natural sleep.
- *Kinetics*. About 94% is protein bound, but this has been reported to be significantly decreased in patients with hepatic impairment. Dexmedetomidine is almost completely metabolized by direct glucuronidation or by cytochrome P450 isoenzymes. It is excreted mainly as metabolites in the urine and feces. The terminal elimination half-life is about 2 h.

- *Dose.* Loading dose of 1 μg/kg over 10 min, followed by a maintenance infusion of 0.2–0.7 μg/kg/min:
  - Reduced doses may be necessary in patients with hepatic impairment and in the elderly.
- Does not depress the respiratory drive.
- The most frequently observed adverse effect with dexmedetomidine is hypotension. Other adverse effects include bradycardia, nausea and vomiting, and fever.
- Unlike clonidine, cessation of administration does not appear to be associated with rebound hypertension or agitation.
- Dexmedetomidine is associated with less delirium than other sedative agents and may also be the drug of choice for the treatment of delirium (see Chapter 47).

Haloperidol

- *Kinetics.* Half-life 18–54 h; onset 5–30 min; duration 4–8 h.
- *Dose.* 2–5 g IV. The dose can be repeated with 5 mg increments every 15 min up to 25 mg.
- Useful for the treatment of delirium.
- *Avoid* in patients with prolonged QTc:
  - Procainamide, quinidine, amiodarone, etc.
  - Monitor QTc with prolonged use.

Fentanyl

- *Kinetics.* Half-life 2–4 h; onset 1–2 min; duration 30–60 min. Fentanyl is a potent opiate which has a rapid time to onset, short duration of action (compared to morphine), is easily titratable, and has minimal hemodynamic effects. These properties make fentanyl the agent of choice for pain control in the ICU.
- *Dose.* 50–100 μg boluses q 2–4 h or an infusion starting at 50 μg/h, titrate up to 200 μg/h in 20 μg increments every 30 min.
- Transdermal fentanyl patches (which deliver 25/50/75 or 100 μg/h) may provide excellent pain control.

Morphine

- *Kinetics.* Half-life 2–3 h; onset 1–2 min, peak effect 20 min, duration 1–2 h.
- *Dose.* 2–5 mg boluses or an infusion starting at 2 mg/h, titrate up to 10 mg/h in 2 mg increments every 30 min.

- Morphine should be *avoided* in patients with renal failure. Morphine has active metabolites (morphine 3-glucuronide and morphine 6-glucuronide) which are renally excreted; these accumulate in renal failure causing "delayed" respiratory depression.

Meperidine

Meperidine should generally be avoided in ICU patients. This drug has an active metabolite normeperidine, which is a CNS stimulant and causes seizures particularly in patients with renal impairment and patients with a history of seizures. This agent is however useful for control shivering/rigors during therapeutic hypothermia (see Chapter 58) and can be used in patients with pancreatitis as it does not cause contraction of the sphincter of Oddi (see Chapter 37).

■ SEDATION PROTOCOLS

The use of continuous vs. intermittent sedation in the ICU is controversial. It has been assumed that because of its smoother pharmacokinetic and pharmacodynamic profile, a continuous infusion would result in smoother sedation without periods of agitation and deep sedation. Furthermore, a continuous infusion requires a smaller cumulative dose. However, Kollef and colleagues[7] in a prospective observational study have suggested that a continuous infusion of sedative agents is associated with prolonged mechanical ventilation. However, it should be noted that lorazepam was the most commonly used sedative in this study. Accumulating data suggest that oversedation is associated with increased complications and prolonged mechanical ventilation. Therefore, intermittent boluses of sedatives titrated to a target level of sedation are preferred. This applies only to the use of benzodiazepines and opiates as propofol and dexmedetomidine are administered as a continuous infusion titrated to a target level of sedation. While in previous years, sedation in mechanically ventilated patients was titrated to deep levels of sedation (RASS −4 to −5), this practice is no longer recommended.[8] Ideally, patients should receive minimal sedation to achieve a state of "alertness and calm" (RASS 0). In patients on the "ARDSnet protocol" or receiving pressure-controlled ventilation, deeper levels of sedation may be required. Airway pressure release ventilation (APRV) is a mode of ventilation that is very well tolerated with minimal sedation; indeed deep sedation should be avoided with this mode of ventilation (see Chapter 14).

Delirium is a very common and serious complication in ICU patients; ICU delirium is associated with increased morbidity and mortality.[9-11]

Benzodiazepines have been reported to be independent predictors for the development of delirium.[11,12] Based on these data, benzodiazepines can no longer be considered the agents of choice for sedation in the ICU (see Chapter 47).

An additional important concept is that the sedative properties of agents of different classes are usually synergistic; this is especially true for the combination of a "sedative" and an opiate. This allows smaller doses of each agent to be used with fewer drug side effects. Furthermore, it should be noted that neither propofol nor benzodiazepines have analgesic properties; these agents should therefore be combined with an opiate (fentanyl). In addition, dexmedetomidine should be combined with fentanyl to achieve "deeper" sedation in patients receiving mechanical ventilation.

A number of randomized controlled studies have compared dexmedetomidine (± open-label fentanyl/midazolam) vs. midazolam (± open-label propofol/fentanyl) for sedation in critically ill ICU patients requiring mechanical ventilation.[13–15] These studies have demonstrated a significantly lower incidence of delirium and a shorter time to extubation with dexmedetomidine as compared to the comparator group. In the study by Pandharipande and colleagues[15] the dexmedetomidine group had a lower mortality. The cost effectiveness of dexmedetomidine in this setting remains to be determined.

No one sedation protocol is ideal for all ICU patients; therefore, the choice of agents should be individualized based on the patient's disease state and associated comorbidities. The target RASS should be dynamically determined (at least daily) with sedation titrated to achieve this goal. Due to the rapid emergence once discontinued, propofol is recommended in neurosurgical patients (head injury, SAH, etc); this allows for frequent neurological examinations.[16] In addition, propofol has neuroprotective effects and lowers ICP (see Chapter 49). Furthermore, due to its favorable pharmacokinetic profile, propofol is recommended in patients with liver failure. The following are suggested sedation protocols:

ALERT

Treat (control) pain (with an opiate) before sedating the patient.

- Do not use sedatives for control of pain.
- Ask the patient does he/she have pain. For intubated patients, use a visual analogue or a diagrammatic (smiling face to crying face) scale.
- Avoid NSAIDs for pain control (renal effects and gastric mucosa).
- Can use acetaminophen as an adjunct for pain control (max. dose 3,200 mg/day).
- Consider a regional block for surgical patients.

Protocol for Ventilated Patients

- Preferred (see Figure 9-1)
  - Propofol infusion 10–100 μg/kg/min
  - Fentanyl 25–200 μg/kg/min (added for pain control and for synergetic "sedative" properties)
  - Dexmedetomidine can be used during weaning and extubation (see below)
- Alternative
  - Dexmedetomidine 1 μg/kg over 10 min, followed by a maintenance infusion of 0.2–0.7 μg/kg/min (up to a max. of 1.5 μg/kg/min)
  - Fentanyl 50–200 μg/kg/min
  - Boluses of lorazepam (1–2 mg) can be added if adequate sedation is not achieved
- "Second"-line protocol
  - Lorazepam 2–10 mg q 4–6 h
  - Fentanyl 50–200 μg/kg/min
  - Lorazepam infusion (2–10 mg/h) can be used if adequate sedation is not achieved.

Prolonged high-dose administration of lorazepam can result in the accumulation of the vehicle, propylene glycol, resulting in worsening renal function, metabolic acidosis, and altered mental status.[17,18] Toxicity is typically observed after prolonged (>7 days), high-dose (average 14 mg/h), continuous lorazepam infusion and can be recognized by an increased osmolal gap.[19] Similarly, prolonged high-dose propofol (>100 μg/kg/min) is rarely associated with the "propofol infusion syndrome" characterized by rhabdomyolysis, metabolic acidosis, renal, and cardiac failure.[16]

Sedation Vacation

Observational and randomized trials have demonstrated that protocols directed at minimizing the use of sedative infusions shorten the weaning process. Specifically, approaches intended to avoid oversedation by limiting the use of continuous infusions either through sedation assessment scoring or by daily cessation of sedation decrease duration of mechanical ventilation and duration of ICU stay.[20–22]

Girard et al.[23] recently published the results of a trial that employed a "wake up and breathe" strategy (the ABC trial). Patients randomized to a daily awakening trial followed by an SBT (vs. SBT alone) experienced increased time off mechanical ventilation, decreased time in coma, decreased ICU and hospital length of stay, and improved survival at 1

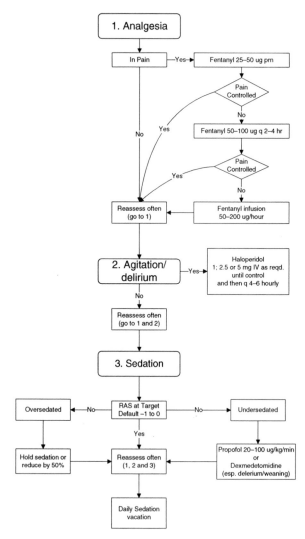

Figure 9-1. Analgesia/sedation protocol for mechanically ventilated patients. Adapted with permission from Vanderbilt University, Drs Girard, Pandharipande, and Ely. Copyright © Vanderbilt University.

year. Based on these data, the sedation should be stopped (or the dose significantly reduced) each morning; this allows for neurological assessment of the patient, performance of an SBT, reassessment of the goals of sedation, and an individualized exercise/occupational program (see below).

Schweickert and colleagues[24] performed an RCT in which patients who remained ventilator dependant for more than 3 days were randomized to early physical and occupational therapy which was coupled with daily awakenings. Patients in the intervention group had shorter duration of delirium and more ventilator-free days with significantly more patients returning to an independent functional status.

Protocol For Non-Ventilated Patients

Control of pain and anxiety is important in intubated as well as non-intubated patients. Continuous infusions of opiates, benzodiazepines, and propofol should be avoided in non-intubated patients. Small doses of lorazepam and fentanyl given at regularly scheduled times are recommended. Dexmedetomidine should be considered in agitated and delirious patients as well as in those undergoing non-invasive ventilation.[25]

Non-Pharmacological Interventions

- Minimize sleep deprivation related to noise and light.
- Establish a "normal" day–night cycle.
- Orient the patient (place, day, time) as frequently as possible.
- Communicate goals of treatment with patient (if possible).
- Music therapy.
- Ensure comfort by turning and positioning.
- Ensure ventilator synchrony.
- Early tracheotomy.

■ NEUROMUSCULAR BLOCKADE

Neuromuscular junction blocking agents (NMBAs) have historically been used in the operating room to augment surgical anesthesia, where they have been found to be remarkably safe. These agents have, however, found their way into ICU, where they have been used for prolonged periods of time to facilitate mechanical ventilation. The safety of these drugs has, however, been questioned due to the increasing number of case reports of prolonged paralysis following their use. In particular, the concomitant use of non-depolarizing NMBAs and high-dose corticosteroids has been linked to the syndrome variously known as "acute quadriplegic myopathy," "acute necrotizing myopathy," and "thick filament myopathy." This syndrome may occur after use for as short as 8 h and without the concomitant use of corticosteroids. Acute quadriplegic myopathy has been associated with the use of both steroid and non-steroid based NMBAs, and is probably a class-related phenomenon. The use of neuromuscular blocking agents is associated with additional complications including increased risk of VAP, skin breakdown, DVTs, etc. NMBA should be used only when absolutely indicated (and only when high-dose propofol has failed) and only for the shortest possible period of time. Due to its favorable pharmacokinetic and pharmacodynamic profile, cisatracurium is currently the favored NMBA in the ICU.[26]

In patients requiring advanced modes of ventilation (PCV, HFO, etc.) or induced hypothermia where deep sedation is required, high-dose propofol + fentanyl should be attempted before paralyzing the patient. The ongoing need for paralysis should be frequently assessed, with the NMBA stopped as soon as feasible.

Neuromuscular Blocking Agents

Cisatracurium

- Duration of action 30–90 min.
- Intubation: initial 0.15–0.20 mg/kg IV bolus.
- Maintenance: 2–3 μg/kg/min (infusion range of 0.5–10.2 μg/kg/min).
- The metabolism and excretion of cisatracurium is not dependent upon renal function, but rather upon organ-independent Hofmann elimination, and dosing reductions are not required in renal failure (and hepatic failure).

Vecuronium

- Duration 60–75 min
- Intubation: 0.07–0.1 mg/kg
- Maintenance: 4–10 mg/h

Atracurium

- Duration 45–60 min
- Intubation: 0.4–0.5 mg/kg
- Maintenance: 20–50 mg/h

Doxacurium

- Duration 30–160 min
- Intubation: 0.015–0.03 mg/kg
- Maintenance: 0.005–0.03 mg/kg/h

Rocuronium (For Intubation Only)

- Duration: Acts within 1 min with duration of action up to 30 min.
- Intubation: 0.6–1.2 mg/kg.

Succinylcholine (For Intubation Only)

- Duration 5–15 min
- Intubation 1 mg/kg
- Beware of bradycardia with repeated doses
- Contraindications to the use of succinylcholine include the following:
  - Renal failure
  - Burns
  - Severe trauma with muscle injury
  - Severe sepsis
  - Ocular injuries

To prevent excessive and prolonged neuromuscular blockade, all patients receiving neuromuscular blocking agents should be monitored using a nerve stimulator. For practical purposes, the train of four (TOF) should be used to access the degree of neuromuscular blockade. The goal is to achieve one to two twitches (see below). CPKs should be monitored daily (NB). In addition, a BIS (bispectral index) monitor should be used to assess the level of hypnosis/sedation in *all* patients receiving an NMBA; target BIS of 20–40.

Train-of-Four (TOF) Monitoring and Dosage Adjustments

The train of four (four stimuli 0.5 s apart) is a convenient way of monitoring the degree of neuromuscular blockade and roughly correlates with the degree of neuromuscular junction receptor occupation:

- 4 twitches: 0–70% receptors occupied
- 3 twitches 70–80% receptors occupied
- 2 twitches 80–90% receptors occupied
- 1 twitch >95% receptors occupied
- 0 twitches 100% receptors occupied

In principle, any superficially located peripheral motor nerve can be stimulated. The ulnar nerve is however the most popular site. The electrodes are best applied on the volar side of the wrist. The distal electrode should be placed about 1 cm proximal to the point at which the proximal flexion crease of the wrist crosses the radial side of the tendon to the flexor carpi ulnaris muscle. The proximal electrode should be placed

2–3 cm proximal to the distal electrode. With this placement of electrodes, electrical stimulation normally elicits finger flexion and thumb adduction.

Because different muscle groups have different sensitivities to neuromuscular blocking agents, results obtained for one muscle cannot be extrapolated automatically to other muscles. The diaphragm is the most resistant of all muscles to neuromuscular blockade. In general, the diaphragm requires 1.4–2 times as much muscle relaxant as the adductor pollicis muscle for an identical degree of blockade. From a practical point of view, one to two twitches (of train of four) of the adductor pollicis muscle will result in sufficient diaphragmatic paralysis to prevent the patient from coughing, hiccoughing, and breathing during mechanical ventilation.[26]

Prior to paralysis the supramaximal stimulation (SMS) must be determined. The SMS is defined as the level at which additional stimulation current does not increase the twitch response. It is important to note that each nerve may have a different SMS and inadequate stimulation may lead the clinician to overestimate the degree of neuromuscular blockade present. The SMS is usually in the range of 20–60 mA. Starting at 10 mA, the TOF current is increased by 10 mA until four equal responses are obtained. The current is increased until the intensity of the response does not increase any further. When this occurs the prior setting will be the SMS for that nerve. Once the patient is paralyzed the TOF is then performed using the SMS.

The TOF test should be performed hourly until the goal is achieved (1–2 twitches) and then 4–6 h. The rate of the infusion should be adjusted as follows:

- 0 twitches: Stop infusion, restart when two twitches are present. Restart infusion rate at
  - 80% if it takes 1 h for 2 twitches
  - 75% if it takes 2 h for 2 twitches
  - 50% if it takes 3 h for 2 twitches
  - 25% if it takes 4 h for 2 twitches
- 1 twitch: Reduce to 80% of the present infusion rate
- 2 twitches: Maintain present infusion rate
- 3 twitches: Reload with 25% of loading dose; increase infusion rate by 25%
- 4 twitches: Reload with 50% of loading dose; increase infusion rate by 50%.

■ CLINICAL PEARLS

- Ask your patient "Do you have pain?" If yes, treat with analgesics.
- Assess the degree of sedation with a sedation–agitation scale.

- Titrate sedative/hypnotic agents to target on sedation scale.
- Benzodiazepines are associated with delirium; minimize their use.
- Avoid NMBA like "the plague."

■ REFERENCES

1. Treggiari-Venzi M, Borgeat A, Fuchs-Buder T, et al. Overnight sedation with midazolam or propofol in the ICU: effects on sleep quality, anxiety and depression. *Intensive Care Med.* 1996;22:1186–1190.
2. Jacobi J, Fraser GL, Coursin DB, et al. Clinical practice guidelines for the sustained use of sedatives and analgesics in the critically ill adult. *Crit Care Med.* 2002;30:119–141.
3. Ramsay MA, Savege TM, Simpson BR, et al. Controlled sedation with alphaxalone–alphadolone. *Br Med J.* 1974;2:656–659.
4. De Jonghe B, Cook D, Appere-De-Vecchi C, et al. Using and understanding sedation scoring systems: a systematic review. *Intensive Care Med.* 2000;26:275–285.
5. Sessler CN, Gosnell MS, Grap MJ, et al. The Richmond Agitation–Sedation Scale: validity and reliability in adult intensive care unit patients. *Am J Respir Crit Care Med.* 2002;166:1338–1344.
6. Ely EW, Truman B, Shintani A, et al. Monitoring sedation status over time in ICU patients: reliability and validity of the Richmond Agitation–Sedation Scale (RASS). *JAMA.* 2003;289:2983–2991.
7. Kollef MH, Levy NT, Ahrens TS, et al. The use of continuous i.v. sedation is associated with prolongation of mechanical ventilation. *Chest.* 1998;114:541–548.
8. Treggiari MM, Romand JA, Yanez ND, et al. Randomized trial of light versus deep sedation on mental health after critical illness. *Crit Care Med.* 2009;37:2517–2534.
9. Gunther ML, Jackson JC, Ely EW. The cognitive consequences of critical illness: practical recommendations for screening and assessment. *Crit Care Clin.* 2007;23:491–506.
10. Ely EW, Shintani A, Truman B, et al. Delirium as a predictor of mortality in mechanically ventilated patients in the intensive care unit. *JAMA.* 2004;291:1753–1762.
11. Pandharipande P, Cotton BA, Shintani A, et al. Prevalence and risk factors for development of delirium in surgical and trauma intensive care unit patients. *J Trauma.* 2008;65:34–41.
12. Pandharipande P, Shintani A, Peterson J, et al. Lorazepam is an independent risk factor for transitioning to delirium in intensive care unit patients. *Anesthesiology.* 2006;104:21–26.
13. Riker RR, Shehabi Y, Bokesch PM, et al. Dexmedetomidine vs. midazolam for sedation of critically ill patients. *JAMA.* 2009;301:489–499.

14. Ruokonen E, Parviainen I, Jakob SM, et al. Dexmedetomidine versus propofol/midazolam for long-term sedation during mechanical ventilation. *Intensive Care Med.* 2009;35:282–290.

15. Pandharipande PP, Pun BT, Herr DL, et al. Effect of sedation with dexmedetomidine vs. lorazepam on acute brain dysfunction in mechanically ventilated patients. The MENDS randomized controlled trial. *JAMA.* 2007;298:2644–2653.

16. Marik PE. Propofol: therapeutic indications and side effects. *Curr Pharm Design.* 2004;10:3639–3649.

17. Arroliga AC, Shehab N, McCarthy K, et al. Relationship of continuous infusion lorazepam to serum propylene glycol concentration in critically ill adults. *Crit Care Med.* 2004;32:1709–1714.

18. Yaucher NE, Fish JT, Smith HW, et al. Propylene glycol-associated renal toxicity from lorazepam infusion. *Pharmacotherapy.* 2003;23:1094–1099.

19. Yahwak JA, Riker RR, Fraser GL, et al. Determination of a lorazepam dose threshold for using the osmol gap to monitor for propylene glycol toxicity. *Pharmacotherapy.* 2008;28:984–991.

20. Brook AD, Ahrens TS, Schaiff R, et al. Effect of a nursing-implemented sedation protocol on the duration of mechanical ventilation. *Crit Care Med.* 1999;27:2609–2615.

21. Arias-Rivera S, Sanchez-Sanchez MM, Santos-Diaz R, et al. Effect of a nursing-implemented sedation protocol on weaning outcome. *Crit Care Med.* 2008;36:2054–2060.

22. Kress JP, Pohlman AS, O'Connor MF, et al. Daily interruption of sedative infusions in critically ill patients undergoing mechanical ventilation. *N Engl J Med.* 2000;342:1471–1477.

23. Girard TD, Kress JP, Fuchs BD, et al. Efficacy and safety of a paired sedation and ventilator weaning protocol for mechanically ventilated patients in intensive care (Awakening and Breathing Controlled trial): a randomised controlled trial. *Lancet.* 2008;371:126–134.

24. Schweickert WD, Pohlman MC, Pohlman AS, et al. Early physical and occupational therapy in mechanically ventilated, critically ill patients: a randomised controlled trial. *Lancet.* 2009;373:1874–1882.

25. Akada S, Takeda S, Yoshida Y, et al. The efficacy of dexmedetomidine in patients with noninvasive ventilation: a preliminary study. *Anesth Analg.* 2008;107:167–170.

26. Lagneau F, D'honneur G, Plaud B, et al. A comparison of two depths of prolonged neuromuscular blockade induced by cisatracurium in mechanically ventilated critically ill patients. *Intensive Care Med.* 2002;28:1735–1741.

10

Sepsis

Sepsis is among the most common reasons for admission to ICUs throughout the world. Over the last two decades, the incidence of sepsis in the United States has tripled and is now the 10th leading cause of death.[1,2] Advances in medical technologies, the increasing use of immunosuppressive agents, and the aging of the population have contributed to the exponential increase in the incidence of sepsis. In the United States alone, approximately 750,000 cases of sepsis occur each year, at least 225,000 of which are fatal.[1,2] Septic patients are generally hospitalized for extended periods, rarely leaving the ICU before 2–3 weeks. Despite the use of anti-microbial agents and advanced life support, the case fatality rate for patients with sepsis has remained between 20 and 30% over the last two decades.[1,2]

■ DEFINITIONS

Sepsis originally meant "putrefaction," decomposition of organic matter by bacteria and fungi. Since then, a wide variety of definitions have been applied to sepsis, including sepsis syndrome, severe sepsis, septicemia, and septic shock. In 1991, the American College of Chest Physicians/Society of Critical Care Medicine developed a new set of terms and definitions to define "sepsis" in a more precise manner.[3,4] The term "systemic inflammatory response syndrome" (SIRS) was coined to describe the common systemic response to a wide variety of insults. It is characterized by two or more of the following clinical manifestations:

- A body temperature of >38°C or <36°C
- A heart rate greater than 90 beats/min
- A respiratory rate of greater than 20 breaths/min
- WBC >12,000 cells/mm^3, less than 4,000 cells/mm^3, or >10% bands

P.E. Marik, *Handbook of Evidence-Based Critical Care*,
DOI 10.1007/978-1-4419-5923-2_10,
© Springer Science+Business Media, LLC 2010

Sepsis

When the systemic inflammatory response syndrome is the result of a confirmed infectious process, it is termed "sepsis."

Severe Sepsis

Severe sepsis is defined as sepsis plus either organ dysfunction or evidence of hypoperfusion or hypotension.

Septic Shock

Septic shock is a subset of severe sepsis and is defined as sepsis-induced hypotension, persisting despite adequate fluid resuscitation (2,000 ml), along with the presence of hypoperfusion abnormalities or organ dysfunction.[5]

■ BACTERIOLOGY AND SITES OF INFECTION

Bacteriologic data from the large sepsis trials published during the last two decades indicate the following pattern of culture results:

- Gram positives 25%
- Gram negatives 25%
- Gram-positive + gram-negative organisms 15%
- Fungal pathogens 3–5%
- Anaerobes 2%
- Culture negative 25%

The most common sites of infection are the following:

- Lung 50%
- Abdomen/pelvis 25%
- Primary bacteremia 15%
- Urosepsis 10%
- Vascular access 5%

■ PATHOGENESIS OF SEPSIS

The pathogenesis of sepsis is exceeding complex and involves an interaction between multiple microbial and host factors. Indeed, after exposure to both gram-negative and gram-positive bacteria, macrophages upregulate the expression of over 1,000 genes (and proteins) and down-regulate in excess of 300 genes, the net result depending on the complex interrelated interaction of these factors.[6] With advances in molecular biology, many of the mysteries of sepsis are being unraveled; however, we have only just embarked on our journey along the "sepsis super-highway." The reader is referred to many excellent reviews on this topic.[7-12] Essentially, as noted by William Osler in 1921, "except on a few occasions the patient appears to die from the body's response to infection rather than from it."[13] Sepsis can be viewed as an excessively exuberant pro-inflammatory response with increased production of pro-inflammatory mediators with activation of leukocytes, mononuclear cells, and the coagulation cascade. The end result is widespread microvascular and cellular injury. The cellular injury results in alteration of cellular and sub-cellular membranes and receptors, activation of intracellular enzymes, increased apoptosis, and mitochondrial dysfunction. The systemic microvascular injury is a defining characteristic of sepsis and is believed to play a major pathophysiological role in the progressive organ dysfunction of sepsis. The microvascular injury is characterized by the following:

- Endothelial activation
- Endothelial injury with edema and increased permeability
- Marked reduction in microvascular flow
- Redistribution of organ blood flow
- Intravascular pooling
- Tissue edema formation
- Opening of AV shunts
- DIC with in vitro thrombosis
- Decreased RBC deformability

It is important to note that volume-resuscitated patients with severe sepsis/septic shock usually have a high cardiac output (and oxygen delivery) yet have impaired oxygen utilization. The impaired oxygen utilization results from both the microvascular injury and the altered cellular metabolism. The decreased oxygen utilization together with the AV shunting results in a normal or high mixed venous oxygen saturation ($SmvO_2$/$ScvO_2$) and muscle oxygen tension (StO_2). It is therefore not surprising that both these parameters have proven to be poor end points of resuscitation in patients with sepsis.

The Hemodynamic Derangements of Sepsis

Sepsis is characterized by a complex combination of cardiovascular derangements, including vasodilation, hypovolemia, myocardial depression, and altered microvascular flow. In volume-resuscitated patients with septic shock, systemic vascular resistance is usually low, contractility and biventricular ejection fractions are reduced, while ventricular dimensions and heart rate are increased. Despite these changes, volume-resuscitated patients typically have a hyperdynamic circulation with a high cardiac output. However, recent data suggest that up to 60% of patients with septic shock may have a hypodynamic circulation with a deceased ejection fraction (<45%) and global left ventricular hypokinesia.[14] Furthermore, increasing evidence suggests that patients with sepsis develop structural injury to the contractile apparatus of the heart that may contribute to the myocardial dysfunction. This is evident by elevated levels of troponins and B-type natriuretic peptide in patients with sepsis.[15-17] In addition, estimates of left ventricular ejection fraction correlate negatively with increased levels of cardiac troponin in patients with septic shock. These data suggest that all patients with sepsis should undergo *serial echocardiography* to characterize the hemodynamic pattern, as this impacts on the approach to the use of vasopressor and inotropic agents.[14] In addition, cardiac troponins should be measured to assess the degree of myocardial injury.

Coagulation Activation

Activation of the coagulation cascade with the generation of fibrin is a pathological and physiological hallmark of sepsis that occurs in both the intravascular and the extravascular compartments (see Chapter 52).[18] Intravascular coagulation is characterized by diffuse microvascular thrombosis which contributes to widespread ischemic organ damage. Activation of coagulation during sepsis is primarily driven by the tissue factor (TF) pathway. Fibrin formation in sepsis likely results from both increased fibrin generation and impaired fibrin degradation. Inhibition of fibrinolysis is primarily due to increases in plasminogen activator inhibitor-1 (PAI-1). Downregulation of the anti-coagulant protein C pathway also plays an important role in the modulation of coagulation and inflammation in sepsis. Due to activation of the coagulation cascade, almost all septic patients are thrombocytopenic (or have a falling platelet count), and indeed a normal platelet count makes the diagnosis of severe sepsis less likely. In the majority of patients with severe sepsis, D-dimer, thrombin–anti-thrombin complexes, and prothrombin time are increased, while anti-thrombin, protein C, and protein S levels are significantly decreased.[19] Replacement of coagulation factors with fresh frozen plasma (and cryoprecipitate if the fibrinogen is less than 100 mg/dl) is indicated only in patients with clinical evidence of bleeding. While it had previously been assumed that such therapy "fuels the fire of DIC," there is no evidence that the infusion of plasma products stimulates the ongoing activation of coagulation.[20]

Clinical Features and Diagnosis of Sepsis

Sepsis is a systemic process with a variety of clinical manifestations. The initial symptoms of sepsis are non-specific and include malaise, tachycardia, tachypnea, fever, and sometimes hypothermia. The manifestations of sepsis can sometimes be quite subtle, particularly in the very young, the elderly, and those patients with chronic debilitating or immunosuppressing conditions. These patients may present with normothermia or hypothermia. An altered mental state or an otherwise unexplained respiratory alkalosis may be the presenting feature of sepsis.

Organ Dysfunction in Severe Sepsis/Septic Shock

Cardiovascular

- *Tachycardia*
- Hypotension
- Decreased contractility
- Vasodilatation

Respiratory

- *Tachypnea*
- *Decreased PaO$_2$/FiO$_2$*
- ALI/ARDS

Hematologic

- *Thrombocytopenia*
- Increased PTT/PT
- Decreased protein C
- Increased D-dimer

Neurological

- *Confusion*
- Agitation
- Altered consciousness
- Neuropathy
- Myopathy
- Cerebral edema

Renal

- *Oliguria*
- Increased S-creatinine

Hepatic

- Increase in transaminases
- Decreased albumin

Metabolic/endocrine

- *AG acidosis*
- *Lactic acidosis*
- *CIRCI (adrenal insufficiency)*
- Hyperglycemia/hypoglycemia
- Hypophosphatemia

The signs and symptoms of systemic inflammation are not useful in distinguishing infectious from non-infectious causes of SIRS. Furthermore, a bacterial pathogen is not isolated in all patients with sepsis. Consequently, a number of markers have been evaluated as more specific indicators of infection, including procalcitonin (PCT) and TREM-1.

PCT, a 114-amino-acid polypeptide, is the precursor of calcitonin, a hormone produced in the medullary C cells of the thyroid gland. Upon systemic infection, PCT is produced and secreted by virtually all parenchymal cells. The circulating levels of several calcitonin precursors, including PCT, but not mature calcitonin, increase several thousand-fold in microbial infections. In healthy individuals, PCT levels are very low (<0.1 ng/ml). In patients with sepsis, however, PCT levels increase dramatically, sometimes to more than several hundred nanograms per milliliter.[21] This increase, specifically the time course, correlates with the severity of the infection and mortality.

Nakamura et al.[22] demonstrated that PCT levels were significantly higher (6.2 vs. 0.3 µg/l) in patients who tested positive for either blood culture or PCR for bacteria with a sensitivity and specificity greater than 90%. Ruiz-Alvarez evaluated the diagnostic value of PCT in patients admitted to the ICU. The mean PCT was 0.3 µg/l in non-infected patients with SIRS, 1.1 µg/l in those with sepsis, 1.9 µg/l in those with severe sepsis, and 9.1 µg/l in those with septic shock.[23] Similarly, Charles et al. reported significantly higher PCT levels (5.5 vs. 0.7 µg/l) in patients who developed nosocomial infection (VAP- or ICU-acquired bacteremia) as compared to a non-infected patients.[24] Schuetz et al.[25] demonstrated that PCT enabled the discrimination of blood contamination from bloodstream infection due to coagulase-negative staphylococci. However, other investigators have reported that PCT had a poor sensitivity and specificity for the diagnosis of infection and did not discriminate SIRS from sepsis or severe sepsis.[26] Furthermore, Tang et al.[27] performed a meta-analysis to assess the diagnostic accuracy of PCT and concluded that "PCT cannot reliably differentiate sepsis from other non-infectious causes of SIRS in critically ill adult patients." The Procalcitonin and Survival Study (PASS) is a randomized, multi-center trial to investigate whether daily measurements of PCT and therapeutic responses to abnormal PCT can improve survival in ICU patients.[28]

Changes in PCT levels may also be useful in determining the appropriateness of antibiotic therapy. Charles reported that appropriate first-line empiric antibiotic therapy was associated with a significantly greater decrease in PCT than inappropriate initial therapy.[29] Similarly, Seligman demonstrated that a decline in PCT was the best predictor of survival in patients with VAP.[30]

The triggering receptor expressed on myeloid cells (TREM-1) is a member of the immunoglobulin superfamily, and its expression on phagocytes is specifically upregulated by microbial products. A soluble form of TREM-1 (sTREM-1) is released from activated phagocytes and can be found in body fluids of infected patients (see Chapter 17).[31,32] It is likely that these and "other biomarkers" will prove to be useful adjuncts in the diagnosis of patients with bacterial infections.

Blood cultures are considered to provide the clinical gold standard for the diagnosis of infections. However, blood cultures are only positive in between 20 and 30% of patients with sepsis and moreover it takes 2–3 days before the results become available. Molecular methods based on polymerase chain reaction (PCR) technology have been developed for infection diagnosis and pathogen identification. These methods offer a new approach based on detection and recognition of pathogen DNA in the blood, or indeed other clinical samples, with the potential to obtain results in a much shorter time frame (hours) than is possible with conventional culture. PCR-based pathogen detection depends on the ability of the reaction to selectively amplify specific regions of DNA, allowing even minute amounts of pathogen DNA in clinical samples to be detected and analyzed. This technique holds great promise and may revolutionize our approach to the diagnosis of bacterial, fungal, and viral infections.

■ MANAGEMENT OF SEPSIS

ALERT

The clock is ticking

- Appropriate broad-spectrum antibiotics within 2 h
- Lactated Ringer's or normal saline (1L) over 20 min on presentation
  - A further liter of lactated Ringer's or normal saline over 20 min if hypotensive

- Full fluid resuscitation within 6 h (up to 5L of crystalloids)
- Norepinephrine if hypotensive after 2 l lactated Ringer's
- Consider stress-dose corticosteroids
- Consider activated protein C
• Source control.

The management of patients with severe sepsis and septic shock is complex requiring multiple concurrent interventions with close monitoring and frequent re-evaluations (see Figure 10-1 and Table 10-1).

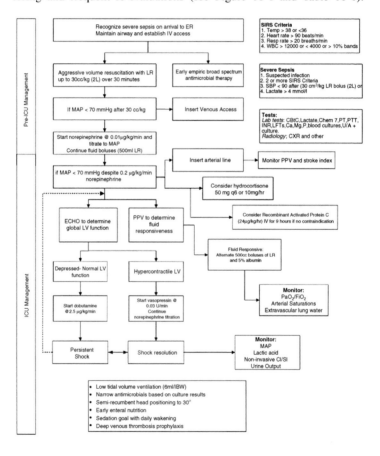

Figure 10-1. Sepsis Management Protocol.

Table 10-1. Advances in the treatment of sepsis.

Modality	Specific Intervention
Antibiotics	Early (<4 h) appropriate antibiotics
Fluids	Early aggressive (<6 h), then conservative approach
	Albumin and crystalloid solutions
	assess volume responsiveness with PPV
Vasopressors	Norepinephrine, epinephrine, and vasopressin are equivalent
Inotropic agents	LV dysfunction common; treat with dobutamine
Coagulation	Activated protein C (APC) in patients at high risk of death
Corticosteroids	Reduce vasopressor dependency; mortality benefit unclear; may be beneficial in patients at high risk of death
Immunoglobulins	Polyclonal IgGAM in patients at high risk of death
Nutrition	Omega-3 enteral nutrition within 24 h

These patients are best managed in ICU's by physicians experienced in the management of critically ill septic patients. The current strategy for the management of patients with sepsis is largely based on treating or eliminating the source of infection, timely and appropriate usage of anti-microbial agents, hemodynamic optimization, and other physiological organ-supportive measures. Attempts at downregulating the pro-inflammatory response with novel agents directed at specific pro-inflammatory mediators have uniformly met with failure. However, both activated protein C (APC) and glucocorticoids (stress dose) are immunomodulators which have been demonstrated to improve the outcome of patients with severe sepsis and septic shock.

It has become increasingly apparent that in many patients there is a long delay in both the recognition of sepsis and the initiation of appropriate therapy. This has been demonstrated to translate into an increased incidence of progressive organ failure and a higher mortality. A significant and causal relationship appears to exist between antibiotic timing and improved outcomes. Kumar and colleagues[33] investigated the relationship between the duration of shock prior to anti-microbial administration in 2,600 patients with sepsis-induced hypotension. They reported that the risk of dying increased progressively with time to receipt of the first dose of antibiotic. Furthermore, there was a 5–15% decrease in survival with every hour delay over the first 6 h. In the ENHANCE study, the morality was 33% if activated drotrecogin alpha (APC) was given within the first 24 h of admission as compared to 52% if it was given on day 3 or after.[34]

Levy et al.[35] retrospectively analyzed the sequential organ failure assessment (SOFA) scores during the first 48 h in 1,036 severely septic patients. From baseline to day 1, the direction of change in cardiovascular, renal, respiratory, hematologic, and hepatic functions independently predicted 28-day mortality. The implications of this study is that if organ dysfunction is not improving during the first day of severe sepsis, the mortality risk is significantly increased, underscoring the importance of early recognition and therapeutic intervention to prevent sequential organ dysfunction.[36] Similarly, Rivers et al. demonstrated that early (within 6 h) clearance of lactate is associated with improved outcome in severe sepsis and septic shock.[37]

The concept that early aggressive treatment (within the first 6 h of admission to hospital) of patients with severe sepsis and sepsis shock reduces sequential organ failure and improves survival has been demonstrated in the study by Rivers and colleagues.[38] In this study, early aggressive therapy that optimized cardiac preload and afterload in patients with severe sepsis and septic shock improved survival. The patients in the early therapy group received, on average, approximately 1,500 ml more total fluids in the first 6 h of treatment than did the standard-therapy group and had a significantly higher mean arterial pressure [mean ($\pm$SD), 95 ± 19 vs. $81+/-18$ mmHg; $p<0.001$]. Mortality was 30.5% in the group receiving early goal-directed treatment, as compared with 46.5% in the control group ($p = 0.009$). This strategy for managing patients with severe sepsis and septic shock has been called "early goal-directed therapy" (EGDT).

ALERT

All is not what it appears to be!!

One has to be very careful in the interpretation of the Rivers et al.'s EGDT trial.[39]

- Data published in the *Wall Street Journal* suggests "errors" in the statistical analysis of the data.[40]
- The "central" tenant of EGDT is based on $ScvO_2$.
  - As discussed above the use of $ScvO_2$ as the end point of resuscitation in patients with sepsis just does not make sense.
  - In the Rivers' study, the mean $ScvO_2$ was 49% with 65% of patients having an $ScvO_2$ less than 70%; no other sepsis study has reproduced this finding; the mean $ScvO_2$ in most sepsis studies was about 70%.[41]
  - Blood was used to increase $ScvO_2$; blood simply does not increase oxygen uptake in sepsis, particularly within the first 6 h.[42]
- The mortality of 60% in the control arm of the study is higher than that of any sepsis study published to date. [43–47]
- The Australian MRC (ARISE) and the NIH (ProCESS) are multi-center RCTs to test "EGDT" in patients with severe sepsis; so stay tuned.

Antibiotics

Broad-spectrum antibiotics should be administered within 2 h of the diagnosis of sepsis (see Chapter 12).

Fluid Resuscitation: Less Is More

In the first hours of severe sepsis, venodilatation, transudation of fluid from the vascular space into the tissues, reduced oral intake, and increased insensible loss combine to produce hypovolemia. Along with ventricular dysfunction and arteriolar dilation, volume depletion contributes to impaired global perfusion and organ dysfunction. Treating hypovolemia is the most important component of the early management of severe sepsis. However, once the patient has received an adequate fluid challenge (3–5 l), further fluid challenges may not increase cardiac output and global perfusion (see Chapter 8). Additional fluid may increase interstitial edema and further comprise the microvascular dysfunction which characterizes severe sepsis. The current paradigm of fluid management in patients with sepsis is one of adequate initial fluid resuscitation followed by a conservative late fluid management strategy. Conservative late fluid management is defined as even-to-negative fluid balance measured on at least two consecutive days during the first 7 days after septic shock onset. In a retrospective cohort study, Murphy and colleagues[48] demonstrated that an approach which combines both adequate initial fluid resuscitation and conservative late fluid management was associated with improved survival. Additional studies have demonstrated that those patients who have a smaller cumulative fluid balance have improved clinical outcomes.[44,49,50]

Type of Fluid

While the type of fluid used in the resuscitation of patients with sepsis has not been definitively shown to affect outcome, subgroup analysis of the SAFE study suggested a trend toward a more favorable outcome in patients who received albumin (see Chapter 8).[51] Albumin has a number of properties that may be advantageous in patients with sepsis, including the maintenance of the endothelial glycocalyx and endothelial function as well as having anti-oxidant and anti-inflammatory properties that may translate into less "third"-space fluid loss. Hydroxyethyl starch (HES) solutions were previously recommended in patients with sepsis; however, these synthetic colloids have recently been demonstrated to be associated with an increased risk of renal failure (and death) and should therefore be avoided in patients with sepsis.[52]

Despite differences in composition, normal saline and lactated Ringer's (LR) solution are frequently considered equivalent and lumped under the term "balanced salt solution." However, both experimental and clinical data have demonstrated that these fluids are not equivalent (see Chapter 8). Normal saline is associated with both a hyperchloremic and dilutional metabolic acidosis. While the clinical implications of this finding is unclear, the additional loss (renal) of HCO_3 in the setting of reduced buffering capacity only adds to the acid–base burden characteristic of hypoperfused states.[53] In addition to its effects on acid–base balance, solutions high in chloride have been shown both experimentally and clinically to reduce the GRF (due to tubuloglomerular feedback).[54] The effects of NS on acid–base balance and renal function may be dose related. These data suggest that in patients with sepsis (except those with hyperkalemia), LR solution may be preferable to normal saline. There is however, no outcome data to support this recommendation.

Based on the composite of these data, we recommend initial resuscitation with NS or LR (30 ml/kg). Patients who respond poorly to this initial bolus (±2 l) may best be fluid resuscitated with alternating boluses (500 ml) of albumin and LR solution until the hemodynamic goals are achieved (see "end points of resuscitation" and Figure 10-1). The goal of this approach is to maintain normal acid–base balance, achieve adequate intravascular volume and yet limit the total amount of fluid given.

Vasopressors, Inotropes, and Cardiac Function

The optimal timing of the initiation of vasopressor agents has not been rigorously studied. Many patients with severe sepsis will respond to a 2 l fluid challenge and require little additional hemodynamic support. Others will remain hypotensive despite 10 l of fluid (fluid does not increase vascular tone!!!). The goal of fluid resuscitation is rapid early restoration of intravascular volume followed by a conservative fluid strategy. We have therefore recommended that a vasopressor agent (norepinephrine) be started once the patient has received 2 l of crystalloid.[5,55] At this point, norepinephrine (starting at 0.01 μg/kg/min) should be titrated upward while fluid resuscitation continues (albumin and LR solution; guided by pulse pressure variation, etc.) (see Chapter 8).

While there is little data to suggest that one vasopressor results in better outcomes than another (norepinephrine, epinephrine, vasopressin), we favor norepinephrine as the first-line agent followed by dobutamine or epinephrine in patients with poor LV function and vasopressin (fixed dose of 0.03 U/min) in patients with "preserved" LV function and a low SVR (see Figure 10-1). In patients with sepsis, norepinephrine increases blood pressure, as well as cardiac output, renal, splanchnic, cerebral, and microvascular blood flow while minimally increasing heart rate.[56,57] Norepinephrine would therefore appear to be the ideal first-line agent for the management of septic shock; additional agents should be considered in patients who remain hypotensive or display evidence of inadequate tissue or organ perfusion despite doses of norepinephrine of up to 0.2 μg/kg/min. The second-/third-line agents should be chosen based on the patient's hemodynamic profile as determined by ECHO and non-invasive assessment of cardiac index.

Dopamine has a number of theoretical disadvantages in patients with sepsis, including the following:

- Tachycardia (increases myocardial oxygen demands)
- Splanchnic mucosal ischemia
- Inhibits T and B lymphocytes (via dopamine receptors)
- Decreases secretion of prolactin, growth hormone, and TSH

The SOAP study suggested that septic patients who received dopamine had an increased mortality when compared to other vasopressors.[58] This drug should therefore be avoided in patients with sepsis. Similarly, phenylephrine is not recommended, as in experimental models, it decreases cardiac output as well as renal and splanchnic blood flow.[59] Furthermore, this agent has not been rigorously tested in any RCT.

The End Points of Resuscitation

The optimal "hemodynamic" end point of resuscitation in patients with sepsis is unknown (see Chapter 8). Similarly, the target MAP is somewhat controversial. Traditional teaching suggests that we should achieve a MAP above 60 mmHg. However, this pressure is below the autoregulatory range of a number of organs, particularly in elderly patients with atherosclerotic disease. The *Surviving Sepsis Campaign* guidelines suggest targeting a MAP above 65 mmHg.[60] In a dose escalation study, Jhanji and colleagues[57] incrementally increased the dose of norepinephrine to achieve a MAP of 60 mmHg, then 70 mmHg, then 80 mmHg, and lastly 90 mmHg. In this study, global oxygen delivery, cutaneous microvascular flow, and tissue oxygenation increased with each sequential increase in MAP. However, LeDoux et al.[61] demonstrated that increasing the MAP from 65 to 85 mmHg with norepinephrine did not significantly affect systemic oxygen metabolism, skin microcirculatory blood flow, urine output, or splanchnic perfusion. Dubin[62] demonstrated that increasing mean arterial pressure from 65 to 75 and 85 mmHg did not improve microcirculatory blood flow. Similarly, Bourgoin et al.[63] demonstrated that increasing MAP from 65 to 85 mmHg with norepinephrine neither affected metabolic variables nor improved renal function. However, Deruddre et al.[64] demonstrated that in patients with septic shock, when the MAP was increased from 65 to 75 mmHg, urinary output increased significantly, while the renal resistive index significantly decreased. This somewhat contradictory data suggest that while the end point of resuscitation should be individualized, a MAP of 65–70 mmHg may be a reasonable initial target.

■ ADJUNCTIVE THERAPIES

While antibiotics, fluid resuscitation, vasopressors/inotropic agents, and source control form the basic elements of the management of severe sepsis/septic shock, a number of adjunctive agents have been demonstrated to improve outcome or hold promise in improving the outcome of patients with sepsis. These agents should be considered in all patients with severe sepsis/septic shock. The benefit of these agents is also time dependent and they should be started as soon as possible and always within the first 24 h of ICU admission.

Adjunctive Therapies of Proven Benefit

Corticosteroids

Hydrocortisone in a dose of 50 mg q 6 h or a 100 mg bolus followed by an infusion at 10 mg/h should be considered in patients who require in excess of 0.1–0.2 μg/kg/min of norepinephrine (see Chapter 40).

Activate Protein C

The PROWESS study demonstrated a significant improvement in mortality in patients with severe sepsis and septic shock when started within the first 24 h of ICU admission.[47] APC should be considered in patients with septic shock and those with sepsis and at least one-organ failure who are at high risk of death, particularly patients with severe community-acquired pneumonia.[65] The use of APC in patients with sepsis has however become a very controversial and charged issue. This is largely driven by the high rate of serious bleeding that has been reported in retrospective cohort studies.[66] APC should be avoided in patients at high risk of bleeding, including patients with a platelet count of <30,000/ml^3. Although APC increases the PTT in vitro, the PROWESS study demonstrated an increased risk of bleeding when the PTT increased above 75 s.

Based on these data, we monitor the PTT in patients on APC and hold the infusion (for a few hours) and transfuse FFP when the PTT exceeds 80 s (anecdotal experience only). DIC is not a contraindication to APC;

indeed in PROWESS the risk reduction was greater in patients with overt DIC than those without DIC (RR of 0.6 vs. 0.85).[67]

Patients with purpura fulminans and multi-organ failure due to meningococcal infection have significantly higher plasma PAI-1 levels as well as lower protein C levels than do patients with meningococcal infection, but without purpura or organ failure.[68] In view of the low protein C levels in purpura fulminans, numerous case reports as well as open-label studies have been published suggesting a benefit of treatment with APC.[68–70] Many of these cases concomitantly received FFP, fibrinogen, and platelets. APC has also been used for the treatment of purpura fulminans associated with streptococcal and staphylococcal infections.[71]

Enteral Nutrition Supplemented with Omega-3 Fatty Acids

An enteral nutritional formula high in omega-3 fatty acids should be initiated within 24 h of admission to the ICU (see Chapter 31). Patients are best fed gastrically via an OG/NG tube. The use of vasopressor agents is not a contraindication to the initiation of enteral nutrition.

Polyclonal Immunoglobulins

Two meta-analyses have demonstrated that polyclonal immunoglobulins, particularly those preparations enriched with IgA and IgM (IgGAM), reduce the mortality in patients with septic shock.[72,73] It is not clear which patient subgroups would benefit from this therapy; clearly, asplenic patients as well as those patients at high risk of death should receive IgGAM.

Adjunctive Therapies of Possible Benefit

Statins

HMG-CoA reductase inhibitors (statins) are a group of drugs with anti-inflammatory, immunomodulating, anti-oxidant, anti-proliferative, anti-apoptotic, anti-thrombotic, and endothelial stabilizing effects. Statins increase the expression of endothelial nitric oxide (eNOS) while down-regulating inducible nitric oxide (iNOS).[74] Furthermore, statins interfere with leukocyte–endothelial interactions by decreasing the expression of adhesion molecules and have anti-thrombotic effects. Experimental sepsis studies have demonstrated improved outcome with the use of statins and clinical studies have demonstrated that patients taking statins have a better outcome when they become septic.[74–76] Our practice is to use high-dose statins in patients with severe sepsis; statins should however be avoided in patients taking azole anti-fungal drugs as well as calcineurin inhibitors; monitor for rhabdomyolysis.

Selenium

Sepsis is associated with an increase in reactive oxygen species and a low endogenous anti-oxidative capacity. The selenium-dependent glutathione peroxidases (GPx's) as well as thioredoxin reductases are important compounds responsible for the maintenance of the redox system in all cells including the immune-competent cells. The activity of these enzymes is mainly regulated by the availability of selenium. The Selenium in Intensive Care (SIC) study demonstrated that high-dose intravenous selenium improved the outcome of patients with severe SIRS, sepsis, and septic shock.[77] Selenium supplementation should be considered in patients with severe sepsis and septic shock. While the optimal dose and the route remain to be established, we use a dose of 400–600 μg p.o. daily.

Zinc

Zinc is required for normal function of both the innate and the acquired immune systems. Zinc deficiency results in marked abnormalities of immune function with zinc supplementation restoring natural killer cell activity, lymphocyte production, mitogen responses, wound healing, and resistance to infection. Stress, trauma, and sepsis have been associated with very low serum zinc levels.[78,79] In an experimental sepsis model, mortality was significantly increased with zinc deficiency, while zinc supplementation normalized the inflammatory response, diminished tissue damage, and reduced mortality.[80] The benefit of zinc supplementation in patients with sepsis has yet to be determined.

■ ADJUNCTIVE THERAPIES OF NO PROVEN BENEFIT

- Tight glycemic control
- TPN
  - Avoid at all costs
  - Increases risk of death
- FFP and platelets
  - Only indicated in bleeding patients
  - May be given in combination with APC in non-bleeding patients with severe coagulopathy and in patients with purpura fulminans
- Blood
- EGDT . . . ala Rivers et al., remains unproven

■ CLINICAL PEARLS

- Fluid challenge with LR or NS 2l bolus is the first step in the resuscitation of patients with severe sepsis/septic shock.
- Ongoing fluid resuscitation with alternating 500 ml boluses of 5% albumin and LR solution.
- Norepinephrine is the initial vasopressor of choice; start if response to 2l crystalloid bolus is poor.
- Patients who require in excess of 0.2 μg/kg/min of norepinephrine require assessment of LV function:
    - Hypodynamic – dobutamine or epinephrine.
    - Hyperdynamic – fixed dose vasopressin.

■ REFERENCES

1. Martin GS, Mannino DM, Eaton S, et al. The epidemiology of sepsis in the United States from 1979 through 2000. *N Engl J Med.* 2003;348:1546–1554.
2. Angus DC, Linde-Zwirble WT, Lidicker J, et al. Epidemiology of severe sepsis in the United States: analysis of incidence, outcome and associated costs of care. *Crit Care Med.* 2001;29:1303–1310.
3. Society of Critical Care Medicine Consensus Conference Committee. American College of Chest Physicians/Society of Critical Care Medicine Consensus Conference: definitions for sepsis and organ failure and guidelines for the use of innovative therapies in sepsis. *Crit Care Med.* 1992;20:864–874.
4. Bone RC. The Sepsis Syndrome: definition and general approach to management. *Clin Chest Med.* 1996;17:175–182.
5. Marik PE, Lipman J. The definition of septic shock: implications for treatment. *Crit Care Clin.* 2007;9:101–103.
6. Nau GJ, Richmond JF, Schlesinger A, et al. Human macrophage activation programs induced by bacterial pathogens. *Proc Natl Acad Sci USA.* 2002;99:1503–1508.
7. Cinel I, Opal SM. Molecular biology of inflammation and sepsis: a primer. *Crit Care Med.* 2009;37:291–304.
8. O'Brien JM Jr., Ali NA, Aberegg SK, et al. Sepsis. *Am J Med.* 2007;120:1012–1022.
9. Mackenzie I, Lever A. Management of sepsis. *BMJ.* 2007;335:929–932.
10. Abraham E, Singer M. Mechanisms of sepsis-induced organ dysfunction. *Crit Care Med.* 2007;35:2408–2416.
11. Singer M. Mitochondrial function in sepsis: acute phase versus multiple organ failure. *Crit Care Med.* 2007;35:S441–S448.
12. Russell JA. Management of sepsis. *N Engl J Med.* 2006;355:1699–1713.

13. Osler W. *The Evolution of Modern Medicine*. New Haven, CT: Yale University Press; 1921.
14. Vieillard-Baron A, Caille V, Charron C, et al. Actual incidence of global left ventricular hypokinesia in adult septic shock. *Crit Care Med*. 2008;36:1701–1706.
15. McLean AS, Huang SJ, Hyams S, et al. Prognostic values of B-type natriuretic peptide in severe sepsis and septic shock. *Crit Care Med*. 2007;35:1019–1026.
16. Favory R, Neviere R. Significance and interpretation of elevated troponin in septic patients. *Crit Care*. 2006;10:224.
17. Mehta NJ, Khan IA, Gupta V, et al. Cardiac troponin I predicts myocardial dysfunction and adverse outcome in septic shock. *Internat J Cardiol*. 2004;95:13–17.
18. Wang L, Bastarache JA, Ware LB. The coagulation cascade in sepsis. *Curr Pharm Des*. 2008;14:1860–1869.
19. Kinasewitz GT, Yan SB, Basson B, et al. Universal changes in biomarkers of coagulation and inflammation occur in patients with severe sepsis, regardless of causative micro-organism. *Crit Care*. 2004;8:R82–R90.
20. Levi M, Toh CH, Thachil J, et al. Guidelines for the diagnosis and management of disseminated intravascular coagulation. British Committee for Standards in Haematology. *Br J Haematol*. 2009;145:24–33.
21. Jones AE, Fiechtl JF, Brown MD, et al. Procalcitonin test in the diagnosis of bacteremia: a meta-analysis. *Ann Emerg Med*. 2007;50:34–41.
22. Nakamura A, Wada H, Ikejiri M, et al. Efficacy of procalcitonin in the early diagnosis of bacterial infections in a critical care unit. *Shock*. 2009;31:586–591.
23. Ruiz-Alvarez MJ, Garcia-Valdecasas S, de PR, et al. Diagnostic efficacy and prognostic value of serum procalcitonin concentration in patients with suspected sepsis. *J Intensive Care Med*. 2009;24:63–71.
24. Charles PE, Kus E, Aho S, et al. Serum procalcitonin for the early recognition of nosocomial infection in the critically ill patients: a preliminary report. *BMC Infect Dis*. 2009;9:49.
25. Schuetz P, Mueller B, Trampuz A. Serum procalcitonin for discrimination of blood contamination from bloodstream infection due to coagulase-negative staphylococci. *Infection*. 2007;35:352–355.
26. Suprin E, Camus C, Gacouin A, et al. Procalcitonin: a valuable indicator of infection in a medical ICU? *Intensive Care Med*. 2000;26:1232–1238.
27. Tang BM, Eslick GD, Craig JC, et al. Accuracy of procalcitonin for sepsis diagnosis in critically ill patients: a systematic review and meta-analysis. *Lancet Infect Dis*. 2007;7:210–217.
28. Jensen JU, Lundgren B, Hein L, et al. The Procalcitonin And Survival Study (PASS) – a randomised multi-center investigator-initiated trial to investigate whether daily measurements biomarker Procalcitonin and pro-active diagnostic and therapeutic responses to abnormal Procalcitonin levels, can improve survival in intensive care unit patients.

Calculated sample size (target population): 1000 patients. *BMC Infect Dis.* 2008;8:91.

29. Charles PE, Tinel C, Barbar S, et al. Procalcitonin kinetics within the first days of sepsis: relationship with the appropriateness of antibiotic therapy and outcome. *Crit Care.* 2009;13:R38.

30. Seligman R, Meisner M, Lisboa TC, et al. Decreases in procalcitonin and C-reactive protein are strong predictors of survival in ventilator-associated pneumonia. *Crit Care.* 2006;10:R125.

31. Gibot S, Cravoisy A, Levy B, et al. Soluble triggering receptor expressed on myeloid cells and the diagnosis of pneumonia. *N Engl J Med.* 2004;350:451–458.

32. Gibot S, Cravoisy A, Kolopp-Sarda MN, et al. Time-course of sTREM (soluble triggering receptor expressed on myeloid cells)-1, procalcitonin, and C-reactive protein plasma concentrations during sepsis. *Crit Care Med.* 2005;33:792–796.

33. Kumar A, Kazmi M, Roberts D, et al. Duration of shock prior to antimicrobial administration is the critical determinant of survival in human septic shock. *Crit Care Med.* 2004;32(suppl):41.

34. Bernard GR, Margolis BD, Shanies HM, et al. Extended evaluation of recombinant human activated protein C United States Trial (ENHANCE US): a single-arm, phase 3B, multicenter study of drotrecogin alfa (activated) in severe sepsis. *Chest.* 2004;125:2206–2216.

35. Levy MM, Macias WL, Russell JA, et al. Failure to improve during the first day of therapy is predictive of 28-day mortality in severe sepsis. *Chest.* 2004;124 (Suppl):120S.

36. Guidet B, Aegerter P, Gauzit R, et al. Incidence and impact of organ dysfunctions associated with sepsis. *Chest.* 2005;127:942–951.

37. Ajemian MS, Nirmul GB, Anderson MT, et al. Routine fiber-optic endoscopic evaluation of swallowing following prolonged intubation: implications for management. *Arch Surg.* 2001;136:434–437.

38. Rivers E, Nguyen B, Havstad S, et al. Early goal-directed therapy in the treatment of severe sepsis and septic shock. *N Engl J Med.* 2001;345:1368–1377.

39. Marik PE, Varon J. Early Goal Directed Therapy (EGDT): on terminal life support? *Am J Emerg Med.* 2010;28:243–245.

40. Burton TM. New therapy for sepsis infection raises hope but many questions (lead article). *Wall St J.* 2008;14 Aug.

41. van Beest PA, Hofstra JJ, Schultz MJ, et al. The incidence of low venous oxygen saturation on admission the intensive care unit: a multi-center observational study in the Netherlands. *Crit Care.* 2008;12:R33-doi:10.1186/cc6811.

42. Marik PE, Sibbald WJ. Effect of stored-blood transfusion on oxygen delivery in patients with sepsis. *JAMA.* 1993;269:3024–3029.

43. The outcome of patients with sepsis and septic shock presenting to emergency departments in Australia and New Zealand. *Crit Care Resus.* 2007;9:8–18.

44. Vincent JL, Sakr Y, Sprung CL, et al. Sepsis in European intensive care units: results of the SOAP study. *Crit Care Med.* 2006;34:344–353.
45. Russell JA, Walley KR, Singer J, et al. Vasopressin versus norepinephrine infusion in patients with septic shock. *N Engl J Med.* 2008;358: 877–887.
46. Annane D, Vignon P, Renault A, et al. Norepinephrine plus dobutamine versus epinephrine alone for management of septic shock: a randomised trial. *Lancet.* 2007;370:676–684.
47. Bernard GR, Vincent JL, Laterre PF, et al. Efficacy and safety of recombinant human activated protein C for severe sepsis. *N Engl J Med.* 2001;344:699–709.
48. Murphy CV, Schramm GE, Doherty JA, et al. The importance of fluid management in acute lung injury secondary to septic shock. *Chest.* 2009;136:102–109.
49. Alsous F, Khamiees M, DeGirolamo A, et al. Negative fluid balance predicts survival in patients with septic shock: a retrospective pilot study. *Chest.* 2000;117:1749–1754.
50. Comparison of two fluid-management strategies in acute lung injury. *N Engl J Med.* 2006;354:2564–2575.
51. Finfer S, Bellomo R, Boyce N, et al. A comparison of albumin and saline for fluid resuscitation in the intensive care unit. *N Engl J Med.* 2004;350:2247–2256.
52. Brunkhorst FM, Engel C, Bloos F, et al. Intensive insulin therapy and pentastarch resuscitation in severe sepsis. *N Engl J Med.* 2008;358: 125–139.
53. Kellum JA, Bellomo R, Kramer DJ, et al. Etiology of metabolic acidosis during saline resuscitation in endotoxemia. *Shock.* 1998;9:364–368.
54. Wilcox CS. Regulation of renal blood flow by plasma chloride. *J Clin Invest.* 1983;71:726–735.
55. Raghavan M, Marik PE. Management of sepsis during the early golden hours. *J Emerg Med.* 2006;31:185–199.
56. Treggiari MM, Romand JA, Burgener D, et al. Effect of increasing norepinephrine dosage on regional blood flow in a porcine model of endotoxin shock. *Crit Care Med.* 2002;30:1334–1339.
57. Jhanji S, Stirling S, Patel N, et al. The effect of increasing doses of norepinephrine on tissue oxygenation and microvascular flow in patients with septic shock. *Crit Care Med.* 2009;37:1961–1966.
58. Sakr Y, Reinhart K, Vincent JL, et al. Does dopamine administration in shock influence outcome? Results of the Sepsis Occurrence in Acutely Ill Patients (SOAP) Study. *Crit Care Med.* 2006;34:589–597.
59. Malay MB, Ashton JL, Dahl K, et al. Heterogeneity of the vasoconstrictor effect of vasopressin in septic shock. *Crit Care Med.* 2004;32: 1327–1331.
60. Dellinger RP, Levy MM, Carlet JM, et al. Surviving sepsis Campaign: International guidelines for management of severe sepsis and septic shock: 2008. *Crit Care Med.* 2008;36:296–327.

61. Ledoux D, Astiz M, Carpati CM, et al. Effects of perfusion pressure on tissue perfusion in septic shock. *Crit Care Med*. 2000;28:2729–2732.
62. Dubin A, Pozo M, Casabella CA, et al. Increasing arterial pressure with norepinephrine does not improve microcirculatory blood flow: a prospective study. *Crit Care*. 2009;13:R92.
63. Bourgoin A, Leone M, Delmas A, et al. Increasing mean arterial pressure in patients with septic shock: effects on oxygen variables and renal function. *Crit Care Med*. 2005;33:780–786.
64. Deruddre S, Cheisson G, Mazoit JX, et al. Renal arterial resistance in septic shock: effects of increasing mean arterial pressure with norepinephrine on the renal resistive index assessed with Doppler ultrasonography. *Intensive Care Med*. 2007;33:1557–1562.
65. Laterre PF, Garber G, Levy H, et al. Severe community-acquired pneumonia as a cause of severe sepsis: data from the PROWESS study. *Crit Care Med*. 2005;33:952–961.
66. Eichacker PQ, Natanson C. Increasing evidence that the risks of rhAPC may outweigh its benefits. *Intensive Care Med*. 2007;33:396–399.
67. Dhainaut JF, Yan SB, Joyce DE, et al. Treatment effects of drotrecogin alfa (activated) in patients with severe sepsis with or without overt disseminated intravascular coagulation. *J Throm Haemo*. 2004;2: 1924–1933.
68. White B, Livingstone W, Murphy C, et al. An open-label study of the role of adjuvant hemostatic support with protein C replacement therapy in purpura fulminans-associated meningococcemia. *Blood*. 2000;96: 3719–3724.
69. Wcisel G, Joyce D, Gudmundsdottir A, et al. Human recombinant activated protein C in meningococcal sepsis. *Chest*. 2002;121:292–295.
70. Hasin T, Leibowitz D, Rot D, et al. Early treatment with activated protein C for meningococcal septic shock: case report and literature review. *Intensive Care Med*. 2005;31:1002–1003.
71. Rintala E, Kauppila M, Seppala OP, et al. Protein C substitution in sepsis-associated purpura fulminans. *Crit Care Med*. 2000;28:2373–2378.
72. Kreymann KG, de HG, Nierhaus A, et al. Use of polyclonal immunoglobulins as adjunctive therapy for sepsis or septic shock. *Crit Care Med*. 2007;35:2677–2685.
73. Laupland KB, Kirkpatrick AW, Delaney A. Polyclonal intravenous immunoglobulin for the treatment of severe sepsis and septic shock in critically ill adults: a systematic review and meta-analysis. *Crit Care Med*. 2007;35:2686–2692.
74. Terblanche M, Almog Y, Rosenson RS, et al. Statins: panacea for sepsis? *Lancet Infect Dis*. 2006;6:242–248.
75. Novack V, Terblanche M, Almog Y. Do statins have a role in preventing or treating sepsis? *Crit Care*. 2006;10:113.
76. Merx MW, Liehn EA, Janssens U, et al. HMG-CoA reductase inhibitor simvastatin profoundly improves survival in a murine model of sepsis. *Circulation*. 2004;109:2560–2565.

77. Angstwurm MW, Engelmann L, Zimmermann T, et al. Selenium in Intensive Care (SIC): results of a prospective randomized, placebo-controlled, multiple-center study in patients with severe systemic inflammatory response syndrome, sepsis, and septic shock. *Crit Care Med.* 2007;35:118–126.
78. Gaetke LM, McClain CJ, Talwalkar RT, et al. Effects of endotoxin on zinc metabolism in human volunteers. *Am J Physiol.* 1997;272: E952–E956.
79. Wong HR, Shanley TP, Sakthivel B, et al. Genome-level expression profiles in pediatric septic shock indicate a role for altered zinc homeostasis in poor outcome. *Physiol Genomics.* 2007;30:146–155.
80. Knoell DL, Julian MW, Bao S, et al. Zinc deficiency increases organ damage and mortality in a murine model of polymicrobial sepsis. *Crit Care Med.* 2009;37:1380–1388.

11

Catheter-Related Bloodstream Infection

Intravascular catheters are a major source of infection in the ICU. Catheter-related bloodstream infection (CRBI) may be caused by the following:

- Non-tunneled central venous catheters (CVCs)
- Tunneled CVCs
- Peripherally inserted central venous catheters (PICCs)
- Arterial lines
- Non-tunneled hemodialysis catheters
- Tunneled hemodialysis catheters
- Subcutaneous ports

Generally, tunneled/cuffed CVCs and PICCs have a lower risk of CRBI than do non-tunneled CVCs. Tunneled hemodialysis catheters have a lower risk of CRBI than do non-tunneled hemodialysis catheters. Similarly, the risk of CRBI is lower for arterial lines as compared to non-cuffed CVCs. The incidence of CVC-related bloodstream infection is reported to vary from about 1 to 5 per 1,000 catheter-days (mean about 3 per 1,000 catheter-days); for arterial lines the incidence varies from about 1 to 2 per 1,000 catheter-days.[1,2]

The pathogenesis of non-tunneled CVC infections is usually due to extraluminal colonization of the catheter by skin commensal flora. In comparison, in tunneled CVCs or implantable devices, contamination of the catheter hub and intraluminal infection are the most common routes of infection. A number of factors have been identified as increasing the risk of CRBI including the length of time in situ, the number of lumens in the CVC, the number of stopcocks, the transfusion of blood and blood products, parenteral nutrition, and an open infusion system. While the

P.E. Marik, *Handbook of Evidence-Based Critical Care*,
DOI 10.1007/978-1-4419-5923-2_11,
© Springer Science+Business Media, LLC 2010

risk of CRBI increases with time, the catheter remains in situ; changing catheters at regularly scheduled interval has not been shown to reduce the risk of CRBI. Furthermore, guidewire exchanges may increase the risk of infection.[3]

The risk of CRBI due to CVCs appears to depend on the site of placement. While the data are somewhat contradictory,[3,4] the risk of infection appears to be lowest with subclavian catheters, followed by the internal jugular and femoral sites.[5,6] However, the risk of CRBI for the femoral site may be related to the patient's BMI, with the risk of infection being higher in obese patients (BMI >30).[4]

Coagulase-negative staphylococci account for up to 40% of cases. Other common causes of CRBI include the following:

- *Staphylococcus aureus*
- Enterococci
- *Candida* species
- Aerobic gram-negative bacilli

Methicillin-resistant *S. aureus* (MRSA) and vancomycin-resistant enterococci are becoming important causes of CRBI. The implicated pathogens vary somewhat with the site of catheter placement, with the incidence of *Candida* species and gram negatives being higher for femoral catheters.[5,7]

The diagnosis of CRBI can be challenging. Routine culture of blood withdrawn from the catheter is not recommended; however, the catheter exit site should be inspected daily for evidence of erythema or pus. The absence of local infection, however, does not exclude CRBI. In a patient with an indwelling CVC who develops a fever, two sets of peripheral blood cultures should be drawn. If the patient has systemic signs of infection and no other identifiable source of infection, the catheter should be removed and empiric antibiotics commenced, pending culture results. The tip of the removed catheter should be cultured (semi-quantitative) in patients with suspected infection. In patients with limited venous access, the central catheter may be replaced with a new catheter over a guidewire; however, both the catheter tip and the intracutaneous portion of the catheter should be sent for culture. If the catheter culture returns positive (>15 cfu) or the blood cultures are consistent with a CRBI, the line that was changed over a guidewire must be removed and replaced with a new catheter at a clean site. Follow-up blood cultures should be obtained in patients with CRBI. If blood cultures remain positive, a thorough investigation for septic thrombosis, infective endocarditis, and other metastatic infections should be pursued.

In a number of patients, the fever defervesces after removal of the catheter, yet the blood cultures remain negative. These patients are considered to have "culture-negative" CRBI; presumably the bacteremia was intermittent or below the threshold required for a positive culture. Antibiotics are generally not required in these cases.

The usual approach to patients with suspected CRBI involves removal of the catheter. However, only about 20% of patients who have a CVC removed due to suspected CRBI are proven to have CRBI. This subjects patients with negative cultures to the added risk of line placement. To avoid this problem, a number of methods which do not require removal of the CVC have been investigated for the diagnosis of CRBI.[8] Comparison of blood cultured from the CVC with that from a peripheral venous site is currently the most useful technique. In patients with CRBI, time to positivity is shorter (more than 2 h) for blood withdrawn from the catheter as opposed to the peripheral site.

■ MANAGEMENT OF CRBI

In patients with suspected CRBI (see Chapter 13), all indwelling catheters should be removed (and cultured) and empiric antibiotic therapy commenced. The initial choice of antibiotics will depend on the severity of the patient's clinical disease, the risk factors for infection, and the likely pathogens associated with the specific intravascular device. Vancomycin is usually recommended because of its activity against coagulase-negative staphylococci and *S. aureus*. Additional empiric coverage for enteric gram-negative bacilli and *Pseudomonas aeruginosa* with the use of a third- or fourth-generation cephalosporin, such as ceftazidime or cefepime, may be needed for severely ill or immunocompromised patients.

Patients with CRBI should be classified into those with uncomplicated bacteremia and those with complicated infections, in which there are the following:

- Septic thrombosis
- Endocarditis
- Osteomyelitis
- Possible metastatic seeding

If there is a prompt response to initial antibiotic therapy, most patients who are not immunocompromised without valvular heart disease or an intravascular prosthetic device should receive 10–14 days of antimicrobial therapy. A more prolonged course of therapy (4–6 weeks) should be considered if there is persistent bacteremia or fungemia after catheter removal or if there is evidence of endocarditis or septic thrombosis, and 6–8 weeks of therapy should be considered for the treatment of osteomyelitis. Echocardiography including transesophageal ECHO should be considered in patients with persistent bacteremia/fungemia or lack of clinical improvement to exclude endocarditis.

Coagulase-negative staphylococci are the most common cause of CRBI. CRBI due to coagulase-negative staphylococci usually presents with fever alone, rarely developing "frank sepsis."[9] While coagulase-negative staphylococci CRBI may resolve with the removal of the catheter and no antibiotic therapy, most experts believe that such infections should be treated with antibiotics (vancomycin).[9]

Antibiotic Lock Therapy

In patients with CRBI, removal of all indwelling vascular catheters is recommended. This may be problematic in patients with tunneled catheters and infusion ports; this necessitates removal of the device and reinsertion once the infection is cleared. A potential solution to this problem is based on the fact that the majority of infections in tunneled catheters originate in the catheter hub and then spread to the catheter lumen. This fact has prompted the "antibiotic lock" technique, where the catheter lumen is filled with pharmacological concentrations of antibiotics where they are allowed to dwell for hours or days. Antibiotic lock therapy, with or without concomitant parental therapy, has a reported response with a catheter salvage rate of about 80%.[9]

■ PREVENTION OF CRBI

While CRBI is an inevitable complication of being sick in the ICU, the risk can be significantly reduced by specific interventions.[10,11] When inserting a new catheter, the following precautions should be followed:

- Full drapes and strict sterile precautions
- Use of a line cart
- Skin cleansing with chlorhexidine
- ICU nurse for observation (sterility not broken) and assistance

Additional measures include the following:

- Clear adhesive dressings.
- Limit blood draws from CVCs.
- Limit "breaks" in the circuit.
- Remove the catheter when no longer required.
- Avoid femoral catheterization if possible (see Chapter 6).
- All catheters inserted in clinically urgent situations without maximal sterile barrier precautions should be replaced as soon as possible.

- Before accessing catheter hubs or injection ports, clean them with an alcoholic chlorhexidine preparation or 70% alcohol to reduce contamination.
- Replace administration sets not used for blood, blood products, or lipids at intervals not longer than 96 h.
- Povidone–iodine or polysporin ointment should be applied to hemodialysis catheter insertion sites in patients with a history of recurrent *S. aureus* CRBI.
- Guidewire exchanges are strongly discouraged.[3]

Anti-microbial-coated/-impregnated CVCs have been demonstrated to reduce the risk of colonization and CRBI.[12,13] These catheters should be considered in ICUs when

- the incidence of CRBI is >3 per 1,000 catheter-days despite all the precautions listed above,
- patients have limited venous access and a history of recurrent CRBI,
- patients are at heightened risk for severe sequelae from a CRBI (e.g., patients with recently implanted intravascular devices, such as a prosthetic heart valve or an aortic graft).

Do not routinely replace CVCs or arterial catheters. As the risk of infection is less with tunneled dialysis catheters, a tunneled catheter should be placed as soon as feasible (patients with ARF generally will require 2–6 weeks of renal replacement therapy).

The role of PICCs in the ICU is unclear. Safdar and Maki demonstrated that the risk of infection with PICCs in ICU patients approaches that with CVCs placed in the subclavian or internal jugular veins.[14] However, Garnacho-Montero et al.[3] demonstrated a lower incidence of CRBI with the use of PICCs. PICCs should be considered in patients who will require prolonged venous access.

■ REFERENCES

1. Lorente L, Santacreu R, Martin MM, et al. Arterial catheter-related infection of 2,949 catheters. *Crit Care*. 2006;10:R83.
2. Koh DB, Gowardman JR, Rickard CM, et al. Prospective study of peripheral arterial catheter infection and comparison with concurrently sited central venous catheters. *Crit Care Med*. 2008;36:397–402.
3. Garnacho-Montero J, Aldabo-Pallas T, Palomar-Martinez M, et al. Risk factors and prognosis of catheter-related bloodstream infection in critically ill patients: a multicenter study. *Intensive Care Med*. 2008;34: 2185–2193.

4. Parienti JJ, Thirion M, Megarbane B, et al. Femoral vs jugular venous catheterization and risk of nosocomial events in adults requiring acute renal replacement: a randomized controlled trial. *JAMA*. 2008;299: 2413–2422.
5. Gowardman JR, Robertson IK, Parkes S, et al. Influence of insertion site on central venous catheter colonization and blood stream infection rates. *Intensive Care Med*. 2008;34:1038–1045.
6. Lorente L, Henry C, Martin MM, et al. Central venous catheter-related infection in a prospective and observational study of 2,595 catheters. *Crit Care*. 2005;9:R631–R635.
7. Lorente L, Jimenez A, Santana M, et al. Microorganisms responsible for intravascular catheter-related bloodstream infection according to the catheter site. *Crit Care Med*. 2007;35:2424–2427.
8. Bouza E, Alvarado N, Alcala L, et al. A randomized and prospective study of 3 procedures for the diagnosis of catheter-related bloodstream infection without catheter withdrawal. *Clin Infect Dis*. 2007;44:820–826.
9. Mermel LA, Farr BM, Sherertz RJ, et al. Guidelines for the management of intravascular catheter-related infections. *CID*. 2001;32:1249–1272.
10. Pratt RJ, Pellowe CM, Wilson JA, et al. epic2: National evidence-based guidelines for preventing healthcare-associated infections in NHS hospitals in England. *J Hosp Infect*. 2007;65(Suppl 1):S1–S64.
11. Marschall J, Mermel LA, Classen D, et al. Strategies to prevent central line-associated bloodstream infections in acute care hospitals. *Infect Control Hosp Epidemiol*. 2008;29(Suppl 1):S22–S30.
12. Ramritu P, Halton K, Collignon P, et al. A systematic review comparing the relative effectiveness of antimicrobial-coated catheters in intensive care units. *Am J Infect Control*. 2008;36:104–117.
13. Casey AL, Mermel LA, Nightingale P, et al. Antimicrobial central venous catheters in adults: a systematic review and meta-analysis. *Lancet Infect Dis*. 2008;8:763–776.
14. Safdar N, Maki DG. Risk of catheter-related bloodstream infection with peripherally inserted central venous catheters used in hospitalized patients. *Chest*. 2005;128:489–495.

12

Antibiotics

■ GENERAL CONCEPTS

- Antibiotics are not anti-pyretic agents; they should be used only when bacterial infection is strongly suspected! (see Chapters 10 and 13).
- Initial appropriate anti-microbial coverage is the most important factor affecting outcome in patients with sepsis.
- Combination anti-microbial therapy is the most effective mechanism of providing empiric broad coverage in critically ill septic patients.
  - Once a pathogen has been isolated and its sensitivity determined, monotherapy is appropriate for most patients except for those patients who are neutropenic or have abdominal sepsis. This is known as de-escalation.
- One should not use the same "combo" for all patients; this encourages anti-microbial resistance:
  - Antibiotic heterogeneity is advocated as a strategy for reducing the emergence of anti-microbial resistance. This is preferred over antibiotic cycling.
- There is enormous variability in bacteriology from one hospital to another, specific sites within the hospital, and from one time period to another. Current site-specific data must be used to guide the choice of antibiotics.
- In patients with a catheter-related bloodstream infection (CRBI) due to *Staphylococcus aureus*, the catheter must be removed (this is regardless of whether the catheter is tunneled or not).
- Serious hospital-acquired infection due to suspected gram-negative bacteria should be treated empirically with dual coverage that includes an aminoglycoside and then de-escalated.[1]

P.E. Marik, *Handbook of Evidence-Based Critical Care*,
DOI 10.1007/978-1-4419-5923-2_12,
© Springer Science+Business Media, LLC 2010

- The inappropriate use of antibiotics is the most important factor leading to multi-drug-resistant bacteria (MDR).
- All attempts must be made to limit the use of antibiotics to patients with bacterial infections and to limit the duration of treatment (Table 12-1).

Table 12-1. Outcomes in patients with MDR and drug-susceptible gram-negative infections.[2]

Outcome	Drug Susceptible	MDR
Hospital cost (US$)	29,604	80,500[a]
Hospital mortality (%)	11	23[a]
Hospital LOS	13	29[a]
ICU LOS	1	13[a]

[a]$p<0.001$.

ALERT

In patients with suspected hospital-acquired infection, the empiric anti-microbial regimen should be broad (Toti-mycin); however, therapy must be de-escalated once microbiological data are obtained and consider stopping all antibiotics if cultures are negative.

Duration of Antibiotic Therapy Guided by Biomarkers (Procalcitonin)

Clinical studies performed over the last decade have demonstrated that the most important factor affecting the outcome of patients with bacterial infections is the early initiation of appropriate antibiotic therapy. In addition, studies have demonstrated that the excessive, inappropriate, and prolonged use of antibiotics increases the likelihood of inducing bacterial resistance. The increasing prevalence of multi-drug-resistant (MDR) organisms, largely due to the excessive use of antibiotics, has necessitated that our empiric anti-microbial regimens become broader and broader, perpetuating this vicious cycle. One mechanism to limit the excessive use of antibiotics is that of antibiotic de-escalation once a pathogen is identified. The second is reducing the duration of a "course" of antibiotics. Until recently the duration of a "course" of antibiotics was based on clinical folklore rather than evidence-based investigations, and patients with hospital-acquired infections were treated for up to 21 days. Theoretically, a course of antibiotics should continue until no viable bacteria are present at the site of infections. In patients with ventilator-associated pneumonia (VAP) who are treated with appropriate antibiotics, serial quantitative BAL cultures demonstrate that the colony counts fall rapidly (over 2–3 days) with negative cultures by day 5.[3] Dennesen[4] investigated 27 patients with VAP treated with appropriate antibiotics; in this study clinical response to therapy occurred within the first 6 days of therapy. Based on these observations, Chastre and colleagues[5] compared the outcome of patients with VAP treated with antibiotics for 8 days as compared to 15 days. Among patients who had received appropriate initial empiric therapy, with the possible exception of those developing non-fermenting gram-negative bacillus infections, comparable clinical effectiveness against VAP was obtained with the 8-day and 15-day treatment regimens. However, it is likely that empirical rules guiding the duration of antibiotics will not apply to all patients in all circumstances but rather will depend on host factors (immune status, age, genotypes, etc.), pathogen factors (species, virulence factors, etc.), and the site and severity of infection. Traditional clinical parameters lack specificity in guiding the duration of a course of antibiotics. However, biomarkers which reflect ongoing infection or resolution of infection hold out promise as a guide in determining when to stop a course of antibiotics. Procalcitonin (PCT) is a specific marker for severe bacterial infection in patients presenting with suspected sepsis (see Chapter 19).[6] Prospective, randomized clinical trials have demonstrated that in patients with community-acquired pneumonia, abdominal sepsis and ICU patients with sepsis, serial PCT levels allow for the discontinuation of antibiotics 2–4 days early when compared to standard guidelines.[7–11] This approach was associated with similar adverse outcomes (treatment failures, etc.) but with fewer antibiotic-associated adverse effects. This approach holds great promise in determining when to discontinue antibiotic therapy. (See Chapter 10; PCT as an adjunct to guide the diagnosis of sepsis and to monitor the response to treatment.)

■ ANTIBIOTIC CHOICES FOR SPECIFIC "ICU" INFECTIONS*

Febrile Neutropenia

- Ceftazidime
- Cefepime
- Imipenem

---

*These general guidelines should be taken together with the clinical context of the patient (underlying disease and comorbidities, severity of illness, previous antibiotics, allergies, etc.) as well as the nature of the local flora.

- Meropenem
- Doripenem
- Piperacillin/tazobactam
- *Add* vancomycin if suspected IV access infection.

Septic Shock (Source Unclear)

- Imipenem
- Meropenem
- Doripenem
- Piperacillin/tazobactam
- Cefepime
- *Plus* vancomycin
- *Plus* aminoglycoside (in most settings)

Catheter-Related Bloodstream Infection

- Vancomycin
- Caspofungin if receiving TPN
- Plus gram-negative coverage if femoral catheter and/or immuno-compromised

Abdominal Sepsis/Peritonitis/Abscess/Diverticulitis
Moderate-to-Severe Disease

- Piperacillin/tazobactam
- Ampicillin/sulbactam
- Ertapenem
- Moxifloxacin
- Tigecycline

Severe Life-Threatening Disease

- Imipenem
- Meropenem
- Doripenem
- Ampicillin + metronidazole + ciprofloxacin

Spontaneous Bacterial Peritonitis

- Ceftriaxone/cefotaxime
- Piperacillin/tazobactam
- Ampicillin/sulbactam
- Ertapenem
- Fluoroquinolone

Cholangitis

- Piperacillin/tazobactam
- Ampicillin/sulbactam

- Ertapenem
- Meropenem

Urosepsis
Uncomplicated

- Quinolone
- Ceftriaxone/cefotaxime
- Ampicillin/sulbactam
- Ertapenem

Complicated (Obstruction, Tubes etc.)

- Piperacillin/tazobactam
- Imipenem
- Meropenem
- Doripenem

COPD Exacerbation

- Azithromycin/clarithromycin
- Levofloxacin/moxifloxacin

Necrotizing Fasciitis

- Penicillin and clindamycin
- Meropenem or imipenem if polymicrobial
- Add vancomycin if MRSA suspected

Ventilator-Associated Pneumonia (See Chapter 17)

Community-Acquired Pneumonia (See Chapter 18)

Aspiration Pneumonia (See Chapter 20)

■ ANTIBIOTIC CHOICES FOR SPECIFIC "ICU" PATHOGENS

Pseudomonas aeruginosa

- *P. aeruginosa* has the capacity to rapidly develop resistance to all known classes of antibiotics and resistance can develop in 30–50% of patients receiving monotherapy.
- No data that combination therapy reduces emergence of resistance.
- No data that clinical outcome is improved by combination therapy (unless patient is bacteremic).
- Drugs of choice include the following:
    - Anti-pseudomonal cephalosporin (cefepime or ceftazidime).
    - Carbapenem (imipenem, doripenem, and meropenem).

- Resistance to quinolones develops rapidly; these drugs should not be used as first-line therapy.
- Aminoglycosides may be used as second-line therapy.
- Colistin should be considered in multi-drug-resistant pseudomonas.

Acinetobacter **spp**.

- The antibiotic armamentarium for treatment of *Acinetobacter* is limited because of native resistance to many classes of antibiotics.
- The most effective antibiotics are the following:
  - Carbapenems.
  - Ampicillin/sulbactam.
  - Polymyxin.

ESBL-Producing *Enterobacteriaceae*

- Third (and fourth)-generation cephalosporins should be avoided.
- Carbapenems are the drugs of choice.

Stenotrophomonas maltophilia

- TMP-SMX

Methicillin-Resistant *Staphylococcus aureus* (MRSA)

- The MIC of MRSA against vancomycin is increasing.
- Vancomycin is a large molecule which penetrates tissue poorly.
- Evidence of increasing treatment failures with vancomycin.
- Linezolid may be the treatment of choice for proven MRSA infection.

See Section "Is Vancomycin Obsolete?"

Community-Acquired MRSA (CA-MRSA)

- TMP-SMX
- Doxycycline
- Vancomycin (serious infection)
- Linezolid (serious infection)

S. aureus

- Oxacillin/nafcillin
- Cefazolin

Staphylococcus epidermidis

- Vancomycin

Enterococcus faecalis

- Vancomycin
- Linezolid

■ IS VANCOMYCIN OBSOLETE?

Many consider vancomycin to be an obsolete drug for the treatment of MRSA pneumonia.[1] Linezolid (LZD), the first oxazolidinone antibiotic, has demonstrated excellent activity against MRSA and has demonstrated a mean penetration in epithelial lining fluid of approximately 100–450% compared with serum. Retrospective analyses of two prospective, double-blind, randomized studies of nosocomial pneumonia including VAP showed that LZD therapy was associated with higher clinical cure and survival rates compared with vancomycin therapy in the subset of patients with documented MRSA pneumonia.[12] In a small prospective study of patients with VAP, due to proven MRSA, there was a trend toward a higher microbiological cure rate and secondary clinical outcomes with LZD as compared to vancomycin; however these end points did not reach statistical significance.[13]

If vancomycin is used to treat MRSA, the MICs must be determined. For patients with pneumonia caused by MRSA strains with vancomycin MICs >1.0 mg/ml, treatment with linezolid is advised.[14]

■ USUAL DOSAGES[a]

- Anti-pseudomonal cephalosporin
  - Cefepime 1–2 g every 8–12 h or 4 g as 24-h infusion[15]
  - Ceftazidime 2 g every 8 h
- Anti-pseudomonal carbapenem
  - Imipenem 500 mg every 6 h or 1 g every 8 h
  - Meropenem 1 g every 8 h
  - Doripenem 500 mg every 8 h
- β-Lactam/β-lactamase inhibitor
  - Piperacillin–tazobactam 4.5 g every 6 h or 18 g as 24-h infusion[16]
- Aminoglycoside[b]
  - Gentamicin 7 mg/kg/day
  - Tobramycin 7 mg/kg/day
  - Amikacin 20 mg/kg/day

---

[a] Based on normal renal and hepatic function.

[b] Trough levels for gentamicin and tobramycin should be less than 1 μg/ml and for amikacin they should be less than 4–5 μg/ml.

- Anti-pseudomonal fluoroquinolone
  - Levofloxacin 750 mg every 24 h
  - Ciprofloxacin 400 mg every 8 h
- Other quinolones
  - Moxifloxacin 400 mg every 24 h
- Vancomycin 15 mg/kg every 12 h or 10 mg/kg every 8 h[c]
- Linezolid 600 mg every 12 h

■ REFERENCES

1. Kollef MH, Napolitano LM, Solomkin JS, et al. Health care-associated infection (HAI): a critical appraisal of the emerging threatproceedings of the HAI Summit. *Clin Infect Dis*. 2008;47(Suppl 2):S55–S99.
2. Evans HL, Lefrak SN, Lyman J, et al. Cost of Gram-negative resistance. *Crit Care Med*. 2007;35:89–95.
3. A'Court CH, Garrard CS, Crook D, et al. Microbiological lung surveillance in mechanically ventilated patients, using non-directed bronchial lavage and quantitative culture. *Q J Med*. 1993;86:635–648.
4. Dennesen PJ, Kessels AG, Ramsay G, et al. Resolution of infectious parameters after antimicrobial therapy in patients with ventilator-associated pneumonia. *Am J Respir Crit Care Med*. 2001;163: 1371–1375.
5. Chastre J, Wolff M, Fagon JY, et al. Comparison of 8 vs 15 days of antibiotic therapy for ventilator-associated pneumonia in adults: a randomized trial. *JAMA*. 2003;290:2588–2598.
6. Marik PE. Definition of sepsis: not quite time to dump SIRS? *Crit Care Med*. 2002;30:706–708.
7. Nobre V, Harbarth S, Graf GD, et al. Use of procalcitonin to shorten antibiotic treatment duration in septic patients. A randomized trial. *Am J Respir Crit Care Med*. 2008;177:498–505.
8. Hochreiter M, Kohler T, Schweiger AM, et al. Procalcitonin to guide duration of antibiotic therapy in the intensive care patients: a randomized prospective controlled trial. *Crit Care*. 2009;13:R83.
9. Schuetz P, Christ-Crain M, Thomann R, et al. Effect of procalcitonin-based guidelines vs standard guidelines on antibiotics use in lower respiratory tract infections. The ProHOSP randomized controlled trial. *JAMA*. 2009;302:1059–1066.
10. Schroeder S, Hochreiter M, Koehler T, et al. Procalcitonin (PCT)-guided algorithm reduces length of antibiotic treatment in surgical intensive care

---

[c] Trough levels of vancomycin should be 15–20 μg/ml.

patients with severe sepsis: results of a prospective randomized study. *Langenbecks Arch Surg.* 2009;394:221–226.

11. Isakow W, Kollef MH. Preventing ventilator-associated pneumonia: an evidence-based approach of modifiable risk factors. *Semin Resp Crit Care Med.* 2006;27:5–17.

12. Wunderink RG, Rello J, Cammarata SK, et al. Linezolid vs vancomycin: analysis of two double-blind studies of patients with methicillin-resistant *Staphylococcus aureus* nosocomial pneumonia. *Chest.* 2003;124: 1789–1797.

13. Wunderink RG, Mendelson MH, Somero MS, et al. Early microbiological response to linezolid vs vancomycin in ventilator-associated pneumonia due to methicillin-resistant *Staphylococcus aureus. Chest.* 2008;134:1200–1207.

14. Rubinstein E, Kollef MH, Nathwani D. Pneumonia caused by methicillin-resistant *Staphylococcus aureus. Clin Infect Dis.* 2008;46(Suppl 5):S378–S385.

15. Boselli E, Breilh D, Duflo F, et al. Steady-state plasma and intrapulmonary concentrations of cefepime administered in continuous infusion in critically ill patients with severe pneumonia. *Crit Care Med.* 2003;31:2102–2106.

16. Boselli E, Breilh D, Rimmele T, et al. Alveolar concentrations of piperacillin/tazobactam administered in continuous infusion to patients with ventilator-associated pneumonia. *Crit Care Med.* 2008;36: 1500–1506.

13

Fever

■ COMMON MISCONCEPTION AND FABLES

- Normal body temperature is fairly constant and is usually 37°C (98.6°F)[1]:
  - Normal oral temperature ranges from 35.6°C (96.1°F) to 38.2°C (100.8°F) with marked diurnal variations.[2]
- Fever is a bad thing and suppressing a fever will eliminate its bad effects.
- Fever should be treated because fever makes patients uncomfortable.
- Fever should be treated empirically with antibiotics.
- Reducing core temperature in febrile patients has no ill effects.
- Atelectasis is the most common cause of fever in the first few postoperative days.

Fever is a common problem in the ICU. A prospective observational study in a general ICU reported fever (core temperature >38.3°C) in 70% of patients, caused equally by infective and non-infective processes.[3] In a large retrospective cohort study (24,204 ICU admission), Laupland et al.[4] reported that 44% of patients developed a fever of >38.2°C during their ICU stay; 17% of these patients had positive cultures. The presence of a fever on an ICU patient has a significant impact on health-care costs, as blood cultures, radiological imaging, and antibiotics routinely follow. It is therefore important to have a good understanding of the mechanisms and etiology of fever in ICU patients, how and when to initiate a diagnostic workup, and when initiation of antibiotics is indicated.

The *Society of Critical Care Medicine* and the *Infectious Disease Society of America* considers a temperature of 38.3°C or greater (101°F) as a fever in an ICU patient which warrants further evaluation.[5] This does not necessarily imply that a temperature below 38.3°C (101°F) does

P.E. Marik, *Handbook of Evidence-Based Critical Care*,
DOI 10.1007/978-1-4419-5923-2_13,
© Springer Science+Business Media, LLC 2010

not require further investigation, as many variables determine a patient's febrile response to an insult. In addition, it should be recognized that there is a daily fluctuation of temperature by 0.5–1.0°C, with women having wider variations in temperature than do men. Furthermore, with aging the maximal febrile response decreases by about 0.15°C/decade.

Accurate and reproducible measurement of body temperature is important in detecting disease and in monitoring patients with an elevated temperature. A variety of methods are used to measure body temperature, combining different sites, instruments, and techniques.[6,7] Infrared ear thermometry has been demonstrated to provide values that are a few tenths of a degree below the temperature in the pulmonary artery and brain. Rectal temperatures obtained with a mercury thermometer or electronic probe are often a few tenths of a degree higher than core temperatures. However, patients perceive having rectal temperatures taken as unpleasant and intrusive. Furthermore, access to the rectum may be limited by patient position with an associated risk of rectal trauma. Many tachypneic patients are unable to keep their mouth closed to obtain an accurate oral temperature. Axillary measurements substantially underestimate core temperature and lack reproducibility. Body temperature is therefore most accurately measured by an intravascular thermistor; however, measurement by infrared ear thermometry or with an electronic probe in the rectum is an acceptable alternative.

■ PATHOGENESIS OF FEVER

Cytokines released by monocytic cells play a central role in the genesis of fever.[8,9] The cytokines primarily involved in the development of fever include interleukin-1 (IL-1), interleukin-6 (IL-6), and tumor necrosis factor-α. These cytokines bind to their own specific receptors located in close proximity to the preoptic region of the anterior hypothalamus. Here the cytokine receptor interaction activates phospholipase A2, resulting in the liberation of plasma membrane arachidonic acid as substrate for the cyclooxygenase pathway. Some cytokines appear to increase cyclooxygenase expression directly, leading to the liberation of prostaglandin E2 (PGE2).

Fever appears to be a preserved evolutionary response within the animal kingdom.[10,11] With few exceptions, reptiles, amphibians, fish, and several invertebrate species have been shown to manifest fever in response to challenge with microorganisms. Increased body temperature has been shown to enhance the resistance of animals to infection. Although fever has some harmful effects, it appears to be an adaptive response which has evolved to help rid the host of invading pathogens. Temperature elevation has been shown to enhance several parameters of immune function including antibody production, T-cell activation, production of cytokines, and enhanced neutrophil and macrophage function. Furthermore, some pathogens such as *Streptococcus pneumoniae* are inhibited by febrile temperatures.

ALERT

Fever from an infectious cause should not be treated (with antipyretics) unless the patient has limited cardiorespiratory reserve or the temperature exceeds 40°C (104°F).

Schulman et al.[12] investigated whether it was beneficial to treat the fever of hospitalized patients admitted to a trauma ICU. Patients were randomized to an active treatment group in which acetaminophen and cooling blankets were used to aggressively cool patients as compared to a permissive group in which fever was treated only once it reached 40°C. In this study there was a strong trend toward increased mortality in the active treatment group; all the patients who died in the aggressive treatment group had an infectious etiology as the cause of the fever. Doran et al. demonstrated that children with varicella who were treated with acetaminophen had a more prolonged illness.[13] Weinstein and colleagues[14] reported that patients with spontaneous bacterial peritonitis had improved survival if they had a temperature greater than 38°C. These data suggest that fever from an infectious cause should not be treated unless the patient has limited cardiorespiratory reserve. In contrast to patients with infectious disorders, patients with cerebral ischemia or head trauma have worse outcomes with increased temperature. For these patients the current recommendation is to maintain the patient's temperature in the normothermic range. Anti-pyresis must always include an anti-pyretic agent, as external cooling alone increases heat generation and catecholamine production.[15] Acute hepatitis may occur in ICU patients with reduced glutathione reserves (alcoholics, malnourished, etc.) who have received regular therapeutic doses of acetaminophen (see Chapter 59).

ALERT

Cooling blankets should only be used for induced hypothermia and *never* for the treatment of a fever.

■ CAUSES OF FEVER IN THE ICU

Any disease process that results in the release of the pro-inflammatory cytokines IL-1, IL-6, and TNF-α will result in the development of fever. While infections are common causes of fever in ICU patients, many non-infectious inflammatory conditions cause the release of pro-inflammatory cytokines and induce a febrile response. Similarly, it is important to appreciate that not all patients with infections are febrile. Approximately 10% of septic patients are hypothermic and 35% are normothermic at presentation. Septic patients who fail to develop a fever have a significantly higher mortality than do febrile septic patients. The reason that patients with established infections fail to develop a febrile response is unclear; however, preliminary evidence suggests that this aberrant response is not due to diminished cytokine production.[16]

The presence of fever in an ICU patient frequently triggers a battery of diagnostic tests that are costly, expose the patient to unnecessary risks, and often produce misleading or inconclusive results. It is therefore important that fever in ICU patients be evaluated in a systematic, prudent, clinically appropriate, and cost-effective manner.

■ INFECTIOUS CAUSES OF FEVER

The prevalence of nosocomial infection in ICUs has been reported to vary from 3 to 31%. The most common infectious causes of fever in ICU patients are listed below[17,18]:

- Ventilator-associated pneumonia (VAP)
- Catheter-related bloodstream infection (CRBI)
- Primary septicemia
- Sinusitis
- Surgical site/wound infection
- *Clostridium difficile* colitis
- Cellulitis/infected decubitus ulcer
- Urinary tract infection (urosepsis)
- Suppurative thrombophlebitis
- Endocarditis
- Diverticulitis
- Septic arthritis
- Abscess/empyema

Catheter-Related Bloodstream Infection

See Chapter 11

Ventilator-Associated Pneumonia

See Chapter 17

Urinary Tract Infection

Most ICU patients require an indwelling urinary catheter for monitoring fluid balance and renal function. Urinary tract infections (UTIs), according to some studies, are the third most common infection found in the intensive care unit. In a study of 4,465 patients who were admitted to the ICU for at least 48 h, 6.5% developed a "UTI" with an overall incidence of 9.6/1,000 ICU days.[19] However, the incidence of bacteremia and fungemia was only 0.1/1,000 catheter days. Risk factors include duration of catheterization, severity of illness, age, and prior use of anti-microbials. Gram-negative bacteria, especially *Escherichia coli* and *Pseudomonas aeruginosa*, account for more than half of the pathogens. Gram positives, especially enterococcus and candida, account for remaining cases. Risk factors for funguria include immunosuppression, diabetes, renal failure, structural or functional abnormalities of the urinary tract, recent surgery, chronic illness, and broad-spectrum antibiotics.[20]

The significance of "UTIs" in catheterized ICU patients is unclear and appears unlikely to lead to increased morbidity or mortality. It is likely that most patients have "asymptomatic bacteriuria" rather than true infections of the urinary tract. The treatment of patients with "asymptomatic bacteriuria" is based on a single study performed in the early 1980s that may not be applicable today.[21] Platt and colleagues demonstrated that in hospitalized patients, bacteriuria with greater than >10^5 colony forming units (CFU) of bacteria per milliliter of urine during bladder catheterization was associated with a 2.8-fold increase in mortality. Based on this study, thousands of ICU patients with urinary tract colonization have been treated with antibiotics.

In patients with indwelling urinary catheters, colonic flora rapidly colonizes the urinary tract. Stark and Maki[22] have demonstrated that in catheterized patients, bacteria rapidly proliferate in the urinary system to exceed 10^5 cfu/ml over a short period of time. Bacteriuria defined as a quantitative culture of >10^5 cfu/ml has been reported in up to 30% of catheterized hospitalized patients. The terms bacteriuria and UTI are generally incorrectly used as synonyms. Indeed, most studies in ICU patients have used bacteriuria to diagnose a UTI. Bacteriuria implies colonization of the urinary tract without bacterial invasion and an acute inflammatory response. Urinary tract infection implies an infection of the urinary tract. Criteria have not been developed for differentiating asymptomatic colonization of the urinary tract from symptomatic infection. Furthermore, the presence of white cells in the urine is not useful for differentiating colonization from infection, as most catheter-associated bacteriurias have accompanying pyuria. It is therefore unclear how many catheterized patients with >10^5 cfu/ml actually have urinary tract infections.

While catheter-associated bacteriuria is common in ICU patients, data from the early 1980s indicate that less than 3% of catheter-associated bacteriuric patients will develop bacteremia caused by organisms in the urine.[23] Therefore, the surveillance for and treatment of isolated bacteriuria in most ICU patients is currently not recommended.[24] Bacteriuria should, however, be treated following urinary tract manipulation or surgery in patients with kidney stones and in patients with urinary tract obstruction.

ALERT

The routine culture (and treatment) of urine in ICU patients is not warranted.

Sinusitis

Sinusitis is an underappreciated cause of fever in the ICU. The diagnosis is usually not made until other more common infectious causes of fever have been excluded. Sinusitis if not diagnosed and treated in timely fashion can lead to nosocomial pneumonia and sepsis. Nasal colonization with enteric gram-negative rods, nasoenteric tubes, and a Glasgow Coma Scale of <7 are all risk factors of acquiring nosocomial sinusitis.[25] Patients that are orally intubated are less prone to develop sinusitis than those who are nasotracheally intubated. Indeed, up to 85% of patients that are nasally intubated will develop sinusitis within a week.

In patients with radiological evidence of sinusitis, aspiration of the sinuses is required to confirm the diagnosis and to identify the causative pathogen.[26] Several radiological tests have been described to screen for sinusitis. A CT scan of the sinuses is considered the gold standard. If a patient is too critically ill to be transported out of the ICU, plain films of the sinuses can be obtained. In order to maximize the chances of making the diagnosis, multiple views of the sinuses are required. Bedside ultrasound has been gaining popularity in European countries over the last decade and studies have suggested that it is at least equivalent to CT scanning.

Once sinusitis is diagnosed, all nasal tubes should immediately be removed with early sinus drainage. Broad-spectrum antibiotics should be commenced with coverage that includes *Pseudomonas* and MRSA. The antibiotics should then be de-escalated once culture data are available. Topical decongestants and vasoconstrictors alone or combined with systemic decongestants and anti-histamines are also recommended.

Clostridium difficile Colitis

In patients that develop fever with concurrent diarrhea, *C. difficile* must be considered. It is crucial to diagnose this disease early as it can lead to severe sepsis, multi-organ failure, and death. Patients with *C. difficile* often present with a leukemoid reaction having impressive white blood cell counts, frequently reaching greater than $35,000/mm^3$. A leukemoid reaction or an unexplained leukocytosis may be the first presenting sign of *C. difficile* even in the absence of diarrheal symptoms.[27] Leukemoid reactions are associated with a worse prognosis and a higher mortality rate. Concurrent or prior antibiotic use is a strong risk factor for developing *C. difficile* colitis. Clindamycin, β-lactam (especially cephalosporins), and more recently quinolones have been the most frequently implicated antibiotics. Many patients in the ICU receive GI prophylaxis, usually with a proton pump inhibitor. Proton pump inhibitors have recently been associated with a higher risk of *C. difficile* infection (see Chapter 32). Recently epidemics of an extremely virulent strain of *C. difficile* have been reported in the United States and Canada.[28] It has been suggested that the increasing use of fluoroquinolones has played a role. This strain is associated with higher morbidity and mortality as it produces significantly more toxins than do the other strains.

The diagnosis of *C. difficile* colitis is usually made by immunoassays of stool against both toxin A and toxin B.[29] The presence of *C. difficile* antigen in the absence of the toxin suggests colonization rather than infection with *C. difficile*. Due to the low sensitivity of the toxin assay, two stool specimens should be examined. The cytotoxic assay is more sensitive and specific than the immunoassay; however, this test is not readily available and takes longer to perform. In patients where the diagnosis is still in doubt, a colonoscopy may be performed to look for pseudomembranes. CT scans can also be helpful as 50% of patients will have changes that can be seen on imaging. Positive CT scans are associated with leukocytosis, abdominal pain, and diarrhea. If *C. difficile* colitis is suspected, empiric treatment should be started until the diagnosis is excluded. It is important to note that alcohol-based hand hygiene which has rapidly gained popularity in hospitals does not kill spore-forming organisms such as *C. difficile* and should not replace hand washing with soap when exposed to these patients.

Skin Infections

Skin infections, especially infected pressure ulcers, may be a source of infection in ICU patients. Several factors increase the risk of ICU patients developing pressure ulcers including emergent admissions, severity of illness, extended ICU length of stay, malnutrition, age, diabetes, infusion of vasopressor agents, anemia, and fecal incontinence. Protocols for the prevention of pressure ulcers should be routinely instituted in the ICU. In addition, physician and nurses should routinely examine their patient's skin, particularly high pressure areas such as the sacrum and heels, to detect early signs of skin breakdown.

Other Infections

Nosocomial meningitis is exceedingly uncommon in hospitalized patients who have not undergone a neurosurgical procedure. Lumbar puncture, therefore, does not need to be performed routinely in ICU patients (non-neurosurgical) who develop a fever unless they have meningeal signs or contiguous infection. In patients who have undergone abdominal surgery and develop a fever, intra-abdominal infection must always be excluded. CT scanning of the abdomen is indicated in these patients. Similarly, in patients who have undergone other operative procedures, wound infection must be excluded.

■ NON-INFECTIONS CAUSES OF FEVER IN THE ICU

A large number of non-infectious conditions result in tissue injury with inflammation and a febrile reaction. Those non-infectious disorders which should be considered in ICU patients are listed below. For reasons that are not entirely clear, most non-infectious disorders usually do not lead to a fever in excess of 38.9°C (102°F); therefore, if the temperature increases above this threshold, the patient should be considered to have an infectious etiology as the cause of the fever.[30] However, patients with drug fever may have a temperature >102°F. Similarly, fever secondary to blood transfusion may exceed 102°F. In patients with a temperature above 40°C (104°F), neuroleptic malignant syndrome, malignant hyperthermia, the serotonin syndrome, and sub-arachnoid hemorrhage must always be considered. Most of those clinical conditions listed below are clinically obvious and do not require additional diagnostic tests to confirm their presence. However, a few of these disorders require special consideration.

Non-infectious Causes of Fever

- Drug related
  - Drug fever
  - Neuroleptic malignant syndrome
  - Malignant hyperthermia
  - Serotonin syndrome (see Chapter 61)
  - Drug withdrawal (including alcohol and recreational drugs)
  - IV contrast reaction
- Post-transfusion fever
- Neurological
  - Intracranial hemorrhage
  - Cerebral infarction
  - Sub-arachnoid hemorrhage
  - Seizures
- Endocrine
  - Hyperthyroidism
  - Pheochromocytoma
  - Adrenal insufficiency
- Rheumatologic
  - Crystal arthropathies
  - Vasculitis
  - Collagen vascular diseases
- Hematologic
  - Phlebitis
  - Hematoma
- Gastrointestinal/hepatic
  - Acalculous cholecystitis
  - Ischemic bowel
  - Cirrhosis
  - Hepatitis
  - Gastrointestinal bleed
  - Pancreatitis
- Pulmonary
  - Aspiration pneumonitis
  - Acute respiratory distress syndrome
  - Thromboembolic disease
  - Fat embolism syndrome
- Cardiac
  - Myocardial infarction
  - Dressler's syndrome
  - Pericarditis
- Oncological
  - Neoplastic syndromes

Drug Fever

Most ICU patients receive numerous medications. All drugs have side effects, including fever. It is estimated that about 10% of inpatients develop drug fever during their hospital stay.[31] The diagnosis of drug fever in ICU patients is challenging as the onset of fever can occur immediately after administration of the drug or it can occur days, weeks, months, or even years after the patient has been on the offending medication. Furthermore, once the implicated medication is discontinued, the fever can take up to 3–4 days to resolve. Associated rashes and leukocytosis occur in less than 20% of cases. Penicillins, cephalosporins, anti-convulsants, heparin, and histamine 2-blockers are commonly used medications in the ICU that are associated with drug fevers.

Malignant Hyperthermia

Malignant hyperthermia is a rare genetic disorder of the muscle membrane causing an increase of calcium ions in the muscle cells. This can cause a variety of clinical problems, most commonly a dangerous hypermetabolic state after the use of anesthetic agents such as succinylcholine and halothane. This reaction typically occurs within 1 h of anesthesia but can be delayed for up to 10 h. Patients present with continually increasing fevers, muscle stiffness, and tachycardia. They can rapidly develop hemodynamic instability with progression into multi-organ failure. Since the introduction of dantrolene, the mortality of malignant hyperthermia has decreased from 80% in the 1960s to <10% today.

Neuroleptic Malignant Syndrome

Neuroleptic malignant syndrome is characterized by high fevers, a change in mental status, muscle rigidity, extrapyramidal symptoms, autonomic nervous system disturbances, and altered levels of consciousness. Symptoms usually begin within days to weeks of starting the offending drug. Patients typically have very high creatinine kinase levels. Neuroleptic malignant syndrome is caused by excessive dopaminergic blockade causing a dopamine deficiency in the central nervous system. Agents that are most commonly implicated include neuroleptic medications and certain anti-emetics. Withdrawal of certain medications, which will be discussed later in this chapter, can cause this syndrome as well. Treatment includes discontinuing the offending drug, aggressive supportive care, and close hemodynamic monitoring. Drug treatment of neuroleptic malignant syndrome is controversial. A case-controlled analysis and a retrospective analysis of published cases suggested that dantrolene, bromocriptine, and amantadine may be beneficial.

Serotonin Syndrome

See Chapter 61.

Alcohol and Drug Withdrawal

Withdrawal from alcohol and medications is a common cause of non-infectious fever in hospitalized patients and usually presents within the first few days of hospital admission. See Chapter 60.

Acalculous Cholecystitis

Acute acalculous cholecystitis is a condition of inflammation of the gallbladder in the absence of calculi.[32] It is a disease with significant morbidity and mortality as it can lead to empyema, gallbladder gangrene, and gallbladder perforation. A high index of suspicion is required as this can be a difficult diagnosis to make, especially in the intubated and sedated patient. Initially patients present with very few symptoms. Clinical features include fever, leukocytosis, abnormal liver function tests, a palpable right upper quadrant mass, vague abdominal discomfort, and jaundice. Untreated, bacterial superinfection may occur and this can progress to empyema, peritonitis, and septic shock.

The pathophysiology of acalculous cholecystitis is complex and involves hypoperfusion and biliary stasis. Risk factors include trauma, surgery, intermittent positive-pressure ventilation, coronary heart disease, cholesterol emboli, fasting, total parental nutrition, immunosuppression, transfusions of blood products, hypotension, multi-organ dysfunction, sedation, opiates, diabetes, infections, childbirth, and renal failure.

Ultrasound is usually the first diagnostic test performed because of the ability to perform this at the bedside. In addition, a bedside ultrasound can readily image the other abdominal organs. Ultrasound for acute acalculous cholecystitis, however, has been found to be inferior to morphine cholescintigraphy and CT. One study showed ultrasound to have a sensitivity of 50% compared to 67% for morphine cholescintigraphy with a specificity of 94 and 100%, respectively.[33] Another study reported a sensitivity of 90% for cholescintigraphy, 67% for CT, and only 29% for ultrasound.[32] An abnormal ultrasound can be seen in 50% of ICU patients even if they are not suspected of having acalculous cholecystitis. As soon as the diagnosis is suspected, blood cultures should be drawn, broad-spectrum antibiotics initiated, and a surgical consult requested. In unstable patients, percutaneous drainage may be preferable to surgical intervention.

Postoperative Fever

Surgery alone can cause fever which is self-limited and resolves spontaneously.[34–36] In the early postoperative period, a patient's temperature may increase up to 1.4°C with the peak occurring approximately 11 h after surgery.[34] Fifty percent of postoperative patients will develop a fever greater than or equal to 38°C with 25% reaching 38.5°C or higher. The fever typically lasts for 2–3 days. Postoperative fever is believed to be caused by tissue injury and inflammation with associated cytokine release.[34] The invasiveness of the procedure, as well as genetic factors, influences the degree of cytokine release and the febrile response. A good physical examination and the history of the timing and sequence of events are crucial to help to differentiate postoperative fever from other infectious and non-infectious causes of fever. Reactions to medications (especially anesthesia), blood products, and infections that might have existed prior to the surgery should also be considered during a patient's early postoperative course. Nosocomial and surgical site infections usually develop 3–5 days following surgery.

Atelectasis

Atelectasis is commonly implicated as a cause of fever.[35] Standard ICU texts list atelectasis as a cause of fever, although they provide no primary source. Indeed a major surgery text states that "fever is almost always present (in patients with atelectasis)."[37] During rounds, many medical students and house staffs have been taught that atelectasis is one of the "five" main causes of postoperative fever. However, there is very little data to support this widely held belief (myth).

Engoren studied 100 postoperative cardiac surgery patients and was unable to demonstrate a relationship between atelectasis and fever.[38] Furthermore, when atelectasis is induced in experimental animals by ligation of a main stem bronchus, fever does not occur.[39] The role of atelectasis as a cause of fever is unclear; however, atelectasis probably does not cause fever in the absence of pulmonary infection.

Blood Transfusions

A large number of patients in the ICU will receive transfusions of blood products. Febrile non-hemolytic transfusion reactions are exceedingly common following transfusion of blood and blood products. This is likely mediated by the transfusion of cytokines such as IL-1, IL-6, IL-8, and TNF-α, which accumulate with increasing length of blood storage.[40,41]

Febrile non-hemolytic reactions normally present within the first 6 h after transfusion and are self-limiting. They can present with chills and rigors in addition to fever. It is crucial to differentiate these from febrile acute hemolytic transfusion reactions which can be life threatening. Leukoreduction has been shown to reduce the risk of febrile non-hemolytic transfusion reactions.

Thromboembolic Disease

Fever has been reported in 14–18% of patients with thromboembolic disease and is generally an uncommon cause of fever in hospitalized patients. Typically the fever is low grade (37.5–38°C).[42]

■ AN APPROACH TO THE CRITICALLY ILL PATIENT WITH FEVER

ALERT

The term *pan-culture* is meaningless, quite impolite and should *never* be uttered in the ICU.

See Figure 13-1. The following approach is suggested in ICU patients who develop a fever. Due to the frequency, excess morbidity and mortality associated with bacteremia, blood cultures are recommenced in all ICU patients who develop a fever. A comprehensive physical examination and review of the chest radiograph is essential. Non-infectious causes of fever should be excluded. In patients with an obvious focus of infection (e.g., purulent nasal discharge, abdominal tenderness, profuse green diarrhea), a focused diagnostic workup is required. If there is no clinically obvious source of infection and unless the patient is clinically deteriorating (falling blood pressure, decreased urine output, increasing confusion, rising serum lactate concentration, falling platelet count, or worsening coagulopathy) or the temperature is in excess of 39°C (102°F), it may be prudent to perform blood cultures and then observe the patient before embarking on the further diagnostic tests and commencing empiric antibiotics. However, all neutropenic patients with fever and patients with severe or progressive signs of sepsis should be started on broad-spectrum anti-microbial therapy immediately after obtaining appropriate cultures.

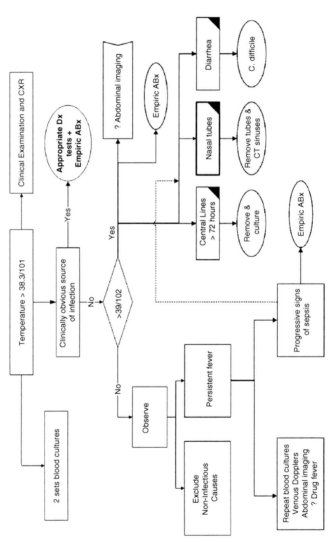

Figure 13-1. Fever management protocol.

In patients whose clinical picture is consistent with infection and in whom no clinically obvious source has been documented, removal of all central lines greater than 48 h old (with semi-quantitative or quantitative culture) as well as stool examination for *C. difficile* toxin (in those patients with loose stools) and a CT scan of the sinuses with removal of all nasal tubes is recommended. Urine culture is indicated only in patients with abnormalities of the renal system or following urinary tract manipulation. If the patient is at risk of abdominal sepsis or has any abdominal signs (tenderness, distension, unable to tolerate enteral feeds), CT scan of abdomen is indicated. Patients with right upper quadrant tenderness require an abdominal ultrasound or CT examination.

Re-evaluation of the patient's status after 48 h using all available results and the evolution of the patient's clinical condition are essential. If fever persists despite empiric antibiotics and no source of infection has been identified, empiric anti-fungal therapy may be indicated in patients with risk factors for candidal infection. Additional diagnostic tests may be appropriate at this time including venous Doppler, differential blood count for eosinophils (diagnosis of drug fever), and abdominal imaging.

■ CLINICAL PEARLS

- All patients with a fever >38.3°C (101°F) require blood cultures and a clinical evaluation to determine the source of fever.
- Urine and sputum cultures should not be routinely performed in patients with a fever.
- Atelectasis does not cause a fever.
- Antibiotics are not anti-pyretic agents and should therefore be used only in patients with suspected or proven bacterial infection.
- As a general rule, anti-pyretics should not be used to treat a fever.
- A cooling blanket should never be used to treat a fever.

■ REFERENCES

1. Barone J. Fever: fact and fiction. *J Trauma*. 2009;67:406–409.
2. Sund-Levander M, Forsberg C, Wahren LK. Normal oral, rectal, tympanic and axillary body temperature in adult men and women: a systematic literature review. *Scand J Caring Sci*. 2002;16:122–128.
3. Circiumaru B, Baldock G, Cohen J, et al. A prospective study of fever in the intensive care unit. *Intensive Care Med*. 1999;25:668–673.
4. Laupland KB, Shahpori R, Kirkpatrick AW, et al. Occurrence and outcome of fever in critically ill adults. *Crit Care Med*. 2008;36: 1531–1535.

5. O'Grady NP, Barie PS, Bartlett JG, et al. Guidelines for evaluation of new fever in critically ill adult patients: 2008 update from the American College of Critical Care Medicine and the Infectious Diseases Society of America. *Crit Care Med.* 2008;36:1330–1349.

6. Sund-Levander M, Forsberg C, Wahren LK. Normal oral, rectal, tympanic and axillary body temperature in adult men and women: a systematic literature review. *Scand J Care Sci.* 2002;16:122–128.

7. Erickson RS, Kirklin SK. Comparison of ear-based, bladder, oral, and axillary methods for core temperature measurement. *Crit Care Med.* 1993;21:1528–1534.

8. Saper CB, Breder CD. The neurologic basis of fever. *N Engl J Med.* 1994;330:1880–1886.

9. Kluger MJ, Kozak W, Leon LR, et al. The use of knockout mice to understand the role of cytokines in fever. *Clin Exp Pharmacol Physiol.* 1998;25:141–144.

10. Kluger MJ, Ringler DH, Anver MR. Fever and survival. *Science.* 1975;188:166–168.

11. Kluger MJ, Kozak W, Conn CA, et al. The adaptive value of fever. *Infect Dis Clin North Am.* 1996;10:1–20.

12. Schulman CI, Namias N, Doherty J, et al. The effect of antipyretic therapy upon outcomes in critically ill patients: a randomized, prospective study. *Surg Infect.* 2005;6:369–375.

13. Doran TF, De AC, Baumgardner RA, et al. Acetaminophen: more harm than good for chickenpox? *J Pediatr.* 1989;114:1045–1048.

14. Weinstein MP, Iannini PB, Stratton CW, et al. Spontaneous bacterial peritonitis. A review of 28 cases with emphasis on improved survival and factors influencing prognosis. *Am J Med.* 1978;64:592–598.

15. Lenhardt R, Negishi C, Sessler DI, et al. The effects of physical treatment on induced fever in humans. *Am J Med.* 1999;106:550–555.

16. Marik PE, Zaloga GP. Hypothermia and cytokines in septic shock. Norasept II Study Investigators. North American study of the safety and efficacy of murine monoclonal antibody to tumor necrosis factor for the treatment of septic shock. *Intensive Care Med.* 2000;26:716–721.

17. Vincent JL, Bihari DJ, Suter PM, et al. The prevalence of nosocomial infection in intensive care units in Europe. Results of the European Prevalence of Infection in Intensive Care (EPIC) Study. EPIC International Advisory Committee. *JAMA.* 1995;274:639–644.

18. Richards MJ, Edwards JR, Culver DH, et al. Nosocomial infections in medical intensive care units in the United States. National Nosocomial Infections Surveillance System. *Crit Care Med.* 1999;27:887–892.

19. Laupland KB, Bagshaw SM, Gregson DB, et al. Intensive care unit-acquired urinary tract infections in a regional critical care system. *Crit Care.* 2005;9:R60–R65.

20. Leone M, Albanese J, Garnier F, et al. Risk factors of nosocomial catheter-associated urinary tract infection in a polyvalent intensive care unit. *Intensive Care Med.* 2003;29:1077–1080.
21. Platt R, Polk BF, Murdock B, et al. Mortality associated with nosocomial urinary tract infection. *N Engl J Med.* 1982;307:637–642.
22. Stark RP, Maki DG. Bacteriuria in the catheterized patient. What quantitative level of bacteriuria is relevant? *N Engl J Med.* 1984;311:560–564.
23. Krieger JN, Kaiser DL, Wenzel RP. Urinary tract etiology of bloodstream infections in hospitalized patients. *J Infect Dis.* 1983;148:57–62.
24. Garibaldi RA, Mooney BR, Epstein BJ, et al. An evaluation of daily bacteriologic monitoring to identify preventable episodes of catheter-associated urinary tract infection. *Infect Control.* 1982;3:466–470.
25. George DL, Falk PS, Umberto MG, et al. Nosocomial sinusitis in patients in the medical intensive care unit: a prospective epidemiological study. *Clin Infect Dis.* 1998;27:463–470.
26. Holzapfel L, Chevret S, Madinier G, et al. Influence of long-term oro- or nasotracheal intubation on nosocomial maxillary sinusitis and pneumonia: results of a prospective, randomized, clinical trial. *Crit Care Med.* 1993;21:1132–1138.
27. Wanahita A, Goldsmith EA, Marino BJ, et al. *Clostridium difficile* infection in patients with unexplained leukocytosis. *Am J Med.* 2003;115: 543–546.
28. McDonald LC, Killgore GE, Thompson A, et al. An epidemic, toxin gene-variant strain of *Clostridium difficile.* *N Engl J Med.* 2005;353:2433–2441.
29. Kuipers EJ, Surawicz CM. *Clostridium difficile* infection. *Lancet.* 2008;371:1486–1488.
30. Marik PE. Fever in the ICU. *Chest.* 2000;117:855–869.
31. Johnson DH, Cunha BA. Drug fever. *Infect Dis Clin North Am.* 1996;10:85–91.
32. Kalliafas S, Ziegler DW, Flancbaum L, et al. Acute acalculous cholecystitis: incidence, risk factors, diagnosis, and outcome. *Am Surg.* 1998;64:471–475.
33. Mariat G, Mahul P, Prevt N, et al. Contribution of ultrasonography and cholescintigraphy to the diagnosis of acute acalculous cholecystitis in intensive care unit patients. *Intensive Care Med.* 2000;26:1658–1663.
34. Frank SM, Kluger MJ, Kunkel SL. Elevated thermostatic setpoint in postoperative patients. *Anesthesiology.* 2000;93:1426–1431.
35. Dionigi R, Dionigi G, Rovera F, et al. Postoperative fever. *Surg Infect.* 2006;7(Suppl 2):S17–S20.
36. Lenhardt R, Negishi C, Sessler DI, et al. Perioperative fever. *Acta Anaesthesiol Scand Suppl.* 1997;111:325–328.
37. Hiyama DT, Zinner MJ. Surgical complications. In: Schwartz SI, Shires GT, Sencer FC, Cowles Husser W, eds. *Principles of Surgery.* 6th ed. New York: McGraw-Hill; 1994:455–487.

38. Engoren M. Lack of association between atelectasis and fever. *Chest.* 1995;107:81–84.
39. Shields RT. Pathogenesis of postoperative pulmonary atelectasis an experimental study. *Arch Surg.* 1949;48:489–503.
40. Snyder EL. The role of cytokines and adhesive molecules in febrile non-hemolytic transfusion reactions. *Immunol Invest.* 1995;24:333–339.
41. Hendrickson JE, Hillyer CD. Noninfectious serious hazards of transfusion. *Anesth Analg.* 2009;108:759–769.
42. Stein PD, Afzal A, Henry JW, et al. Fever in acute pulmonary embolism. *Chest.* 2000;117:39–42.

Part II

Respiratory

14

Mechanical Ventilation 101

A landmark study published by the ARDSNet group (NIH ARDS Network) in 2000 demonstrated that volume-assisted ventilation (AC) with a low tidal volume (6 ml/kg of predicted body weight) was associated with a significant reduction in 28-day all-cause mortality as compared to AC ventilation with traditional tidal volumes (12 ml/kg of PBW) in patients with ARDS.[1] Such an approach is now considered the standard of care and applies to all mechanically ventilated patients, not just those with ARDS.[2–4]

ALERT

The predicted body weight (PBW) should be calculated on all patients undergoing mechanical ventilation (see Table 14-1).

- Men: PBW = 50.0 + 0.91 (height in centimeters – 152.4).
- Women: PBW = 45.5 + 0.91 (height in centimeters – 152.4).

ALERT

Regardless of the mode of mechanical ventilation, the tidal volume (V_t) of all patients undergoing mechanical ventilation should not exceed 6–8 ml/kg IBW[1] (see Table 14-1).

P.E. Marik, *Handbook of Evidence-Based Critical Care*,
DOI 10.1007/978-1-4419-5923-2_14,
© Springer Science+Business Media, LLC 2010

Table 14-1. IBW and tidal volume at 8 ml/kg PBW.

Height	IBW (kg) Male/Female	V_t at 8 ml/kg	
		Male	Female
6'6"	91.4/86.9	731	695
6'5"	89.1/84.6	712	676
6'4"	86.8/82.3	694	658
6'3"	84.5/80.0	676	640
6'2"	82.2/77.7	657	621
6'1"	79.9/75.4	639	603
6'0"	77.6/73.1	620	584
5'1"	75.3/70.8	602	566
5'10"	73.0/68.5	584	548
5'9"	70.7/66.2	565	529
5'8"	68.4/63.9	547	511
5'7"	66.1/61.6	528	492
5'6"	63.8/59.3	510	474
5'5"	61.5/57	492	456
5'4"	59.2/54.7	473	437
5'3"	56.9/52.4	455	419
5'2"	54.6/50.1	436	400
5'1"	52.3/47.8	418	382
5'0"	50.0/45.5	400	364
4'11"	47.7/43.2	381	345
4'10"	45.4/40.9	363	327
4'9"	43.1/38.6	344	308
4'8"	40.8/36.7	326	290
4'7"	38.5/34.4	308	278

■ ALVEOLAR OVERDISTENSION

Alveolar overdistension has clearly been shown to damage normal as well as injured lungs. It is therefore critically important that low V_t be used in all patients undergoing mechanical ventilation. Furthermore, it is important to use the predicted body weight (PBW) and not actual body weight for these calculations. The concept underlying this approach is that it normalizes the V_t to lung size, since lung size has been shown to depend most strongly on height and sex. For example, a person who ideally weighs 70 kg and who then gains 35 kg has essentially the same lung size as he or she did when at a weight of 70 kg and should not receive ventilation with a higher V_t because of the weight gain.

Alveolar Overdistension Damages Normal Lungs

In an observational cohort study, Gajic et al.[5] reported that of patients ventilated for 2 days or longer who did not have ALI/ARDS at the onset of mechanical ventilation, 25% developed ALI/ARDS within 5 days of mechanical ventilation. In a multi-variate analysis, the main risk factors associated with the development of lung injury were the use of large V_t and transfusion of blood products. The odds ratio of developing ALI was 1.3 for each milliliter above 6 ml/kg PBW. Interestingly, female patients were ventilated with larger V_t (per predicted body weight) and tended to develop lung injury more often. Women are generally shorter than men; this may have accounted for this finding. Similarly, in a large prospective international study on mechanical ventilation, a large V_t and a high peak airway pressure were independently associated with the development of ARDS in patients who did not have ARDS at the onset of mechanical ventilation.[6]

The strongest evidence for the benefit of protective lung ventilation in patients without ALI/ARDS comes from a randomized clinical trial in postoperative patients.[7] Intubated mechanically ventilated patients in the surgical intensive care unit were randomly assigned to mechanical ventilation with V_t of 12 ml/kg or lower V_t of 6 ml/kg. The incidence of pulmonary infection tended to be lower, and duration of intubation and duration of ICU stay tended to be shorter for non-neurosurgical and non-cardiac surgical patients randomly assigned to the lower VT strategy, suggesting that morbidity may be decreased.

■ INDICATIONS FOR INTUBATION AND MECHANICAL VENTILATION

- Hypoxic respiratory failure
  - Deliver a high FiO_2
  - Reduce shunt
  - Apply PEEP
- Hypercapnic respiratory acidosis
  - Reduce the work of breathing and thus prevents respiratory muscle fatigue
  - Maintain adequate alveolar ventilation
- Unprotected and unstable airways (e.g., coma)
  - Secure the airway
  - Reduce the risk of aspiration
  - Maintain adequate alveolar ventilation
- Others
  - To facilitate procedure (bronchoscopy), bronchial suctioning

Think of Respiration as Two Separate Processes

- Ventilation (alveolar ventilation is indirectly proportional to $PaCO_2$)
- Oxygenation (assessed by PaO_2 and percent saturation)

Mechanisms of Hypoxemia

- Ventilation/perfusion (VA/Q) mismatching:
  - High VA/Q.
  - Low VA/Q.
- Shunting:
  - If significant shunting is present, the FiO_2 requirement is typically >60% and increased PEEP is required.
- Hypoventilation.
- Impaired diffusion.
- Reduced FiO_2 (e.g., toxic fumes, altitude).

Causes of Hypercapnia

- Inadequate minute ventilation (VE)
- Increased dead space ventilation (V_d/V_t)
- Increased CO_2 production (VCO_2)

Problems Associated with Positive-Pressure Ventilation

- Heart and circulation
  - Reduced venous return
  - Increased RV afterload
- Lungs
  - Barotrauma
  - Ventilator-induced lung injury
  - Air trapping
- Gas exchange
  - May increase dead space (compression of capillaries)
  - Shunt (e.g., unilateral lung disease – the increase in vascular resistance in the normal lung associated with PPV tends to redirect blood flow in the abnormal lung)

Ventilator Basics Defined

- FiO_2 – fraction of inspired oxygen
- Rate – number of breaths per minute
- Tidal volume (V_t) – volume of each breath
- Sensitivity – how responsive the ventilator is to the patient's efforts
- Peak flow – the maximum flow rate used to deliver each breath to the patient
- Inspiratory time – the time spent in the inspiratory phase of the ventilatory cycle
- $I:E$ ratio – the inspiratory time compared to the expiratory time; $I + E$ = total cycle time
- Flow pattern – the shape of the curve representing the breath delivery; it can be square wave of decelerating

- Mode – the manner or the method of support provided by the ventilator
- Cycling – volume, time, pressure, flow – what cycles, or changes, the ventilator from one phase of the respiratory cycle to the other
- Limiting – volume, pressure, time – what limits the delivery of gas to the patient during the inspiratory phase
- Trigger: variable initiating breath (patient effort sensed by change in flow/pressure)

■ MODE OF VENTILATION AND INITIAL SETTINGS

The intensivist should be familiar with a number of modes of ventilation all of which have specific indications. Assist-controlled (volume-controlled) ventilation is the most common mode of mechanical ventilation in the ICU and should be considered the "default mode" (see Figure 14-1). AC-PC (AC pressure controlled) can be used as the default/standard mode in those ICUs that have a *respiratory therapy-driven protocol* in which the tidal volumes (exhaled) are closely monitored. Pressure-support (PS) ventilation is the most frequently used mode used during "weaning" and is commonly used in ventilator-dependent patients with chronic respiratory failure.

Pressure-controlled ventilation (PCV) and airway pressure release ventilation (APRV) should be considered in patients with severe ARDS who have "failed" conventional low V_t AC ventilation. In some centers, APRV is considered the default mode for ALI/ARDS as well as cardiogenic pulmonary edema. APRV is a useful mode in patients with atelectasis. Synchronized intermittent mandatory ventilation (SIMV) has a limited role, mainly in patients with asthma and when weaning patients who have been oversedated (low drive).

Initial (Default) Ventilator Settings

- Mode: AC (see Figure 14-1)
- V_t: 8 ml/kg IBW (see Table 14-1)
- Rate: 16 breaths/min
- PEEP: 5 cm H_2O
- FiO$_2$: 100%
- Flow rate: 80 l/min
- Waveform: decelerating

These settings should then be dynamically adjusted according to the following:

Standard Ventilator Protocol

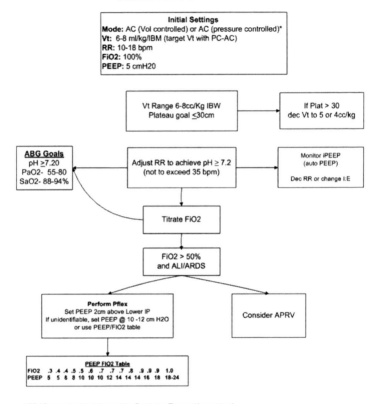

* PC-AC mode should only be used in a Respiratory Therapy driven protocol
in which the exhaled tidal volumes are closely monitored

Figure 14-1. "Standard" ventilator protocol.

- Plateau pressures (keep less than 30 cm H_2O)
- Arterial saturation-pulse oximetry (92–96%)
- pH and $PaCO_2$
- iPEEP (intrinsic PEEP)
- Flow and pressure waveforms

■ VENTILATOR VARIABLES

Phase Variables

See Figure 14-2.

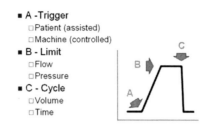

- A -Trigger
  - □ Patient (assisted)
  - □ Machine (controlled)
- B - Limit
  - □ Flow
  - □ Pressure
- C - Cycle
  - □ Volume
  - □ Time

Figure 14-2. Phase variables.

Cycling

Ventilators have traditionally been classified according to the cycling method (cycling from inhalation to exhalation). However, modern ventilators have microprocessors, which allow them to function in many different modes with enormous versatility.

- *Volume cycled*: The ventilator delivers fresh gas until the preselected volume of gas is delivered. The rise in alveolar pressures is to pulmonary compliance and the volume of gas delivered. See Figures 14-2 and 14-3.
- *Pressure cycled*: Inspiration continues until a predetermined peak airway pressure is reached. The tidal volume is variable (from breath to breath) and depends on the following:
  - – Pulmonary compliance.
  - – Respiratory rate.
  - – Inspiratory time and flow rate.

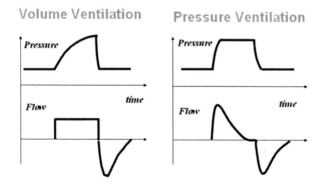

Figure 14-3. Volume- and pressure-limited ventilation.

- *Time cycled*: Inspiration continues for a preset interval, with exhalation beginning when this time interval has elapsed, regardless of airway pressure or volume delivered.

Inspiratory Waveforms

Most ventilators offer at least three different types of inspiratory flow patterns in the SIMV and AC modes of ventilation (see Figure 14-4). These include the following:

- A *square wave*: The inspiratory flow rises rapidly to a preset level and then stays at that level until the end of inspiration.
- A *sinusoidal wave*: The flow gradually increases and then decreases toward the end of inspiration.
- A *descending ramp wave*: The flow increases very rapidly and then decreases gradually until the end of inspiration. This pattern most closely mimics the normal inspiratory pattern.

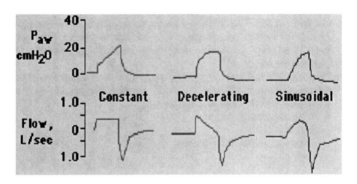

Figure 14-4. Inspiratory waveforms.

In addition, the inspiratory wave can be modified by adjusting the inspiratory flow rate, inspiratory time, and by providing an inspiratory pause (i.e., changing the *I:E* ratio).

Inspiratory-to-Expiratory Ratio

Some ventilators allow the operator to set the *I:E* ratio directly. Other ventilators allow adjustment of the I:E ratio by altering the flow rate, respiratory rate, and inspiratory time (including an inspiratory pause). For most adults, a normal *I:E* ratio of 1:2 or 1:3 is used. In patients with chronic obstructive lung disease and asthma, longer *I:E* ratios are necessary to allow the lungs time to exhale to resting FRC and to avoid hyperinflation.

Patients who are hypoxemic secondary to ARDS require increased mean airway pressure to increase the FRC and allow more surface area for gas transfer to occur. This is achieved using both PEEP and inverse ratio ventilation. In addition, studies have demonstrated that prolonging inspiration can result in a more homogeneous distribution of ventilation within abnormal lungs. When the *I:E* ratio is increased to 1:1 or more, the inspiratory pressure is maintained for a longer period of time; however, the peak inspiratory pressure does not increase.

Ventilator Trigger Variables

With most commonly used modes of mechanical ventilation (AC, SIMV, PSV) and CPAP, a set trigger sensitivity has to be reached before the ventilator delivers flow. Pressure and flow triggering are the most commonly used trigger variables.

With pressure triggering, a set negative pressure must be attained for the ventilator to deliver fresh gas into the inspiratory circuit [both a spontaneous breath (CPAP and SIMV) and a patient-triggered ventilator breath]. This is usually set at -2 cm H_2O. The higher (more negative) the trigger sensitivity, the harder the patient has to work to trigger a breath.

With flow triggering, two variables need to be set: the base flow rate and the flow sensitivity. The base flow consists of fresh gas that circulates continuously within the inhalation and the exhalation circuit. The base flow for adults can be set between 5 and 20 l/min. The flow sensitivity can be set at a minimum of 1 l/min to one half the base flow. The initial demand for flow is satisfied by the base flow, while at the same time generating the inspiratory flow signal according to the set flow sensitivity.

In both the healthy subject and the intubated patient, the inspiratory muscle work has been demonstrated to be significantly higher with pressure-triggered CPAP (without PSV) than with flow-triggered CPAP. However, pressure support of 5 cm H_2O has been demonstrated to reduce the inspiratory muscle work of pressure-triggered CPAP to a level comparable with that of flow-triggered CPAP.

■ MODES OF VENTILATION (SEE TABLE 14-2)

Assist Control (AC)

In the AC mode, the ventilator senses an inspiratory effort by the patient and responds by delivering a preset tidal volume. The trigger threshold is

Table 14-2. Modes of mechanical ventilation.

Mode	Trigger	Limit	Cycle
AC	Patient	Flow	Volume
PCV	Patient	Pressure	Time
PSV	Patient	Pressure	Flow
APRV	Time	Pressure	Time

the negative force that the patient must generate to trigger the ventilator. This trigger threshold can be adjusted, determining how hard the patient must work to trigger the ventilator. The trigger threshold is usually set at -2 cm H_2O. To prevent hypoventilation, a control mode backup rate is set on the ventilator. If the time between two spontaneous inspiratory efforts is greater than the interval corresponding to the backup rate, a breath of the same tidal volume is delivered.

Controlled Mechanical Ventilation (CMV)

The respiratory rate and the tidal volume are preset. The patient cannot trigger the ventilator or move air through the ventilator circuit. The minute volume is therefore dependent on the preset respiratory rate and tidal volume. The CMV mode of ventilation is used only in paralyzed patients.

Pressure-Support Ventilation (PSV)

PSV was developed to reduce the work of spontaneous breathing in the SIMV and continuous positive airway pressure (CPAP) modes (see Figure 14-5). Each time the patient inhales, the ventilator delivers a pressure-limited breath, which continues until a predetermined end point is reached (usually flow). PSV compensates for the inherent impedance of the ventilator circuit and the endotracheal tube, enabling the patient to establish a more natural breathing pattern. A PSV of between 5 and 10 cm H_2O will overcome the resistance of the ventilator circuit and the endotracheal tube.

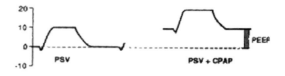

Figure 14-5. Pressure support ventilation (PSV) and CPAP.

- Advantages:
  - Patient controls rate, volume, and duration of breaths.
  - Patient comfort.
  - May overcome WOB.
- Disadvantages:
  - May not be enough ventilatory support if patient condition changes.
  - Support level remains constant regardless of patient drive.
- Patient assessment:
  - Monitor exhaled V_t.
  - Monitor RR.

Pressure-Controlled Ventilation (PCV)

This is a form of AC ventilation; however, following patient or automatic triggering, the ventilator delivers a pressure-limited breath (see Figure 14-3 and Chapter 19). The pressure above end-expiratory pressure is set, and the ventilator delivers a breath until this pressure is reached. As the pressure difference falls with progression of inspiration, the flow rate has a decelerating pattern. This inspiratory waveform has been shown to result in a more homogeneous distribution of gas flow in patients with the acute respiratory distress syndrome (ARDS). The tidal volume varies (from breath to breath), being dependent upon the set pressure, the compliance of the respiratory system, and the inspiratory time.

- Key set variables
  - Pressure (driving pressure or Delta P)
  - Inspiratory time
  - Frequency
  - PEEP
  - FiO_2
- Mandatory breaths
  - Ventilator generates a predetermined pressure for a preset time

Advantages

- Limits risk of barotrauma
- May recruit collapsed and flooded alveoli
- Improved gas distribution

Disadvantages

- Tidal volumes vary when patient compliance changes (i.e., ARDS, pulmonary edema).
- With increases in I time, patient may require sedation and/or chemical paralysis.

Monitoring

- Tidal volume.
  - A pneumothorax or other adverse change in the mechanics of the respiratory system will not trigger a high alarm pressure but a low tidal volume alarm instead.
- Minute ventilation.
- End-tidal CO_2:
  - As noted above a fall in tidal volume may be "obscured"; it is therefore very important to monitor end-tidal CO_2 as an index of alveolar ventilation.
- iPEEP.

Synchronized Intermittent Mandatory Ventilation (SIMV)

In the SIMV mode, the patient breathes spontaneously through the ventilator circuit at a tidal volume and rate that he/she determines according to the need. The patient, however, must open (trigger) a demand valve to breathe through the circuit, increasing the work of breathing. At regular intervals, the ventilator delivers breaths based on a preset tidal volume and rate, which are synchronized with the patient's respiratory efforts. The degree of respiratory support is determined by the SIMV rate (see Figure 14-6).

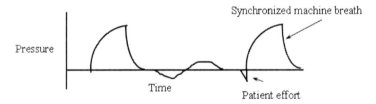

Figure 14-6. Synchronized intermittent mandatory ventilation (SIMV).

Airway Pressure Release Ventilation (APRV)

APRV is a time-triggered, pressure-limited, time-cycled mode of ventilation that allows unrestricted spontaneous breathing throughout the entire ventilatory cycle (see Figure 14-7). It is an alternative approach to the "open-lung" ventilation strategy.[8] Although recruitment maneuvers may be effective in improving gas exchange and compliance, these effects are

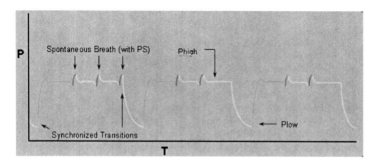

Figure 14-7. Airway pressure release ventilation (APRV).

not sustained; APRV may be viewed as a nearly continuous recruitment maneuver.[9] The ventilator maintains a high-pressure setting for the bulk of the respiratory cycle (P_{High}), which is followed by a periodic release to a low pressure (P_{Low}).[10] The periodic releases aid in carbon dioxide elimination (CO_2). The release periods (T_{Low}) are kept short (0.7–1 s); this prevents derecruitment and enhances spontaneous breathing during T_{High}.[8,11] The advantages of APRV over volume-controlled ventilation include an increase in mean alveolar pressure with alveolar recruitment, the hemodynamic and ventilatory benefits associated with spontaneous breathing, and the reduced requirement for sedation.

Indications for APRV

- ALI/ARDS with
  - $FiO_2 \geq 60\%$
  - Peep ≥ 10
- Cardiogenic pulmonary edema
- Morbid obesity with basal atelectasis[12]
- Segmental/lobar atelectasis[13]
- Pregnancy[14]

Exclusion

- COPD/asthma
- Contraindication to permissive hypercapnia

Potential Advantages of APRV

- Lung protective – minimizes VILI
  - Alveolar recruitment
  - Decreases overinflation
  - Enhanced gas exchange

- Improves hemodynamic profile
  - Reduced need for pressors
  - Enhanced venous return
  - Increased cardiac output
  - Reduced myocardial work
- Provides benefit from spontaneous breathing
  - Improves V/Q mismatching
  - Preferentially aerates dependent lung
  - Limited adverse effects on cardiopulmonary function
- Decreased work of breathing
- Decreased need for sedation

Initial Settings

- Release rate (frequency) 12–14 breaths/min
- P_{High} 20–25 cm H_2O (75% of P_{plat} on AC)
- P_{Low} 5–10 cm H_2O (75% of orig. PEEP)
- TLow 0.7–1 s
- PS 5 cm H_2O

An alternative method of setting up and adjusting APRV is by measuring transalveolar pressures using an esophageal balloon (see Chapter 19). P_{Low} is set such that transalveolar end-expiratory pressure (release pressure) is 0–5 cm H_2O and the transalveolar inspiratory pressure is <30 cm H_2O (see Figure 14-8):

$$Transalveolar\ pressure = airway\ pressure - esophageal\ pressure$$

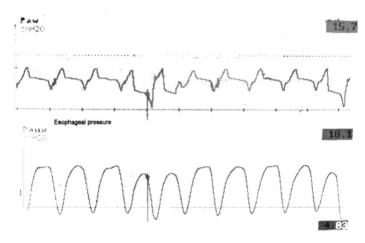

Figure 14-8. Effect of PEEP.

Monitoring on APRV

- Minute ventilation
- Tidal volume
  - APRV (release volume)
  - Spontaneous
- SaO_2
- Patient rate
- $PaCO_2$

In order to prevent alveolar overdistension, the release volume should be monitored and should be kept below 8 ml/kg PBW. If the release volumes are excessive, this can be corrected by either reducing P_{High} or increasing P_{Low}.

Weaning from APRV

Decrease FiO_2.
Decrease P_{High}.
Increase TimeL.
The goal is to arrive at straight CPAP usually at 12 cm H_2O.

■ POSITIVE END-EXPIRATORY PRESSURE

- PEEP provides positive end-expiratory pressure above atmospheric pressure (see Figure 14-9). The mean airway pressure increases in proportion to the level of PEEP. In patients with pulmonary edema, PEEP shifts the pressure–volume inflation curve toward normal, increasing compliance, recruiting alveoli, and increasing functional residual capacity (FRC). It is thought that PEEP redistributes lung water. In patients with a large shunt, increasing FiO_2 has little effect on arterial PaO_2 (see Figure 14-10). Increased PEEP is required to increase PaO_2 in patients with a large shunt.

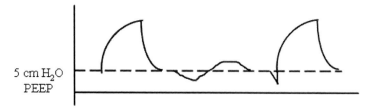

5 cm H_2O
PEEP

Figure 14-9. APRV and transalveolar pressures.

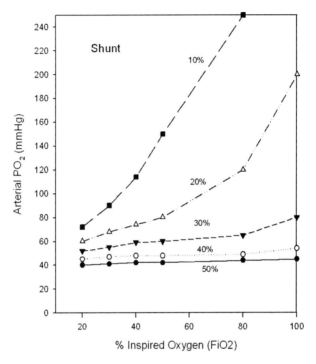

Figure 14-10. Effect of increasing FiO_2 according to shunt fraction.

- PEEP is "good" for left ventricular function:
  - Decreases preload.
  - Decreases afterload.
  - Improves pulmonary compliance and therefore decreases work of breathing.
- PEEP is "bad" for right ventricular (RV) function:
  - Increases RV afterload; RV may acutely fail in patients with severe pulmonary hypertension and patients with RV infarction.
- *Physiological PEEP*: Some intensivists use "physiological" or prophylactic PEEP (5 cm H_2O) to prevent atelectasis/pneumonia. Manzano et al.[15] randomized 131 mechanically ventilated patients with normal chest radiograph and PaO_2/FiO_2 above 250 to receive mechanical ventilation with 5–8-cm-H_2O PEEP or no-PEEP. Ventilator-associated pneumonia was detected in 16 (25.4%) patients in the control group and 6 (9.4%) patients in the PEEP

group. The number of patients who developed hypoxemia was significantly higher in the control group (34 of 63 patients, 54%) than in the PEEP group (12 of 64 patients, 19%).

Indications for PEEP

- Cardiogenic pulmonary edema
- Acute lung injury and ARDS
- Postoperative patients (decreased FRC)
- Prevent basal atelectasis in morbidly obese patients (see Chapter 56)

Contraindications

- Bullous lung disease and emphysema
- Unilateral lung disease (relative contraindication)

Best PEEP

The level of PEEP that should be used is "Best PEEP." In patients with large intrapulmonary shunts, increasing the FiO_2 will not increase the PaO_2. However, excessive PEEP will overinflate compliant lungs and increase V/Q mismatching as well as reduce cardiac output and impair RV function. A PEEP trial should be performed daily to determine the lowest level of PEEP that provides adequate arterial saturation and maximal oxygen delivery. Patients with ARDS generally require a PEEP of 10–15 cm H_2O (see Chapter 19).

PEEP valve: When using >5-cm-H_2O PEEP, a PEEP valve should be used when suctioning the patient. Disconnecting the endotracheal tube will result in a loss of PEEP, a rapid reduction in the FRC, and alveolar flooding.

Detrimental Effects of PEEP

- Reduced venous return and cardiac output
- Reduction in hepatic and renal blood flow
- Barotrauma
- Increased intra-abdominal pressure
- Fluid retention
- Increased inspiratory workload
- Increased extravascular lung water
- Alveolar overdistension
- Ileus
- RV dysfunction

Auto-PEEP

As with spontaneous ventilation, exhalation during mechanical ventilation is a passive event and continues until the FRC is achieved. In patients with airflow limitation (asthma and chronic obstructive pulmonary disease) and in patients ventilated with reversed inspiratory/expiratory ($I:E$) ratios, a positive-pressure breath may be initiated before exhalation is complete. This process leads to air trapping and intrinsic PEEP or auto-PEEP (see Figure 14-11). Auto-PEEP is common in mechanically ventilated patients. Auto-PEEP increases intrathoracic pressure, thereby exacerbating the effects of positive-pressure ventilation. In patients with severe airflow limitation, severe auto-PEEP may develop. Patients may present with hemodynamic collapse similar to that of a tension pneumothorax. Auto-PEEP is treated by disconnecting the patient from the ventilator to "vent" the trapped air and then changing the I:E ratio, allowing more time for exhalation. The presence of auto-PEEP cannot be detected unless the exhalation port venting to the atmosphere is occluded at end expiration (using a one-way valve). Some ventilators have an expiratory hold valve, enabling the auto-PEEP to be measured directly.

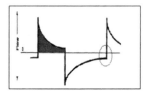 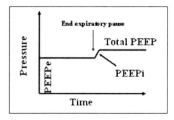

Figure 14-11. Auto-PEEP.

■ MONITORING VENTILATED PATIENTS

- All patients receiving mechanical ventilation should be monitored by pulse oximetry.
- Arterial blood gas analysis should be performed during the initial ventilator adjustments and then when clinically indicated. The arterial saturation as measured by pulse oximetry provides adequate information for managing most ventilated patients. Patients with CO_2 retention and patients with complex metabolic derangements generally require regular arterial blood gases. It is not necessary to perform an arterial blood gas analysis after every ventilator change.
- All the ventilator parameters, including peak airway and plateau pressures, should be recorded hourly on the patient's flowchart.
- The following formulas are useful in evaluating patients in respiratory failure:

- Age-predicted PaO_2 = expected PaO_2 – 0.3 (age 25) [expected PaO_2 at sea level is 100 mg/Hg].
- As a rough rule of thumb, expected $PaO_2 \approx FiO_2$ (%) × 5.
- $AaDO_2$ = (FiO_2 × [BP–47]) – (PaO_2 + $PaCO_2$), where BP = barometric pressure.
- The PaO_2/FiO_2 ratio is a better indicator of the degree of intrapulmonary shunting than is the $AaDO_2$.
- V_d/V_t = ($PaCO_2–PECO_2$)/$PaCO_2$ (N = 0.2–0.4).

Sudden Increase in Airway Pressure and/or Fall in Arterial Saturation

Causes

- Blocked endotracheal tube
- Herniated endotracheal tube cuff
- Tension pneumothorax
- Kinked endotracheal tube
- Tube migration (right mainstem bronchus)
- Mucous plug with lobar atelectasis
- Patient biting down on tube
- Patient ventilator synchrony

Management

- Bag the patient with 100% oxygen.
- Check position of endotracheal tube.
- Suction through the endotracheal tube; if unable to pass catheter, then reintubate.
- Listen for tension pneumothorax; place chest drain if silent and deviated trachea.
- Urgent chest X-ray.

■ TRACHEOSTOMY IN THE CRITICALLY ILL

The decision to perform a tracheostomy in critically patients should be adapted to each patient and his/her pathology – balancing the patient's wishes, expected recovery course, risk of continued translaryngeal intubation, and surgical risks of the procedure. Medical indications for tracheostomy include the following:

- Failure of extubation
- Upper airway obstruction

- Airway protection
- Airway access for secretion removal
- Avoidance of serious oropharyngeal and laryngeal injury from prolonged translaryngeal intubation

ACCP guidelines suggest that tracheostomy should be considered after an initial period of stabilization on the ventilator (generally, within 3–7 days) when it becomes apparent that the patient will require prolonged ventilator assistance.[16]

Proposed beneficial effects of tracheostomy include the following:

- Improved patient comfort through allowance of speech, oral nutrition, and easier nursing care.
- The need for less sedation and analgesia requirements.
- Reduced airway resistance is thought to facilitate the weaning process.
- Ventilator-associated pneumonia may also be reduced by substituting a tracheostomy for translaryngeal intubation.

Timing of Tracheostomy in the Critically Ill

Optimal timing for tracheostomy (early vs. late) remains a subject of debate and continued investigation. Furthermore, there is no consensus in the literature about the definition of what constitutes "early" tracheostomy.

Rumbak et al.[17] studied 120 patients in a prospective, randomized trial comparing early (within 48 h) vs. delayed tracheostomy (14–16 days). These authors demonstrated a significantly decreased time on mechanical ventilation (7.6 ± 4.0 vs. 17.4 ± 5.3 days) and a 50% reduction in mortality rate after early tracheostomy compared with delayed tracheostomy (19% vs. 37%). More patients died of ventilator-associated pneumonia in the delayed tracheostomy group than in the early tracheostomy group (nine vs. two). This confirms the findings of Kollef et al.[18] with mortality rates of 13.7% vs. 26.4%. Flaatten et al.[19] showed a decreased median number of days on the ventilator after early tracheostomy (4.7 vs. 14.7 days) in their retrospective analysis of 461 patients receiving tracheostomy during their ICU stay. The overall ICU, hospital, and 1-year survival rates were lower in patients receiving early tracheostomy compared with patients receiving mechanical ventilation for more than 24 h without a tracheostomy. Barquist et al.,[20] however, randomized 60 trauma patients to tracheostomy placement before day 8 or after day 28. There was no significant difference between groups in any outcome variable including length of ventilator support, pneumonia rate, or death.

Despite inconclusive data, "early" (2–5 days) tracheostomy in patients likely to require long-term ventilation (>14 days) is associated with better outcomes.

■ CLINICAL PEARLS

- Monitor tidal volume and plateau pressures in all patients undergoing mechanical ventilation.
- PEEP is required to improve oxygenation in patients with a large shunt.
- Patients tolerate permissive ventilation (pH >7.2) with "low" saturations (85–90%) just fine; do not kill them with the ventilator.
- Consider an "early" tracheostomy.

■ REFERENCES

1. Ventilation with lower tidal volumes as compared with traditional tidal volumes for acute lung injury and the acute respiratory distress syndrome. *N Engl J Med*. 2000;342:1301–1308.
2. Girard TD, Bernard GR. Mechanical ventilation in ARDS: a state-of-the-art review. *Chest*. 2007;131:921–929.
3. Wheeler AP, Bernard GR. Acute lung injury and the acute respiratory distress syndrome: a clinical review. *Lancet*. 2007;369:1553–1565.
4. Malhotra A. Low-tidal-volume ventilation in the acute respiratory distress syndrome. *N Engl J Med*. 2007;357:1113–1120.
5. Gajic O, Dara SI, Mendez JL, et al. Ventilator-associated lung injury in patients without acute lung injury at the onset of mechanical ventilation. *Crit Care Med*. 2004;32:1817–1824.
6. Gajic O, Frutos-Vivar F, Esteban A, et al. Ventilator settings as a risk factor for acute respiratory distress syndrome in mechanically ventilated patients. *Intensive Care Med*. 2005;31:922–926.
7. Lee PC, Helsmoortel CM, Cohn SM, et al. Are low tidal volumes safe? *Chest*. 1990;97:430–434.
8. Myers TR, MacIntyre N. Does airway pressure release ventilation offer important new advantages in mechanical ventilator support? *Resp Care*. 2007;52:452–458.
9. Hemmila MR, Napolitano LM. Severe respiratory failure: advanced treatment options. *Crit Care Med*. 2006;34:S278–S290.
10. Rose L, Hawkins M. Airway pressure release ventilation and biphasic positive airway pressure: a systematic review of definitional criteria. *Intensive Care Med*. 2008;34:1766–1773.

11. Neumann P, Golisch W, Strohmeyer A, et al. Influence of different release times on spontaneous breathing pattern during airway pressure release ventilation. *Intensive Care Med*. 2002;28:1742–1749.
12. Hirani A, Cavallazzi R, Shnister A, et al. Airway pressure release ventilation (APRV) for treatment of severe life-threatening ARDS in a morbidly obese patient. *Crit Care Shock*. 2008;11:132–136.
13. Gilbert C, Marik PE, Varon J. Acute lobar atelectasis during mechanical ventilation: to beat, suck or blow? *Crit Care Shock*. 2009;12:67–70.
14. Hirani A, Plante LA, Marik PE. Airway pressure release ventilation in pregnant patients with ARDS: a novel strategy. *Resp Care*. 2009; 54:1405–1408.
15. Manzano F, Fernandez-Mondejar E, Colmenero M, et al. Positive-end expiratory pressure reduces incidence of ventilator-associated pneumonia in nonhypoxemic patients. *Crit Care Med*. 2008;36:2225–2231.
16. MacIntyre NR, Cook DJ, Ely EW Jr., et al. Evidence-based guidelines for weaning and discontinuing ventilatory support: a collective task force facilitated by the American College of Chest Physicians; the American Association for Respiratory Care; and the American College of Critical Care Medicine. *Chest*. 2001;120:375S–395S.
17. Rumbak MJ, Newton M, Truncale T, et al. A prospective, randomized, study comparing early percutaneous dilational tracheotomy to prolonged translaryngeal intubation (delayed tracheotomy) in critically ill medical patients. *Crit Care Med*. 2004;32:1689–1694.
18. Kollef MH, Ahrens TS, Shannon W. Clinical predictors and outcomes for patients requiring tracheostomy in the intensive care unit. *Crit Care Med*. 1999;27:1714–1720.
19. Flaatten H, Gjerde S, Heimdal JH, et al. The effect of tracheostomy on outcome in intensive care unit patients. *Acta Anaesthesiol Scand*. 2006;50:92–98.
20. Barquist ES, Amortegui J, Hallal A, et al. Tracheostomy in ventilator dependent trauma patients: a prospective, randomized intention-to-treat study. *J Trauma*. 2006;60:91–97.

15

Non-invasive Positive-Pressure Ventilation

NIPPV can be delivered nasally or by face mask, using either a conventional mechanical ventilator or a machine designed specifically for this purpose. NIPPV has two major modes of supplying ventilatory support, namely continuous positive airway pressure (CPAP) and bilevel positive airway pressure (BiPAP). CPAP provides continuous positive pressure throughout the respiratory cycle. CPAP recruits underventilated alveoli by increasing lung volume at the end of expiration, resulting in improved gas exchange. CPAP is also effective in decreasing the work of breathing compared with unsupported ventilation.[1]

NIPPV is usually delivered either by portable positive-pressure BiPAP ventilators or critical care ventilators designed to deliver invasive mechanical ventilation. No study has shown better NIPPV success rates for one type of ventilator than the other, but the ventilator mode used and specific settings are important for patient comfort and decreased work of breathing. Generally, pressure-support ventilation is rated as more tolerable by patients than are assist-control modes when using a conventional ventilator.[2]

BiPAP ventilators provide high-flow positive airway pressure that cycles between high-positive pressure and low-positive pressure. In the spontaneous mode, BiPAP responds to the patient's own flow rate and cycles between high-pressure inspiration and low-pressure exhalation. BiPAP reliably senses the patient's breathing efforts and even air leaks that occur within the unit. When inspiration is detected, the inspiratory pressure is known as inspiratory positive airway pressure (IPAP). During this cycle, higher pressures are delivered for a fixed time or until the

P.E. Marik, *Handbook of Evidence-Based Critical Care*, 175
DOI 10.1007/978-1-4419-5923-2_15,
© Springer Science+Business Media, LLC 2010

gas flow rate falls below a threshold level, usually 25% of the expiratory volume. At this point in time, the expiratory positive airway pressure (EPAP) cycle begins delivering a lower positive pressure that splints and maintains a fixed alveolar pressure. BiPAP is similar to pressure-support ventilation. The terminology differs, however; for BiPAP, the expiratory pressure is equivalent to the sum of the positive end-expiratory pressure and the inspiratory pressure. Thus, a BiPAP setting of 12 cm of inspiratory pressure and 5 cm of expiratory pressures is equivalent to a standard ventilator setting of 7 cm for pressure support and 5 cm for positive end-expiratory pressure (PEEP).

The advantages of NIPPV include improved patient comfort, reduced need for sedation, avoidance of the complications of endotracheal intubation, including upper airway trauma, sinusitis, and nosocomial pneumonia. Furthermore, airway defense mechanisms, and speech and swallowing are left intact, and the patient remains alert and communicative. NIPPV has been used successfully to treat acute respiratory failure in postoperative patients and in those with pulmonary edema, chronic obstructive pulmonary disease, and obstructive sleep apnea. NIPPV has also been used to facilitate weaning. However, NIPPV appears to be particularly effective in patients with an exacerbation of COPD who are alert and cooperative.

The most common complication with the use of NIPPV is facial trauma related to the use of tight-fitting masks. The problem of skin necrosis, particularly over the bridge of the nose, makes it difficult for patients to be ventilated continuously for more than 1–2 days. Retention of secretions and gastric distension may be problematic in some patients.

■ SETUP

NIPPV works best in patients relaxed and prepared. The first few seconds should be used to fit the mask and familiarize the patient with equipment. Patients may feel claustrophobic, especially when increasing respiratory drive and when difficult breathing is present. NIPPV is tolerated best when pressures are increased gradually as the work of breathing and respiratory drive eases.

■ INITIAL SETTINGS

- Spontaneous trigger mode with backup rate.
- Start with low pressures:
  - IPAP 8–12 cm H_2O .
  - PEEP 3–5 cm H_2O.

- Adjust inspired O_2 to keep saturated O_2 >90%.
- Increase IPAP gradually up to 20 cm H_2O (as tolerated) to
  - alleviate dyspnea,
  - decrease respiratory rate,
  - increase tidal volume,
  - establish patient–ventilator synchrony.

■ INDICATIONS FOR NIPPV

Many applications of NIPPV have been tried in the critical care setting, but as of yet, only five are supported by multiple randomized controlled trials and meta-analyses (see below).[3] In addition to these indications, NIPPV can be useful in selected patients with asthma (see Chapter 23) and in extubation failure (see Chapter 16).

COPD Exacerbations

The strongest level of evidence supports the use of NIPPV to treat exacerbations of COPD. NIPPV results in more rapid improvements in vital signs and gas exchange, reduction in the need for intubation, decreased mortality, and decreased hospital length of stay.[4,5] Based on these findings, NIPPV should now be considered the ventilatory modality of first choice to treat acute respiratory failure caused by exacerbations of COPD.

Acute Cardiogenic Pulmonary Edema

Strong evidence supports the use of NIPPV to treat acute cardiogenic pulmonary edema. Both CPAP and BiPAP lower intubation and mortality rates compared to conventional therapy with oxygen. CPAP should be considered as the first-line intervention as it is as efficacious as BiPAP and CPAP is cheaper and easier to implement in clinical practice.[6,7]

Facilitating Extubation in COPD Patients

NIPPV has been successfully used to facilitate extubation in patients with hypercapnic respiratory failure and to avoid the complications of prolonged intubation (see Chapter 22).

Immunocompromised Patients

NIPPV has traditionally not been considered in the management strategy of patients with malignancy; however, this mode of ventilatory support may be appropriate in three specific situations[8]:

- For avoiding endotracheal intubation in patients with hematologic malignancy or following bone marrow transplant
- In patients with malignancy who have refused invasive mechanical ventilation (DNI) but who still desire aggressive treatment
- For the relief of disabling dyspnea

In neutropenic patients, mechanical ventilation is associated with significant mortality and morbidity, with in-hospital mortality rates as high as 90–97%.[9,10] Ewig and colleagues[9] demonstrated that endotracheal intubation and mechanical ventilation increase the risk of death by 43-fold in patients with hematologic malignancy. Consequently, any less invasive method of ventilatory support which is able to avoid the use of endotracheal ventilation would appear to be particularly useful in these high-risk patients. Hilbert and colleagues[11] randomized 52 immunosuppressed patients with early hypoxic acute respiratory failure to NIPPV or standard treatment with supplemental oxygen and no ventilatory support. In this study, fewer patients in the NIPPV group required endotracheal intubation (46% vs. 77%), had serious complications (50% vs. 81%), or died in hospital (50% vs. 81%). NIPPV should be considered in the management strategy in immunocompromised patients who develop respiratory failure.[8] However, careful patient selection is crucial and early identification of patients likely improves outcome.

Postoperative Patients

Due to pain, poor cough, delayed ambulation, and underlying comorbidities, postoperative pulmonary complications have been reported in up to 50% of patients undergoing abdominal surgery. A meta-analysis by Ferreyra and colleagues[12] demonstrated that CPAP used prophylactically reduced the risk of postoperative respiratory complications in patients undergoing abdominal surgery. Similarly, Squadrone and colleagues[13] demonstrated that CPAP reduced the incidence of endotracheal intubation and other severe complications in patients who developed hypoxemia after elective major abdominal surgery.

■ WHEN TO USE NIPPV

Hypercapnic Respiratory Failure

- Severe dyspnea at rest
- Respiratory rate >25 breaths/min
- Use of accessory muscle of respiration
- Acute respiratory acidosis (pH <7.30)
- An alert and cooperative patient

Hypoxemic Respiratory Failure

- Respiratory rate >30 breaths/min
- PaO_2/FiO_2 <200 mmHg
- Increased use of accessory muscle or $PaCO_2$ retention
- Alert and cooperative patient

Contraindications to NIPPV

- Hemodynamic or electrocardiographic instability
- Patient at risk for aspiration
- Inability to clear copious secretions
- Cardiac or respiratory arrest
- Non-respiratory organ failure
- Severe encephalopathy (e.g., GCS <10)
- Severe upper gastrointestinal bleeding
- Facial surgery, trauma, or deformity
- Upper airway obstruction
- Inability to cooperate/protect the airway
- Inability to clear respiratory secretions
- Obtunded or uncooperative patient

Success and Failure Criteria for NIPPV

- Improvements in pH and PCO_2 occurring within 2 h predict the eventual success of NIPPV.
- If stabilization or improvement has not been achieved during this time period, the patient should be considered an NIPPV failure and intubation must be strongly considered.
- Other criteria for a failed NIPPV trial include the following:
  - Worsened encephalopathy or agitation.
  - Inability to clear secretions.
  - Inability to tolerate any available mask.
  - Hemodynamic instability.
  - Worsened oxygenation.

■ CLINICAL PEARLS

- BiPAP is considered the treatment of choice for COPD.
- CPAP is considered the treatment of choice for cardiogenic pulmonary edema.
- NIPPV is best applied to alert cooperative patients.

■ REFERENCES

1. Katz JA, Marks JD. Inspiratory work with and without continuous positive airway pressure in patients with acute respiratory failure. *Anesthesiology.* 1985;63:598–607.
2. Vitacca M, Rubini F, Foglio K, et al. Non-invasive modalities of positive pressure ventilation improve the outcome of acute exacerbations in COLD patients. *Intensive Care Med.* 1993;19:450–455.
3. Garpestad E, Brennan J, Hill NS. Noninvasive ventilation for critical care. *Chest.* 2007;132:711–720.
4. Keenan SP, Sinuff T, Cook DJ, et al. Which patients with acute exacerbation of chronic obstructive pulmonary disease benefit from noninvasive positive-pressure ventilation? A systematic review of the literature. *Ann Intern Med.* 2003;138:861–870.
5. Ram FS, Picot J, Lightowler J, et al. Non-invasive positive pressure ventilation for treatment of respiratory failure due to exacerbations of chronic obstructive pulmonary disease. *Cochrane Database Syst Rev.* 2004;3:CD004104.
6. Winck JC, Azevedo LF, Costa-Pereira A, et al. Efficacy and safety of non-invasive ventilation in the treatment of acute cardiogenic pulmonary edema – a systematic review and meta-analysis. *Crit Care.* 2006;10:R69.
7. Ho KM, Wong K. A comparison of continuous and bi-level positive airway pressure non-invasive ventilation in patients with acute cardiogenic pulmonary oedema: a meta-analysis. *Crit Care.* 2006;10:R49.
8. Marik PE. Non-invasive positive-pressure ventilation in patients with malignancy. *Am J Hosp Palliat Care.* 2007;24:417–421.
9. Ewig S, Torres A, Riquelme R, et al. Pulmonary complications in patients with haematological malignancies treated at a respiratory ICU. *Eur Respir J.* 1998;12:116–122.
10. Paz HL, Crilley P, Weinar M, et al. Outcome of patients requiring medical ICU admission following bone marrow transplantation. *Chest.* 1993;104:527–531.
11. Hilbert G, Gruson D, Vargas F, et al. Noninvasive ventilation in immunosuppressed patients with pulmonary infiltrates, fever, and acute respiratory failure. *N Engl J Med.* 2001;344:481–487.

12. Ferreyra GP, Baussano I, Squadrone V, et al. Continuous positive airway pressure for treatment of respiratory complications after abdominal surgery: a systematic review and meta-analysis. *Ann Surg.* 2008;247:617–626.
13. Squadrone V, Coha M, Cerutti E, et al. Continuous positive airway pressure for treatment of postoperative hypoxemia: a randomized controlled trial. *JAMA.* 2005;293:589–595.

16

Weaning (Liberation)

■ GENERAL CONCEPTS

Weaning is the process by which a patient is removed from the ventilator. This process has also been referred to as separation, liberation, and withdrawal from the ventilator, as well as discontinuation of mechanical ventilation. The currently popular term is liberation from mechanical ventilation.

Early weaning studies suggested that physicians did not initiate weaning early enough and this increased time spent on the ventilator as well as ICU length of stay. Furthermore, the weaning process was extended over many days by gradually reducing the rate (on IMV) or the degree of ventilator support (PS).[1] This concept of weaning was replaced by the concept of "liberation" whereby the patient was either ready (and hence *readiness testing* was done) or not ready for extubation and the "classic weaning" method slowed the process and may have further compromised respiratory muscle fatigue. Furthermore, a number of respiratory therapy/nurse-driven "weaning protocols" which screen patients daily for "readiness to wean" who then undergo a spontaneous breathing trial (SBT) followed by a decision to extubate have been demonstrated to significantly reduce the weaning time.[2–5] Daily readiness screening is coupled with "sedation vacations" to expedite the process.[6] This is now the preferred method of weaning.

The factors that need to be evaluated when considering weaning a patient from mechanical ventilation include the patient's underlying disease process, the reasons for intubation and mechanical ventilation in the first instance, the patient's level of consciousness, the ability to protect his/her airway, pulmonary mechanics, and oxygenation defect. In many patients, ventilatory assistance need not be decreased gradually; mechanical ventilation and artificial airways can simply be removed (liberated).

P.E. Marik, *Handbook of Evidence-Based Critical Care*,
DOI 10.1007/978-1-4419-5923-2_16,
© Springer Science+Business Media, LLC 2010

According to this thesis, patients can simply be removed from the ventilator once the disease process that led to intubation and mechanical ventilation has improved or resolved; a prolonged weaning process is therefore not required. Treatment of reversible factors and "medical optimization" should be performed in those patients who fail an SBT (see below). A daily SBT should be performed until the patient is ready for extubation. The practice of respiratory muscle training with a gradual reduction of ventilatory support has fallen out of favor. A randomized trial showed no benefit to inspiratory muscle training.[7]

Effect of Weaning on Oxygen Consumption and Cardiac Function

It has been demonstrated that oxygen consumption increases by about 15% when critically ill patients are switched from assist-control mechanical ventilation to spontaneous breathing (continuous positive airway pressure). The increased oxygen consumption is likely due to the increased mechanical load and the inefficiency of the respiratory muscles. This increased oxygen consumption must be met by an increased oxygen delivery. In patients who are unable to increase oxygen delivery, this may result in tissue hypoxia in vital organs due to a redistribution of blood flow. Mohsenifar and colleagues[8] demonstrated the development of gastric intramucosal acidosis in patients who failed to be weaned from mechanical ventilation.

Positive-pressure ventilation (PPV) decreases left ventricular preload as well as left ventricular afterload. Therefore, PPV may improve left ventricular performance. Removing PPV results in both an increased cardiac demand and an increased workload on the heart. In patients with coronary artery disease (CAD), this may result in myocardial ischemia and pulmonary edema (which further increases pulmonary workload). Chatila et al.[9] detected electrocardiographic evidence of cardiac ischemia in 10% of patients with a history of CAD who were being weaned. Evidence of myocardial ischemia was associated with a failure to wean in 22% of these patients. Anti-anginal medication and diuretics may be useful in preventing both myocardial ischemia and cardiac failure when weaning patients with CAD from the ventilator.

■ THE WEANING PROCESS

Recognizing that respiratory failure and respiratory muscle function have improved and the patient is capable of spontaneous breathing is termed *readiness testing*. Most patients satisfying readiness criteria tolerate *spontaneous breathing* (with no or minimal ventilator support) indicating that mechanical ventilation is no longer necessary.

The weaning process is best classified as follows[10]:

- *Simple weaning*: Patient tolerates first spontaneous breathing trial (SBT) and is successfully extubated (70% of all patients).
- *Difficult weaning*: Patient fails to tolerate initial SBT; successful weaning requires up to three SBTs or up to 7 days from first SBT.
- *Prolonged weaning*: Patient fails at least three SBTs or takes more than 7 days after first SBT.

"Readiness" Testing

Over 50 physiological tests (weaning parameters) have been studied to assess the patients' readiness for spontaneous breathing. Of these tests, only five have been demonstrated to be able to predict weaning success or failure; however, the predictive capacity was only modest: These include (readiness criteria) the following:

- Negative inspiratory force.
- Minute ventilation.
- Respiratory frequency.
- Tidal volume.
- Frequency–tidal volume ratio (Tobin index). Of these the Tobin index has proven to be the most accurate.

Once a patient meets the following criteria (liberal readiness criteria)

- Underlying disease has improved
- Patient off sedative agents
- Hemodynamically stable
- Awake and responsive
- SaO_2 >88% on $FiO_2 \leq 50\%$
- PEEP <8 cm H_2O

the patient is placed on unassisted breathing and the "readiness parameters" measured (usually Tobin index and minute ventilation). If the Tobin index <105 breaths/min and the MV <10 l/min, the patient is considered ready for a spontaneous breathing trial (SBT). A 30–120-min SBT is then performed. Patients who "pass" the SBT are then extubated.

Tanios and colleagues[11] randomized 304 ventilated patients to a daily readiness screen (PaO_2/FiO_2, PEEP, hemodynamic stability, mental status, cough) that included or excluded the Tobin index. The group randomized to use the Tobin index took longer to wean. The results of this study are supported by the ABC trial in which greater than 50% passed an

SBT when readiness was assessed using the "liberal criteria" and weaning predictors were not used.[6] Recent consensus guidelines do not recommend the routine application of weaning predictors for weaning decision making.[10,12] Rather patients are considered for an SBT when there is evidence of clinical improvement, oxygenation is adequate, hemodynamics are stable, and spontaneous breathing efforts are present (i.e., liberal criteria).

Spontaneous Breathing Trials

Direct extubation after satisfying readiness criteria alone is unwise, as 40% of such patients require reintubation.[13] Therefore, a trial of spontaneous breathing carried out on low-level pressure support (PSV 5–10 cm H_2O), CPAP, or unassisted through a T-piece is indicated. RCTs indicate that these techniques are equivalent.[14,15]

Theoretically, PSV more effectively counterbalances endotracheal tube-related resistive workload, but a given level may either overcompensate or undercompensate for imposed work.[16,17] This limitation might be overcome by using automatic tube compensation (ATC), a technique that continuously adjusts PSV on the basis of tube characteristics.[18] In a non-randomized study of patient failing a 30-min T-tube trial, immediate conversion to PSV 7 cm H_2O for additional 30 min led to weaning success in 21 of 31 patients, suggesting that the endotracheal tube can contribute to iatrogenic weaning failure.[19] For this reason as well as its simplicity, we prefer PSV over a T-tube trial. Optimal SBT duration has been examined in two studies suggesting that 30 min is equivalent to 120 min.[20,21] The SBT is usually terminated if the patient meets any of the following criteria:

- Respiratory rate >35 breaths/min
- Arterial saturation <90%
- Heart rate >140 beats or heart rate change (either direction) >20% or arrhythmias
- Systolic blood pressure >180 or <90 mmHg
- Increased anxiety and diaphoresis

Should the patient "pass" the SBT, he/she should be placed on increased ventilator support (PSV of 10–12 cm H_2O) to prevent excessive fatigue. If the patient is at risk for postextubation stridor, a cuff leak test should be performed (see below). Tube feeds should be stopped and a D5 1/2 NS infusion started (to prevent hypoglycemia). The stomach should be emptied and the OG/NG tube removed to reduce the risk of aspiration. Once these preparations have been performed, the patient can be extubated to a face mask or nasal cannulae.

Causes of Weaning Failure

- Critical illness polyneuropathy (see Chapter 7). This is one of the most common causes of failure to wean. An EMG should be performed.
- Adrenal insufficiency.[22] An ACTH test should be performed.
- Electrolyte disturbances:
  - Hypophosphatemia.
  - Hypokalemia.
  - Hypomagnesemia.
  - Hypocalcemia (ionized).
- Malnutrition.
- Myocardial ischemia.
- Cardiac failure.[23] Check BNP after trial[24] and ECHO.
- Volume overload/positive fluid balance[25].

Early Extubation Followed by NIPPV in COPD

Nava and colleagues[26] reported a novel method of weaning COPD patients who required mechanical ventilation for respiratory failure. These authors provided intensive medical management for 48 h, followed by extubation at 48 h, regardless of the patient's respiratory parameters. These early extubated patients were then treated with non-invasive positive-pressure ventilation (NIPPV) until their respiratory function returned to baseline. The authors reported a high success rate with a shortened length of ICU stay, lower mortality, and decreased complication rate using this approach.

NIPPV for Persistent Weaning Failure

Two RCT have explored the use of NIPPV in patients having difficulty in weaning from mechanical ventilation.[27,28] The most recent study randomized 43 patients who had failed three SBTs, 77% of whom had chronic lung disease.[27] This study was stopped at an interim analysis finding that NIPPV was associated with shorter duration of mechanical ventilation, shorter ICU and hospital stay, fewer tracheotomies, higher ICU survival, and a lower incidence of nosocomial pneumonia and septic shock. These studies indicate that NIPPV can facilitate weaning in a highly selected group of patients with acute-on-chronic lung disease. Important caveats include the following: SBT readiness criteria must be satisfied, extubation criteria must be satisfied, and the candidate must be a good candidate for NIPPV and not be a difficult candidate for reintubation.

Extubation Failure

Despite advances is predicting extubation failure, between 25 and 40% of patients develop signs of respiratory distress after extubation. Extubation failure, when defined as reintubation within the subsequent 24–72 h, occurs in 5–20% of patients, depending on the patient population. Extubation failure often results from the inability to protect the airway and manage secretions as well as from postextubation stridor. Salam et al.[29] demonstrated that cough strength, volume of respiratory secretions, and mental status were major determinants of reintubation.

Randomized trials in heterogeneous populations (few with COPD) with overt or early signs of extubation failure found that NIPPV does not reduce the need for reintubation or improve survival.[30,31] However, two recent RCTs suggest that the immediate postextubation application of NIPPV in patients at highest risk for extubation failure is effective in preventing reintubation and may reduce mortality.[32,33]

Patients at High Risk for Extubation Failure

- Chronic heart failure
- Age >65 years
- More than one failed weaning trial
- More than one comorbidity
- $PaCO_2$ >45 mmHg after extubation
- Weak cough
- Voluminous secretions

■ THE CUFF LEAK TEST

The cuff leak test is performed in patients suspected of having laryngeal edema. The cuff of the endotracheal tube is deflated; if there is no laryngeal edema, the patient should be able to breathe around the tube. A patient with a positive cuff leak test (i.e., no leak) has approximately a 30% chance of developing postextubation stridor; however, the risk is negligible in patients with a negative cuff leak test.[34] The degree of leak can be quantified by comparing the returned tidal volume before and after the cuff is deflated. A cuff leak of less than 110 ml or <24% has been shown to be associated with an increased risk of postextubation stridor.[35,36]

The cuff leak test should be performed before extubation in the following circumstances:

- Traumatic intubation
- Prolonged intubation, i.e., longer than 7 days
- Patients with head and neck trauma

- Head and neck surgery
- Patients with previous failed extubation accompanied by stridor
- Patients with airway edema (e.g., angioedema)

Corticosteroids for the Prevention of Postextubation Stridor

RCTs have demonstrated that systemic corticosteroids reduce the risk of postextubation stridor.[37] Cheng et al. randomized 128 high-risk patients with a cuff leak volume <24% to placebo or methylprednisolone injection (multi-dose or single dose) during the 24 h prior to extubation. Treatment with methylprednisolone significantly reduced the risk of postextubation stridor and the need for reintubation.[36] Lee et al. demonstrated similar findings using a cuff leak volume of <110 ml.[38]

■ CLINICAL PEARLS

- All ventilated patients should have a daily "sedation vacation" as well as a "readiness" assessment.
- Those patients deemed "ready" for weaning should undergo a 30 min spontaneous breathing trial.
- The cuff leak should be determined prior to extubation; those with a low leak volume should be treated with at least one dose of 40 mg methylprednisolone prior to extubation.
- NIPPV can be used as a weaning adjunct in patients with acute-on-chronic respiratory failure.

■ REFERENCES

1. Brochard L, Rauss A, Benito S, et al. Comparison of three methods of gradual withdrawal from ventilatory support during weaning from mechanical ventilation. *Am J Respir Crit Care Med.* 1994;150:896–903.
2. Arias-Rivera S, Sanchez-Sanchez MM, Santos-Diaz R, et al. Effect of a nursing-implemented sedation protocol on weaning outcome. *Crit Care Med.* 2008;36:2054–2060.
3. Dries DJ, McGonigal MD, Malian MS, et al. Protocol-driven ventilator weaning reduces use of mechanical ventilation, rate of early reintubation, and ventilator-associated pneumonia. *J Trauma.* 2004;56:943–951.
4. Ely EW, Bennett PA, Bowton DL, et al. Large scale implementation of a respiratory therapist-driven protocol for ventilator weaning. *Am J Respir Crit Care Med.* 1999;159:439–446.

5. Ely EW, Meade MO, Haponik EF, et al. Mechanical ventilator weaning protocols driven by nonphysician health-care professionals: evidence-based clinical practice guidelines. *Chest*. 2001;120: 454S–463S.
6. Girard TD, Kress JP, Fuchs BD, et al. Efficacy and safety of a paired sedation and ventilator weaning protocol for mechanically ventilated patients in intensive care (Awakening and Breathing Controlled trial): a randomised controlled trial. *Lancet*. 2008;371:126–134.
7. Caruso P, Denari SD, Ruiz SA, et al. Inspiratory muscle training is ineffective in mechanically ventilated critically ill patients. *Clinics*. 2005;60:479–484.
8. Mohsenifar Z, Hay A, Hay J, et al. Gastric intramural pH as a predictor of success or failure in weaning patients from mechanical ventilation. *Ann Intern Med*. 1993;119:794–798.
9. Chatila W, Ani S, Guaglianone D, et al. Cardiac ischemia during weaning from mechanical ventilation. *Chest*. 1996;109:1577–1583.
10. Boles JM, Bion J, Connors A, et al. Weaning from mechanical ventilation. *Eur Respir J*. 2007;29:1033–1056.
11. Tanios MA, Nevins ML, Hendra KP, et al. A randomized, controlled trial of the role of weaning predictors in clinical decision making. *Crit Care Med*. 2006;34:2530–2535.
12. MacIntyre NR, Cook DJ, Ely EW Jr., et al. Evidence-based guidelines for weaning and discontinuing ventilatory support: a collective task force facilitated by the American College of Chest Physicians; the American Association for Respiratory Care; and the American College of Critical Care Medicine. *Chest*. 2001;120:375S–395S.
13. Zeggwagh AA, Abouqal R, Madani N, et al. Weaning from mechanical ventilation: a model for extubation. *Intensive Care Med*. 1999;25: 1077–1083.
14. Esteban A, Alia I, Gordo F, et al. Extubation outcome after spontaneous breathing trials with T-tube or pressure support ventilation. The Spanish Lung Failure Collaborative Group. *Am J Respir Crit Care Med*. 1997;156:459–465.
15. Jones DP, Byrne P, Morgan C, et al. Positive end-expiratory pressure vs T-piece. Extubation after mechanical ventilation. *Chest*. 1991;100: 1655–1659.
16. Brochard L, Rua F, Lorino H, et al. Inspiratory pressure support compensates for the additional work of breathing caused by the endotracheal tube. *Anesthesiology*. 1991;75:739–745.
17. Brochard L, Harf A, Lorino H, et al. Inspiratory pressure support prevents diaphragmatic fatigue during weaning from mechanical ventilation. *Am Rev Respir Dis*. 1989;139:513–521.
18. Cohen JD, Shapiro M, Grozovski E, et al. Extubation outcome following a spontaneous breathing trial with automatic tube compensation versus continuous positive airway pressure. *Crit Care Med*. 2006;34:682–686.

19. Ezingeard E, Diconne E, Guyomarc'h S, et al. Weaning from mechanical ventilation with pressure support in patients failing a T-tube trial of spontaneous breathing. *Intensive Care Med.* 2006;32:165–169.
20. Esteban A, Alia I, Tobin MJ, et al. Effect of spontaneous breathing trial duration on outcome of attempts to discontinue mechanical ventilation. Spanish Lung Failure Collaborative Group. *Am J Respir Crit Care Med.* 1999;159:512–518.
21. Perren A, Domenighetti G, Mauri S, et al. Protocol-directed weaning from mechanical ventilation: clinical outcome in patients randomized for a 30-min or 120-min trial with pressure support ventilation. *Intensive Care Med.* 2002;28:1058–1063.
22. Huang CJ, Lin HC. Association between adrenal insufficiency and ventilator weaning. *Am J Respir Crit Care Med.* 2006;173:276–280.
23. Richard C, Teboul JL. Weaning failure from cardiovascular origin. *Intensive Care Med.* 2005;31:1605–1607.
24. Grasso S, Leone A, De MM, et al. Use of N-terminal pro-brain natriuretic peptide to detect acute cardiac dysfunction during weaning failure in difficult-to-wean patients with chronic obstructive pulmonary disease.[see comment]. *Crit Care Med.* 2007;35:96–105.
25. Upadya A, Tilluckdharry L, Muralidaran V, et al. Fluid balance and weaning outcomes. *Intensive Care Med.* 2005;31:1642–1647.
26. Nava S, Ambrosino N, Clini E, et al. Noninvasive mechanical ventilation in the weaning of patients with respiratory failure due to chronic obstructive pulmonary disease. A randomized, controlled trial. *Ann Intern Med.* 1998;128:721–728.
27. Ferrer M, Esquinas A, Arancibia F, et al. Noninvasive ventilation during persistent weaning failure: a randomized controlled trial. *Am J Respir Crit Care Med.* 2003;168:70–76.
28. Girault C, Daudenthun I, Chevron V, et al. Noninvasive ventilation as a systematic extubation and weaning technique in acute-on-chronic respiratory failure: a prospective, randomized controlled study. *Am J Respir Crit Care Med.* 1999;160:86–92.
29. Salam A, Tilluckdharry L, Amoateng-Adjepong Y, et al. Neurologic status, cough, secretions and extubation outcomes. *Intensive Care Med.* 2004;30:1334–1339.
30. Esteban A, Frutos-Vivar F, Ferguson ND, et al. Noninvasive positive-pressure ventilation for respiratory failure after extubation. *N Engl J Med.* 2004;350:2452–2460.
31. Keenan SP, Powers C, McCormack DG, et al. Noninvasive positive-pressure ventilation for postextubation respiratory distress: a randomized controlled trial. *JAMA.* 2002;287:3238–3244.
32. Nava S, Gregoretti C, Fanfulla F, et al. Noninvasive ventilation to prevent respiratory failure after extubation in high-risk patients. *Crit Care Med.* 2005;33:2465–2470.

33. Ferrer M, Valencia M, Nicolas JM, et al. Early noninvasive ventilation averts extubation failure in patients at risk: a randomized trial. *Am J Respir Crit Care Med.* 2006;173:164–170.
34. Marik PE. The cuff-leak test as a predictor of postextubation stridor: a prospective study. *Resp Care.* 1996;41:509–511.
35. Miller RL, Cole RP. Association between reduced cuff leak volume and postextubation stridor. *Chest.* 1996;110:1035–1040.
36. Cheng KC, Hou CC, Huang HC, et al. Intravenous injection of methylprednisolone reduces the incidence of postextubation stridor in intensive care unit patients. *Crit Care Med.* 2006;34:1345–1350.
37. Francois B, Bellissant E, Gissot V, et al. 12-h pretreatment with methylprednisolone versus placebo for prevention of postextubation laryngeal oedema: a randomised double-blind trial. *Lancet.* 2007;369:1083–1089.
38. Lee CH, Peng MJ, Wu CL. Dexamethasone to prevent postextubation airway obstruction in adults: a prospective, randomized, double-blind, placebo-controlled study. *Crit Care.* 2007;11:R72.

17

Ventilator-Associated Pneumonia

Ventilator-associated pneumonia (VAP) is defined as a pneumonia which develops after 48 h of mechanical ventilation. VAP is the commonest nosocomial infection in the ICU and an important cause of morbidity. While the incidence varies according to the diagnostic criteria used and the patient population, it complicates the hospital course of about 20% of patients receiving mechanical ventilation or about five episodes per 1,000 ventilator days.[1] VAP increases the number of days requiring mechanical ventilation as well as ICU and hospital length of stay; however, it is unclear if VAP independently increases mortality.

In mechanically ventilated patients, colonization of the oropharynx with potentially pathogenic organisms (PPOs) occurs within 36 h of intubation with colonization of the endotracheal biofilm within 96 h.[2] Furthermore, endotracheal intubation compromises the patient's natural anatomic barriers (glottis, larynx, ciliated epithelium, and mucus). Subglottic pooling of colonized oropharyngeal secretions with subsequent leakage of secretions around the endotracheal cuff allows PPO to gain entry into the lower respiratory tract.[3] Patients are unable to cough and the mucociliary escalator is rendered ineffective by endotracheal intubation. Patients are therefore unable to clear these colonized secretion from the lower respiratory tract predisposing to both infection and atelectasis. The "aspiration" of colonized oropharyngeal secretions is therefore believed to be the major pathogenic mechanism causing VAP.[4] Using molecular biotyping, Bahrani-Mougeot and colleagues[5] demonstrated that 88% of patients with VAP had the same bacteria isolated from the lung (by bronchoalveolar lavage) as their oral cavity. Hematogenous spread from infected catheters or bacterial translocation from the gastrointestinal tract is considered a very rare cause of VAP.

P.E. Marik, *Handbook of Evidence-Based Critical Care*,
DOI 10.1007/978-1-4419-5923-2_17,
© Springer Science+Business Media, LLC 2010

The major risk factors for VAP include factors that increase oropharyngeal colonization, increase the risk or degree of aspiration as well as factors that impair local defense mechanisms. The major risk factors include the following:

- Supine positioning
- Previous antibiotics (esp. broad spectrum)
- Ventilation lasting greater than 7 days
- Reintubation
- Intrahospital patient transport
- Chronic obstructive pulmonary disease
- ARDS
- Thoracoabdominal surgery
- Trauma
- Burns
- Central nervous system disease

■ MICROBIOLOGY

The common pathogens causing VAP include the following:

- *Pseudomonas aeruginosa*
- Methicillin-resistant *Staphylococcus aureus* (MRSA)
- *Klebsiella pneumoniae*
- *Acinetobacter* species
- *Stenotrophomonas maltophilia*
- *Streptococcus pneumoniae* (early VAP)
- *Haemophilus influenzae* (early VAP).

Less common pathogens include the following:

- *Escherichia coli*
- *Enterobacter* spp.
- *Citrobacter* spp.
- *Serratia* spp.
- *Legionella* spp.

Colonization (often extensive) of the respiratory tract with *Candida* species is common in mechanically ventilated patients.[6] Invasive *Candida* pneumonia is extremely rare. Quantitative culture of BAL fluid has poor diagnostic value for *Candida* pneumonia. Respiratory tract colonization with *Candida* species has been reported to be an independent predictor of mortality; this is likely related to the fact that colonization is associated with severity of illness, the number of comorbidities, and prior use of broad-spectrum antibiotics rather than being a direct contributor to excess mortality.[7] At this time there is no data to suggest that coloniza-tion of the respiratory tract with *Candida* species or its presence in high concentration in quantitative culture requires treatment with anti-fungal agents. *Aspergillus fumigatus* may occur in organ transplant, immuno-compromised, and neutropenic patients; an environmental source such as contaminated air ducts or hospital construction should be suspected.

Polymicrobial infection is common. Importantly, the incidence of VAP caused by multi-drug-resistant (MDR) organisms is increasing.[8] VAP caused by MDR organism(s) is associated with increased mortality.[3,9,10] Risk factors for infection by MDR organisms include the following:

- Intubation for longer than 7 days
- Previous broad-spectrum antibiotics
- Hemodialysis
- Hospitalization for 2 days or more (in the last 90 days)
- Prior admission to the ICU
- Nursing home residence
- Immunosuppression
- Chronic wound care

Taking these factors into account, patients with suspected VAP should be divided into two groups, namely those at high and low risk of having an infection with multi-resistant pathogens.[11] This classification is more useful than the traditional distinction between early and late VAP.[12,13]

■ DIAGNOSIS OF VAP

The clinical criteria that have "traditionally" been used to diagnose VAP include the following:

- A new or progressive pulmonary infiltrate
- Fever
- Leukocytosis
- Tracheobronchial secretions

These clinical criteria are however non-specific and of little clinical utility in the diagnosis of VAP.[14,15] An autopsy investigation demon-strated that only 52% of patients with pneumonia at autopsy had a localized infiltrate on their chest radiograph and that 40% did not have a leukocytosis close to their death.[16] The clinical pulmonary infection score (CPIS) was developed as a "non-invasive" method to diagnose VAP and uses a combination of clinical features together with the culture of a tracheal aspirate to diagnose pneumonia.[17] The CPIS assigns 0–12 points based on six clinical criteria:

- Fever
- Leukocyte count
- Oxygenation
- Quantity and purulence of secretions
- Type of radiographic abnormality
- Results of sputum (tracheal aspirate) gram stain and culture

Both the original CPIS and the modified CPIS have, however, proven unreliable for the diagnosis of VAP, with a low sensitivity and specificity with considerable interobserver variability in the calculation of the score.[15,18–20] It should be emphasized that the upper respiratory tract of intubated patients are rapidly colonized with PPO and that gram stain and culture of tracheal aspirates are unable to distinguish between upper airway colonization and lower respiratory tract infection (pneumonia).

As the clinical criteria of VAP lack specificity, a number of diagnostic techniques have been reported which attempt to distinguish between patients with lung infection and those colonized with potentially pathogenic organisms or those with a tracheobronchitis. Lower respiratory tract sampling is based on the premise that

- the lower respiratory tract is normally sterile:
- there is a good correlation between the concentration of bacteria in the lung and the severity of the pulmonary inflammatory process, and
- bronchoalveolar lavage (BAL) quantitative culture closely correlates with the concentration of bacteria in the lung.[21]

Chastre and colleagues[22] documented the similarity between BAL quantitative cultures obtained from patients who were dying with VAP and quantitative cultures obtained soon after their death. Fagon and colleagues[23] compared a diagnostic approach based on lower respiratory tract sampling and quantitative culture with the "standard approach" using clinical criteria and tracheal aspirates. Compared with the noninvasive strategy, the invasive strategy was associated with fewer deaths at 14 days, earlier resolution of organ dysfunction, and less antibiotic use in patients suspected of having VAP. A meta-analysis of randomized controlled trial of invasive diagnostic strategies demonstrated that this technique led to a change in antibiotics in over 50% of patients.[24]

Several factors limit the routine use of bronchoscopy-directed BAL in the clinical setting; bronchoscopy is expensive, time consuming, and not readily available in many ICUs. A number of investigators have demonstrated a high concordance between the results of quantitative culture of BAL fluid performed by bronchoscopy and that performed "blindly" (m-BAL).[17,25] The advantages of m-BAL are that bronchoscopy is not required and that sampling can readily and safely be performed by trained respiratory care practitioners.[26,27]

The Canadian Critical Care Trials Group randomized patients with suspected VAP to undergo either BAL and quantitative culture or endotracheal aspiration with non-quantitative culture of the aspirate.[28,29] Patients were further randomized to therapy with meropenem or meropenem and ciprofloxacin. There was no difference in any of the outcome measures between the invasive and non-invasive groups nor between antibiotic treatment with combination or monotherapy. This study is often cited to support the use of a non-invasive approach to diagnose VAP as well as to support monotherapy in the treatment of suspected VAP.[30] It should, however, be noted that patients suspected of being infected with MRSA, *P. aeruginosa,* or other MDR organisms were excluded from this study. This is a critical issue in interpreting the results of this study as *S. aureus* and *P. aeruginosa* are the two most common pathogens causing VAP, and infection with an MDR organism is an independent predictor of mortality. Furthermore, all patients received a broad-spectrum carbapenem (meropenem) making it unlikely to detect any difference in outcome between any of the groups of patients infected with highly susceptible pathogens.

The major limitation of BAL with quantitative culture are false-negative results which have been reported to occur between 3 and 30%.[31-34] The incidence of false negatives is partly related to the diagnostic threshold used. The lower the diagnostic threshold, the lower the incidence of false-negative results; however, the specificity declines sharply as the threshold is decreased. The initial diagnostic threshold of 10^4 was based on postmortem histology and bronchoscopic BAL. This threshold has been used in most studies which have examined the utility of quantitative culture of BAL fluid.[23,25,35] More recent data in trauma patients suggest that a threshold of 10^5 has the best diagnostic performance.[32-34] Effective antibiotic therapy causes a rapid decline in the BAL bacterial load within 24 h. False-negative results are therefore more common in patients who have had a new antibiotic instituted within 72 h of sampling. To lower the risk of not treating patients with VAP (false negatives), we suggest a diagnostic threshold of 10^4.

The major limitations of BAL include the false-negative results and the delay in obtaining the culture results (typically 48–72 h). Due to these limitations, attempts have been made to find a biomarker that might reflect the presence of an infection. Serum procalcitonin levels are increased in patients with bacterial infection and have proven to be of value in the evaluation of patients with suspected sepsis (see Chapter 10). The role of PCT in the diagnosis of VAP is controversial with studies showing conflicting results.[36-40] The triggering receptor expressed on myeloid cells (TREM-1) is a member of the immunoglobulin superfamily, and its expression on phagocytes and neutrophils is specifically unregulated by microbial products.[41] Gibot and colleagues[42] measured TREM-1 in the BAL fluid (mini-BAL) of patients receiving mechanical ventilation in whom an infectious pneumonia was suspected. The diagnostic sensitivity and specificity of TREM-1 were 98 and 90%, respectively, with TREM-1 being the strongest independent predictor of pneumonia. In this study, there was no difference between the levels of procalcitonin in those patients with and without pneumonia. Determann[43] reported similar plasma levels of TREM-1 in the plasma of patients with and without VAP but higher levels in the BAL fluid of patients with VAP. These authors followed mini-BAL TREM-1 levels over time and demonstrated that the TERM-1 levels rose significantly before the diagnosis of VAP. Similarly, Huh and colleagues demonstrated that TREM-1 was an independent predictor of bacterial pneumonia in patients with bilateral lung infiltrates.[44] It is likely that diagnostic algorithms which incorporate quantitative cultures together with biomarkers (PRCT and TREM-1) will improve the diagnostic accuracy of VAP.

■ TREATMENT

Multiple studies have demonstrated that the most important factor determining the outcome of VAP is the early initiation of appropriate antibiotic therapy.[45–48] In order to initiate appropriate initial anti-microbial coverage, two factors are crucial:

ALERT

- Is the patient at risk for infection with an MDR organism?
- Local ICU bacteriology.
- What is your local (ICU) bacteriology.

Due to the spectrum of potential pathogens and the increasing prevalence of MDR organisms, a broad-spectrum, multi-drug, empiric antibiotic protocol is required in most patients with suspected VAP (except those at low risk of infection with a MDR organism). BAL and quantitative culture allows for the de-escalation of antibiotics once a pathogen(s) is identified. Furthermore, negative lower respiratory tract cultures can be used to stop antibiotic therapy in a patient who had cultures obtained in the absence of an antibiotic change in the past 72 h.[11]

General Concepts of Anti-microbial Treatment

- An empiric therapy regimen should include agents that are from a different class than the patient has recently received.

- Linezolid should be considered the drug of choice for proven MRSA infection. The role of vancomycin for the initial empiric coverage until microbiological data is available is controversial.
- De-escalation of antibiotics should be considered once data on the results of lower respiratory tract cultures and the patient's clinical response are available.
- Once a pathogen has been isolated and its sensitivity determined, monotherapy is appropriate for most patients with VAP (including *Pseudomonas*) except for those patients who are neutropenic or bacteremic.[49]
- Aerosolized antibiotics have not been proven to have value in the therapy of VAP.
- An 8-day course of antibiotics is recommended for patients with uncomplicated VAP who have received initially appropriate therapy and have had a good clinical response, with no evidence of infection with non-fermenting gram-negative bacilli.
- There is enormous variability of bacteriology from one hospital to another, specific sites within the hospital, and from one time period to another. Current site-specific data must be used to guide the choice of antibiotics.

Empiric Antibiotic Choices

No Risk Factors for MDR Pathogens (Single-Agent Rx)

- Ceftriaxone[11] or
- Levofloxacin or moxifloxacin or
- Ampicillin/sulbactam or
- Ertapenem or
- Piperacillin/tazobactam

Risk Factors for MDR Pathogens (Combination Rx)

- Anti-pseudomonal cephalosporin (cefepime, ceftazidime)[11] or
- Anti-pseudomonal carbapenem (imipenem or meropenem) or
- β-Lactam/β-lactamase inhibitor

Plus

- Anti-pseudomonal fluoroquinolone (ciprofloxacin or levofloxacin) or
- Aminoglycoside (amikacin, gentamicin, or tobramycin)

Plus

- Linezolid or
- Vancomycin

■ STRATEGIES FOR PREVENTING VAP

- Head up 30–45°.[36,50,51]
- Oral care and chlorhexidine mouth wash.[52]
- Use orogastric rather than nasogastric tubes.
- Avoid unnecessary changes of ventilator circuit.
- Routinely empty condensate in the ventilator circuit.
- Implement weaning and wake-up protocols.
- Avoid unnecessary blood transfusion.
- Maintain endotracheal cuff pressure >20 cm H_2O.
- Limit the use of proton pump inhibitors.[53]
- "Prophylactic PEEP" of 5 cm H_2O.[54]
- Chest therapy.[55]
- Avoid gastric overdistention.
- Avoid unplanned extubation and reintubation.
- Kinetic/rotating beds in high-risk patient.[56]
- Early tracheotomy.[57]
- General infection control measures (hand hygiene, isolate MDR pathogens, etc).

■ CLINICAL PEARLS

- Culture of tracheal aspirate is a "waste of time" and leads to excessive and inappropriate antibiotic use.
- At this time, VAP is best diagnosed by BAL and quantitative culture.
- Initial appropriate anti-microbial therapy is the most important factor determining the outcome of VAP.

■ REFERENCES

1. Safdar N, Dezfulian C, Collard HR, et al. Clinical and economic consequences of ventilator-associated pneumonia: a systematic review. *Crit Care Med.* 2005;33:2184–2193.
2. Feldman C, Kassel M, Cantrell J, et al. The presence and sequence of endotracheal tube colonization in patients undergoing mechanical ventilation. *Eur Respir J.* 1999;13:546–551.
3. Chastre J, Fagon JY. Ventilator-associated pneumonia. *Am J Respir Crit Care Med.* 2002;165:867–903.
4. Dobbins BM, Kite P, Wilcox MH. Diagnosis of central venous catheter related sepsis – a critical look inside. *J Clin Pathol.* 1999;52: 165–172.

5. Bahrani-Mougeot FK, Paster BJ, Coleman S, et al. Molecular analysis of oral and respiratory bacterial species associated with ventilator-associated pneumonia. *J Clin Microbiol.* 2007;45:1588–1593.

6. el-Ebiary M, Torres A, Fabregas N, et al. Significance of the isolation of Candida species from respiratory samples in critically ill, non-neutropenic patients. An immediate postmortem histologic study. *Am J Respir Crit Care Med.* 1997;156:583–590.

7. Delisle MS, Williamson DR, Perreault MM, et al. The clinical significance of Candida colonization of respiratory tract secretions in critically ill patients. *J Crit Care.* 2008;23:11–17.

8. Trouillet JL, Chastre J, Vuagnat A, et al. Ventilator-associated pneumonia caused by potentially drug-resistant bacteria. *Am J Respir Crit Care Med.* 1998;157:531–539.

9. Rello J, Jubert P, Valles J, et al. Evaluation of outcome for intubated patients with pneumonia due to *Pseudomonas aeruginosa. Clin Infect Dis.* 1996;23:973–78.

10. Rello J, Torres A, Ricart M, et al. Ventilator-associated pneumonia by *Staphylococcus aureus.* Comparison of methicillin-resistant and methicillin-sensitive episodes. *Am J Respir Crit Care Med.* 1994;150:1545–1549.

11. Niederman MS, Craven DE, Bonten MJ, et al. Guidelines for the management of adults with hospital-acquired, ventilator-associated, and healthcare-associated pneumonia. *Am J Respir Crit Care Med.* 2005;171:388–416.

12. Mandelli M, Mosconi P, Langer M, et al. Is pneumonia developing in patients in intensive care always a typical "nosocomial" infection? *Lancet.* 1986;2:1094–1095.

13. Giard M, Lepape A, Allaouchiche B, et al. Early- and late-onset ventilator-associated pneumonia acquired in the intensive care unit: comparison of risk factors. *J Crit Care.* 2008;23:27–33.

14. Mabie M, Wunderink RG. Use and limitations of clinical and radiologic diagnosis of pneumonia. *Semin Resp Infect.* 2003;18:72–79.

15. Lauzier F, Ruest A, Cook D, et al. The value of pretest probability and modified clinical pulmonary infection score to diagnose ventilator-associated pneumonia. *J Crit Care.* 2008;23:50–57.

16. Fabregas N, Ewig S, Torres A, et al. Clinical diagnosis of ventilator associated pneumonia revisited: comparative validation using immediate post-mortem lung biopsies. *Thorax.* 1999;54:867–873.

17. Pugin J, Auckenthaler R, Mili N, et al. Diagnosis of ventilator-associated pneumonia by bacteriologic analysis of bronchoscopic and nonbronchoscopic "blind" bronchoalveolar lavage fluid. *Am Rev Respir Dis.* 1991;143:1121–1129.

18. Schurink CA, Van Nieuwenhoven CA, Jacobs JA, et al. Clinical pulmonary infection score for ventilator-associated pneumonia: accuracy and inter-observer variability. *Intensive Care Med.* 2004;30:217–224.

19. Croce MA, Swanson JM, Magnotti LJ, et al. The futility of the clinical pulmonary infection score in trauma patients. *J Trauma*. 2006;60: 523–527.

20. Pham TN, Neff MJ, Simmons JM, et al. The clinical pulmonary infection score poorly predicts pneumonia in patients with burns. *J Burn Care Res*. 2007;28:76–79.

21. Johanson WG Jr., Seidenfeld JJ, Gomez P, et al. Bacteriologic diagnosis of nosocomial pneumonia following prolonged mechanical ventilation. *Am Rev Respir Dis*. 1988;137:259–264.

22. Chastre J, Fagon JY, Bornet-Lecso M, et al. Evaluation of bronchoscopic techniques for the diagnosis of nosocomial pneumonia. *Am J Respir Crit Care Med*. 1995;152:231–240.

23. Fagon JY, Chastre J, Wolff M, et al. Invasive and non-invasive strategies for management of suspected ventilator-associated pneumonia. *Ann Intern Med*. 2000;132:621–630.

24. Shorr AF, Sherner JH, Jackson WL, et al. Invasive approaches to the diagnosis of ventilator-associated pneumonia: a meta-analysis. *Crit Care Med*. 2005;33:46–53.

25. Kollef MH, Bock KR, Richards RD, et al. The safety and diagnostic accuracy of minibronchoalveolar lavage in patients with suspected ventilator-associated pneumonia. *Ann Intern Med*. 1995;122:743–748.

26. Marik PE, Brown WJ. A comparison of bronchoscopic vs blind protected specimen brush sampling in patients with suspected ventilator-associated pneumonia. *Chest*. 1995;108:203–207.

27. Marik PE, Careau P. A comparison of mini-bronchoalveolar lavage and blind -protected specimen brush sampling in ventilated patients with suspected pneumonia. *J Crit Care*. 1998;13:67–72.

28. Heyland D, Dodek P, Muscedere J, et al. A randomized trial of diagnostic techniques for ventilator-associated pneumonia. *N Engl J Med*. 2006;355:2619–2630.

29. Heyland DK, Dodek P, Muscedere J, et al. Randomized trial of combination versus monotherapy for the empiric treatment of suspected ventilator-associated pneumonia. *Crit Care Med*. 2008;36:737–744.

30. Muscedere J, Dodek P, Keenan S, et al. Comprehensive evidence-based clinical practice guidelines for ventilator-associated pneumonia: diagnosis and treatment. *J Crit Care*. 2008;23:138–147.

31. Nseir S, Marquette CH. Diagnosis of hospital-acquired pneumonia: postmortem studies. *Infect Dis Clin North Am*. 2003;17:707–716.

32. Malhotra AK, Riaz OJ, Duane TM, et al. Subthreshold quantitative bronchoalveolar lavage: clinical and therapeutic implications. *J Trauma*. 2008;65:580–588.

33. Miller PR, Meredith JW, Chang MC. Optimal threshold for diagnosis of ventilator-associated pneumonia using bronchoalveolar lavage. *J Trauma*. 2003;55:263–267.

34. Croce MA, Fabian TC, Mueller EW, et al. The appropriate diagnostic threshold for ventilator-associated pneumonia using quantitative cultures. *J Trauma*. 2004;56:931–934.

35. Stryjewski ME, Sczech LA, Benjamin DK, et al. Use of vancomycin or first-generation cephalosporins for the treatment of hemodialysis-dependent patients with methicillin-susceptible *Staphylococcus aureus* Bacteremia. *Clin Infect Dis*. 2007;44:190–196.

36. Luyt CE, Combes A, Reynaud C, et al. Usefulness of procalcitonin for the diagnosis of ventilator-associated pneumonia. *Intensive Care Med*. 2008;34:1434–1440.

37. Pelosi P, Barassi A, Severgnini P, et al. Prognostic role of clinical and laboratory criteria to identify early ventilator-associated pneumonia in brain injury. *Chest*. 2008;134:101–108.

38. Duflo F, Debon R, Monneret G, et al. Alveolar and serum procalcitonin: diagnostic and prognostic value in ventilator-associated pneumonia. *Anesthesiology*. 2002;96:74–79.

39. Ramirez P, Garcia MA, Ferrer M, et al. Sequential measurements of procalcitonin levels in diagnosing ventilator-associated pneumonia. *Eur Respir J*. 2008;31:356–362.

40. Charles PE, Kus E, Aho S, et al. Serum procalcitonin for the early recognition of nosocomial infection in the critically ill patients: a preliminary report. *BMC Infect Dis*. 2009;9:49.

41. Gibot S, Massin F, Le RP, et al. Surface and soluble triggering receptor expressed on myeloid cells-1: expression patterns in murine sepsis. *Crit Care Med*. 2005;33:1787–1793.

42. Gibot S, Cravoisy A, Levy B, et al. Soluble triggering receptor expressed on myeloid cells and the diagnosis of pneumonia. *N Engl J Med*. 2004;350:451–458.

43. Determann RM, Millo JL, Gibot S, et al. Serial changes in soluble triggering receptor expressed on myeloid cells in the lung during development of ventilator-associated pneumonia. *Intensive Care Med*. 2005;31:1495–1500.

44. Huh JW, Lim CM, Koh Y, et al. Diagnostic utility of the soluble triggering receptor expressed on myeloid cells-1 in bronchoalveolar lavage fluid from patients with bilateral lung infiltrates. *Crit Care*. 2008; 12:R6.

45. Kollef KE, Schramm GE, Wills AR, et al. Predictors of 30-day mortality and hospital costs in patients with ventilator-associated pneumonia attributed to potentially antibiotic-resistant gram-negative bacteria. *Chest*. 2008;134:281–287.

46. Iregui M, Ward S, Sherman G, et al. Clinical importance of delays in the initiation of appropriate antibiotic treatment for ventilator-associated pneumonia. *Chest*. 2002;122:262–268.

47. Garnacho-Montero J, Garcia-Garmendia JL, Barrero-Almodovar A, et al. Impact of adequate empirical antibiotic therapy on the outcome of

patients admitted to the intensive care unit with sepsis. *Crit Care Med.* 2003;31:2742–2751.

48. Garnacho-Montero J, Ortiz-Leyba C, Fernandez-Hinojosa E, et al. *Acinetobacter baumannii* ventilator-associated pneumonia: epidemiological and clinical findings. *Intensive Care Med.* 2005;31:649–655.

49. Paul M, Benuri-Silbiger I, Soares-Weiser K, et al. Beta lactam monotherapy versus beta lactam–aminoglycoside combination therapy for sepsis in immunocompetent patients: systematic review and meta-analysis of randomised trials. *Br Med J.* 2004;328:668.

50. Coffin SE, Klompas M, Classen D, et al. Strategies to prevent ventilator-associated pneumonia in acute care hospitals. *Infect Control Hosp Epidemiol.* 2008;29(Suppl 1):S31–S40.

51. Drakulovic MB, Torres A, Bauer TT, et al. Supine body position as a risk factor for nosocomial pneumonia in mechanically ventilated patients: a randomised trial. *Lancet.* 1999;354:1851–1858.

52. Koeman M, van der Ven AJ, Hak E, et al. Oral decontamination with chlorhexidine reduces the incidence of ventilator-associated pneumonia. *Am J Respir Crit Care Med.* 2006;173:1348–1355.

53. Miano TA, Reichert MG, Houle TT, et al. Nosocomial pneumonia risk and stress ulcer prophylaxis. A comparison of pantoprazole vs Ranitidine in cardiothoracic surgery patients. *Chest.* 2009;136:440–447.

54. Manzano F, Fernandez-Mondejar E, Colmenero M, et al. Positive-end expiratory pressure reduces incidence of ventilator-associated pneumonia in nonhypoxemic patients. *Crit Care Med.* 2008;36:2225–2231.

55. Ntoumenopoulos G, Presneill JJ, McElholum M, et al. Chest physiotherapy for the prevention of ventilator-associated pneumonia. *Intensive Care Med.* 2002;28:850–856.

56. Marik PE, Fink MP. One good turn deserves another! *Crit Care Med.* 2002;30:2146–2148.

57. Rumbak MJ, Newton M, Truncale T, et al. A prospective, randomized, study comparing early percutaneous dilational tracheotomy to prolonged translaryngeal intubation (delayed tracheotomy) in critically ill medical patients. *Crit Care Med.* 2004;32:1689–1694.

18

Community-Acquired Pneumonia

In the United States, community-acquired pneumonia (CAP) in adults results in approximately 600,000 hospital admissions annually and ranks as the sixth leading cause of death. The mortality rate from CAP varies dramatically depending on the patient's severity of illness at presentation and underlying comorbid conditions. In the outpatient setting, the mortality rate is <1–5%; however, once patients require hospitalization, the mortality rate approaches 12%. Of those patients with CAP hospitalized, between 18 and 36% require treatment in an ICU. The mortality of these patients is about 35%. While approximately 20% of patients admitted to the ICU with CAP are in septic shock, the mortality of these patients may be as high as 60%.

The presence of underlying comorbid conditions such as

- chronic obstructive pulmonary disease (COPD)
- asthma
- diabetes mellitus
- renal insufficiency
- congestive heart failure
- coronary artery disease
- malignancy
- alcoholism
- age >70 years
- chronic neurological disease
- chronic liver disease

not only contribute significantly to CAP morality but also may alter the etiologic organisms underlying the infection (see below).

P.E. Marik, *Handbook of Evidence-Based Critical Care*,
DOI 10.1007/978-1-4419-5923-2_18,
© Springer Science+Business Media, LLC 2010

■ ICU ADMISSION CRITERIA

Major Criteria

- Requirement for mechanical ventilation[1] or
- Septic shock (SBP <90 despite fluids)

Minor Criteria (Three or More)

- 30 < white blood cell count <4 × 10^9/l
- Blood urea nitrogen >20 mg/dl
- PaO_2/FiO_2 <250
- Multi-lobe involvement
- Respiratory rate >30 breaths/min
- Platelet count <100,000 × 10^9/l
- Confusion/disorientation
- Hypothermia (temperature <36°C)
- Hypotension requiring fluid resuscitation

A review of those studies that have investigated the etiologic diagnosis in patients with *severe CAP* have isolated a pathogen in approximately 60% of patients, with the infection being polymicrobial in about 17% of patients. In these studies the most common pathogens were the following:

- *Streptococcus pneumoniae* (15–46%)
- *Legionella* species (0–23%)
- *Staphylococcus aureus* (0–22%)
- *Haemophilus influenzae* (0–14%)
- Gram-negative bacilli (4–25%)

The classically described "atypical" pathogens that cause CAP include *Chlamydia pneumoniae*, *Mycoplasma pneumoniae*, and *Legionella* species. The "atypical" moniker is an inaccurate description of the clinical features of the pneumonia associated with these organisms and is retained more as a classification than as a specific descriptor of the disease process or the clinical presentation. *Mycoplasma pneumoniae* has been shown to be the most common of the atypical pathogens and accounts for 17–37% of outpatient CAP and 2–33% of CAP requiring hospitalization. *Chlamydia pneumoniae* is more common than *Legionella* species; however, *Legionella* species can lead to rapidly progressive and fatal pneumonia.

■ PATHOGENS ASSOCIATED WITH UNDERLYING COMORBID CONDITION

- *S. pneumoniae*
  - Dementia
  - Congestive heart failure
  - COPD
  - Cerebrovascular disease
  - Institutional crowding
  - Seizures
- Penicillin-resistant and drug-resistant pneumococcus
  - Age >65 years
  - Alcoholism
  - Immunomodulating illness or therapy (including steroids)
  - Previous β-lactam therapy within 3 months
  - Multiple medical comorbidities
  - Exposure to child in day care center
- Enteric gram negatives
  - Residence in long-term facility
  - Underlying cardiopulmonary disease
  - Recent antibiotic therapy
  - Multiple medical comorbidities
- *Pseudomonas aeruginosa*
  - Broad-spectrum antibiotics for >7 days in the past month
  - Structural lung disease (bronchiectasis)
  - Corticosteroid therapy
  - Malnutrition
  - Undiagnosed HIV infection
  - Neutropenia
- Legionnaires' disease
  - AIDS
  - Hematologic malignancy
  - End-stage renal disease

■ DIAGNOSTIC TESTING

Patients with severe CAP should have the following:

- Blood cultures.
- Urinary antigen tests for *Legionella pneumophila* and *S. pneumoniae.*
- Expectorated sputum for culture.
- Intubated patients require endotracheal aspirate (fresh) or m-BAL.
- Screening for HIV.
- Nasopharyngeal swab for influenza during seasonal influenza (rapid Ag test and viral PCR)

The only randomized controlled trial evaluating a diagnostic strategy in CAP demonstrated no statistically significant differences in mortality or LOS between patients receiving pathogen-directed therapy and patients receiving empiric therapy.[2] However, pathogen-directed therapy was associated with lower mortality among the patients admitted to the ICU.

Non-infectious diseases masquerading as CAP should be excluded, namely:

- Cryptogenic organizing pneumonia (COP)
- Eosinophilic pneumonia
- Hypersensitivity pneumonia
- Drug-induced pneumonitis: methotrexate, nitrofurantoin, gold, amiodarone, etc
- Pulmonary vasculitis
- Pulmonary embolism/infarction
- Pulmonary malignancy
- Radiation pneumonitis
- Tuberculosis

■ ANTIBIOTIC TREATMENT (ICU PATIENTS)

First Choice

- β-Lactam[1]
  - Cefotaxime
  - Ceftriaxone
  - Ampicillin–sulbactam

PLUS

- Azithromycin or fluoroquinolone

Penicillin Allergy

- Fluoroquinolone

PLUS

- Aztreonam

Pseudomonal Infection

- Anti-pneumococcal, anti-pseudomonal β-lactam
  - Piperacillin–tazobactam
  - Cefepime
  - Imipenem
  - Meropenem

PLUS

- Ciprofloxacin or levofloxacin (750 mg)

OR

- Anti-pneumococcal, anti-pseudomonal β-lactam

PLUS

- Aminoglycoside and azithromycin

OR

- Anti-pneumococcal, anti-pseudomonal β-lactam

PLUS

- Aminoglycoside and anti-pneumococcal fluoroquinolone

Penicillin allergic

- Aztreonam

PLUS

- Aminoglycoside and anti-pneumococcal fluoroquinolone

Community-Acquired MRSA

Add vancomycin or linezolid
See Chapter 12.

■ INFLUENZA (COEXISTENT OR INFLUENZA PNEUMONIA)

- Early treatment (within 48 h of the onset of symptoms) with oseltamivir or zanamivir is recommended for influenza A.
- Use of oseltamivir and zanamivir is not recommended for patients with uncomplicated influenza with symptoms for >48 h, but these drugs may be used to reduce viral shedding in hospitalized patients or for influenza pneumonia.
- *Streptococcus pneumoniae* and *S. aureus* are the most common causes of secondary bacterial pneumonia in patients with influenza.

Supportive Care

See Chapter 10.

■ SPECIAL CONSIDERATIONS

Double Cover for CAP

Although monotherapy is considered as standard for CAP, a survival benefit of the combination of β-lactam and macrolide has been suggested. Waterer[3] found that patients with bacteremic pneumococcal CAP who receive at least two effective antibiotic agents within the first 24 h after presentation to hospital have a significantly lower mortality than do patients who receive only one effective antimicrobial agent. The most common combination was a third-generation cephalosporin with a macrolide or a quinolone. Using a large hospital database, Brown et al.[4] demonstrated a lower mortality, shorter LOS, and lower hospital charges for patients with CAP treated with dual therapy using macrolides as the second agent. Rodriguez et al. undertook a secondary analysis of data obtained from a prospective observational cohort study of cases in 33 ICUs in Spain. Overall, 270 patients required vasoactive drugs and were characterized as having shock. In the cases with shock, combination antibiotic therapy was associated with a significantly higher adjusted 28-day in-ICU survival (hazard ratio 1.69; 95% CI 1.09–2.60; $p = 0.01$).[5] Another study investigated the outcome of patients with severe CAP, comparing patients treated with β-lactam/macrolide combination vs. those treated with fluoroquinolone monotherapy.[6] Lower 30-day mortality rates were seen for those treated with β-lactam/macrolide combination (18.4% vs. 36.6%, $p = 0.05$).

The possible explanations for the benefits of dual coverage (esp. with a macrolide) include antibiotic synergy, coverage of unrecognized atypical pathogens, immunomodulating effects, and the effect on bacterial quorum sensing. Macrolides, at sub-minimum inhibitory concentrations (MIC), are potent inhibitors of the production of pneumolysin (a potent virulence factor) by macrolide-susceptible strains of the pneumococcus, whereas the β-lactam agent ceftriaxone, as well as amoxicillin, ciprofloxacin, moxifloxacin, and tobramycin, is relatively ineffective.[7] Although they also antagonize various pro-inflammatory activities of neutrophils, macrolides primarily target the synthesis of interleukin (IL)-8 by bronchial epithelial cells, eosinophils, monocytes, fibroblasts, and airway smooth muscle cells.[8] While there is no definitive evidence that combination therapy improves outcome, dual therapy with a macrolide and a third-generation cephalosporin should be considered in patients with severe CAP.

Community-Acquired MRSA Pneumonia (CA-MRSA)

Recently, an increasing incidence of pneumonia due to CA-MRSA has been observed.[9–11] CA-MRSA appears in two patterns: the typical hospital-acquired strain and a strain that is epidemiologically, genotypically, and phenotypically distinct from hospital-acquired strains. Many of the former may represent health-care-associated CAP (HCAP). The latter are resistant to fewer anti-microbials than are hospital-acquired MRSA strains and often contain a novel type IV *SCCmec* gene. In addition, most contain the gene for Panton-Valentine leucocidin, a toxin associated with clinical features of necrotizing pneumonia, shock, and respiratory failure, as well as the formation of abscesses and empyemas. This strain should also be suspected in patients who present with cavitary infiltrates without risk factors for anaerobic aspiration pneumonia. Diagnosis is usually straightforward, with high yields from sputum and blood cultures in this characteristic clinical scenario. CA-MRSA CAP remains rare in most communities but is expected to be an emerging problem in CAP treatment.

Health-Care-Associated Pneumonia

Patients who develop pneumonia in the setting of an acute or a chronic health-care facility must be distinguished from those who develop pneumonia in the community; these patients are referred to as having health-care-associated pneumonia, which includes hospital-acquired pneumonia and ventilator-associated pneumonia. (See Chapter 17.) This distinction is important as these patients are at high risk for having infection with MRSA and multi-drug-resistant (MDR) bacterial pathogens. The MDR pathogens include *P. aeruginosa*, extended-spectrum β-lactamase-producing *Klebsiella pneumoniae*, *Acinetobacter baumannii*, *Enterobacter* species and *Enterococcus* species. Early broad-spectrum anti-microbial coverage with multiple antibiotics is recommended in these patients, with de-escalation once the implicated pathogen has been identified In general, this requires the combination of an anti-pseudomonal cephalosporin (cefepime, ceftazidime), carbapenem (imipenem, meropenem), or penicillin (piperacillin/tazobactam) plus either an anti-pseudomonal fluoroquinolone or aminoglycoside.

Persistent Temperature/Failure to Respond to Rx

A common misconception is that the patient's temperature should settle within 24 h of commencing antibiotic therapy. It has been demonstrated that it may take up to 72 h for the temperature to normalize in a patient with pneumococcal pneumonia. However, in a patient with a widely swinging temperature, it would be prudent to exclude a complication within this time frame. The following are the major reasons for a failure to respond to anti-microbial agents:

- Wrong antibiotic: wrong spectrum or drug resistance
- Exclude masquerader
- Wrong dosage
- Viral, fungal, or opportunistic pathogen
- Unusual pathogens (see below)
- Superadded complication
- Complicated pleural effusion/empyema
- Endocarditis
- Purulent pericarditis
- Septic arthritis
- Meningitis, etc.

Unusual Pathogens

- *Coxiella burnetii*
  - Cats, goats, sheep, cattle
- Tularemia
  - Rabbits, ticks
- Leptospirosis
  - Rats
- Hantavirus
  - Rats
- SARS
- Psittacosis
  - Birds
- *Nocardia*
  - Steroids
- *Aspergillus*
  - Steroids
- *Pneumocystis jiroveci*
  - Immunosuppression
- Dimorphic fungi
  - Recent travel
- *Burkholderia pseudomallei*
  - Recent travel
- TB

Complicated Pleural Effusion/Empyema

When pleural fluid is detected in a patient with pneumonia, a diagnostic thoracocentesis should always be performed to rule out pleural space infection (except if the effusion is very small). Pleural fluid studies differentiate between a benign parapneumonic effusion and an early empyema (complicated pleural effusion). Drainage is necessary when the pleural fluid is grossly purulent or if pleural fluid studies show any of the following:

- pH <7.2 (most sensitive indicator)
- Glucose <40 mg/dl
- White blood cell count >10,000/ml

■ CLINICAL PEARLS

- The combination of a third-generation cephalosporin and a macrolide is the preferred treatment option for patients with severe CAP.
- Always exclude conditions that may masquerade as CAP.
- Always obtain travel history and history of contacts with animals, i.e., unusual pathogens.
- Consider community-acquired MRSA in toxic patients and those with severe disease.
- Consider *P. aeruginosa* risk factors.

■ REFERENCES

1. Mandell LA, Wunderink RG, Anzueto A, et al. Infectious diseases society of America/American thoracic society consensus guidelines on the management of community-acquired pneumonia in adults. *Clin Infect Dis.* 2007;44(Suppl 2):S27–S72.
2. van der Eerden MM, Vlaspolder F, de Graaff CS, et al. Comparison between pathogen directed antibiotic treatment and empirical broad spectrum antibiotic treatment in patients with community acquired pneumonia: a prospective randomised study. *Thorax.* 2005;60:672–678.
3. Waterer GW, Somes GW, Wunderink RG. Monotherapy may be suboptimal for severe bacteremic pneumococcal pneumonia. *Arch Intern Med.* 2001;161:1837–1842.
4. Brown RB, Iannini P, Gross P, et al. Impact of initial antibiotic choice on clinical outcomes in community-acquired pneumonia: analysis of a hospital claims-made database. *Chest.* 2003;123:1503–1511.
5. Rodriguez A, Mendia A, Sirvent JM, et al. Combination antibiotic therapy improves survival in patients with community-acquired pneumonia and shock. *Crit Care Med.* 2007;35:1493–1498.
6. Lodise TP, Kwa A, Cosler L, et al. Comparison of beta-lactam and macrolide combination therapy versus fluoroquinolone monotherapy in hospitalized Veterans Affairs patients with community-acquired pneumonia. *Antimicrob Agents Chemother.* 2007;51:3977–3982.

7. Anderson R, Steel HC, Cockeran R, et al. Comparison of the effects of macrolides, amoxicillin, ceftriaxone, doxycycline, tobramycin and fluoroquinolones, on the production of pneumolysin by *Streptococcus pneumoniae* in vitro. *J Antimicrob Chemother*. 2007;60:1155–1158.

8. Simpson JL, Powell H, Boyle MJ, et al. Clarithromycin targets neutrophil airway inflammation in refractory asthma. *Am J Respir Crit Care Med*. 2008;177:148–155.

9. Dufour P, Gillet Y, Bes M, et al. Community-acquired methicillin-resistant *Staphylococcus aureus* infections in France: emergence of a single clone that produces Panton-Valentine leukocidin. *Clin Infect Dis*. 2002;35:819–824.

10. Deresinski S. Methicillin-resistant *Staphylococcus aureus*: an evolutionary, epidemiologic, and therapeutic odyssey. *Clin Infect Dis*. 2005;40:562–573.

11. Fridkin SK, Hageman JC, Morrison M, et al. Methicillin-resistant *Staphylococcus aureus* disease in three communities. *N Engl J Med*. 2005;352:1436–1444.

19

ARDS

ALERT

Lung protective ventilation strategies, which include low tidal volumes (approximately 6 ml/kg), high PEEP (>10 cm H_2O or 1–2 cm H_2O above the lower inflection point on the pressure–volume loop), and a plateau airway pressure of approximately 28–30 cm H_2O, are currently accepted as the standard of care for ventilating patients with ALI/ARDS.[1]

■ DEFINITION, CAUSES, AND ASSESSMENT OF SEVERITY

Acute respiratory distress syndrome (ARDS) was initially described by Ashbaugh and Petty[2] as a syndrome characterized by diffuse pulmonary infiltrates, with decreased pulmonary compliance and hypoxemia. It has however been recognized that "ARDS" is a spectrum varying from mild acute lung injury (ALI) at one end to ARDS at the other. The diagnosis of ARDS should be reserved for patients with ALI who have severe disease (see criteria below). The outcome of ALI is largely dependent on both the severity of ALI and the causative factors. It should be emphasized that in most cases ALI is a multi-system disease; the microcirculatory changes which occur in the lung occur in all organs; the pathophysiological derangements, however, are most evident in the lung.

P.E. Marik, *Handbook of Evidence-Based Critical Care*,
DOI 10.1007/978-1-4419-5923-2_19,
© Springer Science+Business Media, LLC 2010

Definition of ALI

A condition involving[3]

- an oxygenation defect with bilateral alveolar infiltrates,
- a patient who has suffered an acute catastrophic event, and
- a patient who has a pulmonary capillary wedge pressure ≤18 mmHg or no clinical evidence of an elevated left atrial pressure.

A patient is defined as having ALI when the $PO_2/FiO_2 \leq 300$ (regardless of the amount of PEEP).

Definition of ARDS

A patient is said to have ARDS when the $PO_2/FiO_2 \leq 200$ (regardless of the amount of PEEP).

Causes of ALI

ALI may result from either direct or indirect lung injury.[4,5] It is likely that the severity of ALI and the outcome are related to the causation of ALI. The common causes include the following:

- Direct lung injury
  - Pneumonia
  - Aspiration pneumonitis
  - Smoke inhalation
  - Chemical inhalation
  - Drowning
- Indirect lung injury
  - Sepsis and sepsis syndrome
  - Polytrauma
  - Transfusion of blood and blood products (TRALI)
  - Pancreatitis
  - Drug induced (heroin, tricyclic anti-depressants, etc.)
  - Fat embolism
  - Burns

■ MANAGEMENT OF THE ACUTE PHASE

The management of ARDS is essentially supportive and includes cardiorespiratory and nutritional support, the prevention of further lung injury, and the prevention of complications while waiting for the acute inflammatory response to resolve and lung function to improve.[4,5]

Ventilation Strategy

ALERT

The most important "recent" advance in the management of patients with ARDS (indeed in critical care medicine) is the realization that overdistension of alveoli causes acute lung injury. Hence a "lung protective strategy" is the standard of care and the cornerstone of the management of patients with ARDS.[1] Tidal volumes (V_t) should not exceed 6 ml/kg PBW (see Chapter 14).

The chest radiographs of patients with ARDS classically show widespread involvement of all lung fields. It was therefore assumed that ARDS was a homogenous process. However, high-resolution computed tomographic scans performed in patients with ARDS have demonstrated areas of normal, consolidated, and overinflated lung. The large area of consolidated and collapsed lung is predominantly distributed in the dependent areas and participates minimally in gas exchange. The normal lung is usually anterior and often markedly overdistended. In addition, in the early stages of ARDS, consolidated lung units can be "recruited" with the application of modest distending pressures. Consequently, patients with ARDS typically have three functionally distinct lung zones, namely

- that portion of the lung that is diseased and not recruitable,
- that portion of the lung that is diseased but recruitable, and
- that portion of the lung that is normal.

Because a significant portion of the lung is consolidated and not recruitable, only a small amount of aerated lung receives the total tidal volume – ARDS leads to "baby lungs."[6] The use of traditional tidal volumes (12–15 ml/kg) in these patients will result in high inspiratory pressures with overdistension of the normally aerated lung units. A growing body of experimental evidence has demonstrated that mechanical ventilation that results in high transpulmonary pressure gradients and overdistension of lung units will cause acute lung injury, characterized by hyaline membranes, granulocytic infiltration, pulmonary hypertension, and increased pulmonary and systemic vascular permeability. Animal studies have demonstrated that a transpulmonary pressure in excess of 35 cm H_2O will lead to alveolar damage.[7] These studies have demonstrated that ventilation with low tidal volumes preserves pulmonary

ultrastructure. Furthermore, it has been postulated that the cyclic opening and closing of lung units (recruitment and derecruitment) in patients
with ARDS who are ventilated with insufficient PEEP may further potentiate this iatrogenic lung injury.[4,5,8] It has therefore been suggested that
ventilatory strategies that avoid regional or global overdistension of lung
units and also avoid end-expiratory alveolar collapse may limit the degree
of lung injury in ARDS: the open-lung approach.[9]

The Acute Respiratory Distress Syndrome Network randomized
patients with ARDS to receive traditional volume-controlled ventilation
(an initial tidal volume of 12 ml/kg and a plateau pressure of ≤ 50 cm of
water) or low tidal volume ventilation (an initial tidal volume of 6 ml/kg
and a plateau pressure of ≤ 30 cm of water).[1] In the low V_t group,
V_t was reduced further to 5 or 4 ml/kg PBW if necessary to maintain
plateau pressure (P_{plat}) at less than 30 cm H_2O. The trial was stopped
after the enrollment of 861 patients because mortality was lower in the
group treated with lower tidal volumes (31.0% vs. 39.8%, $p = 0.007$).
This study has provided convincing evidence that a strategy that avoids
alveolar overdistension in ARDS improves outcome (see Figure 19-1).

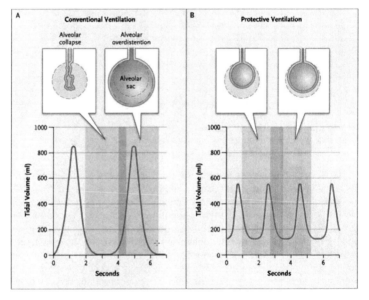

Figure 19-1. Conventional as compared with protective lung ventilation.
Reproduced with permission from Ref. 8 Copyright © 2007 Massachusetts
Medical Society. All rights reserved.

The response to low tidal volume ventilation should be assessed initially on the basis of plateau airway pressure. The goal should be to maintain a plateau airway pressure (i.e., the pressure during an end-inspiratory pause) of 30 cm of water or less; if this target is exceeded, the tidal volume should be further reduced to a minimum of 4 ml/kg of predicted body weight. An important caveat relates to patients who have stiff chest walls (for example, those with massive ascites). In such patients, it is reasonable to allow the plateau pressure to increase to values greater than 30 cm of water, since the pleural pressures are elevated and hence the transpulmonary pressures are not elevated (i.e., there is not necessarily alveolar overdistension).

ALERT

The available data do not support the commonly held view that inspiratory plateau pressures of 30–35 cm H_2O are safe.[10] There is no safe upper limit for plateau pressures in patients with ALI/ARDS. The lower the plateau pressure, the lower the mortality (see Figure 19-2), i.e. a V_t of 6 ml/kg PBW should be used even if the plateau pressures are less than 28 cm H_2O.

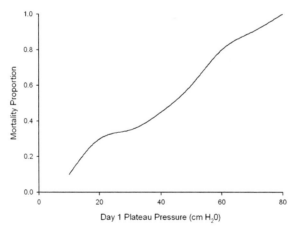

Figure 19-2. Relationship between day 1 plateau pressure and mortality. Reproduced with permission from Ref. 10.

While sepsis and multi-system organ failure (MSOF) remain the most common causes of death in patients with ARDS, up to 20% of deaths are attributable to progressive respiratory failure.[11] A number of interventions have been attempted in this group of patients including inhaled nitric oxide, nebulized prostacyclin and surfactant, recruitment maneuvers, liquid ventilation, and prone positioning with little evidence that these interventions improve outcome.[5,12-14] Pressure-controlled ventilation (PCV), high-frequency oscillation, and airway pressure release ventilation (APRV) have been used in these patients. APRV has recently emerged as an alternative ventilatory strategy in patients with severe ARDS (see Chapter 14).[15-17]

PCV and APRV have, however, yet to be carefully compared with volume-cycled ventilation in patients with ARDS in terms of morbidity, length of mechanical ventilation, and ultimate patient outcome in an RCT. It is unlikely that such a trial will be performed; however, from the forgoing, it is likely that ventilation strategies that achieve the same end points (i.e., prevent alveolar overdistension and limit airway pressures) will have similar outcomes.

Pressure-Controlled Ventilation

To prevent alveolar overdistension and reduce the transpulmonary pressure gradients, the inspiratory pressure is set such that the peak inspiratory pressure is less than 30 cm H_2O (i.e., applied PEEP + inspiratory pressure <30 cm H_2O) when possible and always less than 35 cm H_2O. An inspiratory pressure of 20 cm H_2O (plus PEEP of 10 cm H_2O) with a respiratory rate of 16 breaths/min are convenient starting points.

The inspiratory and expiratory times (or *I:E* ratio) and respiratory rate are best determined by analyzing the flow vs. time waveform (see Figure 19-3). Flow will initially enter the lung rapidly because the ventilator attempts to reach the set airway pressure as quickly as it can

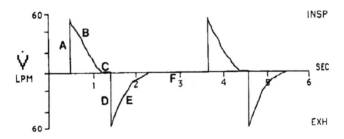

Figure 19-3. Pressure-controlled ventilation, flow vs. time waveform.

(point A, Figure 19-3). Airways that are open and have the least resistance will receive the greatest amount of gas flow and reach equilibrium with the preset pressure more quickly than airways with greater resistance. As the open airways fill and the lung pressure reaches equilibrium with the preset pressure, flow will decelerate as the airways with higher resistance continue to fill with gas (point B, Figure 19-3). Flow into the lung will continue until one of the following two events occur:

- The preset pressure reaches equilibrium throughout all lung units (indicated by the flow pattern decelerating to zero).
- The preset inspiratory time ends inspiration before pressure has equilibrated throughout all lung units (indicated by the flow pattern not reaching zero).

When inspiratory flow reaches zero, it means that the pressure in the lung is equal to the pressure set on the ventilator (point C, Figure 19-3). It is essential that adequate inspiratory time be given so that all the airways, both healthy and diseased, have time to reach the preset pressure level. In ARDS, much of the airway bed may take a relatively long time to open. For this reason, it may be necessary to lengthen the inspiratory time, sometimes to the point that the inspiratory time is longer than the expiratory time. If air trapping is not present, this approach will increase mean airway pressure without increasing maximal end-expiratory pressure. In patients with ARDS, oxygenation is primarily a function of mean airway pressure. This strategy will therefore increase alveolar ventilation and improve oxygenation. The inspiratory time can be lengthened in two ways:

- If the ventilator allows for the adjustment of inspiratory time, then simply increase the inspiratory time until the inspiratory flow reaches zero (recommended method).
- If the ventilator allows adjustment of the I/E ratio, then reducing the "E" part of the ratio will increase "I."

If flow reaches zero and there is a long inspiratory pause, this is an indication that inspiratory time is too long. There is little benefit of having a prolonged inspiratory pause. Setting inspiratory time longer than that which is required to open recruitable airways increases the likelihood of significant auto-PEEP with its attendant hemodynamic complications.

To evaluate the adequacy of the expiratory time, the flow vs. time waveform (Figure 19-3) needs to be studied again. This waveform shows whether the patient has enough time to exhale to the preset PEEP level before the ventilator gives the next breath. In Figure 19-3, point D represents the beginning of exhalation. When exhalation begins, gas will exit the lungs quickly at first because a large pressure gradient exists between the lungs and the atmosphere. As gas continues to exit the lungs, the pressure gradient will become smaller and flow will decelerate (point E, Figure 19-3). Exhalation will continue until one of the following two events occur:

- The pressure in the lung reaches atmospheric pressure plus the set PEEP pressure (point F, Figure 19-3).
- The set inspiratory time mandates that inhalation begin before exhalation of the previous breath is complete, thus causing auto-PEEP/intrinsic PEEP (iPEEP).

Figure 19-4 demonstrates gas trapping as inhalation begins before expiratory flow is allowed to reach zero. Should gas trapping be evident on the flow vs. time waveform, either the respiratory rate or the inspiratory time should be reduced, allowing time for complete exhalation and thereby minimizing iPEEP. Both the respiratory rate and the inspiratory time should be independently and sequentially reduced in order to determine which maneuver affects ventilation the least.

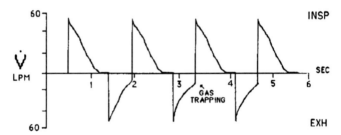

Figure 19-4. Pressure-controlled ventilation, flow vs. time waveform demonstrating air trapping.

It is essential that the level of iPEEP be measured in all patients receiving PCV. There is no data that iPEEP has any advantage over extrinsic (i.e., applied) PEEP. However, the unrecognized development of iPEEP may result in hemodynamic compromise, leading to the inappropriate use of fluid and vasopressor therapy. The flow vs. time waveform should be monitored regularly. As the patients' pulmonary mechanics change, the inspiratory time and the respiratory rate may need to be altered. Once the patients' condition has stabilized, attempts should be made to reduce the level of PEEP (and FiO_2).

Permissive Hypercapnia

The strategy to reduce volume-induced lung injury by using small tidal volumes may lead to CO_2 retention. The term "permissive hypercapnia" has been used to describe this ventilatory strategy. Hypercapnic acidosis is generally well tolerated by the patients, especially when it develops gradually over 1–2 days. The intracellular acidosis is corrected rapidly during sustained hypercapnia, whereas the extracellular acidosis may persist for much longer. The lowest pH that can be safely tolerated in unknown; however, a pH >7.2 is generally recommended. Some patients, however, have tolerated a pH as low as 7.05 without obvious adverse effects. It has been suggested that bicarbonate should be used to correct the pH. However, the administration of bicarbonate may paradoxically increase intracellular acidosis. Permissive hypercapnia should not be used in patients with acute intracranial pathology as this may cause a precipitous increase in intracranial pressure. Furthermore in patients with ischemic heart disease, arrhythmias, and patients requiring high doses of inotropic drugs, hypercapnia should be allowed to develop gradually. Surprisingly, permissive hypercapnia itself has anti-inflammatory effects and has been shown to attenuate lung injury in animal models.[18,19] Furthermore, permissive hypercapnia has beneficial hemodynamic effects.[19]

Best PEEP

Positive end-expiratory pressure (PEEP) appears to be protective against ventilator-induced lung injury in animal studies, perhaps by recruiting more aerated lung and preventing shear forces produced during repetitive opening of closed airways or alveoli. Low tidal volume ventilation has been demonstrated to cause a decline in compliance in healthy subjects as well as patients in respiratory failure. It has been suggested that the smaller the tidal volume, the higher the PEEP level need to optimize lung mechanics. It is generally believed that PEEP set below 10 cm H_2O will probably keep healthy alveoli open at end exhalation but will not be enough to distend diseased airways. These airways will then continually open and collapse throughout the ventilator cycle. The goal is to set PEEP at a level that does not overdistend healthy alveoli but at the same time does not let diseased airways collapse. The term "open-lung approach" has been used to describe this method of ventilation.[9] It has been reported that in patients with ARDS, a mean PEEP level of 15 cm H_2O is required to keep the airways "open" at end expiration.[9]

While the beneficial effects of a low tidal volume strategy are largely accepted, the role of PEEP as part of the "lung protective strategy" is more controversial.[20–22] However, a meta-analysis demonstrated a trend toward improved mortality with high PEEP, even though the difference did not reach statistical significance, with the pooled cumulative risk of 0.90 (95% CI 0.72–1.02, $p = 0.077$).[23] The reduction in absolute risk of death was approximately 4%. There was no evidence of a significant increase in barotrauma in patients receiving high PEEP, with a pooled risk of 0.95 (95% CI 0.62–1.45, $p = 0.81$).

"Best PEEP" can be estimated by plotting a static pressure/volume curve and measuring airway pressure at each incrementally higher tidal volume. This curve classically demonstrates an upper and a lower inflection point (Figure 19-5). PEEP should be set above the lower inflection point such that the sum of the PEEP and the inspiratory pressure should be below 30 cm H_2O (a plateau pressure of up to 35 cm H_2O may be acceptable) or the upper inflection point. Should an inflection point not be present on the pressure/volume curve or not be possible to perform this maneuver, the initial PEEP should be set between 10 and 15 cm H_2O.

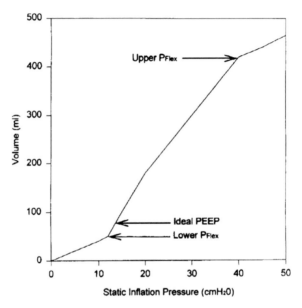

Figure 19-5. Static pressure–volume *curve* showing *upper* and *lower* inflection points.

PEEP Guided by Esophageal Pressures

Ideally, both tidal volume and PEEP should be adjusted according to transpulmonary pressures (airway pressure minus pleural pressure) to maintain oxygenation while minimizing repeated alveolar collapse (negative end-expiratory transpulmonary pressure) and minimizing alveolar overdistension (high end-inspiratory transpulmonary pressure). While pleural pressure is very difficult to measure clinically, it can be estimated using esophageal pressures. According to this approach, in patients with high estimated pleural pressure, raising PEEP to maintain a positive transpulmonary pressure might improve aeration and oxygenation without causing overdistension. Conversely, in patients with low pleural pressure, maintaining low PEEP would keep transpulmonary pressure low, preventing overdistension and minimizing the adverse hemodynamic effects of high PEEP. Talmor and colleagues[24] performed a RCT in which PEEP and V_t were set according to the measurement of esophageal pressures or according to the ARDSNet "protocol." In this pilot study, oxygenation and respiratory compliance were significantly better in the esophageal pressure group with a trend toward improved survival.

Recruitment Maneuvers

Recruitment refers to the dynamic process of reopening unstable airless alveoli through an intentional transient increase in transpulmonary pressure. The rationale for the use of recruitment maneuvers (RMs) in ALI is to promote alveolar recruitment, leading to increased end-expiratory lung volume. An increase in end-expiratory lung volume may improve gas exchange and attenuate ventilator-induced lung injury by preventing repetitive opening and closing of unstable lung units. However, RMs may directly overdistend aerated lung units and could, paradoxically, lead to increased lung injury. Clinical studies of RMs in ALI have yielded variable results. A systematic review on the topic concluded that "given the uncertain benefit of transient oxygenation improvements in patients with ALI and the lack of information on their influence on clinical outcomes, the routine use of RMs cannot be recommended or discouraged at this time."[25]

Non-ventilatory Adjuncts to Gas Exchange

Inhaled Nitric Oxide

Nitric oxide is an endogenous vasodilator. When administered by inhalation at concentrations up to 20 parts per million, it reduces pulmonary vascular resistance. Although about 60% of patients with acute lung injury have an initial noticeable improvement in oxygenation, the effect is transient (48 h) and does not confer mortality benefit or reduction in the duration of mechanical ventilation.[12] Nitric oxide should not be used routinely but be reserved for patients in whom adequate oxygenation cannot be achieved by lung protective mechanical ventilation and prone positioning.

Nebulized Prostacyclin

Prostacyclin is an endogenous vasodilator with similar physiological effects to nitric oxide. When nebulized, it has an equivalent effect on pulmonary vasodilation and oxygenation but is easier to administer, has harmless metabolites, and requires no special monitoring. However, no large randomized controlled trials in acute respiratory distress syndrome have been conducted.

Surfactant

Although patients with acute respiratory distress syndrome have decreased and dysfunctional surfactant, no benefit has been found after the administration of both natural and synthetic formulations – in terms either of mortality or of the need for mechanical ventilation.

Prone Positioning

Moving patients with acute respiratory distress syndrome into the prone position has consistently been shown to improve oxygenation initially in about 60% of cases. However, prone positioning does not reduce mortality or duration of ventilation in patients with ARDS.[26] However, a sustained improvement in oxygenation may support the use of prone positioning in patients with very severe hypoxemia.

ECMO

Extracorporeal CO_2 removal with apneic oxygenation (ECMO) has been used to avoid additional ventilator-induced lung injury in patients with severe ARDS. Until recently the use of ECMO in adults with ARDS has been controversial with no compelling data that it improves outcome. The most important results regarding the use of ECMO are expected from the *Conventional Ventilatory Support vs. Extracorporeal Membrane Oxygenation for Severe Adult Respiratory Failure* (CESAR) study, a randomized clinical trial assessing the effectiveness of extracorporeal lung assist in ARDS patients.[27] Although not yet formally published, the results of this study represent the first positive randomized clinical trial on adult ECMO in ARDS patients. This trial was conducted in the United Kingdom; a particular design modeled on the template of the previous successful ECMO study in neonates was used. Patients randomized to ECMO were transferred to the ECMO center in Leicester; control patients either were transferred to or remained in a hospital selected for its capability of providing advanced care and continued the conventional treatment according to the best available clinical practice. In most of the patients assigned to the treatment group, venovenous ECMO via percutaneous cannulation was applied. Blood was drained from the jugular or the femoral vein and returned to the contralateral femoral vein. The system was designed to provide full substitution of pulmonary gas exchange under normothermia, with high blood flow capabilities (>5 l/min) and high gas exchange surfaces. The average duration of bypass was 9 days. Most importantly, during ECMO, the ventilator settings were gradually reduced to allow lung rest, limiting the peak inspiratory pressure to 20 cm H_2O and using an end-expiratory pressure of 10 cm H_2O, a respiratory rate of 10 breaths/min, and an FiO_2 of 30%. As customary, heparin was infused to keep the activated clotting time between 160 and 220 s. From July 2001 to August 2006, 180 patients were enrolled into the study, 90 in each arm. Survival at 6 months or the absence of severe disability was achieved in 63% of the ECMO patients, comparing very favorably against 47% of the control group.

ECMO is very labor intensive, expensive, associated with additional complications, and should be undertaken only by centers with experience in this technique.

Hemodynamic Support

The optimal fluid strategy in patients with ARDS has until recently been a hotly debated topic with a "wet lung" and a "dry lung" camp. The ARDSNet group compared a "conservative" vs. a "liberal" strategy of fluid management using explicit protocols in a large RCT of patients with ALI/ARDS (FACCT Trial).[28] The mean ($\pm$SE) cumulative fluid balance during the first 7 days was -136 ± 491 ml in the conservative-strategy group and $6,992 \pm 502$ ml in the liberal-strategy group ($p<0.001$). As compared with the liberal strategy, the conservative strategy was associated with a significantly improved

- oxygenation index
- lung injury score
- number of ventilator-free days
- ICU LOS

Although this study did not demonstrate a survival advantage in favor of the conservative group, this approach is now the favored and is supported by studies in surgical patients and patients with sepsis (see Chapter 8). The amount of intravenous fluids (lactated Ringer's) should be minimized; this may require vasopressor and/or inotropic agents to maintain adequate cardiac output. The BUN should be closely monitored allowing it to creep up to about 40 mg/dl.[28] However, do not allow the patient to progress to acute renal failure. The combination of furosemide and albumin may be useful to achieve a negative fluid balance without compromising renal function.[29]

Corticosteroids

The use of corticosteroids in ARDS is a very controversial and politically charged topic (see Chapter 40).[30] However, a number of meta-analyses have demonstrated that stress-dose corticosteroids[31–33]

- improved PaO_2/FiO_2
- improved MODS score
- improved lung injury score
- increased the number of ventilator-free days
- reduced ICU LOS
- reduced mortality (RR 0.62; 95% CI 0.43–0.91)
- did not increase the risk of infection or neuromyopathy

It is likely that both the dose and the dosing schedule are major determinants of the outcome of patients with ARDS treated with corticosteroids (see Chapter 40). The recommended dosing schedule is methylprednisolone in a dose not to exceed 1 mg/kg/day for 14 days followed by a slow taper.[30,34] We recommend the use of corticosteroids within 72 h of admission to the ICU in patients with severe and progressive ALI.

Omega-3 Enteral Nutrition

Omega-3 fatty acids have important anti-inflammatory and immunomodulating properties (see Chapter 31). Three RCTs have demonstrated that an enteral formula high in omega-3 fatty acids[35,36]

- improves PaO_2/FiO_2
- improves lung injury score
- increases the number of ventilator-free days
- reduces ICU LOS
- reduces mortality

All patients with ALI/ARDS should be fed enterally with a formula supplemented with fish oil (see Chapter 31).

Other Supportive Measures

- DVT prophylaxis (see Chapter 21).
- Adequate sedation is required to facilitate "low-volume ventilation" (see Chapter 9).
- β-Agonists accelerate alveolar fluid clearance and may decrease lung inflammation and extravascular lung water. The efficacy and safety of aerosolized β-agonist therapy in patients with ALI has yet to be determined.

Pulmonary Infection in ARDS

Patients with ALI/ARDS have a high incidence of "secondary" pulmonary infection. Pulmonary sepsis (i.e., VAP) should therefore be aggressively diagnosed and treated (see Chapter 17).

"Our" Approach to Refractory Hypoxemia

All patients with ALI/ARDS should initially be ventilated using volume-controlled ventilation with a V_t of 6 ml/kg PBW and a PEEP of 10–15 cm H_2O. They should be kept "dry" and receive an enteral formula high in omega-3 fatty acids. Corticosteroids should be added within 72 h in patients with progressive ALI. The following sequential interventions should be attempted (and withdrawn if no response) in patients with refractory hypoxemia:

- Nebulized prostacyclin
- APRV/PCV
- Prone positioning
- ECMO

ECMO should be considered only in suitable candidates with single-organ failure (lung failure) and no associated comorbidities.

■ CLINICAL PEARLS

- Ensure that V_t does not exceed 6 ml/kg PBW.
- Use adequate PEEP (10–15 cm H_2O).
- Keep them "dry."
- Give them fish.

■ REFERENCES

1. Ventilation with lower tidal volumes as compared with traditional tidal volumes for acute lung injury and the acute respiratory distress syndrome. *N Engl J Med.* 2000;342:1301–1308.
2. Ashbaugh DG, Bigelow DB, Petty TL, et al. Acute respiratory distress in adults. *Lancet.* 1967;1:319–323.
3. Bernard GR, Artigas A, Brigham KL. The American–European Consensus Conference on ARDS: definitions, mechanisms, relevant outcomes, and clinical trial coordination. *Am J Respir Crit Care Med.* 1994;149:818–824.

4. Ware LB, Matthay MA. The acute respiratory distress syndrome. *N Engl J Med*. 2000;342:1334–1349.

5. Leaver SK, Evans TW. Acute respiratory distress syndrome. *BMJ*. 2007;335:389–394.

6. Gattinoni L, Pesenti A. The concept of "baby lung". *Intensive Care Med*. 2005;31:776–784.

7. Dreyfuss D, Basset G, Soler P, et al. Intermittent positive-pressure hyperventilation with high inflation pressures produces pulmonary microvascular injury in rats. *Am Rev Respir Dis*. 1985;132:880–884.

8. Malhotra A. Low-tidal-volume ventilation in the acute respiratory distress syndrome. *N Engl J Med*. 2007;357:1113–1120.

9. Amato MB, Barbash CS, Medeiros DM, et al. Beneficial effects of the "Open lung approach" with low distending pressures in acute respiratory distress syndrome: a prospective randomized study on mechanical ventilation. *Am J Respir Crit Care Med*. 1995;152:1835–1846.

10. Hager DN, Krishnan JA, Hayden DL, et al. Tidal volume reduction in patients with acute lung injury when plateau pressures are not high. *Am J Respir Crit Care Med*. 2005;172:1241–1245.

11. Stapleton RD, Wang BM, Hudson LD, et al. Causes and timing of death in patients with ARDS. *Chest*. 2005;128:525–532.

12. Adhikari NK, Burns KE, Friedrich JO, et al. Effect of nitric oxide on oxygenation and mortality in acute lung injury: systematic review and meta-analysis. *BMJ*. 2007;334:779.

13. Girard TD, Bernard GR. Mechanical ventilation in ARDS: a state-of-the-art review. *Chest*. 2007;131:921–929.

14. Wheeler AP, Bernard GR. Acute lung injury and the acute respiratory distress syndrome: a clinical review. *Lancet*. 2007;369:1553–1565.

15. Habashi NM. Other approaches to open-lung ventilation: airway pressure release ventilation. *Crit Care Med*. 2005;33:S228–S240.

16. Habashi N, Andrews P. Ventilator strategies for posttraumatic acute respiratory distress syndrome: airway pressure release ventilation and the role of spontaneous breathing in critically ill patients. *Curr Opin Crit Care*. 2004;10:549–557.

17. Dart BW, Maxwell RA, Richart CM, et al. Preliminary experience with airway pressure release ventilation in a trauma/surgical intensive care unit. *J Trauma*. 2005;59:71–76.

18. Laffey JG, Honan D, Hopkins N, et al. Hypercapnic acidosis attenuates endotoxin-induced acute lung injury. *Am J Respir Crit Care Med*. 2004;169:46–56.

19. Wang Z, Su F, Bruhn A, et al. Acute hypercapnia improves indices of tissue oxygenation more than dobutamine in septic shock. *Am J Respir Crit Care Med*. 2008;177:178–183.

20. Meade MO, Cook DJ, Guyatt GH, et al. Ventilation strategy using low tidal volumes, recruitment maneuvers, and high positive end-expiratory

pressure for acute lung injury and acute respiratory distress syndrome: a randomized controlled trial. *JAMA*. 2008;299:637–645.

21. Brower RG, Lanken PN, MacIntyre N, et al. Higher versus lower positive end-expiratory pressures in patients with the acute respiratory distress syndrome. *N Engl J Med*. 2004;351:327–336.

22. Mercat A, Richard JC, Vielle B, et al. Positive end-expiratory setting in adults with acute lung injury and acute respiratory distress syndrome. A randomized controlled trial. *JAMA*. 2008;299:646–655.

23. Phoenix SI, Paravastu S, Columb M, et al. Does a higher positive end expiratory pressure decrease mortality in acute respiratory distress syndrome? A systematic review and meta-analysis. *Anesthesiology*. 2009;110:1098–1105.

24. Talmor D, Sarge T, Malhotra A, et al. Mechanical ventilation guided by esophageal pressure in acute lung injury. *N Engl J Med*. 2008;359: 2095–2104.

25. Fan E, Wilcox ME, Brower RG, et al. Recruitment maneuvers for acute lung injury: a systematic review. *Am J Respir Crit Care Med*. 2008;178:1156–1163.

26. Sud S, Sud M, Friedrich JO, et al. Effect of mechanical ventilation in the prone position on clinical outcomes in patients with acute hypoxemic respiratory failure: a systematic review and meta-analysis. *CMAJ*. 2008;178:1153–1161.

27. Peek GJ, Clemens F, Elbourne D, et al. CESAR: conventional ventilatory support vs extracorporeal membrane oxygenation for severe adult respiratory failure. *BMC Health Serv Res*. 2006;6:163.

28. Comparison of two fluid-management strategies in acute lung injury. *N Engl J Med*. 2006;354:2564–2575.

29. Martin GS, Moss M, Wheeler AP, et al. A randomized, controlled trial of furosemide with or without albumin in hypoproteinemic patients with acute lung injury. *Crit Care Med*. 2005;33:1681–1687.

30. Meduri GU, Marik PE, Annane D. Prolonged glucocorticoid treatment in acute respiratory distress syndrome: evidence supporting effectiveness and safety. *Crit Care Med*. 2009;37:1800–1803.

31. Tang BM, Craig JC, Eslick GD, et al. Use of corticosteroids in acute lung injury and acute respiratory distress syndrome: A systematic review and meta-analysis. *Crit Care Med*. 2009;37:1595–1603.

32. Meduri GU, Marik PE, Chrousos GP, et al. Steroid treatment in ARDS: a critical appraisal of the ARDS network trial and the recent literature. *Intensive Care Med*. 2008;34:61–69.

33. Peter JV, John P, Graham PL, et al. Corticosteroids in the prevention and treatment of acute respiratory distress syndrome (ARDS) in adults: meta-analysis. *BMJ*. 2008;336:1006–1009.

34. Meduri GU, Golden E, Freire AX, et al. Methylprednisolone infusion in patients with early severe ARDS: results of a randomized trial. *Chest*. 2007;131:954–963.

35. Marik PE, Zaloga GP. Immunonutrition in critically ill patients: a systematic review and analysis of the literature. *Intensive Care Med.* 2008;34:1980–1990.
36. Pontes-Arruda A, DeMichele S, Srth A, et al. The use of an inflammation modulating diet in patients with acute lung injury or acute respiratory distress syndrome: a Meta-analysis evaluation of outcome data. *JPEN.* 2008;32(6):596–605.

20

Aspiration Pneumonia and Pneumonitis

Aspiration is defined as the misdirection of oropharyngeal or gastric contents into the larynx and the lower respiratory tract.[1] An assortment of pulmonary syndromes may occur following aspiration depending on the quantity and nature of the aspirated material, the frequency of aspiration, as well as the nature of the host defense mechanisms and the host's response to the aspirated material. The most important syndromes include *aspiration pneumonitis* or Mendelson's syndrome, which is a chemical pneumonitis caused by the aspiration of gastric contents and *aspiration pneumonia*, an infectious process caused by the aspiration of oropharyngeal secretions colonized by pathogenic bacteria.[1] While there is some overlap between these two syndromes, they are distinct clinical entities.

■ ASPIRATION PNEUMONIA

Aspiration pneumonia develops after the aspiration of colonized oropharyngeal contents. Aspiration of pathogens from a previously colonized oropharynx is the primary pathway by which bacteria gain entry into the lungs. Indeed, *Haemophilus influenzae* and *Streptococcus pneumoniae* first colonize the naso/oropharynx before being aspirated and causing community-acquired pneumonia (CAP). However, when the term aspiration pneumonia is used, it refers to the development of a radiographic infiltrate in the setting of patients with risk factors for increased oropharyngeal aspiration. Any condition which increases the volume and/or the bacterial burden of oropharyngeal secretion in the setting of impaired host defense mechanism may lead to aspiration pneumonia. Indeed, in stroke

P.E. Marik, *Handbook of Evidence-Based Critical Care*,
DOI 10.1007/978-1-4419-5923-2_20,
© Springer Science+Business Media, LLC 2010

patients undergoing swallow evaluation, there is a strong correlation between the volume of the aspirate and the development of pneumonia.[2] The clinical setting in which pneumonia develops largely distinguishes aspiration pneumonia from other forms of pneumonia.

Aspiration pneumonia has been reported to be the second most frequent principle diagnosis among hospitalization of Medicare patients.[3] Several studies list "aspiration pneumonia" as the cause of CAP in 5–15% of cases. CAP is the major cause of morbidity and mortality in the elderly and it is likely that aspiration is the major cause of pneumonia in these cases. Epidemiological studies have demonstrated that the incidence of pneumonia increases with aging, with the risk being almost six times higher in those over the age of 75 compared to those less than 60 years of age. Furthermore, the mortality from pneumonia increases strikingly with aging. The attack rate for pneumonia is highest among those in nursing homes.

Risk Factors for Dysphagia and Aspiration Pneumonia

Dysphagia is particularly common following a stroke. In patients with an acute stroke, the incidence of dysphagia ranges from 40 to 70%.[4] Approximately 40–50% of stroke patients with dysphagia aspirate. Dysphagic patients who aspirate are at an increased risk of developing pneumonia. Specifically, the development of pneumonia is seven times greater in stroke patients who aspirate, as compared to those who do not. Although dysphagia improves in most patients following a stroke, in many, the swallowing difficulties follow a fluctuating course with 10–30% continuing to have dysphagia with aspiration. Elderly patients are at risk of silent cerebral infarction. Nakagawa et al. demonstrated that elderly patients with silent cerebral infarction have a fivefold higher risk of developing pneumonia than do elderly patients with normal head computed tomographic scans.[5]

Almost all patients with degenerative diseases of the central nervous system develop dysphagia. In patients with Alzheimer's disease, amyotrophic lateral sclerosis (ALS), and Parkinson's disease, dysphagia usually occurs early in the course of the disease and the severity of dysphagia does not necessarily relate to the overall severity of the neurological disease. Considering the high incidence of cerebrovascular and degenerative neurological diseases in nursing home residents, it is not surprising that the reported incidence of dysphagia in this population is between 50 and 75% and explains the extremely high attack rate of pneumonia in these patients.

Patients who have undergone major surgical procedures particularly cardiothoracic surgery are at a high risk for aspiration and should undergo routine swallow evaluation.[6] Similarly, ICU patients after tracheal extubation are at high risk for aspiration because of swallowing dysfunction related to alterations of upper airway sensitivity, glottic injury, and laryngeal muscular dysfunction. Alteration in the swallow reflex can be detected in patients who have been intubated for as short as 24 h. This abnormality usually recovers within 48 h. We recommend withholding feeding for at least 6 h after extubation (in case reintubation is required), followed by a pureed and then soft diet for at least 48 h. A formal swallow evaluation is suggested in cases of traumatic intubations and in patients with anatomical or functional abnormalities of the upper airway.

Some types of malignancy, especially esophageal and head and neck cancer, are associated with an increased risk of aspiration, which may be due to an obstructive lesion or a treatment complication. Almost half of the patients who undergo concurrent chemotherapy and radiation for head and neck cancer develop severe dysphagia, leading to an increased risk of aspiration pneumonia. The manifestations of aspiration in this group may be insidious because of the depressed cough reflex.

Factors Which Increase the Risk of Pneumonia in Patients who Aspirate

While the presence of dysphagia and the volume of the aspirate are key factors which predispose patients to aspiration pneumonia, a number of other factors play an important role. Colonization of the oropharynx is an important step in the pathogenesis of aspiration pneumonia. The elderly have increased oropharyngeal colonization with pathogens such as *Staphylococcus aureus* and aerobic gram-negative bacilli (e.g., *Klebsiella pneumoniae* and *Escherichia coli*). Although this increased colonization may be transient, lasting less than 3 weeks, it underlies the increased risk of pneumonia with these pathogens. The defects in host defenses that predispose to enhanced colonization with these organisms are uncertain; however, dysphagia with a decrease in salivary clearance and poor oral hygiene may be major risk factors. Edentulous patients have a lower risk of aspiration pneumonia than do dentate patients.

Evaluation and Assessment

In patients with aspiration pneumonia, the episode of aspiration is generally not witnessed. The diagnosis is therefore inferred when a patient with known risk factors for aspiration has an infiltrate in a characteristic bronchopulmonary segment. In patients who aspirate in the recumbent position, the commonest sites of involvement are the posterior segments of the upper lobes and the apical segments of the lower lobes. In patients who aspirate in the upright or semi-recumbent position, the basal segments of the lower lobes are favored. The usual picture is that of an acute pneumonic process which runs a course similar to that of a typical CAP. If untreated, however, these patients appear to have a higher incidence of cavitation and lung abscess formation. Gram-negative pathogens and *S. aureus* are the likely pathogens in patients with CAP due to aspiration pneumonia.

All elderly patients with CAP as well as patients with a recent cerebrovascular accident as well as those with degenerative neurological diseases should be referred to a speech and language pathologist (SLP) for a formal swallow evaluation and for the development and implementation of a management program. A clinician's bedside assessment of the cough and gag reflex is unreliable in screening for patients at risk for aspiration. The SLP can reliably identify those patients who aspirate by performing a bedside swallowing evaluation supplemented by either a videofluoroscopic swallow study or a fiber-optic endoscopic evaluation (FEES). This evaluation identifies those patients who require further behavioral, dietary, and medical management to reduce the risk of aspiration. In hospitalized patients, nasogastric or feeding tubes are frequently removed prior to the swallow evaluation. Due to scheduling difficulties, this may lead to a prolonged period of starvation. However, Leder and Suiter[7] demonstrated that a FEES can be performed with a NG tube in place and that the presence of such a tube does not affect the results of swallow evaluation.

Treatment

Anti-microbial therapy is indicated in patients with aspiration pneumonia. The choice of antibiotics should depend on the setting in which the aspiration occurs as well as the patient's premorbid condition. However, anti-microbial agents with gram-negative activity such as third-generation cephalosporins, fluoroquinolones, and piperacillin are usually required. Penicillin and clindamycin, the "standard" anti-microbial agents for aspiration pneumonia, provide inadequate activity in the majority of patients with aspiration pneumonia. Anti-microbials with specific anaerobic activity are not routinely warranted and may be indicated only in patients with severe periodontal disease, patients expectorating putrid sputum, and patients with a necrotizing pneumonia or lung abscess on chest radiograph.[8]

The management of patients with dysphagia requires the coordinated expertise of a number of health-care professionals, including the patients' primary care physician, pulmonologist, SLP, clinical dietician, occupational therapist, physiotherapist, nurse, oral hygienist, dentist, as well as the patients' primary caregivers. The goal is to optimize the safety, the efficiency, and the effectiveness of the oropharyngeal swallow, to maintain adequate nutrition and hydration, and to improve oral hygiene.

Enhanced quality of life, wherever possible, should direct management. This would be to maximize oral vs. non-oral nutritional intake and hydration.

The management plan is developed according to the clinical and instrumental assessment results. Compensatory strategies for increasing eating and swallowing efficiency, and for reducing the risk of aspiration, may involve modifying food and liquid consistencies and volumes, as well as altering the bolus presentation. Dietary modification is a common management approach. Patients vary in their ability to swallow thin and thick liquids, semisolids, and solids. The consistency of the patients' food should be individualized according to the findings from clinical testing. Dehydration in the elderly is one of the leading problems in nursing homes and long-term care facilities. Caution should therefore be taken with regard to the modification of fluids, as compliance with thickened liquids is often reduced. Treatment techniques include compensatory strategies (postural maneuvers) and indirect therapy (exercises to strengthen swallowing musculature). These techniques alter the physiology of the swallow to achieve improved efficiency or a safer swallow.

Tube Feeding

Tube feeding is not essential in all patients who aspirate. The practice of tube feeding in the end stages of degenerative illnesses in the elderly should be carefully reconsidered. Finucane et al.[9] found no data to suggest that tube feeding of patients with advanced dementia prevented aspiration pneumonia, prolonged survival, reduced the risk of pressure sores or infections, improved function, and provided palliation.

Short-term tube feeding, however, may be indicated in elderly patients with severe dysphagia and aspiration in whom improvement of swallowing is likely to occur. Nakajoh and colleagues[10] demonstrated that the incidence of pneumonia was significantly higher in stroke patients with dysphagia who were fed orally compared to those who received tube feeding (54.3% vs. 13.2%, $p<0.001$) despite the fact that the orally fed patients had a higher functional status (higher Barthel index). The FOOD trials consisted of two large randomized studies that enrolled dysphagic stroke patients.[11] In the first trial, patients enrolled within 7 days of admission were randomly allocated to tube feeding or no tube feeding. Early tube feeding was associated with an absolute reduction in risk of death of 5.8%. The second trial allocated patients to early nasogastric feeding or early feeding via a percutaneous endoscopic gastrostomy (PEG) tube. PEG feeding was associated with an absolute increase in the risk of death of 1% and an increased risk of death or poor outcome of 7.8%. Patients with a PEG were less likely to be transitioned to oral feeding than were the NG group and were more likely to be living in an institution. These two factors may in part explain the higher mortality of the PEG-fed patients. Furthermore, it was interesting to note that PEG-fed patients were more likely to develop pressure sores, suggesting that these patients may have been nursed differently. The FOOD trials clearly demonstrate that dysphagic stroke patients who "fail a swallow examination" should be fed early via a nasogastric or a feeding tube and transitioned to oral feeding as their dysphagia resolves. Those patients whose dysphagia does not resolve may be candidates for placement of a PEG tube.

Colonized oral secretions are a serious threat to dysphagic patients and feeding tubes offer no clear protection. There is no data to suggest that patients fed with gastrostomy tubes have a lower incidence of pneumonia than do patients fed with nasogastric tubes. Similarly, the incidence of aspiration pneumonia has been shown to be similar in stroke patients with postpyloric as compared to intragastric feeding tubes. Over the long term, aspiration pneumonia is the most common cause of death in gastrostomy tube-fed patients.

Pharmacological Management

The neurotransmitter substance P is believed to play a major role in both the cough and swallow sensory pathways. Angiotensin-converting enzyme (ACE) inhibitors prevent the breakdown of substance P and may theoretically be useful in the management of patients with aspiration pneumonia. A number of studies have demonstrated a lower risk of aspiration pneumonia in stroke patients treated with an ACE inhibitor compared to other anti-hypertensive agents. These studies provide supportive evidence that patients with oropharyngeal dysphagia should be considered for treatment with an ACE inhibitor (even if normotensive).[4]

Sedative medication has been demonstrated to increase the risk of pneumonia in residents of long-term care facilities and should therefore be avoided. The prescription of phenothiazines and haloperidol should be very carefully considered, as they reduce oropharyngeal swallow coordination, causing dysphagia. Medications which dry up secretions, including anti-histamines and drugs with anti-cholinergic activity, make it more difficult for patients to swallow and should therefore also be avoided.

Due to the underlying cause of their dysphagia, patients who are hospitalized with aspiration pneumonia will frequently return to or will require treatment in an extended care facility. These patients will require ongoing evaluation and treatment of their swallow dysfunction, as well as ongoing assessment of the necessity for tube feeding. Occupants of residential homes have been shown to have poor oral hygiene and rarely receive treatment from dentists and oral hygienists. An aggressive protocol of oral care will reduce colonization with potentially pathogenic organisms and decrease the bacterial load, measures likely to reduce the risk of pneumonia. Furthermore, a number of studies have demonstrated that a protocol of aggressive daily oral care among elderly nursing home patients resulted in a significant improvement in the swallow and cough reflex with a lower incidence of pneumonia.

■ ASPIRATION PNEUMONITIS

Aspiration pneumonitis is best defined as acute lung injury following the aspiration of regurgitated gastric contents.[1] This syndrome occurs in patients with a marked disturbance of consciousness such as drug overdose, seizures, massive cerebrovascular accident, following head trauma and anesthesia. Drug overdose is the most common cause of aspiration pneumonitis, occurring in approximately 10% of patients hospitalized following a drug overdosage. Adnet and Baut[12] demonstrated that the risk of aspiration increases with the degree of unconsciousness (as measured by the Glasgow Coma Scale). Historically the syndrome most commonly associated with aspiration pneumonitis is Mendelson's syndrome, reported in 1946 in obstetric patients who aspirated while receiving general anesthesia.[13] Mendelson's original report consisted of 44,016 non-fasted obstetric patients whom he studied between 1932 and 1945, of whom more than half received an "operative intervention" with ether by mask without endotracheal intubation. He described aspiration in 66 patients (1:667). Although several of the patients were critically ill from their aspiration, "recovery was usually complete" within 24–36 h and only two patients died (1:22,008).

Although aspiration is a widely feared complication of general anesthesia, clinically apparent aspiration in modern anesthesia practice is exceptionally rare, and in healthy patients the overall morbidity and mortality are low. The risk of aspiration with modern anesthesia is about 1 in 3,000 anesthetics with a mortality of approximately 1:125,000, and accounting for between 10 and 30% of all anesthetic deaths.[14,15] The risk of aspiration is greatly increased in patients intubated emergently in the field, the emergency room, or in the ICU. In these patients, every effort should be made to reduce the risk of aspiration; this includes removing dentures and clearing the airway and in certain circumstances placing a nasogastric tube to empty the stomach prior to intubation. If there is an immediate risk of airway compromise, endotracheal intubation should be performed prior to placement of a nasogastric tube. However, if the patient is likely to have a full stomach (upper GI bleeding, small bowel obstruction, ileus, etc.), it may be prudent to place a nasogastric tube prior to endotracheal intubation. When intubating emergently, suction equipment must be immediately available and rapid-sequence induction using cricoid pressure should be performed. Those factors which are reported to increase the risk of aspiration during endotracheal intubation include the following:

- Emergent situations
- Upper gastrointestinal bleeding
- Difficult intubation/multiple intubation attempts
- Advanced age (>70 years)
- Seizures
- Conditions predisposing to gastroesophageal reflux
  - Bowel obstruction
  - Ileus
  - Hiatal hernia
  - Peptic ulcer disease
  - Gastritis

Mendelson emphasized the importance of acid when he showed that un-neutralized gastric contents introduced into the lungs of rabbits caused severe pneumonitis indistinguishable from that caused by an equal amount of 0.1 N hydrochloric acid.[13,14,16] However, if the pH of the vomitus was neutralized before aspiration, the pulmonary injury was minimal. Experimental studies have demonstrated that the severity of lung injury increases significantly with the volume of the aspirate and indirectly with its pH, with a pH of less than 2.5 being required to cause aspiration pneumonitis. However, the stomach contains a variety of other substances in addition to acid. Several experimental studies have revealed that aspiration of small, particulate food matter from the stomach may cause severe pulmonary damage even if the pH of the aspirate is above 2.5.

Aspiration of gastric contents results in a chemical burn of the tracheobronchial tree and the pulmonary parenchyma with an intense parenchymal inflammatory reaction. The pro-inflammatory cytokines including tumor necrosis factor-α and CXC chemokines are crucial to the development of aspiration pneumonitis by mediating neutrophil recruitment. Once localized to the lung, neutrophils play a key role in the development of lung injury through the release of oxygen radicals and proteases. Gastric acid prevents the growth of bacteria and therefore the contents of the stomach are normally sterile. Bacterial infection, therefore, does not play a significant role in the early stages of acute lung injury following aspiration of gastric contents. However, acid aspiration pneumonitis reduces host defenses against infection, increasing the risk of superinfection.[17] The incidence of this complication has, however, not been well studied. Furthermore, experimental models suggest that acid aspiration pneumonitis "primes the lung" making secondary infection more severe.[17,18]

Colonization of the gastric contents by potentially pathogenic organisms may occur when the gastric pH is increased by the use of antacids, H2-blockers, or proton pump inhibitors. In addition, gastric colonization by gram-negative bacteria occurs in patients receiving gastric enteral feedings, as well as in patients with gastroparesis and small bowel obstruction. In these circumstances, the pulmonary inflammatory response is likely to result from both bacterial infection and the inflammatory response of the gastric particulate matter.

Aspiration of gastric contents can present dramatically with a full-blown picture that includes gastric contents in the oropharynx, wheezing, coughing, shortness of breath, cyanosis, pulmonary edema, hypotension, and hypoxemia, which may progress rapidly to severe ARDS and death. However, many patients may not develop signs or symptoms associated with aspiration, while others may develop a cough or a wheeze. In some patients, aspiration may be clinically silent manifesting only as arterial desaturation with radiological evidence of aspiration. Warner and colleagues[14] studied 67 patients who aspirated while undergoing anesthesia. Forty-two (64%) of these patients were totally asymptomatic, 13 required mechanical ventilatory support for more than 6 h, and four died.

Management of Aspiration Pneumonitis

The upper airway should be suctioned following a witnessed aspiration. Endotracheal intubation should be considered in patients who are unable to protect their airway. While a common practice, the prophylactic use of antibiotics in patients with suspected or witnessed aspiration is not recommended. Similarly, the use of antibiotics shortly after an aspiration episode in a patient who develops a fever, leukocytosis, and a pulmonary infiltrate is discouraged as it may select for more resistant organisms in a patient with an uncomplicated chemical pneumonitis. However, empiric anti-microbial therapy is appropriate in patients who aspirate gastric contents in the setting of small bowel obstruction or in other circumstances associated with colonization of gastric contents. Anti-microbial therapy should be considered in patients with an aspiration pneumonitis which fails to resolve within 48 h. Empiric therapy with broad-spectrum agents is recommended. Anti-microbials with anaerobic activity are not routinely required. Lower respiratory tract sampling (protected specimen brush/bronchoalveolar lavage) and quantitative culture in intubated patients may allow targeted anti-microbial therapy and the discontinuation of antibiotics in culture-negative patients.

Corticosteroids have been used in the management of aspiration pneumonitis since 1955.[19] However, limited data exist on which to evaluate the role of these agents, with only a single prospective, placebo-controlled study having been performed. In this study, Sukumaran and colleagues[20] randomized 60 patients with aspiration pneumonitis to methylprednisolone (15 mg/kg/day for 3 days) or placebo. The patients were subdivided into two groups: a younger group with drug overdose as the predominant diagnosis and an older group with neurological disorders. Eighty-seven percent of the patients in the overdose group had an initial gastric pH below 2.5 as compared to 12.8 in the neurological group; patients (77.6%) in the overdose group were admitted from the community as compared to 12.8% of patients in the neurological group. Radiographic changes improved quicker in the steroid group, as did oxygenation. The number of ventilator and ICU days was significantly shorter in the overdose patients who received corticosteroids; however, these variables were longer in the neurological group. There was no significant difference in the incidence of complications or outcome. The results of this study are somewhat difficult to interpret as it is likely that the patients in the overdose group had true "aspiration pneumonitis," while many patients in the neurological group probably developed "aspiration pneumonia." In addition, patients received a short course of high-dose corticosteroids; current evidence suggests that patients with ARDS may benefit from a prolonged course of low-dose corticosteroids, while a short course of high-dose corticosteroids may be harmful (see Chapters 19 and 40). Wolfe and colleagues[21] performed a case-controlled study of 43 patients with aspiration pneumonitis of whom 25 patients received high-dose corticosteroids (approx. 600 mg prednisolone/day for 4 days. While there was no difference in mortality, secondary gram-negative pneumonia was reported to be more frequent in the steroid group (7/20 vs. 0/13); however, ventilator days tended to be less in this group (4.3 vs. 9.8 days). Based on these limited data, it is not possible to make evidence-based recommendations on the use of corticosteroids in patients with acid aspiration pneumonia. However, as the more recent literature suggest that patients with ARDS may benefit from a prolonged course of low-dose corticosteroids, this approach should be considered.[22]

In animal models, a number of pharmacological interventions including inhaled B_2 agonists, pentoxifylline, anti-platelet drugs, and omega-3 fatty acids have been shown to attenuate the acute lung injury following acid aspiration.[23-28] The role of these interventions in patients remains to be tested; however, due to their inherent safety, these agents should be considered in patients with severe acid aspiration pneumonitis.

■ CLINICAL PEARLS

- An OG/NG or a feeding tube does *not* need to be removed for the SLP to perform a swallow evaluation.
- All elderly patients with CAP as well as patients with a recent cerebrovascular accident require a formal swallow evaluation.

- Patients with dysphagia require a multi-disciplinary approach to swallowing management, aggressive oral care, and consideration for treatment with an ACE inhibitor.
- Patients with acid aspiration pneumonitis do not routinely require treatment with antibiotics; however, they are at an increased risk of superinfection.

■ REFERENCES

1. Marik PE. Aspiration pneumonitis and pneumonia: a clinical review. *N Engl J Med*. 2001;344:665–672.
2. Croghan JE, Burke EM, Caplan S, et al. Pilot study of 12-month outcomes of nursing home patients with aspiration on videofluoroscopy. *Dysphagia*. 1994;9:141–146.
3. Baine WB, Yu W, Summe JP. Epidemiologic trends in the hospitalization of elderly Medicare patients for pneumonia, 1991–1998. *Am J Public Health*. 2001;91:1121–1123.
4. Marik PE, Kaplan D. Aspiration pneumonia and dysphagia in the elderly. *Chest*. 2003;124:328–336.
5. Nakagawa T, Sekizawa K, Nakajoh K, et al. Silent cerebral infarction: a potential risk for pneumonia in the elderly. *J Intern Med*. 2000;247: 255–259.
6. Keeling WB, Lewis V, Blazick E, et al. Routine evaluation for aspiration after thoracotomy for pulmonary resection. *Ann Thorac Surg*. 2007;83:193–196.
7. Leder SB, Suiter DM. Effect of nasogastric tubes on incidence of aspiration. *Arch Phys Med Rehabil*. 2008;89:648–651.
8. El-Sohl AA, Pietrantoni C, Bhat A, et al. Microbiology of severe aspiration pneumonia in institutionalized elderly. *Am J Respir Crit Care Med*. 2003;167:1650–1654.
9. Finucane TE, Christmas C, Travis K. Tube feeding in patients with advanced dementia: a review of the evidence. *JAMA*. 1999;282: 1365–1370.
10. Nakajoh K, Nakagawa T, Sekizawa K, et al. Relation between incidence of pneumonia and protective reflexes in post-stroke patients with oral or tube feeding. *J Intern Med*. 2000;247:39–42.
11. Dennis MS, Lewis SC, Warlow C. Effect of timing and method of enteral tube feeding for dysphagic stroke patients (FOOD): a multicentre randomised controlled trial. *Lancet*. 2005;365:764–772.
12. Adnet F, Baud F. Relation between Glasgow Coma Scale and aspiration pneumonia [letter]. *Lancet*. 1996;348:123–124.
13. Mendelson CL. The aspiration of stomach contents into the lungs during obstetric anesthesia. *Am J Obstet Gynecol*. 1946;52:191–205.

14. Warner MA, Warner ME, Weber JG. Clinical significance of pulmonary aspiration during the perioperative period. *Anesthesiology.* 1993;78: 56–62.
15. Olsson GL, Hallen B, Hambraeus-Jonzon K. Aspiration during anaesthesia: a computer-aided study of 185,358 anaesthetics. *Acta Anaesthesiol Scand.* 1986;30:84–92.
16. Teabeaut JR. Aspiration of gastric contents. An experimental study. *Am J Pathol.* 1952;28:51–67.
17. Rotta AT, Shiley KT, Davidson BA, et al. Gastric acid and particulate aspiration injury inhibits pulmonary bacterial clearance. *Crit Care Med.* 2004;32:747–754.
18. van Westerloo DJ, Knapp S, van't Veer C, et al. Aspiration pneumonitis primes the host for an exaggerated inflammatory response during pneumonia. *Crit Care Med.* 2005;33:1770–1778.
19. Haussmann W, Lunt RL. Problem of treatment of peptic aspiration pneumonia following obstetric anesthesia (Mendelson's syndrome). *J Obstet Gynaecol Br Commonw.* 1955;62:509–512.
20. Sukumaran M, Granada MJ, Berger HW, et al. Evaluation of corticosteroid treatment in aspiration of gastric contents: a controlled clinical trial. *Mt Sinai J Med.* 1980;47:335–340.
21. Wolfe JE, Bone RC, Ruth WE. Effects of corticosteroids in the treatment of patients with gastric aspiration. *Am J Med.* 1977;63:719–722.
22. Tang BM, Craig JC, Eslick GD, et al. Use of corticosteroids in acute lung injury and acute respiratory distress syndrome: a systematic review and meta-analysis. *Crit Care Med.* 2009;37:1595–1603.
23. Kudoh I, Miyazaki H, Ohara M, et al. Activation of alveolar macrophages in acid-injured lung in rats: different effects of pentoxifylline on tumor necrosis factor-alpha and nitric oxide production. *Crit Care Med.* 2001;29:1621–1625.
24. Zarbock A, Singbartl K, Ley K. Complete reversal of acid-induced acute lung injury by blocking of platelet–neutrophil aggregation. *J Clin Invest.* 2006;116:3211–3219.
25. Kinniry P, Amrani Y, Vachani A, et al. Dietary flaxseed supplementation ameliorates inflammation and oxidative tissue damage in experimental models of acute lung injury in mice. *J Nutr.* 2006;136:1545–1551.
26. Terao Y, Nakamura T, Morooka H, et al. Effect of cyclooxygenase-2 inhibitor pretreatment on gas exchange after hydrochloric acid aspiration in rats. *J Anesth.* 2005;19:257–259.
27. Pawlik MT, Schreyer AG, Ittner KP, et al. Early treatment with pentoxifylline reduces lung injury induced by acid aspiration in rats. *Chest.* 2005;127:613–621.
28. Pawlik MT, Schubert T, Hopf S, et al. The effects of fenoterol inhalation after acid aspiration-induced lung injury. *Anesth Analg.* 2009;109: 143–150.

Deep Venous Thrombosis–Pulmonary Embolism

Deep venous thrombosis (DVT) and pulmonary embolism (PE) are in reality one and the same disease, known as *thromboembolic disease*, as a large proportion of patients with DVT have "asymptomatic" PE and about 40% of patients with PE have "asymptomatic DVT." Critically ill ICU patients have many of the risk factors which increase the risk of DVT, including the following:

- Prolonged venous stasis caused by bed rest
- Cardiac failure
- Dehydration
- Obesity
- Sepsis
- Vascular/endothelial injury
- Trauma
- Transfusion of blood products
- Renal failure
- Advanced age
- Femoral catheters
- Surgical interventions

Consequently DVT is common in ICU patients. Unfortunately, there are few prospective studies which have evaluated the incidence of DVT in ICU patients and *no* randomized control trials (RCTs) which have evaluated the efficacy of DVT prophylactic measures in ICU patients. The best study to date is that by Cook and colleagues who prospectively screened 261 patients during their ICU stay (venous Dopplers on admission and

P.E. Marik, *Handbook of Evidence-Based Critical Care*,
DOI 10.1007/978-1-4419-5923-2_21,
© Springer Science+Business Media, LLC 2010

twice weekly).[1] In this study, despite the fact that all patients received DVT prophylaxis (SC heparin 5,000 U q 12 h), 9.6% of patients were diagnosed with DVT. Patients with DVT had a significantly longer duration of mechanical ventilation and ICU stay compared to patients without DVT. This study highlights the fact that DVT is common in ICU patients and that SC heparin alone is inadequate for DVT prophylaxis. Other studies have documented DVT in up to 44% of ICU patients.[2,3] It is important to note that in these studies the majority of DVTs were not suspected clinically. This highlights the fact that PE remains one of the most common unsuspected autopsy findings in critically ill patients.[4] These data suggest that *all ICU* patients require aggressive DVT prophylaxis. Routine screening (lower extremity Dopplers) of all ICU patients is probably not cost effective but should be considered in those patients at highest risk of DVT.

ALERT

All ICU patients require aggressive DVT prophylaxis.

The optimal DVT prophylactic regimen for ICU patients has yet to be determined. DVT prophylaxis should therefore be individualized based on the following factors:

- Risk of DVT (trauma, hip/knee surgery, malignancy, etc.)
- Risk of bleeding (neurosurgery, spinal surgery)
- The patient's platelet count
- The patient's coagulation profile

The reader is referred to the *American College of Chest Physicians Evidence-Based Clinical Practice Guidelines on the Prevention of Venous Thromboembolism (8th Edition)* for a comprehensive review on this topic.[5]

The issue of heparin-induced thrombocytopenia (HIT) is a major concern in patients receiving heparin. While thrombocytopenia is a very common finding in ICU patients, HIT is quite uncommon (see Chapter 53). However, due to the devastating consequences of "missing a case," many patients at low risk of HIT undergo complex diagnostic screening. For this reason I recommend that unfractionated heparin (UH) be avoided in patients at high risk for HIT (cardiac surgery, orthopedic) as well as in patients who are thrombocytopenic (most ICU patients), as this complicates the diagnostic workup. Furthermore, UH alone appears to provide inadequate DVT prophylaxis in ICU patients. It should be noted that in the non-ICU setting, LMWH, fondaparinux, desirudin, and rivaroxaban (oral Xa inhibitor) are more effective than SC heparin in preventing DVT.

Furthermore, while the risk of HIT is much lower with LWMH, to all intents and purposes, this problem does not occur with other agents. It is also important to note that aspirin should not be used for DVT prophylaxis. LMWH, fondaparinux, or desirudin should therefore be considered the agents of choice for DVT prophylaxis in ICU patients. As the half-life of LMWHs, desirudin, and fondaparinux is prolonged in patients with renal dysfunction, UH may be appropriate in these patients. The role of oral Xa inhibitors (and direct thrombin inhibitors) in the ICU setting remains to be determined. Sequential compression devices (SCDs) reduce the risk of DVT when compared to placebo but are less effective than pharmacological prophylaxis.[6,7] However, SCDs improve the efficacy of pharmacological agents. It should be appreciated, however, that the improper use and/or application of SCDs will result in ineffective prophylaxis.

Crudely the efficacy of interventions in preventing DVT can be ranked as the following (from best to worse):

- Rivaroxaban PO
- Fondaparinux daily SC
- Adjusted dose IV UH
- LMWH daily SC
- Coumadin PO (should be avoided in the ICU)
- UH q 8 SC
- UH q 12 SC
- SCDs

It is important to note that LMWHs, fondaparinux, and desirudin are all renally excreted (and therefore should not be used when GFR <35 ml/min), will accumulate in renal failure, and that the anti-coagulant activity of these drugs are not easily reversed. Fondaparinux has a long half-life, which may be problematic in patients at risk of bleeding. Furthermore, the anti-coagulant activity of LMWHs and fondaparinux requires monitoring of factor Xa; this is cumbersome and not readily available. Prophylactic vena caval filters have limited utility for DVT prophylaxis; their use is associated with significant long-term sequela (recurrent DVT and postphlebitic syndrome). However, percutaneous retrievable filters may have a role in very high-risk patients in whom pharmacological prophylaxis is contraindicated. Vena caval filters are frequently placed in trauma patients because of the perceived risk of pharmacological prophylaxis. However, a large randomized clinical trial supports the fact that pharmacological prophylaxis is both safe and effective in these patients.[8] Furthermore, there are no randomized prospective evaluations of temporary IVC interruption in this setting.

■ SUGGESTED DVT PROPHYLAXIS PROTOCOL

As a default, all patients should receive the following:

- Enoxaparin (or equivalent) 40 mg SC once daily or fondaparinux 2.5 mg SC once daily *plus* SCDs.
- Reduce dose of enoxaparin to 30 mg SC once daily with renal impairment.
- In patients with renal failure (GFR <35 ml/min), UFH 5,000 SC q 12 h *plus* SCDs.

■ UPPER EXTREMITY DVT

Upper extremity DVT is not uncommon in the ICU. Risk factors include central venous catheters, malignancy, previous lower extremity DVT, and inherited disorders of coagulation.[9–11] In a prospective study, Merrer and colleagues[12] reported that upper extremity DVT occurred in 1.9% of patients with a subclavian central venous catheter. As is the case with lower extremity DVT, most cases of upper extremity DVT are thought to be asymptomatic. Presenting features include pain and swelling of the extremity. These features should prompt a Doppler ultrasound examination. Complications of upper extremity DVT include pulmonary embolism and postthrombotic syndrome.[10] While there are no RCTs to guide the management of this condition, the "current standard" treatment is anti-coagulation with unfractionated heparin or LWMH followed by Coumadin for 3 months.[13]

■ PULMONARY EMBOLISM

Pulmonary embolism should be suspected in ICU patients with an unexplained deterioration in oxygenation and/or hemodynamic instability. It should also be considered in patients with new-onset atrial fibrillation/flutter. It is important to note that "unsuspected PE" may be the cause of a "COPD exacerbation" or worsening heart failure.[14]

Diagnosis of Pulmonary Embolism

The diagnosis of PE is one of the more challenging dilemmas in clinical medicine. While pulmonary angiography is the gold standard with which to compare other methods, angiography is invasive, costly, not readily available in most hospitals, and associated with significant complications. A contrast-enhanced helical CT (CTPA) is currently the diagnostic test of choice. This allows for the diagnosis of a major PE with a "high diagnostic accuracy" and also allows for the visualization of the lung parenchyma. In the PIOPED II study, a CTPA had a sensitivity 83% and a specificity of 96%; this increased to 90% and 95%, respectively, with CT venography (of the lower limbs).[15] Lower extremity Dopplers increase the diagnostic yield by about 10% and should be performed in patients with a negative CT scan (when CT venography is not performed). A V/Q scan is indicated in patients with a dye allergy and those with moderate to severe renal dysfunction. In ICU patients, positive venous Dopplers negate the need for further diagnostic testing (as the patient needs to be anti-coagulated anyway) and may be a safer first step. A D-dimer has limited diagnostic value in ICU patients; however, a negative D-Dimer (below 500 ng/ml) has a negative predictive value of about 90%.

Patients admitted to the ICU with PE require risk stratification as these patients may be candidates for thrombolytic therapy or mechanical clot extraction. This entails the following:

- Urgent ECHO to assess RV function
- Biomarkers such as BNP and troponins[16]

Data from the ICOPER and French registries have demonstrated that patients with RV dysfunction on ECHO have an increased risk of death.[17,18] RV function would appear to be the most important prognostic factor in PE.

Treatment of Thromboembolic Disease

Immediate anti-coagulation with heparin is the treatment of choice in all patients unless heparin is absolutely contraindicated (see below). Unfractionated heparin (UH) has until recently been considered the treatment of choice. However, with increasing experience with LMWH, this class of drugs is emerging as the drug of choice. LMWHs have a number of practical and therapeutic advantages over UH. The disadvantage of LMWHs includes their long half-life and difficulty in monitoring the degree of anti-coagulation. UH is indicated in "unstable" ICU patients and those at risk for bleeding. The following are the "standard" dosing regimens:

- UFH 80 U/kg IV bolus, 18 U/kg/h infusion; titrated to maintain PTT between 60 and 80 s
- Enoxaparin 1 mg/kg every 12 h or 1.5 mg/kg SC daily
- Tinzaparin 175 IU/kg SC daily
- Fondaparinux 5.0/7.5/10 mg SC daily

Thrombolytic Therapy

Thrombolytic therapy should be considered in patients with acute massive pulmonary embolus who are hemodynamically unstable (hypotension, oliguria) and who have no contraindication to thrombolysis. In hemodynamically stable patients, thrombolysis has not been proven to reduce mortality or the risk of recurrent PE. It has been suggested that in "hemodynamically stable" patients, the presence of right ventricular dysfunction (diagnosed by ECHO) might identify a subset of patients who may benefit from thrombolytic therapy. MAPPETT-3 randomized patients with sub-massive PE (with RV dysfunction) to t-PA plus UH or UH alone. The primary end point (which included escalation of care) occurred in 10.2% of t-PA patients compared to 24.6% of controls ($p = 0.005$). There was however no difference in mortality (3.4% vs. 2.2%, $p = 0.71$). Although no intracerebral bleeds occurred in MAPPETT-3, this remains the biggest concern. In the ICOPER registry, 3% of patients who received lytic therapy suffered an intracerebral bleed as compared to 0.3% treated with other agents.[17] The role of thrombolytic therapy in "hemodynamically stable" patients who demonstrate acute RV dilatation/failure remains controversial at this time.

Catheter-Directed Clot Fragmentation and Aspiration

In patients with sub-massive PE, catheter-directed clot fragmentation and aspiration may be a viable alternative to systemic thrombolysis in centers that have the expertise to perform this procedure.[19–21]

Vena Caval Interruption

No randomized controlled trial has been conducted which has compared heparin to vena caval interruption (alone) in the management of thromboembolic disease. However, the available evidence suggests that venal caval interruption is associated with a higher incidence of complications, particularly recurrent DVT and postphlebitic syndrome. Because of "presumed contraindications" to heparin, vena caval filters have become commonplace for the primary and secondary prevention of pulmonary embolism. This is in spite of lack of data on the relative safety and efficacy of venal caval interruption as compared with anti-coagulant therapy. However, most of the presumed contraindications have never been subject to rigorous analysis to determine whether they are associated with a worse outcome than are those treated with vena caval interruption. For example, intracranial neoplasms have been considered an "absolute" contraindication to anti-coagulation. However, studies have suggested a high complication rate with IVC filters in these patients. Furthermore, in this patient population, anti-coagulation is well tolerated, is associated with a low risk of intracerebral bleeding (if excessive anti-coagulation is avoided), and results in a better quality of life than is an IVC filter.[21]

"Absolute Contraindications" for Anti-coagulation with Heparin

- Recent intracerebral bleed (2–3 weeks).
- Recent gastrointestinal bleeding (2 weeks).
- Patients with heparin-associated thrombocytopenia; these patients can be treated with direct thrombin inhibitors which do not cross-react with heparin.

■ CLINICAL PEARLS

- All ICU patients require DVT prophylaxis.
- Enoxaparin (or equivalent) 40 mg SC once daily *plus* SCDs or fondaparinux 2.5 mg SC once daily *plus* SCDs should be considered as the default DVT prophylaxis regimen in ICU patients.

■ REFERENCES

1. Cook D, Crowther M, Meade M, et al. Deep venous thrombosis in medical–surgical critically ill patients: prevalence, incidence, and risk factors. *Crit Care Med.* 2005;33:1565–1571.
2. Marik PE, Andrews L, Maini B. The incidence of deep venous thrombosis in ICU patients. *Chest.* 1997;111:661–664.
3. Hirsch DR, Ingenito EP, Goldhaber SZ. Prevalence of deep venous thrombosis among patients in medical intensive care. *JAMA.* 1995;274:335–337.
4. Twigg SJ, McCrirrick A, Sanderson PM. A comparison of post mortem findings with post hoc estimated clinical diagnoses of patients who die in a United Kingdom intensive care unit. *Intensive Care Med.* 2001;27: 706–710.
5. Geerts WH, Bergqvist D, Pineo GF, et al. Prevention of venous thromboembolism: American College of Chest Physicians evidence-based clinical practice guidelines (8th Edition). *Chest.* 2008;133:381S–453S.
6. Agu O, Hamilton G, Baker D. Graduated compression stockings in the prevention of venous thromboembolism. *Br J Surg.* 1999;86:992–1004.
7. Phillips SM, Gallagher M, Buchan H. Use of graduated compression stockings postoperatively to prevent deep vein thrombosis. *BMJ.* 2008;336:943–944.
8. Geerts WH, Jay RM, Code KI, et al. A comparison of low-dose heparin with low-molecular-weight heparin as prophylaxis against venous

thromboembolism after major trauma. *N Engl J Med.* 1996;335: 701–707.

9. Mustafa S, Stein PD, Patel KC, et al. Upper extremity deep venous thrombosis. *Chest.* 2003;123:1953–1956.

10. Prandoni P, Polistena P, Bernardi E, et al. Upper-extremity deep vein thrombosis. Risk factors, diagnosis, and complications. *Arch Intern Med.* 1997;157:57–62.

11. Marinella MA, Kathula SK, Markert RJ. Spectrum of upper-extremity deep venous thrombosis in a community teaching hospital. *Heart Lung.* 2000;29:113–117.

12. Merrer J, De Jonghe B, Golliot F, et al. Complications of femoral and subclavian venous catheterization in critically ill patients: a randomized controlled trial. *JAMA.* 2001;286:700–707.

13. Shah MK, Burke DT. Upper-extremity deep vein thrombosis. *South Med J.* 2003;96:669–672.

14. Rizkallah J, Man P, Sin DD. Prevalence of pulmonary embolism in acute exacerbations of COPD. A systematic review and metaanalysis. *Chest.* 2009;135:786–793.

15. Stein PD, Woodard PK, Weg JG, et al. Diagnostic pathways in acute pulmonary embolism: recommendations of The PIOPED II Investigators. *Am J Med.* 2006;119:1048–1055.

16. Cavallazzi R, Nair A, Vasu T, et al. Natriuretic peptides in acute pulmonary embolism: a systematic review. *Intensive Care Med.* 2008;34:2147–2156.

17. Goldhaber SZ, Visani L, De RM, et al. Acute pulmonary embolism: clinical outcomes in the International Cooperative Pulmonary Embolism Registry (ICOPER). *Lancet.* 1999;353:1386–1389.

18. Fremont B, Pacouret G, Jacobi D, et al. Prognostic value of echocardiographic right/left ventricular end-diastolic diameter ratio in patients with acute pulmonary embolism: results from a monocenter registry of 1,416 patients. *Chest.* 2008;133:358–362.

19. Eid-Lidt G, Gasper J, Sandoval J, et al. Combined clot fragmentation and aspiration in patients with acute pulmonary embolism. *Chest.* 2008;134:54–60.

20. Kuo WT, van den Bosch MA, Hofmann LV, et al. Catheter-directed embolectomy, fragmentation, and thrombolysis for the treatment of massive pulmonary embolism after failure of systemic thrombolysis. *Chest.* 2008;134:250–254.

21. Gerber DE, Grossman SA, Streiff MB. Management of venous thromboembolism in patients with primary and metastatic brain tumors. *J Clin Oncol.* 2006;24:1310–1318.

22

COPD Exacerbation

A COPD exacerbation is defined as an increase in the symptoms of COPD (dyspnea, cough, sputum production, and sputum purulence) of a magnitude greater than the normal day-to-day variability.[1,2] An increase in airway inflammation is considered central to the pathogenesis of a COPD exacerbation. A stimulus that acutely increases airway inflammation results in increased bronchial tone, increased bronchial wall edema, and increased mucus production. These processes worsen ventilation–perfusion mismatch and expiratory flow limitation. Corresponding clinical manifestations include worsening gas exchange, dyspnea, cough, sputum production, and sputum purulence, which are the cardinal manifestations of an exacerbation.

Patients with chronic obstructive pulmonary disease (COPD) who acutely decompensate may benefit from admission to the ICU. Patients with COPD admitted to an ICU for an acute exacerbation of COPD have a hospital mortality of between 10 and 25% with a 1-year mortality of about 40%.[3,4] Long-term survival of patients with COPD who required mechanical ventilation for an acute exacerbation of their disease cannot be predicted simply from data available at the time of intubation. Furthermore, the need for mechanical ventilation appears not to influence either short- or long-term outcome; therefore, the need for mechanical ventilation should not be used as a reason for not offering respiratory support.[3,4] Non-invasive positive-pressure ventilation (NIPPV) should be considered prior to endotracheal intubation in suitable candidates (see Chapter 15).

■ COMMON PRECIPITATING EVENTS

Precipitating factors must be determined in patients with COPD who present with an acute deterioration in respiratory status.[3] While chest

P.E. Marik, *Handbook of Evidence-Based Critical Care*,
DOI 10.1007/978-1-4419-5923-2_22,
© Springer Science+Business Media, LLC 2010

infection is the most common precipitating factor, other readily treatable factors (e.g., atrial fibrillation, cardiac failure) should be actively investigated, including the following:

- Upper respiratory tract infection
- Chest infection: acute bronchitis or pneumonia
- Pneumothorax
- Pleural effusion
- Pulmonary embolus
- Heart failure
- Arrhythmias
- Atelectasis/mucous plugging
- Use of sedative agents

Lower airway colonization by bacteria is common in patients with stable COPD. *Haemophilus influenzae*, *Streptococcus pneumoniae,* and *Moraxella catarrhalis* are the most common colonizing organisms. Exacerbations of COPD are frequently associated with viral infections; influenza, parainfluenza, and respiratory syncytial viruses are the most common etiologic agents. Studies using invasive diagnostic testing suggest that between 50 and 70% of exacerbations of COPD are related to bacterial infection.[2] Approximately 25% of patients admitted to hospital with an exacerbation of COPD have coinfection with bacteria and viruses.[5] It is not possible to clinically differentiate those patients whose exacerbation of COPD is caused by a bacterial infection. *H. influenzae*, *S. pneumoniae*, *M. catarrhalis*, and *Chlamydia pneumoniae* are the most common pathogens; however, multi-drug-resistant (MDR) gram-negative rods (including *Pseudomonas aeruginosa*) are not uncommon.[6–8] Risk factors for MDR gram negatives include previous anti-microbial treatment and previous intubation.[6] Gram stain and culture should therefore be performed in all patients admitted to the ICU with an exacerbation of COPD (not to diagnose infection but to identify the potential pathogens).

Pulmonary embolism has been implicated in up to 25% of patients with a COPD exacerbation who require hospitalization.[9] Based on these data, all patients with a COPD exacerbation requiring admission to the ICU should undergo lower extremity Doppler studies. D-Dimer levels have a high-negative but a low-positive predictive value for PE in COPD exacerbations because a multitude of different inflammatory and infectious etiologies can cause blood D-dimers to rise.[10] A CTPA should be considered in those patients with negative Dopplers, a positive D-dimer, and an intermediate-to-high pretest probability of PE.

■ INDICATIONS FOR HOSPITALIZATION

- Comorbid conditions[1]
  - Pneumonia
  - Heart failure
  - Renal or liver failure
- Inadequate response of symptoms to outpatient management
- Marked increase in dyspnea
- Worsening hypoxemia
- Worsening hypercapnia
- Changes in mental status
- Inability for patient to care of her/himself

■ INDICATIONS FOR ICU ADMISSION

- Impending or actual respiratory failure[1]
- Hemodynamic instability
- Increasing confusion or obtundation

■ TREATMENT

- Correct hypoxia; this usually requires only small increases in FiO_2. A high PaO_2 may cause an increase in CO_2; the mechanisms of this phenomenon are complex and include an increase in V/Q mismatching, the Haldane effect, and possibly a suppression of the "hypoxic drive." Patients with severe COPD develop chronic compensatory mechanisms for a low PaO_2 and therefore do not require a "normal" PaO_2; a PaO_2 between 50 and 60 mmHg is usually well tolerated. An elevated $PaCO_2$ is acceptable as long as the patient is alert and cooperative and the arterial pH >7.2.[1]
- The results of RCTs demonstrate that NIPPV reduces the need for intubation, reduces in-hospital mortality, and shortens hospital stay during acute COPD exacerbations.[11] NIPPV should be considered in all patients who are alert and cooperative and able to tolerate NIPPV (see Chapter 15).
- Empiric antibiotics are usually given even in the absence of clinical features of infection. A meta-analysis demonstrated that antibiotics significantly reduced treatment failures in hospitalized patients (RR 0.34; 95% CI 0.20–0.56) and mortality (RR 0.22; 95% CI 0.08–0.62).[11] The antibiotic of choice in a patient with a COPD exacerbation should be guided by knowledge of the local pathogens and their sensitivity patterns. Ampicillin/clavulanate or

respiratory fluoroquinolones (levofloxacin, moxifloxacin) are suitable choices. The antibiotics may need to be changed, guided by sputum/lower respiratory tract sampling culture results. Antipseudomonal/extended-spectrum β-lactams will be required in patients "colonized" with *P. aeruginosa* or other MDR gram negatives and vancomycin/linezolid in those with MRSA.[8]

- Inhaled bronchodilators are usually given to all patients even if the patient does not have measurable reversible airway disease. β2-Agonists and ipratropium bromide should be used.
- A short course of intravenous corticosteroid has been shown to be beneficial even in patients with no demonstrable airway obstruction. In a recent meta-analysis, corticosteroid treatment was associated with a more rapid improvement in FEV1, significantly fewer treatment failures, and a shorter duration of hospitalization as compared to placebo.[12] The initial dose of corticosteroid (first 72 h) varied from 30 to 500 mg prednisone/methylprednisolone (VA study) per day, with no clear dose–response effect. While the optimal dose and the duration of treatment are unclear, methylprednisolone 30–60 mg q 12 h for 7–10 days would be a reasonable compromise between treatment effect and drug-associated complications.
- DVT prophylaxis; LMWH or subcutaneous heparin.
- Do not use sedative drugs unless the patient is on a ventilator:
  - Dexmedetomidine may be a suitable choice in patients with a COPD exacerbation (see Chapter 9).

Indications for NIPPV

- Respiratory rate >30 breaths/min
- PaO_2 <45–50 mmHg (on room air)
- $PaCO_2$ >45–50 mmHg
- pH <7.32

Indications for Endotracheal Intubation

- Somnolence/decreased level of arousal
- Unable to protect airway
- Unable to deal with pulmonary secretions
- Failed trial of NIPPV

■ MECHANICAL VENTILATION IN COPD

Despite the use of NIPPV, as many as 50% of patients with a COPD exacerbation will require intubation and mechanical ventilation. Most of these patients have underlying chronic ventilatory failure with a baseline state of chronic compensated respiratory acidosis (i.e., high baseline PCO_2, high HCO_3 with a low-normal pH). The serum bicarbonate level on admission, or even better, obtained during a recent period of stability, may provide an indirect indication of the patient's baseline $PaCO_2$. Ventilator settings that produce a "normal" $PaCO_2$ will likely lead to renal dumping of bicarbonate, leading to difficulty in weaning from the ventilator since this level will be needed to maintain the status quo off the mechanical ventilator. "Controlled hypoventilation" should guide management, aiming for a $PaCO_2$ at or above the patient's usual baseline with a pH target of 7.32–7.36.

ALERT

Do not aim to normalize blood gasses in patients with COPD; these patients are usually members of the "50–50 club"; so aim to keep $PaCO_2$ and PaO_2 near baseline levels.

Worsened airway inflammation, edema, bronchospasm, and increased secretions cause patients with a COPD exacerbation to experience increased airway obstruction and greater than usual degrees of airway closure and inhomogeneous ventilation. If adequate time is not given for expiration, end-expiratory lung volume increases beyond the normal functional residual capacity (FRC). The result is dynamic hyperinflation of the lung, with positive end-expiratory pressure in the lung due to this trapped gas, referred to as intrinsic PEEP (iPEEP), air trapping, or auto-PEEP. Gas trapping and iPEEP have multiple adverse consequences.

Other than treating the underlying condition with bronchodilators and anti-inflammatory agents, the primary method by which dynamic hyperinflation is reduced is through increasing expiratory time.[13] This is accomplished by reducing the respiratory rate but can also be treated by altering the inspiratory-to-expiratory (*I:E*) ratio. A decelerating waveform results in the lowest peak inspiratory pressure, physiological dead–space ratio, and $PaCO_2$ compared to square and sine wave patterns. Somewhat more controversial is the application of extrinsic PEEP (ePEEP) to decrease air trapping in patients with COPD (see Chapter 23). In most instances ePEEP is best avoided as it may worsen lung hyperinflation and air trapping.

Patients with COPD should not be oversedated as they are likely to lose their respiratory drive. A combination of dexmedetomidine and fentanyl are suggested (see Chapter 9).

Suggested Initial Settings

- Mode: AC
- Rate: 12–14 breaths/min
- Tidal volume: 6–8 ml/kg IBW
- PEEP: 0
- FiO_2: 40–60%

These settings should be dynamically adjusted to achieve an arterial saturation of 88–92% (by pulse oximetry) and a low-normal pH (a venous blood gas is just fine). The time–flow waveform should be monitored to ensure adequate expiratory time and the iPEEP should be measured (see also Chapter 14).

■ CLINICAL PEARLS

- NIPPV should be considered in patients with a COPD exacerbation with impending or overt respiratory failure.
- Patients with a COPD exacerbation admitted to the ICU require treatment with systemic corticosteroids and targeted antibiotics.
- Sputum/tracheal culture, lower extremity Dopplers, and a D-dimer should be performed soon after admission in all patients with a COPD exacerbation admitted to the ICU.
- Do not overventilate patients with a COPD exacerbation.

■ REFERENCES

1. Celli BR, MacNee W, ERS TF, et al. Standards for the diagnosis and treatment of patients with COPD: a summary of the ATS/ERS position paper. *Eur Resp J*. 2004;23:932–946.
2. Sethi S. New developments in the pathogenesis of acute exacerbations of chronic obstructive pulmonary disease. *Curr Opin Infect Dis*. 2004;17:113–119.
3. Afessa B, Morales IJ, Scanlon PD, et al. Prognostic factors, clinical course, and hospital outcome of patients with chronic obstructive pulmonary disease admitted to an intensive care unit for acute respiratory failure. *Crit Care Med*. 2002;30:1610–1615.
4. Ai-Ping C, Lee KH, Lim TK. In-hospital and 5-year mortality of patients treated in the ICU for acute exacerbation of COPD: a retrospective study. *Chest*. 2005;128:518–524.
5. Papi A, Bellettato CM, Braccioni F, et al. Infections and airway inflammation in chronic obstructive pulmonary disease severe exacerbations. *Am J Respir Crit Care Med*. 2006;173:1114–1121.

6. Nseir S, Di PC, Cavestri B, et al. Multiple-drug-resistant bacteria in patients with severe acute exacerbation of chronic obstructive pulmonary disease: prevalence, risk factors, and outcome. *Crit Care Med.* 2006;34:2959–2966.

7. Soler N, Torres A, Ewig S, et al. Bronchial microbial patterns in severe exacerbations of chronic obstructive pulmonary disease (COPD) requiring mechanical ventilation. *Am J Respir Crit Care Med* 1998;157: 1498–1505.

8. Ferrer M, Ioanas M, Arancibia F, et al. Microbial airway colonization is associated with noninvasive ventilation failure in exacerbation of chronic obstructive pulmonary disease. *Crit Care Med.* 2005;33:2003–2009.

9. Rizkallah J, Man P, Sin DD. Prevalence of pulmonary embolism in acute exacerbations of COPD. A systematic review and metaanalysis. *Chest.* 2009;135:786–793.

10. Sohne M, Kruip MJ, Nijkeuter M, et al. Accuracy of clinical decision rule, D-dimer and spiral computed tomography in patients with malignancy, previous venous thromboembolism, COPD or heart failure and in older patients with suspected pulmonary embolism. *J Throm Haemo.* 2006;4:1042–1046.

11. Quon BS, Gan WQ, Sin DD. Contemporary management of acute exacerbations of COPD: a systematic review and metaanalysis. *Chest.* 2008;133:756–766.

12. Walters JA, Gibson PG, Wood-Baker R, et al. Systemic corticosteroids for acute exacerbations of chronic obstructive pulmonary disease. *Cochrane Database Syst Rev.* 2009;1:CD001288.

13. Ward NS, Dushay KM. Clinical concise review: mechanical ventilation of patients with chronic obstructive pulmonary disease. *Crit Care Med.* 2008;36:1614–1619.

23

Acute Severe Asthma

Two distinctive phenotypes of near-fatal asthma have been identified: one with eosinophilic inflammation associated with a gradual onset and a slow response to therapy and a second phenotype with neutrophilic inflammation associated with a rapid onset and a rapid response to therapy.[1] Patients who develop sudden-onset, near-fatal asthma frequently have massive allergen exposure or acute emotional distress.

■ INDICATIONS FOR ADMISSION TO THE ICU

- Difficulty in talking due to breathlessness
- Altered level of consciousness
- Inability to lie supine
- FEV1 and/or peak flow <40% predicted
- Pulsus paradoxus >18 mmHg
- Pneumothorax or pneumomediastinum
- PaO_2 <65 mmHg on 40% O_2
- $PaCO_2$ >40 mmHg
- Patient tiring
- Poor (or no) response to initial bronchodilator therapy (<10% increase in peak expiratory flow rate)
- Heart rate >120 beats/min

Early response to treatment (PEFR or FEV1 at 30 min) in the ED is the most important predictor of outcome and a useful guide for admission to the ICU. PEFR increase over baseline of >50 l/min and PEFR >40% of normal, both measured at 30 min after beginning of treatment, are predictors of good outcome.

P.E. Marik, *Handbook of Evidence-Based Critical Care*,
DOI 10.1007/978-1-4419-5923-2_23,
© Springer Science+Business Media, LLC 2010

The classic signs of wheezing correlate poorly with the degree of airflow limitation. Severely obstructed patients may have a silent chest if there is insufficient alveolar ventilation and airflow for wheezes to occur. In these patients, the development of wheezes generally indicates improved airflow. Localized wheezing or crackles on chest auscultation may represent mucous plugging or atelectasis, but they should prompt consideration of pneumonia, pneumothorax, endobronchial lesions, or a foreign body.

■ INITIAL TREATMENT

- Oxygen mask.
- Short-acting β-2 agonist by nebulization every 15–20 min initially, then 1–4 h.
- Ipratropium bromide nebulization, q 2–4 h, has synergistic bronchodilatory activity with β-2 agonists.
- Corticosteroids: methylprednisolone 60 mg IV q 6 h.
- Do not use sedative drugs unless the patient is on a ventilator. If the patient has a large psychosomatic component to his/her asthma and sedative drugs are deemed necessary, use small doses and observe closely in an ICU.
- Keep the patient well hydrated.

Larger and more frequent doses of β-agonists are needed in acute severe asthma because the dose–response curve and the duration of activity of these drugs are affected adversely by the degree of bronchoconstriction. Recent data suggest that in both non-intubated and intubated patients, metered dose inhalers combined with a spacing device are just as effective as nebulizers, and they are quicker and cheaper to use (four to six puffs of albuterol every 20 min).[2]

Subcutaneously administered epinephrine or terbutaline sulfate has no advantage over inhaled β-agonists. Subcutaneous therapy should be considered, however, in patients not responding to inhaled β-agonists. Furthermore, the available data do not support the routine use of intravenous β-agonists in the treatment of patients with severe asthma.[3] Several studies have demonstrated inhaled therapy to be equal to or better than intravenous therapy in treating airflow obstruction, and less likely to cause cardiac toxicity. However, intravenous β-agonists may be considered in patients who have not responded to inhaled therapy and have life-threatening disease.

■ OTHER THERAPEUTIC OPTIONS

- Leukotriene antagonists. Despite limited data, leukotriene antagonists should be considered in patients who have responded poorly to initial therapy.[4] An RCT of patients with moderate to severe acute asthma treated with intravenous montelukast demonstrated less β-agonist use and patients receiving intravenous montelukast had fewer treatment failures than did patients receiving placebo.[5]
- Intravenous β-2 agonists.
- Theophylline should be reserved only for those patients not responding to standard therapy. A loading dose of 6 mg/kg over 30 min is followed by an infusion of 0.5 mg/kg/h with measurement of theophylline levels (target of 8–12 μg/ml). In patients already receiving theophylline, a serum level should be measured and appropriate dosing continued if deemed necessary.
- Subcutaneous epinephrine 0.3 ml 1:1,000 solution (drug of choice in anaphylactoid asthma). Epinephrine should be avoided in patients with a history of ischemic heart disease and/or hypertension.
- Heliox is a blend of helium and oxygen (80:20, 70:30, or 60:40) with a gas density approximately one-third that of air. In normal subjects, heliox reduces airway resistance (R_{aw}) by about 40% and increases maximum expiratory flows by about 50%. Heliox may be useful in buying time and avoiding intubation in acute attacks of asthma. In mechanically ventilated patients with severe asthma, heliox (60:40) has been demonstrated to reduce peak inspiratory pressure and $PaCO_2$ by up to 50%.
- Mechanically ventilated patients with severe bronchospasm in whom mechanical ventilation has become extremely difficult (cannot get air in or out) may benefit from halothane or enflurane anesthesia. This procedure should be performed only in the operating room by an experienced anesthesiologist.
- Intravenous magnesium has no proven benefit in acute severe asthma.[6]

■ COMPLICATIONS OF ACUTE ASTHMA

- Pneumothorax
- Pneumomediastinum, pneumopericardium
- Myocardial infarction
- Mucous plugging
- Atelectasis
- Theophylline toxicity

- Lactic acidosis
- Myopathy

■ NON-INVASIVE POSITIVE-PRESSURE VENTILATION IN STATUS ASTHMATICUS

Patients with severe asthma have a significant increase in both inspiratory and expiratory indexes of airway obstruction and considerable dynamic compliance. Inspiratory muscle failure and increased physiological dead space lead to ventilatory failure. Endotracheal intubation is associated with a high rate of complications and results in increased airway resistance. In patients with COPD and acute respiratory failure, non-invasive positive-pressure ventilation (NIPPV) has been demonstrated to be very effective in reducing the work of breathing, improving oxygenation, and reducing the need for intubation. Several studies have demonstrated that in severe asthma, mask continuous positive airway pressure (CPAP) causes the following:

- Bronchodilation and decreases airway resistance.
- Re-expands atelectasis and promotes removal of secretions.
- Rests the diaphragm and inspiratory muscles and may offset intrinsic positive end-expiratory pressure (iPEEP).
- Decreases the adverse hemodynamic effects of large negative peak and mean inspiratory pleural pressures.

Meduri et al.[7] have demonstrated that NIPPV can be safely applied to patients with severe asthma and hypercarbia whose condition has failed to improve with aggressive medical management. In their series, only 2 of 17 patients required intubation. Similarly, Fernandez described the successful use of NIPPV in 19 of 22 patients with status asthmatics; the remaining three patients required mechanical ventilation. Soroksky et al., in a prospective, randomized, placebo-controlled study, compared 15 patients with status asthmatics who received NIPPV plus conventional therapy vs. conventional therapy alone. The use of NIPPV significantly improved lung function and decreased hospitalization rate. It may be reasonable to try NIPPV before intubation in alert cooperative patients (see Chapter 15). NIPPV should not be attempted in patients who are rapidly deteriorating or are somnolent or confused.

■ INDICATIONS FOR INTUBATION

Endotracheal intubation is not curative, is associated with significant morbidity, and can increase the degree of airway narrowing and inflammation. The timing of intubation is essentially one of clinical judgment. A high $PaCO_2$ in itself is not an indication for intubation if the patient is alert and cooperative and the arterial pH >7.2. The following are indications for intubation and mechanical ventilation:

- Altered consciousness
- PaO_2 <50 mmHg on a rebreathing mask
- Rising $PaCO_2$ with a falling pH
- Anaphylactic asthma with rapidly deteriorating clinical course
- Patient fatigue

Intubating an asthmatic patient can be extremely difficult and should be performed by an operator with extensive experience in upper airway management. It should be remembered that it may be impossible to ventilate a severe asthmatic with an Ambu bag (air will follow the path of least resistance and go into the stomach). Orotracheal intubation will invariably require rapid-sequence anesthesia.

Sedation Postintubation

Sedation is invariably required postintubation as the settings required to achieve hypoventilation are not tolerated by awake and alert patients. In the past, paralytics were often administered to facilitate synchronization of the asthmatic with the mechanical ventilator, to avoid excessive hyperinflation, to facilitate permissive hypercapnia, and to decrease respiratory muscle activity. However, numerous studies have indicated an unacceptable incidence of postparalytic myopathy in patients with asthma and respiratory failure.[8] In most cases, the myopathy is reversible but may take weeks to resolve. This complication is associated with a significant increase in complications as well as length of ICU and hospital stay. Neuromuscular blockers should therefore be avoided in patients with asthma at all costs. The combination of propofol and fentanyl is suggested to avoid the use of paralytic agents (see Chapter 8). Propofol has the additional advantage of having bronchodilator properties.[9]

■ MECHANICAL VENTILATION

Mechanical ventilation may precipitate cardiorespiratory collapse in patients with severe asthma. Causative factors are pulmonary hyperinflation, hypovolemia, and sedation.[7] In the postintubation period, dangerous levels of pulmonary hyperinflation can develop if patients are "bagged" excessively in a misguided attempt to stabilize or resuscitate the patient. With severe airflow obstruction, even delivery of a normal minute ventilation may cause substantial gas trapping that reduces venous return and hence cardiac output. Concomitantly, hypovolemia related to previous dehydration, sedation, and muscle relaxation all act to decrease mean systemic vascular pressure, further decreasing venous return to the heart.

Mechanical ventilation of patients with severe asthma is fraught with difficulties. Severe airflow obstruction results in a prolonged expiratory time with incomplete exhalation even at low ventilator rates. This results in progressive dynamic hyperinflation and the development of auto-PEEP (iPEEP) until a new equilibrium is reached at some volume above functional residual capacity (FRC). This equilibrium occurs because increasing lung volume increases both the lung elastic recoil pressure driving expiratory flow and reduced airway resistance by expansion of the small airways in parallel with lung volume. If large tidal volumes and rates are used, significant iPEEP will develop. iPEEP acts as an inspiratory threshold load and contributes to the increased work of breathing. Furthermore, iPEEP may be associated with severe hemodynamic compromise. These effects are compounded by the fact that the minute ventilation required for normocapnia is increased to approximately 16 ± 3 l/min in patients with severe asthma. These changes will result in increased morbidity and mortality if patients are ventilated to achieve normocapnia.

The use of PEEP (extrinsic PEEP) in patients with asthma is controversial. PEEP has been demonstrated to reduce the work of breathing and dyspnea in patients with severe COPD and acute respiratory failure. Because flow is limited in the small airways, low levels of pressure applied downstream from the compression site may alter its anatomic location without causing a proportional rise in alveolar pressure. PEEP that is set at a level below iPEEP might then dilate collapsed or severely narrowed airways, enabling decompression of the alveolar units they serve. In addition, this will narrow the gradient between end-expiratory alveolar pressure (total PEEP) and the pressure in the central airways. This would then reduce the effort required to trigger the ventilator. However, PEEP has been demonstrated to increase lung volumes and alveolar pressures with a concomitant fall in venous return and hypotension. A practical method of identifying those patients who may benefit from PEEP may be to observe the response of the ventilator cycling pressures to small increments of PEEP. If little change in peak dynamic and static cycling pressures occurs after PEEP, then extensive dynamic collapse is unlikely and PEEP may be helpful. The level of PEEP should not be set higher than the level of the original iPEEP. On the other hand, if the cycling pressures increase in direct relationship to the level of applied PEEP, additional hyperinflation will develop.

It is rarely a problem to oxygenate the patient with severe asthma; the problem is one of achieving adequate alveolar ventilation. The goals of ventilatory therapy include the following:

- Keep end-inspiratory pressure (plateau) <35 cm H_2O.
- Maintain arterial pH >7.2.
- Limit iPEEP to <5–10 cm H_2O.

Synchronized intermittent mandatory ventilation (SIMV) with no or very low pressure support is recommended. The assist-control ventilation should not be used, because it can lead the patient to generate excessive minute ventilation, resulting in excessive iPEEP. The setting of the inspiratory flow rate remains controversial, with both high and low flow rates being recommended. The weight of evidence appears to favor a high inspiratory flow. However, in patients with severe airway obstruction, a prolonged inspiratory time may be required; a high flow rate will result in excessive pressures in these patients.

Initial Ventilator Settings

- FiO_2 60–80%[10]
- Respiratory rate of 8–12 breaths/min, depending on the degree of airway obstruction
- Peak flow of 80–100 l/min
- Tidal volume of 5–7 ml/kg IBW

The iPEEP and the exhaled tidal volumes must be measured in all patients to avoid significant air trapping and the flow–time waveforms followed closely. A low *I:E* ratio (long expiration) should always be used. Permissive hypoventilation should be used in patients with severe airway obstruction aiming to maintain the arterial pH above 7.2 (if possible). Sodium bicarbonate should be avoided as it is likely to make matter worse (increased intracellular CO_2 and acidosis) due to reduced CO_2 elimination.

- Atelectasis should be treated by chest physiotherapy and airway humidification.
- Bronchoscopy is potentially dangerous in intubated asthmatic patients.
- Maintain adequate hydration.

ALERT

All that wheezes is not asthma.

Paradoxical vocal cord motion disorder (PVCM), also called vocal cord dysfunction, is an important differential diagnosis for asthma.[11] The disorder is often misdiagnosed as asthma leading to unnecessary drug use, very high medical utilization, and occasionally tracheal intubation or tracheostomy. Laryngoscopy is the gold standard for diagnosis of PVCM (during an episode); the diagnosis is usually made based on the clinical features alone. However, it is important to recognize that patients may have both asthma and PVCM, which complicates the management of these very "difficult" patients. Benzodiazepines used to sedate patients and relieve their anxiety have been shown to be effective in terminating acute symptoms of PVCM. However, it is prudent to confirm normal oxygen saturation and exclude hypercapnia before administering these drugs.

■ **CLINICAL PEARLS**

- *Avoid* neuromuscular blockers.
- *Prevent* dynamic hyperinflation; small tidal volumes and low rate.
- Be patient; the "attack" will "brake."

■ **REFERENCES**

1. Restrepo RD, Peters J. Near-fatal asthma: recognition and management. *Curr Opin Pulm Med.* 2008;14:13–23.
2. Colacone A, Afilalo M, Wolkove N, et al. A comparison of albuterol administered by metered dose inhaler (and holding chamber) or wet nebulizer in acute asthma. *Chest.* 1993;104:835–841.
3. Beveridge RC, Grunfeld AF, Hodder RV, et al. Guidelines for the emergency management of asthma in adults. CAEP/CTS Asthma Advisory Committee. Canadian Association of Emergency Physicians and the Canadian Thoracic Society. *CMAJ.* 1996;155:25–37.
4. Ferreira MB, Santos AS, Pregal AL, et al. Leukotriene receptor antagonists (Montelukast) in the treatment of asthma crisis: preliminary results of a double-blind placebo controlled randomized study. *Allerg Immunol.* 2001;33:315–318.

5. Camargo CA Jr., Smithline HA, Malice MP, et al. A randomized controlled trial of intravenous montelukast in acute asthma. *Am J Respir Crit Care Med*. 2003;167:528–533.
6. Rodrigo G, Rodrigo C, Burschtin O. Efficacy of magnesium sulfate in acute adult asthma: a meta-analysis of randomized trials. *Am J Emerg Med*. 2000;18:216–221.
7. Meduri GU, Cook TR, Turner RE, et al. Noninvasive positive pressure ventilation in status asthmaticus. *Chest*. 1996;110:767–774.
8. Adnet F, Dhissi G, Borron SW, et al. Complication profiles of adult asthmatics requiring paralysis during mechanical ventilation. *Intensive Care Med*. 2001;27:1729–1736.
9. Marik PE. Propofol: therapeutic indications and side effects. *Curr Pharm Des*. 2004;10:3639–3649.
10. Rodrigo GJ, Rodrigo C, Hall JB. Acute asthma in adults: a review. *Chest*. 2004;125:1081–1102.
11. Ibrahim WH, Gheriani HA, Almohamed AA, et al. Paradoxical vocal cord motion disorder: past, present and future. *Postgrad Med J*. 2007;83:164–172.

24

Pleural Effusions and Atelectasis

Both pleural effusions and atelectasis are exceedingly common in mechanically ventilated patients.[1] While in some patients the diagnosis is clearly obvious, in many it may be difficult to distinguish these two entities apart. Furthermore, both entities may coexist in the same patient (atelectasis over and above "compression atelectasis" caused by the effusion).[1] Attempting to drain a "pleural effusion" by sticking a needle into an atelectatic lung is a recipe for disaster (potentially fatal bleeding). A bedside ultrasound (or chest CT) is recommended in all circumstances of suspected atelectasis/pleural effusion, except for those patients with obvious lobar lung collapse. Drainage of a pleural effusion must always be performed under ultrasound guidance (see Chapter 6).

■ PLEURAL EFFUSIONS

Pleural effusions are common and related to the following:

- Volume overload in the setting of sepsis/SIRS/ALI
- Left-sided heart failure
- Chronic critical illness and hypoproteinemia
- Cirrhosis
- Pneumonia
- Pancreatitis

P.E. Marik, *Handbook of Evidence-Based Critical Care*,
DOI 10.1007/978-1-4419-5923-2_24,
© Springer Science+Business Media, LLC 2010

Pathophysiology

Experimental studies demonstrate that hydrostatic and permeability pulmonary edema are followed by pleural fluid accumulation that comes from the lung interstitium.[2-4] Furthermore, there is a good correlation between extravascular lung water content and pleural effusion volume. The notion that the major source of hydrostatic effusion is the lung is further supported by clinical studies showing that in patients with chronically elevated hydrostatic pressures, the presence of pleural effusion correlates better with left than right heart filling pressures. These data suggest that the excess fluid exits the lung via the visceral pleura into the pleural space.

Lung collapse associated with pleural effusions may lead to hypoxemia due to ventilation–perfusion mismatch or true shunt. The extent of these abnormalities depends upon the extent of perfusion of the compressed airspace, as determined by local factors such as hypoxic vasoconstriction and vascular compression.

The reduction in lung volume induced by a pleural effusion can be largely attributed to the collapse of the dependent portions of the lung most prominent at end expiration. However, the change in lung volumes is less than the volume of the pleural effusion and is dependent on the compliance of the lungs and the chest wall. The more compliant the lung, the greater the change in lung FRC; the more compliant the chest wall, the greater the thoracic cage adjustment with a smaller impact on lung volume. A number of studies in spontaneously breathing patients with unilateral pleural effusion show a disproportionately small increase in lung volumes after large volume thoracentesis and no or poor relationship between the volume of fluid removed and the increase in lung volume. In mechanically ventilated patients, the effect of pleural fluid drainage on lung volumes and gas exchange has been variable, with some studies demonstrating little improvement in PaO_2/FiO_2 ratio while others demonstrating a significant increase in the PaO_2/FiO_2 ratio.[5-7] The response to fluid drainage may depend on the applied airway pressure. Alveolar pressure generated during the respiratory cycle may not be enough to reopen collapsed lung (see lung recruitment below). Recruitment maneuvers (including bilevel ventilation) should therefore be considered after drainage of a pleural effusion.

Drainage of Pleural Effusion

Pleural fluid may be drained by either thoracentesis or placement of a small bore catheter (pigtail catheter).[5-9] A pigtail catheter is recommended for large effusions. A pigtail catheter may also obviate the need to repeat thoracentesis. Pleural fluid drainage should always be performed under ultrasound guidance (see Chapter 6). Ultrasound allows estimation of the size of the effusion[10,11]; attempts at thoracentesis should be aborted in patients with small effusions (less than 750–1,000 ml). Furthermore, ultrasound allows the procedure to be performed safely, particularly in ventilated patients.[8,9,12]

Not all patients with a pleural effusion require drainage. This should be considered only in patients with a low PaO_2/FiO_2 and in patients who have failed a spontaneous breathing trial. However, in an intriguing study (published in abstract only), Adenigbagbe et al.[13] randomized 168 mechanically ventilated patients with a pleural effusion to standard care or standard care plus pigtail drainage. The average duration of drainage was 2.8 days with 1,220 ml being drained in the first 24 h. The average duration of mechanical ventilation was 3.8 days in the pigtail group compared to 6.5 days in the control group ($p = 0.01$). This study challenges "conventional wisdom" and suggests that it may be a worthwhile exercise to drain all large effusions in patients on mechanical ventilation.

■ HEPATIC HYDROTHORAX

Hepatic hydrothorax is defined as the presence of pleural fluid (usually greater than 500 cm^3) in a patient with cirrhosis in the absence of primary cardiac or pulmonary disease. This complication occurs in approximately 6–10% of patients with advanced cirrhosis and has a predilection for the right hemithorax. The incidence of pleural effusion is much higher with the concomitant presence of ascitic fluid. However, isolated hepatic hydrothorax (usually on the right) may occur. The direct passage of peritoneal fluid via diaphragmatic defects appears to be the most plausible cause in most cases.[14] The composition of the pleural fluid from hepatic hydrothorax, as expected, is similar to that of ascitic fluid and is always transudative.

A diagnostic thoracentesis is indicated in all cases to exclude spontaneous bacterial empyema (SBEM) and other causes including the following[15]:

- Tuberculosis
- Adenocarcinoma
- Parapneumonic empyema
- Undiagnosed exudates

SBEM is defined as an infection of pre-existing pleural fluid (hydrothorax) in a patient with cirrhosis. Pathogenesis, bacteriology, diagnostic criteria, and treatment are similar to those of SBP. Diagnostic criteria include the following:

- PMN count >500 cells/mm^3
- Positive culture with PMN >250 cells/mm^3

The treatment of a hepatic hydrothorax is similar to that of ascites: sodium restriction, cautious dieresis, and treatment of portal hypertension. However, in most patients, this is ineffective and liver transplantation remains the only definitive treatment.

ALERT

Tube thoracostomy (and pigtail drainage) is considered a contraindication for the treatment of hepatic hydrothorax; this may lead to massive fluid shifts, significant protein and electrolyte losses, hemodynamic compromise, and death. A fistulous tract which continues to leak fluid may also develop.[14,16]

■ ATELECTASIS

Mechanically ventilated patients have an ineffective cough reflex and are unable to adequately deal with their respiratory sections. Atelectasis is therefore a common problem in these patients. The risk of atelectasis may be increased with the widespread use of a lung protective strategy utilizing low tidal volumes (6 ml/kg IBW).[17] Atelectasis may worsen hypoxemia through shunting and may predispose to nosocomial pneumonia. Traditionally, the treatment of atelectasis in mechanically ventilated patients has centered on chest therapy (slapping, beating, and vibrating) and endotracheal suctioning.[18] When this fails, bronchoscopy and/or recruitment maneuvers are attempted.[19]

Respiratory Therapy

Respiratory therapy refers to "treatments" provided by the respiratory therapist to aid in lung expansion and mobilizes retained secretions. This includes techniques to loosen and mobilize secretions including saline instillation, endotracheal suctioning and chest clapping/vibration, and recruitment (hyperinflation) maneuvers. Manual hyperinflation delivers a large tidal volume breath over a prolonged inspiratory time, followed by an inspiratory hold and a rapid release of pressure.[18] The goal is to stimulate cough and propel mucous cephalad. There are limited data with respect to the efficacy of manual hyperinflation; however, high airway pressure and large lung volumes may produce adverse homodynamic effects and injure the lung via barotrauma and/or volutrauma. Maa and colleagues[18] performed a randomized controlled trial in which ventilated patients with atelectasis were randomized to manual hyperinflations three times a day or to "standard" care. The manual hyperinflation technique used a rate of 8–13 breaths/min for a period of 20 min in each session. The manual hyperinflations were performed by a single investigator using a predefined protocol which limited peak airway pressure to 20 cm H_2O. Spontaneous tidal volumes, oxygenation, sputum volume, and chest radiographic score increased in the treatment group, whereas these indices remained largely unchanged in the standard care group. The mechanical ventilator can be used to achieve hyperinflation with similar results.[20,21] This approach may be safer as the inflation volumes and pressures can be preset. High-frequency chest wall vibration/compression/oscillation, rib cage compression (or squeezing), and chest wall "clapping/slapping" have been used to loosen and mobilize secretions. There is however no evidence that any of these interventions have any beneficial effects and they are currently not recommended in mechanically ventilated patients.[22,23]

Bronchoscopy

Bronchoscopy is a commonly performed treatment for atelectasis, with reports indicating that more than 50% of bronchoscopies performed in the ICU are for retained secretions and/or atelectasis.[24,25] However, the utility of fiber-optic bronchoscopy for the treatment of atelectasis is unclear. Olopade and Prakash[25] reviewed the experience at the Mayo Clinic over a 4-year period from 1985 to 1988. During this period, 90 fiber-optic bronchoscopies were performed for atelectasis and retained secretions, with only 17 (19%) patients demonstrating an improvement in oxygenation or radiographic changes following the procedure. Stevens and colleagues[26] reported their experience with 297 fiber-optic bronchoscopies in 223 ICU patients. Of the 118 patients in whom FOB was performed for atelectasis, 93 (79%) patients showed an improvement in aeration on examination, oxygenation, or chest radiographic appearance. However, of the 70 patients in whom bronchoscopy was performed for retained secretions, only 31 (44%) patients improved following the procedure. Marini and colleagues,[19] in the only randomized controlled study reported to date, compared an aggressive chest therapy regimen with that of fiber-optic bronchoscopy in 31 patients with acute lobar atelectasis. Forty-three percent of the patients in this study were intubated at the time of treatment. Chest therapy was performed every 4 h in both groups and included deep breathing (non-intubated patients) or manual inflations and endotracheal suctioning, as well as nebulization and chest percussion. In this study, approximately 65% of the volume loss on the chest radiograph was restored by 24 h (and 80% at 48 h) with no difference between groups (ventilated bronchoscopy vs. chest therapy and non-ventilated bronchoscopy vs. chest therapy).

Bilevel/APRV

Non-invasive modes of ventilation which provide positive pressure including continuous positive airway pressure (CPAP), bilevel positive airway pressure, and pressure-support ventilation have been used successfully in surgical patients to both prevent[23,27,28] and treat[29] postoperative atelectasis. We have demonstrated APRV (bilevel ventilation) to be very effective in re-expanding atelectatic lung in patients who have failed traditional approaches.[30] We use a high pressure of 20–25 cm H_2O, a low pressure of 5 cm H_2O, and a low time of 1–1.4 s (see Chapter 14). Although recruitment maneuvers may be effective in improving gas exchange and compliance, these effects are not sustained; APRV may be viewed as a nearly continuous recruitment maneuver. Ventilation modes such as APRV are likely to be more successful than conventional recruitment maneuvers as they provide a more gradual and prolonged recruitment of alveoli. We believe that endotracheal suctioning and APRV may be the preferred approach to the recruitment of collapsed lung in intubated patients.

■ REFERENCES

1. Mattison LE, Coppage L, Alderman DF, et al. Pleural effusions in the medical ICU: prevalence, causes, and clinical implications. *Chest.* 1997;111:1018–1023.
2. Lai-Fook SJ. Pleural mechanics and fluid exchange. *Physiol Rev.* 2004;84:385–410.
3. Broaddus VC, Wiener-Kronish JP, Staub NC. Clearance of lung edema into the pleural space of volume-loaded anesthetized sheep. *J Appl Physiol.* 1990;68:2623–2630.
4. Wiener-Kronish JP, Matthay MA, Callen PW, et al. Relationship of pleural effusions to pulmonary hemodynamics in patients with congestive heart failure. *Am Rev Respir Dis.* 1985;132:1253–1256.
5. Doelken P, Abreu R, Sahn SA, et al. Effect of thoracentesis on respiratory mechanics and gas exchange in the patient receiving mechanical ventilation. *Chest.* 2006;130:1354–1361.
6. Ahmed SH, Ouzounian SP, Dirusso S, et al. Hemodynamic and pulmonary changes after drainage of significant pleural effusions in critically ill, mechanically ventilated surgical patients. *J Trauma.* 2004;57:1184–1188.

7. Talmor M, Hydo L, Gershenwald JG, et al. Beneficial effects of chest tube drainage of pleural effusion in acute respiratory failure refractory to positive end-expiratory pressure ventilation. *Surgery.* 1998;123: 137–143.
8. Liang SSJ, Tu CY, Chen HJ, et al. Application of ultrasound-guided pigtail catheter for drainage of pleural effusions in the ICU. *Intensive Care Med.* 2009;35:350–354.
9. Mayo PH, Goltz HR, Tafreshi M, et al. Safety of ultrasound-guided thoracentesis in patients receiving mechanical ventilation. *Chest.* 2004;125:1059–1062.
10. Balik M, Plasil P, Waldauf P, et al. Ultrasound estimation of volume of pleural fluid in mechanically ventilated patients. *Intensive Care Med.* 2006;32:318–321.
11. Roch A, Bojan M, Michelet P, et al. Usefulness of ultrasonography in predicting pleural effusions > 500 ml in patients receiving mechanical ventilation. *Chest.* 2005;127:224–232.
12. Petersen S, Freitag M, Albert W, et al. Ultrasound-guided thoracentesis in surgical intensive care patients. *Intensive Care Med.* 1999;25:1029.
13. Adenigbagbe A, Kupfer Y, Seneviratne C, et al. Pigtail catheter drainage of transudative pleural effusions hastens liberation from mechanical ventilation {Abstract # 5928]. *Chest.* 2007;132(suppl.):455S.
14. Kiafar C, Gilani N. Hepatic hydrothorax: current concepts of pathophysiology and treatment options. *Ann Hepatol.* 2008;7:313–320.
15. Xiol X, Castellote J, Cortes-Beut R, et al. Usefulness and complications of thoracentesis in cirrhotic patients. *Am J Med.* 2001;111:67–69.
16. Cardenas A, Arroyo V. Management of ascites and hepatic hydrothorax. *Best Pract Res Clin Gastroenterol.* 2007;21:55–75.
17. Kallet RH, Siobal MS, Alonso JA, et al. Lung collapse during low tidal volume ventilation in acute respiratory distress syndrome. *Respir Care.* 2001;46:49–52.
18. Maa SH, Hung TJ, Hsu KH, et al. Manual hyperinflation improves alveolar recruitment in difficult-to-wean patients. *Chest.* 2005;128: 2714–2721.
19. Marini JJ, Pierson DJ, Hudson LD. Acute lobar atelectasis: a prospective comparison of fiberoptic bronchoscopy and respiratory therapy. *Am Rev Respir Dis.* 1979;119:971–978.
20. Savian C, Paratz J, Davies A. Comparison of the effectiveness of manual and ventilator hyperinflation at different levels of positive end-expiratory pressure in artificially ventilated and intubated intensive care patients. *Heart Lung.* 2006;35:334–341.
21. Berney S, Denehy L. A comparison of the effects of manual and ventilator hyperinflation on static lung compliance and sputum production in intubated and ventilated intensive care patients. *Physiother Res Int.* 2002;7:100–108.
22. Branson RD. Secretion management in the mechanically ventilated patient. *Respir Care.* 2007;52:1328–1342.

23. Chatburn RL. High-frequency assisted airway clearance. *Respir Care.* 2007;52:1224–1235.
24. Jolliet P, Chevrolet JC. Bronchoscopy in the intensive care unit. *Intensive Care Med.* 1992;18:160–169.
25. Olopade CO, Prakash UB. Bronchoscopy in the critical-care unit. *Mayo Clin Proc.* 1989;64:1255–1263.
26. Stevens RP, Lillington GA, Parsons GH. Fiberoptic bronchoscopy in the intensive care unit. *Heart Lung.* 1981;10:1037–1045.
27. Ferreyra GP, Baussano I, Squadrone V, et al. Continuous positive airway pressure for treatment of respiratory complications after abdominal surgery: a systematic review and meta-analysis. *Ann Surg.* 2008;247:617–626.
28. Matte P, Jacquet L, Van DM, et al. Effects of conventional physiotherapy, continuous positive airway pressure and non-invasive ventilatory support with bilevel positive airway pressure after coronary artery bypass grafting. *Acta Anaesthesiol Scand.* 2000;44:75–81.
29. Pasquina P, Tramer MR, Granier JM, et al. Respiratory physiotherapy to prevent pulmonary complications after abdominal surgery: a systematic review. *Chest.* 2006;130:1887–1899.
30. Gilbert C, Marik PE, Varon J. Acute lobar atelectasis during mechanical ventilation: to beat, suck or blow? *Crit Care Shock.* 2009;12:67–70.

Part III

Cardiac

25

Hypertensive Crises

Hypertensive emergencies and hypertensive urgencies (see definitions below) are commonly encountered by a wide variety of clinicians. It is estimated that 1–2% of patients with hypertension will develop a hypertensive crisis at some point in their life span. Prompt recognition, evaluation, and appropriate treatment of these conditions are crucial to prevent permanent end-organ damage.

■ DEFINITIONS

The classification and approach to hypertension undergoes periodic review by the Joint National Committee (JNC) on Prevention, Detection, Evaluation, and Treatment of High Blood Pressure, with the most recent report (JNC 7) having been released in 2003.[1] With this report, the classification of blood pressure (BP) was simplified with the recognition of two stages of hypertension (compared to the previous four stages in JNC VI). In addition, a new category called prehypertension was added. Although not specifically addressed in the JNC 7 report, patients with a systolic blood pressure of greater than 179 mmHg or a diastolic that is greater than 109 mmHg are usually defined as having a "hypertensive crisis."

The 1993 report of the JNC proposed an operational classification of hypertensive crises as either "hypertensive emergencies" or "hypertensive urgencies."[2] This classification remains useful today. Severe elevations in BP were classified as follows:

- *Hypertensive emergencies* in the presence of acute end-organ damage or
- *Hypertensive urgencies* in the absence of acute target-organ involvement

P.E. Marik, *Handbook of Evidence-Based Critical Care*,
DOI 10.1007/978-1-4419-5923-2_25,
© Springer Science+Business Media, LLC 2010

Distinguishing hypertensive urgencies from emergencies is critically important in formulating a therapeutic plan. Patients with hypertensive urgency should have their BP reduced within 24–48 h (with PO medication), whereas patients with hypertensive emergencies should have their blood pressure lowered immediately, although not to "normal" levels. The term "malignant hypertension" has been used to describe a syndrome characterized by elevated BP accompanied by encephalopathy or acute nephropathy. This term, however, has been removed from National and International Blood Pressure Control guidelines and is best referred to as a hypertensive emergency.

ALERT

- Hypertensive urgencies are treated with oral anti-hypertensive agents usually on an outpatient basis.

- Hypertensive emergencies are treated in the ICU with a rapidly acting, titratable, intravenous anti-hypertensive agent.

■ PATHOPHYSIOLOGY

The factors leading to the severe and rapid elevation of BP in patients with hypertensive emergencies are poorly understood. The rapidity of onset suggests a triggering factor superimposed on pre-existing hypertension. Non-compliance with anti-hypertensive medication and use of recreational drugs are common initiating factors. Hypertensive emergencies are thought to be initiated by an abrupt increase in systemic vascular resistance likely related to humoral vasoconstrictors.[3] The subsequent increase in BP generates mechanical stress and endothelial injury, leading to increased permeability, activation of the coagulation cascade and platelets, and deposition of fibrin. With severe elevations of BP, endothelial injury and fibrinoid necrosis of the arterioles ensue. This process results in ischemia and the release of additional vasoactive mediators, generating a vicious cycle of ongoing injury. The volume depletion that results from pressure natriuresis further simulates the release of vasoconstrictor substances from the kidney. These collective mechanisms can culminate in end-organ hypoperfusion, ischemia, and dysfunction that manifests as a hypertensive emergency.

■ CLINICAL PRESENTATION

The clinical manifestations of a hypertensive emergency are directly related to the particular end-organ dysfunction that has occurred and include the following:

- Hypertensive encephalopathy (and PRES, see Chapter 63)
- Acute aortic dissection
- Acute myocardial infarction
- Acute coronary syndrome
- Pulmonary edema with respiratory failure
- Severe pre-eclampsia, HELLP syndrome, eclampsia
- Microangiopathic hemolytic anemia
- Acute postoperative hypertension

The signs and symptoms vary from patient to patient depending upon the specific end-organ involved. Zampaglione et al.[4] reported that the most frequent presenting signs in patients with hypertensive emergencies were chest pain (27%), dyspnea (22%), and neurological deficits (21%). No particular BP threshold has been associated with the development of a hypertensive emergency. However, organ dysfunction is uncommon with a diastolic blood pressure (DBP) less than 130 mmHg (except in children and pregnancy). The absolute level of BP may not be as important as the rate of increase. For example, in patients with long-standing hypertension, a systolic blood pressure (SBP) of 200 mmHg or a DBP up to 150 mmHg may be well tolerated without the development of hypertensive encephalopathy, whereas in children and pregnant women, encephalopathy may develop with a DBP of only 100 mmHg. In a recent study by Tisdale and coworkers, the mean SBP and DBP of patients with hypertensive emergency presenting to the emergency department was 197 ± 21 and 108 ± 14 mmHg, respectively.[5]

■ INITIAL EVALUATION

Patients with hypertensive emergency usually present for evaluation as a result of a new symptom complex related to their elevated BP. Patient triage and physician evaluation should proceed expeditiously to prevent ongoing end-organ damage.

A focused medical history should include the following:

- History of hypertension, previous control, current anti-hypertensive medications with dosing, compliance, and time from last dose
- The use of any prescribed or over-the-counter medications

- Use of recreational drugs (amphetamines, cocaine, phencyclidine) or monoamine oxidase inhibitors

Physical examination should

- confirm the elevated BP by measuring the BP in *both* arms with an adequately sized cuff:
  - The appropriate size of the cuff is particularly important as the use of a cuff too small for the arm size has been shown to artificially elevate BP readings in obese patients.
- identify evidence of end-organ damage by
  - assessing pulses in all extremities
  - auscultating the lungs for evidence of pulmonary edema, the heart for murmurs or gallops, and the renal arteries for bruits
  - performing a focused neurological and fundoscopic examination

Headache and altered level of consciousness are the usual manifestations of hypertensive encephalopathy. Focal neurological findings, especially lateralizing signs, are uncommon in hypertensive encephalopathy, being more suggestive of a cerebrovascular accident. Subarachnoid hemorrhage should be considered in patients with a sudden onset of a severe headache. The ocular exam may show evidence of advanced retinopathy with arteriolar changes, exudates, hemorrhages, or papilledema assisting in the identification of hypertensive encephalopathy. Cardiac evaluation should aim to identify angina or myocardial infarction with the focus on clarifying any atypical symptoms such as dyspnea, cough, or fatigue that may be overlooked. Severe renal injury may result in hematuria or oliguria. On the basis of this evaluation, the clinician should be able to distinguish between a hypertensive emergency and an urgency and to formulate the subsequent plan for further diagnostic tests and treatment.

Initial objective evaluation should include the following:

- A metabolic panel to assess electrolytes, creatinine, and blood urea nitrogen.
- A complete blood count (and smear if microangiopathic hemolytic anemia is suspected).
- A urinalysis to look for proteinuria or microscopic hematuria.
- An electrocardiogram to assess for cardiac ischemia.
- Radiographic studies such as a chest radiograph in a patient with cardiopulmonary symptoms or a head computed tomography scan in a patient with neurological symptoms should be obtained in the appropriate clinical scenario.
- If the physical examination or the clinical picture is consistent with aortic dissection (severe chest pain, unequal pulses, widened mediastinum), a contrast computed tomography scan of the chest should

be obtained promptly to rule out aortic dissection. Although trans-esophageal echocardiography has excellent sensitivity and specificity for aortic dissection, this study should not be performed until adequate blood control has been achieved.

- In patients presenting with pulmonary edema, it is important to obtain an echocardiogram to distinguish between diastolic dysfunction, transient systolic dysfunction, or mitral regurgitation. Many patients, particularly the elderly, have a normal ejection fraction and in such patients, heart failure is due to isolated diastolic dysfunction. The management in these patients differs from that of patients with predominant systolic dysfunction and in those with transient mitral regurgitation (see Chapter 29).

■ INITIAL MANAGEMENT OF BLOOD PRESSURE

The majority of patients in whom severe hypertension (SBP >160 mmHg, DBP >110 mmHg) is identified on initial evaluation will have no evidence of acute end-organ damage and thus have a *hypertensive urgency*. Since no acute end-organ damage is present, these patients may present for evaluation of another complaint and the elevated BP may represent an acute recognition of chronic hypertension. In these patients, oral medication to lower the BP gradually over 24–48 h is the best approach to management.[3] Rapid reduction of BP may be associated with significant morbidity in hypertensive urgency due to a rightward shift in the pressure/flow autoregulatory curve in critical arterial beds (cerebral, coronary, renal). Rapid correction of severely elevated BP below the autoregulatory range of these vascular beds can result in marked reduction in perfusion causing ischemia and infarction. Therefore, although the BP must be reduced in these patients, it must be lowered in a slow and controlled fashion to prevent organ hypoperfusion.

ALERT

Examine your patient! An elevated BP without acute end-organ damage implies the patient has a hypertensive urgency and *not* a hypertensive emergency.

Altered autoregulation similarly occurs in patients with hypertensive emergencies and since end-organ damage is already present, rapid and excessive correction of the BP can further reduce perfusion and propagate further injury. Therefore, patients with a hypertensive emergency are best managed with a *continuous infusion of a short-acting, titratable anti-hypertensive agent*. Due to unpredictable pharmacodynamics, the sublingual and intramuscular route should be avoided. Patients with a hypertensive emergency should be managed in an ICU with close monitoring. For those patients with the most severe clinical manifestations or with the most labile BP, intra-arterial BP monitoring may be prudent. There are a variety of rapid-acting intravenous agents that are available for use in patients with hypertensive emergency; the agent of choice depends on the organ system involved:

- Acute pulmonary edema (systolic dysfunction)
  - Nicardipine, clevidipine, or fenoldopam
  - Nitroprusside + nitroglycerin (only if other agents are not available)
- Acute pulmonary edema (diastolic dysfunction)
  - Esmolol, metoprolol, labetalol, or verapamil in combination with low-dose nitroglycerin
- Acute coronary syndrome
  - Labetalol or esmolol in combination with nitroglycerin
- HT encephalopathy (and PRES, see Chapter 63)
  - Nicardipine, clevidipine, labetalol, or fenoldopam
- Aortic dissection
  - Labetalol or
  - Combination of nicardipine/clevidipine and esmolol or
  - Combination of nitroprusside with esmolol/metoprolol
- Pre-eclampsia
  - Labetalol or nicardipine
- ARF/microangiopathic anemia
  - Nicardipine, clevidipine, or fenoldopam
- Sympathetic crisis/cocaine overdose
  - Verapamil, diltiazem, nicardipine, or clevidipine in combination with a benzodiazepine (see Chapter 59)
- Acute ischemic stroke/intracerebral bleed
  - Nicardipine, clevidipine, or labetalol (see Chapter 46)
- Acute postoperative HT
  - Esmolol, clevidipine, nicardipine, or labetalol

ALERT

Patients with a hypertensive urgency should *not* receive intravenous anti-hypertensive agents. If you feel compelled to treat with an IV agent, give yourself or the bedside nurse some Ativan!

Rapid-acting intravenous agents should not be used outside of a monitored ICU setting to prevent precipitous falls of BP, which may cause significant morbidity or mortality. The immediate goal is to reduce DBP by 10–15% or to about 110 mmHg over a period of 30–60 min. In aortic dissection, this goal should be achieved within 5–10 min. Once the BP is controlled with intravenous agents and end-organ damage has ceased, oral therapy can be initiated as the intravenous agents are slowly titrated down. An important consideration prior to initiating intravenous therapy is to assess the patient's volume status (see Chapter 8). Due to pressure natriuresis, patients with hypertensive emergencies may be volume depleted and restoration of intravascular volume with intravenous saline will serve to restore organ perfusion and prevent a precipitous fall in BP when anti-hypertensive regimens are initiated.

Drugs to Avoid

- Clonidine and ACE inhibitors are long acting and poorly titratable; however, these agents are useful in the management of hypertensive urgencies.
- Hydralazine is a direct-acting vasodilator. Following intramuscular or intravenous administration, there is an initial latent period of 5–15 min followed by a progressive and often precipitous fall in BP that can last up to 12 h. Although hydralazine's circulating half-life is only about 3 h, the half-time of its effect on BP is about 10 h. Because of hydralazine's prolonged and unpredictable anti-hypertensive effects and the inability to effectively titrate the drugs' hypotensive effect, hydralazine is best avoided in the management of hypertensive crises.
- Sublingual and intranasal nifedipine may cause a precipitous drop in blood pressure with cerebral and myocardial infarction, renal failure, and death. These complications are best avoided and therefore this approach to BP control is strongly "discouraged."
- Furosemide is a "no-no". Volume depletion is common in patients with hypertensive emergencies and the administration of a diuretic together with a hypertensive agent can lead to a precipitous drop in BP. Diuretics should be avoided unless specifically indicated for volume overload as occurs in renal parenchymal disease or coexisting pulmonary edema.
- Nitroglycerin is a potent venodilator and only at high doses affects arterial tone. It causes hypotension and reflex tachycardia, which are exacerbated by the volume depletion characteristic of hypertensive emergencies. Nitroglycerin reduces BP by reducing preload

and cardiac output, undesirable effects in patients with compromised cerebral and renal perfusion. Low-dose ($\leq$ 60 mg/min) nitroglycerin may, however, be used as an adjunct to intravenous anti-hypertensive therapy in patients with hypertensive emergencies associated with acute coronary syndromes or acute pulmonary edema.

- Sodium nitroprusside is an arterial and venous vasodilator that decreases both afterload and preload. Nitroprusside decreases cerebral blood flow while increasing intracranial pressure, effects that are particularly disadvantageous in patients with hypertensive encephalopathy or following a cerebrovascular accident. Nitroprusside is a very potent agent, with an onset of action of seconds, a duration of action of 1–2 min, and a plasma half-life of 3–4 min. Nitroprusside is a *toxic drug*. Data suggest that nitroprusside infusion rates in excess of 4 μg/kg/min, for as little as 2–3 h, may lead to cyanide levels which are in the toxic range.[6] The usual "recommended" dose of nitroprusside of up to 10 μg/kg/min results in cyanide formation at a far greater rate than human beings can detoxify. Considering the potential for severe toxicity with nitroprusside, this drug should be used only when other intravenous anti-hypertensive agents are not available and then only in specific clinical circumstances and in patients with normal renal and hepatic function. The duration of treatment should be as short as possible and the infusion rate should not exceed 2 μg/kg/min.

ALERT

- Do not administer a loop diuretic (Lasix) unless the patient is in pulmonary edema; rather give fluids.

- Do not use s/l nifedipine or IV hydralazine to treat a hypertensive emergency (or urgency).

Recommended Anti-hypertensive Agents

The pharmacokinetics and dosages of the recommended intravenous anti-hypertensive agents are listed below:

- Labetalol is a combined selective alpha-1 and non-selective β-adrenergic receptor blocker with an alpha- to beta-blocking ratio of 1:7. The hypotensive effect of labetalol begins within 2–5 min after its intravenous administration, reaching a peak at 5–15 min following administration, and lasting for about 2–4 h. Due to its beta-blocking effects the heart rate is either maintained or slightly reduced. Unlike pure β-adrenergic blocking agents which decrease cardiac output, labetalol maintains cardiac output. Labetalol may be given as loading dose of 20 mg, followed by repeated incremental doses of 20–80 mg given at 10 min intervals until the desired BP is achieved. Alternatively, after the initial loading dose, an infusion commencing at 1–2 mg/min and titrated until the desired hypotensive effect is achieved is particularly effective. Bolus injections of 1–2 mg/kg have been reported to produce precipitous falls in BP and should therefore be avoided.

- Nicardipine is a second-generation dihydropyridine derivative calcium channel blocker with high vascular selectivity and strong cerebral and coronary vasodilatory activity. The onset of action of intravenous nicardipine is between 5 and 15 min with a duration of action of 4–6 h. Nicardipine's dosage is independent of the patient's weight, with an initial infusion rate of 5 mg/h, increasing by 2.5 mg/h every 5 min to a maximum of 15 mg/h until the desired BP reduction is achieved.
- Clevidipine is third-generation dihydropyridine calcium channel blocker that has been developed for use in clinical settings where tight BP control is crucial. Clevidipine is an ultra-short-acting selective arteriolar vasodilator. Similar to esmolol, it is rapidly metabolized by red blood cell esterases; thus its metabolism is not affected by renal or hepatic function. The starting dose is 2 mg/h which is doubled every 3 min up to a dose of 32 mg/h until control is achieved. Clevidipine has proven particularly useful in the management of perioperative hypertension (see below).
- Esmolol is an ultra-short-acting cardioselective, β-adrenergic blocking agent. The onset of action of this agent is within 60 s with a duration of action of 10–20 min. Typically, the drug is given as a 0.5–1 mg/kg loading dose over 1 min, followed by an infusion starting at 50 μg/kg/min and increasing up to 300 μg/kg/min as necessary.
- Fenoldopam is unique among the parenteral blood pressure agents as it mediates peripheral vasodilation by acting on peripheral dopamine-1 receptors. The onset of action is within 5 min, with the maximal response being achieved by 15 min. The duration of action is between 30 and 60 min, with the pressure gradually returning to pretreatment values without rebound once the infusion is stopped. An initial starting dose of 0.1 μg/kg/min is recommended.

Acute Hypertension and Cerebrovascular Disease

See Chapter 46.

Pre-eclampsia and HELLP Syndrome

See Chapter 54.

Posterior Reversible Encephalopathy Syndrome (PRES)

See Chapter 63.

Acute Postoperative Hypertension

Acute postoperative hypertension (APH) has been defined as a significant elevation in BP during the immediate postoperative period that may lead to serious neurological, cardiovascular, or surgical-site complications and that requires urgent management. While APH is widely recognized, there is no standardized definition to define this disorder. We consider an increase in the SBP by more than 20% or an increase in the DBP to above 110 mm/Hg to be indicative of APH.[7] APH usually develops within 2 h of surgery and resolves within a few hours. The complications associated with APH include myocardial ischemia, myocardial infarction, cardiac arrhythmias, congestive cardiac failure with pulmonary edema as well as hemorrhagic stroke, cerebral ischemia, and encephalopathy. APH will increase bleeding at the surgical site and compromise vascular anastomoses. The pathophysiological mechanism underlying APH is uncertain and may vary with the surgical procedure and other factors. However, the final common pathway leading to hypertension appears to be activation of the sympathetic nervous system, as evidenced by elevated plasma catecholamine concentrations in patients with APH. The primary hemodynamic alteration observed in APH is an increase in afterload with an increase in SBP and DBP with or without tachycardia. Although APH may occur following any major surgery, it is most commonly associated with cardiothoracic, vascular, head and neck, and neurosurgical procedures.

In cardiac surgery patients, treatment is usually suggested for a BP >140/90 mmHg or a MAP > 105 mmHg. In these patients, meticulous blood pressure control is recommended. In the non-cardiac surgery patient, there is no consensus regarding the treatment threshold. Treatment of these patients is usually a clinical decision based on the degree of blood pressure elevation, the nature of the surgery, the patients' comorbidities, and the risks of treatment.

Pain and anxiety are common contributors to BP elevations and should be treated before administration of anti-hypertensive therapy. The patients' volume status should be carefully assessed. Intravascular volume depletion will increase sympathetic activity and vasoconstriction; in this setting a volume challenge should be considered. Other potentially reversible causes of APH include hypothermia with shivering, hypoxemia, hypercarbia, and bladder distension.

Short-term administration of a short-acting intravenous agent is recommended when there is no identifiable treatable cause of hypertension. As increased sympathetic activity underlies the pathophysiology of APH, an α-/β-blocker or a β-blocker alone would appear to be a rational agent to use. The short-acting intravenous calcium channel-blocking agents also have a role. Labetalol, esmolol, nicardipine, and clevidipine are generally considered the agents of choice for the treatment of APH.

Several trials have shown clevidipine to be very effective in the control of postoperative hypertension.[8] The recently completed ECLIPSE trial demonstrated the efficacy and safety of this agent in the treatment of APH.[9] ECLIPSE randomized 1964 cardiac patients who required treatment for perioperative hypertension to clevidipine or a comparator agent (nitroprusside or nicardipine). Clevidipine was more effective than nitroprusside in controlling BP, with a lower mortality (1.7% vs. 4.7%; $p = 0.045$) and with similar efficacy and safety to nicardipine.

Preoperative Hypertension

Although preoperative hypertension has been found to be a significant predictor of postoperative morbidity, no data have definitively established that preoperative treatment of hypertension reduces postoperative complications. However, ideally, all patients with cardiovascular risk factors undergoing elective surgery should undergo aggressive preoperative optimization, including control of blood pressure, correction of electrolytes, glucose control, cessation of smoking, nutritional optimization (in high-risk patients), and treatment with a statin.[10–13]

Hypertensive patients should continue to receive all their anti-hypertensive drugs preoperatively, except for ACE inhibitors (ACEIs) and angiotensin II receptor antagonists (ARAs). ACEIs and ARAs should be discontinued at least 10 h before surgery.

The management plan in patients who present to the operating room with "poorly" controlled blood pressure should be individualized based on the patient's clinical presentation, comorbidities, and the assumed risks of surgery. Surgery should be deferred in those patients with acute end-organ hypertensive injury, i.e., those with cardiac failure, myocardial ischemia, acute renal dysfunction, and papilledema/encephalopathy. In high-risk patients (previous stroke, active CAD, etc.) with an SBP greater than 180 mmHg and/or a diastolic BP greater than 110 mmHg, it may be prudent to cancel surgery until the patient's blood pressure and cardiovascular status have been optimized. In otherwise low-risk patients with an SBP greater than 180 mmHg and/or a DBP greater than 110 mmHg, it may be reasonable to reduce the blood pressure (by no more than 20%) with a combination of an intravenous β-blocking agent and a benzodiazepine (for anxiolysis) prior to surgery. A β-blocker (metoprolol) or an α–β-blocker (labetalol) is the agent of choice. Patients with adequate β-blockade (low pulse rate) or patients in whom a β-blocker is contraindicated (asthma, conduction defect) may be treated with one of the intravenous dihydropyridine calcium channel blockers (nicardipine or clevidipine). Due to its short half-life, clevidipine is particularly useful in this setting. Agents with unpredictable hypotensive effects, namely nifedipine, hydralazine, and ACEIs, should not be used in this situation.

■ CLINICAL PEARLS

- It is critical to distinguish between a hypertensive urgency and an hypertensive emergency; only patients with a hypertensive emergency require rapid control with an intravenous anti-hypertensive agent.
- s/l nifedipine and IV hydralazine have no role in the management of acute hypertension.
- Avoid diuretics; most patients are volume contorted and require fluid replacement.

■ REFERENCES

1. Chobanian AV, Bakris GL, Black HR, et al. The seventh report of the joint national committee on prevention, detection, evaluation, and treatment of high blood pressure. The JNC 7 Report. *JAMA.* 2003;289: 2560–2572.
2. The fifth report of the joint national committee on detection, evaluation and treatment of high blood pressure. *Arch Intern Med.* 1993;153: 154–183.
3. Marik PE, Varon J. Hypertensive crises: challenges and management. *Chest.* 2007;131:1949–1962.
4. Zampaglione B, Pascale C, Marchisio M, et al. Hypertensive urgencies and emergencies. Prevalence and clinical presentation. *Hypertension.* 1996;27:144–147.

5. Tisdale JE, Huang MB, Borzak S. Risk factors for hypertensive crisis: importance of out-patient blood pressure control. *Fam Pract.* 2004;21:420–424.
6. Pasch T, Schulz V, Hoppenshauser G. Nitroprusside-induced formation of cyanide and its detoxication with thiosulphate during deliberate hypotension. *J Cardiovasc Pharmacol.* 1983;5:77–85.
7. Marik PE, Varon J. Perioperative hypertension: a review of current and emerging therapeutic agents. *J Clin Anesth.* 2009;21:220–229.
8. Singla N, Warltier DC, Gandhi SD, et al. Treatment of acute postoperative hypertension in cardiac surgery patients: an efficacy study of clevidipine assessing its postoperative antihypertensive effect in cardiac surgery-2 (ESCAPE-2), a randomized, double-blind, placebo-controlled trial. *Anesth Analg.* 2008;107:59–67.
9. Aronson S, Dyke CM, Stierer KA, et al. The ECLIPSE trials: comparative studies of clevidipine to nitroglycerin, sodium nitroprusside, and nicardipine for acute hypertension treatment in cardiac surgery patients. *Anesth Analg.* 2008;107:1110–1121.
10. Poldermans D, Bax JJ, Kertai MD, et al. Statins are associated with a reduced incidence of perioperative mortality in patients undergoing major noncardiac vascular surgery. *Circulation.* 2003;107:1848–1851.
11. Tepaske R, Velthuis H, Oudemans-van Straaten HM, et al. Effect of preoperative oral immune-enhancing nutritional supplement on patients at high risk of infection after cardiac surgery: a randomised placebo-controlled trial. *Lancet.* 2001;358:696–701.
12. Schoeten O, Boersma E, Hoeks SE, et al. Fluvastatin and perioperative events in patients undergoing vascular surgery. *N Engl J.* 2009;361: 980–989.
13. Noordzij PG, Boersma E, Schreiner F, et al. Increased preoperative glucose levels are associated with perioperative mortality in patients undergoing noncardiac, nonvascular surgery. *Eur J Endocrinol.* 2007;156:137–142.

26

Acute Coronary Syndromes

In the United States, more than a million people are hospitalized annually with unstable angina or myocardial infarction without ST segment elevation (NSTEMI), so-called acute coronary syndromes (ACS's). For these patients, several treatments have proved to be effective in reducing the incidence of death, infarction or reinfarction, and recurrent ischemia. These treatments include intensive medical therapy and coronary angiography followed by revascularization, if indicated.

Unstable angina (UA) is characterized by the clinical presentation of angina with or without ischemic ECG changes (ST segment depression or new T-wave inversion). NSTEMI is similar to UA but is characterized by positive biomarkers [troponin or creatine kinase-MB (CK-MB)] in the setting of angina or ECG changes. The presence of myonecrosis as evident by positive cardiac markers portends a higher risk than that presenting with just UA. UA and NSTEMI pathophysiologically and clinically are related and initially may be indistinguishable, as biomarkers may not be elevated at presentation. Rupture of an atherosclerotic plaque and subsequent formation of a thrombus usually are the triggering events in the pathogenesis of most cases of ACS.

■ CANADIAN CARDIOVASCULAR CLASSIFICATION OF ANGINA

- Class 1: pain is precipitated only by severe and unusually prolonged exertion.

P.E. Marik, *Handbook of Evidence-Based Critical Care*,
DOI 10.1007/978-1-4419-5923-2_26,
© Springer Science+Business Media, LLC 2010

- Class 2: pain on moderate effort. There is slight limitation of ordinary activity.
- Class 3: marked limitation of ordinary activity; pain occurs on mild exertion, usually restricting daily chores. Patient is unable to walk two blocks on the level at a comfortable temperature and at a normal pace.
- Class 4: chest discomfort on almost any physical activity.

■ TYPES OF PRESENTATIONS OF UNSTABLE ANGINA

- Rest angina
  - Angina occurring at rest and prolonged, usually >20 min
- New-onset angina
  - New-onset angina of at least CCS class III severity
- Increasing angina
  - Previously diagnosed angina that has become distinctly more frequent, longer in duration, or lower in threshold (i.e., increased by ≥1 CCS class to at least CCS class III severity)

■ DIFFERENTIAL DIAGNOSIS

- AMI
- Aortic dissection
- Esophagitis
- Pleurisy
- Leaking or ruptured thoracic aneurysm
- Acute pericarditis
- Pulmonary embolism
- Pneumothorax
- Esophageal rupture

■ ELECTROCARDIOGRAPHY

Most patients who have ACS have some ECG changes. The ECG is important for diagnostic and risk stratification purposes. Specific characteristics and the magnitude of pattern abnormalities increase the likelihood of CAD. ST–T segment depression portends a poorer prognosis than T-wave inversion alone or no ECG changes. The Global Use of Strategies to Open Occluded Coronary Arteries in Acute Coronary Syndromes (GUSTO-IIb) trial demonstrated that the 30-day incidence of death or MI was 10.5% in those who had ST segment depression vs. 5.5% in patients who had T-wave inversion, and a higher mortality was also seen at 6-month follow-up.[1] The sum of ST depression is a strong independent predictor of short-term mortality and the risk increases with the magnitude of depression.[2]

■ TROPONINS

Troponins play a central role in the diagnosis of NSTEMI and risk stratification. The joint statement of the European Society of Cardiology and the American College of Cardiology (ACC) defines myonecrosis as when the peak concentration of troponin T or I exceeds the decision limit (99th percentile for a reference group) on at least one occasion in a 24-h period.[3] This definition has increased the frequency of the diagnosis of NSTEMI in patients who have ACS by 30%. The troponins are detectable approximately 6 h after myocardial injury and are measurable for up to 2 weeks. Mortality risk is directly proportional to troponin levels and the prognostic information is independent of other clinical and ECG risk factors.[4]

■ MANAGEMENT

Risk Stratification

Risk stratification plays a central role in determining the treatment strategy of patients with ACS. Two risk assessment algorithms have been developed for determining whether a patient is at high risk or at relatively low risk for having an ischemic event. Patients with ≥3 TIMI variables are considered to be at high risk. Similarly, patients with >110 total risk score points using the GRACE model have >5% 6-month mortality.

Thrombolysis in Myocardial Infarction (TIMI) Risk Score

- Age >65 years[5]
- Risk factors (≥3) for coronary artery disease
- Prior coronary stenosis of ≥50%
- ST segment deviation on electrocardiogram at presentation
- At least two anginal events in prior 24 h
- Use of aspirin in prior 7 days
- Elevated serum cardiac markers

Global Registry of Acute Coronary Events (GRACE) Risk Model

- Age[6]
- Killip class (a classification of the severity of heart failure)
- Systolic arterial pressure
- ST segment deviation
- cardiac arrest during presentation
- Serum creatinine concentration
- Elevated serum markers for myocardial necrosis
- Heart rate

Each variable is assigned a numerical score on the basis of its specific value, and the eight scores are added to yield a total score, which is applied to a reference nomogram to determine the patient's risk. The GRACE application tool is available at www.outcomes-umassmed.org/grace.

■ TREATMENT STRATEGIES FOR ACS

Low-Risk Patients

Anti-anginal Drug

- β-Blocker (oral or IV)[7,8]:
  - Immediately.
- Nitroglycerin:
  - Immediately
  - Sublingual NTG (0. 4 mg) every 5 min for a total of three doses.
  - Intravenous NTG is indicated in the first 48 h after UA/NSTEMI for treatment of persistent ischemia, heart failure, or hypertension.

Analgesia

- Morphine sulfate (1–5 mg intravenously) is reasonable for patients whose symptoms either are not relieved despite NTG or recur despite adequate anti-ischemic therapy. Hypotension, nausea, and respiratory depression are potential adverse effects of morphine. A large observational registry that included patients with UA/NSTEMI suggested a higher adjusted likelihood of death with morphine use.[9]

Lipid Lowering

- Statin
  - Before hospital discharge

Anti-platelet Drug

- Aspirin

- Immediately
- Clopidogrel

Anti-coagulant Drug

- Unfractionated heparin, enoxaparin, fondaparinux, and bivalirudin
  - Immediately then for 2–5 days

Non-invasive Testing

- Non-invasive stress testing is recommended in low-risk patients who have been free of ischemia at rest or with low-level activity and of heart failure for a minimum of 12–24 h.

High-Risk Patients

Anti-anginal Drug

- β-Blocker
  - Immediately
- Nitroglycerin
  - Immediately

Lipid Lowering

- Statin
  - Before hospital discharge

Anti-platelet Drug

- Aspirin
  - Immediately
- Clopidogrel
  - Immediately
- Glycoprotein IIb/IIIa inhibitor (eptifibatide, tirofiban, or abciximab)
  - At the time of PCI, then for 12–24 h

Anti-coagulant Drug

- Unfractionated heparin, enoxaparin, and bivalirudin
  - Immediately, discontinue after successful PCI

Invasive Management

- Coronary angiography followed by revascularization (if appropriate)
  - Up to 36–80 h after hospitalization
  - Within 24 h in very high risk (GRACE >140)

■ REFERENCES

1. Savonitto S, Ardissino D, Granger CB, et al. Prognostic value of the admission electrocardiogram in acute coronary syndromes. *JAMA.* 1999;281:707–713.
2. Savonitto S, Cohen MG, Politi A, et al. Extent of ST-segment depression and cardiac events in non-ST-segment elevation acute coronary syndromes. *Eur Heart J.* 2005;26:2106–2113.
3. Alpert JS, Thygesen K, Antman E, et al. Myocardial infarction redefined – a consensus document of The Joint European Society of Cardiology/American College of Cardiology Committee for the redefinition of myocardial infarction. *J Am Coll Cardiol.* 2000;36:959–969.
4. Antman EM, Tanasijevic MJ, Thompson B, et al. Cardiac-specific troponin I levels to predict the risk of mortality in patients with acute coronary syndromes. *N Engl J Med.* 1996;335:1342–1349.
5. Antman EM, Cohen M, Bernink PJ, et al. The TIMI risk score for unstable angina/non-ST elevation MI: a method for prognostication and therapeutic decision making. *JAMA.* 2000;284:835–842.
6. Eagle KA, Lim MJ, Dabbous OH, et al. A validated prediction model for all forms of acute coronary syndrome: estimating the risk of 6-month postdischarge death in an international registry. *JAMA.* 2004;291: 2727–2733.
7. Hillis LD, Lange RA. Optimal management of acute coronary syndromes. *N Engl J Med.* 2009;360:2237–2240.
8. Anderson JL, Adams CD, Antman EM, et al. ACC/AHA 2007 guidelines for the management of patients with unstable angina/non-ST-Elevation myocardial infarction: a report of the American College of Cardiology/American Heart Association Task Force on Practice Guidelines – Executive Summary. *J Am Coll Cardiol.* 2007;50:652–726.
9. Meine TJ, Roe MT, Chen AY, et al. Association of intravenous morphine use and outcomes in acute coronary syndromes: results from the CRUSADE Quality Improvement Initiative. *Am Heart J.* 2005;149: 1043–1049.

27

ST Segment Elevation Myocardial Infarction

Over 1.2 million patients suffer from new or recurrent ischemic events annually. This includes an estimated 565,000 cases of first and 300,000 cases of recurrent myocardial infarction. Although mortality from acute myocardial infarction (AMI) has declined in recent years, it still remains high at 25–30%. The most common cause of ST elevation AMI (STEMI) is acute plaque rupture with the resultant thrombosis leading to acute closure of coronary arteries.

■ MANAGEMENT OF PATIENTS IN THE EMERGENCY DEPARTMENT

When the patient with suspected AMI reaches the emergency department (ED), evaluation and initial management should take place promptly. The initial evaluation of the patient ideally should be accomplished within 10 min of his/her arrival in the ED. On arrival in the ED, the patient with suspected AMI should immediately receive the following:

- Oxygen by nasal prongs
- Sublingual nitroglycerin (unless systolic BP <90 mmHg or heart rate <50 or >100 beats/min)
- Aspirin 160–325 mg orally
- Morphine 2–4 mg as required

Effective analgesia should be administered promptly at the time of diagnosis and should not be delayed on the premise that it will

P.E. Marik, *Handbook of Evidence-Based Critical Care*,
DOI 10.1007/978-1-4419-5923-2_27,
© Springer Science+Business Media, LLC 2010

mask symptoms of ongoing ischemia. Long-acting oral nitrates should be avoided. Continuous ECG and pulse oximetry should be initiated. Patients with an arterial saturation of less than <90% should be treated with a venturi or a CPAP mask.

The 12-lead ECG in the ED is at the center of the decision pathway because of the strong evidence that ST segment elevation identifies patients who benefit from reperfusion therapy. Patients with ST segment elevation (equal to or greater than 1 mV) in contiguous leads are candidates for immediate reperfusion therapy, either by fibrinolysis or primary percutaneous coronary intervention (PCI). In contrast, the patient without ST segment elevation should not receive thrombolytic therapy (see Chapter 26).

■ CHOOSING A REPERFUSION STRATEGY

Patients presenting within 12 h should undergo reperfusion therapy. An invasive strategy is preferred for high-risk patients (elderly, large AMI, cardiogenic shock, or those with comorbid conditions) if the door-to balloon time can be achieved within 90 min, or there is contraindication for fibrinolysis or the diagnosis is uncertain.[1] On the other hand, fibrinolytic therapy remains the principal mode of reperfusion globally because of the lack of facilities and accessibility to invasive centers that can perform primary PCI in a timely manner. The National Heart Attack Alert Program Coordinating Committee has established a door-to-needle time (for fibrinolysis) to be less than 30 min and door-to-balloon time (for PCI) to be less than 90 min within which diagnosis is to be completed and reperfusion achieved.

■ FIBRINOLYTIC THERAPY

Fibrinolytic therapy represents one of the major advances in the management of STEMI. The guidelines recommend fibrinolytic therapy within the first hour after symptom onset, since mortality significantly increases every hour thereafter.[1] The benefits of fibrinolytic therapy on STEMI have been well established with overall 18% risk reduction in 30-day mortality relative to control.[2] Furthermore, this reduction in mortality is risk dependent with higher risk subgroups showing the greatest benefit. A major concern with the administration of fibrinolytics is the risk of intracranial hemorrhage.[2] This is because it is fatal in up to one-half to two-thirds of patients and associated with permanent disability in a vast majority of patients who survive this event. Factors identified with increased risks have included increasing age, African-American race, lower body weight, prior transient ischemic attack or stroke, presenting systolic blood pressure, excessive anti-coagulation, and fibrin-specific agents compared with non-fibrin-specific agents.

Contraindications for Thrombolytic Therapy

- Active peptic ulcer, recent bleeding
- Suspected aortic aneurysm
- Recent head injury or cerebral neoplasm
- CVA within 2 months
- Previous hemorrhagic stroke at any time
- Trauma or major surgery within 6 weeks
- Recent prolonged or traumatic CPR
- Diabetic retinopathy or other ophthalmic hemorrhagic lesions
- Acute pancreatitis

Relative Contraindications

- Severe uncontrolled hypertension on presentation (blood pressure >180/110 mmHg)
- History of prior cerebrovascular accident or known intracerebral pathology not covered in contraindications
- Current use of anti-coagulants in therapeutic doses (INR 2–3)
- Known bleeding diathesis
- Non-compressible vascular punctures
- Recent (within 2–4 weeks) internal bleeding
- For streptokinase/anistreplase: prior exposure (especially within 5 days to 2 years) or prior allergic reaction
- Pregnancy
- Active peptic ulcer
- History of chronic severe hypertension

■ PRIMARY PCI

Primary PCI with patency rates greater than 90% and few contraindications is an attractive reperfusion strategy. This mode of reperfusion has been shown to decrease mortality, non-fatal reinfarction, and hemorrhagic stroke when compared with fibrinolytic therapy.[3] Thus, primary PCI is the preferred reperfusion strategy when performed in a timely manner.

Elective PCI of an occluded infarct artery 1–28 days after MI in stable patients has no incremental benefit beyond optimal medical therapy with aspirin, β-blockers, ACE inhibitors, and statins in preserving LV function and preventing subsequent cardiovascular events.[1]

■ ADJUNCTIVE THERAPY

Patients Receiving Thrombolytic Therapy

Anti-platelet Agents

- Aspirin
  - 162–325 mg immediately
- Clopidogrel
  - 75 mg immediately

Anti-thrombotic Agents

- Except those receiving streptokinase
- Unfractionated heparin
  - 60 U/kg bolus (max. 4000), 12 U/kg/h (max. 1,000 U/h; 800 U/h in elderly) or
- LMWH (less than 75 years, no renal dysfunction)
  - 1 mg/kg q 12 h
- Fondaparinux

Other

- Oral β-blocker
  - Immediately
- Statin
  - Before hospital discharge
- ACE
  - EF <40%
  - Anterior MI
  - Within 24 h

Patients Treated by PCI

Anti-platelet Agents

- Aspirin
  - 162–325 mg immediately
- Clopidogrel
  - 600 mg immediately, then 75 mg daily

- G IIb/IIIa inhibitor
  - Immediately

Other

- Oral β-blocker
  - Immediately
- Statin
  - Before hospital discharge
- ACE
  - EF <40%
  - Anterior MI
  - Within 24 h

■ COMPLICATIONS

Recurrent Chest Pain Post-AMI

The two most common causes of recurrent chest pain are acute pericarditis and ischemia. An ECG taken during the recurrent chest pain and compared with the previous ECGs is helpful in distinguishing between these two conditions. Cardiac rupture may also result in recurrent chest pain.

Pericarditis

Pericarditis has been reported to occur in 20% of patients following AMI and occurs with extension of myocardial necrosis through the wall to the epicardium. The pain associated with pericarditis is pleuritic in nature and positional. The ECG features of pericarditis include J point elevation, concave-up ST segment elevation, and PR segment depression. It is not associated with re-elevation of the CK-MB. Aspirin is the treatment of choice, but high doses (650 mg q 4–6 h) may be required.

Ischemia

Reinfarction during the first 10 days postinfarction has been reported to occur in about 10% of patients who have not received thrombolytic therapy compared to approximately 3% of patients who have been thrombolysed. Coronary angiography is indicated in patients with suspected ischemic-type chest pain. Prompt reperfusion using PCI or additional thrombolytic may be feasible.

Mitral Regurgitation

Acute mitral regurgitation is a life-threatening complication that can occur with or without papillary muscle rupture. It is more common with inferior STEMI, usually because of occlusions of the right coronary or left circumflex arteries. Medical management carries a very high mortality (70%). Surgical mortality, although high, is still lower (40%) than medical treatment alone.[4] Diagnosis can be established rapidly by transthoracic and if required transesophageal echocardiography. All patients should be considered for emergent surgery, while stabilization is achieved by IABP, inotropes, and vasodilators. Delay in operation increases the risk of myocardial and other organ injury and subsequent death.

Left Ventricular Failure and Low Output States

Heart failure is present in 15–25% of patients with acute myocardial infarction with an in-hospital mortality rate of 15–40%. The severity of left ventricular dysfunction is proportional to the extent of myocardial injury. Mortality has been reported to vary from 6% in patients with clear lung fields and no third heart sound to up to 60% in patients with cardiogenic shock in the reperfusion era. The Forrester Classification (Table 27-1) is useful in the management of post AMI cardiac dysfunction.

Table 27-1 Forrester Classification of AMI

Class	PCWP (mmHg)	CI (l/min)
I	<18	>2.2
II	>18	>2.2
III	<18	<2.2
IV	>18	<2.2

Adequate Output, Pulmonary Congestion (Forrester Class II)

In the early hours of acute infarction, ischemia often contributes substantially to LV dysfunction. The elevated pulmonary capillary wedge pressure is largely due to the poorly compliant ischemic left ventricle. In patients with a systolic BP greater than 100 mmHg and with adequate tissue perfusion and features of pulmonary congestion, gentle diuresis with furosemide in combination with preload and afterload reduction with intravenous nitroglycerin may improve LV function.

Nitroglycerin may also relieve ischemia by dilating epicardial coronary arteries. Nitroprusside has been demonstrated to cause coronary steal and should be avoided.

Poor Output, Clear Chest (Forrester Class III)

Due to a combination of factors including poor oral intake, sweating, nausea and vomiting, as well as nitrates, left ventricular preload may be reduced. These patients should be treated with repeated fluid challenges (200 ml boluses of lactate Ringer's solution or normal saline). Right ventricular infarction (see below) should also be considered.

Poor Output, Pulmonary Congestion (Forrester IV)

Patients with a systolic blood pressure below 90 mmHg and/or with signs of inadequate tissue perfusion together with pulmonary congestion have significant LV dysfunction with elevated left-sided filling pressures. Intravenous norepinephrine should be administered and titrated to increase the mean arterial pressure (MAP) above 65–70 mmHg. Dobutamine 5–20 μg/kg/min should be added to improve cardiac function. Pulmonary artery catheterization should be considered in these patients to optimize preload and allow the more rational use of vasoactive agents. In addition, consideration should be given to initiating intra-aortic counterpulsation. Reperfusion by PCI or CABG may improve the outcome of these patients.

Right Ventricular Infarction

Right ventricular infarction (RVI) commonly occurs in patients with an inferior myocardial infarction (and very rarely with anterior myocardial infarction). Although RVI is evident in approximately 25% of patients with an inferior STEMI, hemodynamic compromise is evident in fewer than 10% of these patients. EKGs with right-sided precordial leads should be obtained in all patients with an inferior STEMI.

Diagnosis

- Clinical:
  - A raised JVP, with hypotension and a clear chest.
  - Kussmaul's sign may be positive.
- Hemodynamic criteria:
  - RA pressure >10 mmHg or a PA/PCWP >0.8 in patient with no features of cor pulmonale.

- ECG criteria:
  - ST segment elevation in V4R. ST elevation in V1 with ST depression in V2 is said to be characteristic of RV infarction.
- Radionuclide techniques:
  - These are the most sensitive diagnostic methods. MUGA scan or pyrophosphate scan.

Management of RV Infarct

- Fluid administration (despite a raised JVP) is the cornerstone of therapy. The "optimal CVP" is between 10 and 14 mmHg.
- Stop/avoid use of nitrates/diuretics.
- Patients who have not responded to fluid challenges should have a therapeutic trial of dobutamine. A PAC may be useful in these patients.
- High-degree heart block is common in these patients. AV sequential pacing improves right ventricular filling and increase in cardiac output (even in patients who have not improved with ventricular pacing alone).

Atrial Fibrillation

Atrial fibrillation (and flutter) in STEMI is an independent predictor of 30-day mortality. Atrial fibrillation associated with AMI most often occurs within the first 24 h and is usually transient but may recur. The incidence of AF in AMI ranges from 10 to 16%. In the patient with AMI, the appearance of atrial fibrillation is often a manifestation of extensive LV systolic dysfunction. If its occurrence causes hemodynamic compromise or ongoing ischemia, direct-current cardioversion should be performed.

In the absence of CHF, bronchospastic disease, or AV block, the most effective means of slowing the ventricular rate in AF is the use of intra-venous adrenoceptor-blocking agents such as atenolol or metoprolol. Rate slowing may also be achieved with intravenous diltiazem. However, because of the concerns regarding the use of calcium channel blockers in AMI, these agents are not recommended as first-line agents.

The role of class I and class III anti-arrhythmic agents and electric shock for converting persistent AF is unclear as is the role of anti-arrhythmic agents for the prevention of further episodes of AF in patients who convert to sinus rhythm. Anti-coagulation with heparin is indicated in patients who remain in AF for more than 48 h or have recurrent episodes of AF.

Other Arrhythmias

Episodes of ventricular fibrillation and sustained ventricular tachycardia (more than 30 s of causing hemodynamic compromise) should be treated with immediate direct-current countershock; the same is true for episodes of monomorphic ventricular tachycardia associated with angina, pulmonary congestion, or hypotension.

Monomorphic ventricular tachycardia not accompanied by chest pain, pulmonary congestion, or hypotension should be treated with intravenous lidocaine, procainamide, or amiodarone. Infusions of anti-arrhythmic drugs may be used after an episode of VT/VF but should be discontinued after 6–24 h and the need for further arrhythmia management assessed. Electrolyte and acid–base disturbances should be corrected to prevent recurrent episodes once the initial episode has been treated.

An implantable cardioverter defibrillator (ICD) is indicated for patients with VF or hemodynamically significant sustained VT more than 2 days after STEMI, provided the arrhythmia is not judged to be due to transient or reversible ischemia or reinfarction.

Sinus bradycardia occurs in up to 40% of patients with an acute AMI, especially within the first hour of an inferior AMI and with reperfusion of the right coronary artery. Heart block develops in about 6–14% of patients with acute AMI. The increased mortality associated with heart block and intraventricular conduction delay is related more to extensive myocardial damage than to heart block as such. Indeed, pacing has not been shown to reduce mortality in these patients. Atropine is indicated in patients with symptomatic bradycardia (generally heart rate less than 50 beats/min) associated with hypotension, ischemia or ventricular escape rhythm, and symptomatic AV block.

■ REFERENCES

1. Antman EM, Hand M, Armstrong PW, et al. 2007 Focused Update of the ACC/AHA 2004 Guidelines for the management of patients with ST-elevation myocardial infarction. *J Am Coll Cardiol*. 2008;51: 210–247.
2. Indications for fibrinolytic therapy in suspected acute myocardial infarction: collaborative overview of early mortality and major morbidity results from all randomised trials of more than 1000 patients. Fibrinolytic Therapy Trialists' (FTT) Collaborative Group. *Lancet*. 1994;343: 311–322.
3. Keeley EC, Boura JA, Grines CL. Primary angioplasty versus intravenous thrombolytic therapy for acute myocardial infarction: a quantitative review of 23 randomised trials. *Lancet*. 2003;361:13–20.

4. Thompson CR, Buller CE, Sleeper LA, et al. Cardiogenic shock due
   to acute severe mitral regurgitation complicating acute myocardial
   infarction: a report from the SHOCK Trial Registry. SHould we use emergently revascularize Occluded Coronaries in cardiogenic shocK? *J Am
   Coll Cardiol.* 2000;36:1104–1109.

28

Arrhythmias

Sustained arrhythmias occur in approximately 10–15% of general ICU patients.[1,2] As a general rule, the development of arrhythmias is a reflection of the severity of the underlying disease and they do not appear to be independent predictors of death, although they increase the risk of neurological sequela. Atrial arrhythmias (atrial fibrillation/atrial flutter) are the most common arrhythmia. AF/atrial flutter are usually secondary to the underlying disease process (respiratory failure), while ventricular arrhythmias are usually due to pre-existent cardiac disease or acute ischemia. Atrial arrhythmias are usually the consequence of acute respiratory failure (acute cor pulmonale–pulmonary hypertension, right ventricular failure, and atrial distension).[3] Left ventricular systolic dysfunction (sepsis, ARDS, etc.) as well as abnormalities in fluid balance and electrolytes may contribute to the development of sustained arrhythmias in critically ill ICU patients. The management of arrhythmias in acutely ill ICU patients differs from that of patients with primary cardiac disease. Unfortunately, there is little (if any) evidence-based literature to guide the management of these arrhythmias in the ICU.

■ ARRHYTHMIAS AND ELECTROLYTE DISTURBANCES

Intravenous magnesium has been used to prevent and treat many different types of cardiac arrhythmias. It has diverse electrophysiological actions on the conduction system of the heart, including prolonging sinus node recovery time and reducing automaticity, atrioventricular nodal conduction, antegrade and retrograde conduction over an accessory pathway, and His-ventricular conduction. Intravenous magnesium can also homogenize transmural ventricular repolarization. Because of

P.E. Marik, *Handbook of Evidence-Based Critical Care*,
DOI 10.1007/978-1-4419-5923-2_28,
© Springer Science+Business Media, LLC 2010

its unique and diverse electrophysiological actions, intravenous magnesium has been reported to be useful in preventing atrial fibrillation and ventricular arrhythmias after cardiac and thoracic surgery; in reducing the ventricular response in acute-onset atrial fibrillation, including patients with Wolff–Parkinson–White syndrome; and in the treatment of digoxin-induced supraventricular and ventricular arrhythmias, multifocal atrial tachycardia, and polymorphic ventricular tachycardia or ventricular fibrillation from drug overdoses.[4] In addition, magnesium has synergistic activity when combined with other rate- and rhythm-controlling drugs.[5] Magnesium sulfate, when used to supplement other standard rate-reduction therapies, enhances rate reduction and conversion to sinus rhythm in patients with rapid atrial fibrillation.[6] Magnesium has a relatively wide toxic/therapeutic window; the most common reported side effects are a transient sensation of warmth and flushing. Magnesium should be considered the "first-line" agent for the control of arrhythmias in the ICU even in patients with normal serum magnesium (1.8–3.0 mg/dl); aim is to achieve a serum magnesium level of about 3.0 mg/dl.

ALERT

Magnesium is the intensivist's anti-arrhythmic agent of first choice!

Hypokalemia causes cellular hyperpolarity, increases resting potential, hastens depolarization, and increases automaticity and excitability. Hypokalemia appears to be a risk factor for the development of both atrial and ventricular arrhythmias. In the Study of Prevention of Postoperative Atrial Fibrillation (SPPAF), the rate of postoperative AF was 51% in patients with a serum potassium <3.9 mmol/l compared to 33% in patients with a serum potassium >4.3 mmol/l ($p<0.05$).[7]

■ ACUTE ATRIAL FIBRILLATION/ATRIAL FLUTTER

Atrial tachyarrhythmias are the commonest arrhythmias occurring in ICU patients, with a reported prevalence of between 8 and 28%.[1,2] Atrial fibrillation is the commonest atrial arrhythmia, followed by atrial flutter and multi-focal atrial tachycardia (MAT). Since the etiology and management strategies of atrial fibrillation and atrial flutter overlap, for the purposes of this discussion, they will be considered one entity (AF). Patients who develop AF have a worse prognosis than those who remain in sinus rhythm (SR); however, the attributable mortality of AF is unclear. Loss of atrioventricular synchrony will compromise stroke volume and cardiac output to a variable degree depending upon ventricular compliance, venous filling pressure, ventricular rate, and other hemodynamic factors. In the study by Annane and colleagues,[1] the presence of a supraventricular arrhythmia doubled the risk of a neurological sequelae (OR 2.64; 95% CI 1.19–5.84).

AF is particularly common in ICU patients with cardiovascular disorders, respiratory failure, and sepsis. The etiology is largely multifactorial, with hypoxia, electrolyte disturbance, myocardial ischemia, increased sympathetic tone, and atrial distension being implicated. Pulmonary hypertension with right atrial distension may be an important precipitant in patients with respiratory failure and sepsis.

The components of the acute management of AF include the following:

- Assessment of the need for urgent cardioversion
- Correcting treatable precipitating factors
- Controlling the ventricular response rate
- Prophylaxis against thromboembolic events in those patients who remain in AF

Drugs such as aminophylline and dopamine should be stopped. Pain and anxiety, which increase sympathetic activity, should be treated. New-onset atrial fibrillation may occur in patients with pulmonary embolism; this diagnosis should be considered.

Urgent Cardioversion

Electrical cardioversion is a time-honored, highly effective method for converting AF to sinus rhythm. Urgent cardioversion is indicated when the ventricular response is greater than 130 beats/min in association with the following:

- Angina/myocardial ischemia on ECG
- Acute cardiac failure
- Hypotension (MAP <70 mmHg or fall in MAP >15 mmHg)
- Indices of inadequate tissue perfusion

Rate Control

Rate control can improve hemodynamics even if the patient remains in AF. Digoxin is commonly used in the treatment of AF in ICU patients. Yet, in the critically ill ICU patient, digoxin is probably the least effective drug in controlling the ventricular response in AF. Digoxin decreases ventricular response in AF by vagotonic mechanisms. In critically ill patients, AF occurs in the setting of high sympathetic tone and frequently with the use of vasopressors and inotropic agents, a situation in which digoxin is likely to be ineffective. In addition, this drug has a very narrow therapeutic index and should be avoided except in patients with poor LV function.

Diltiazem is an effective agent for rate control in most patients with a response rate of between 93 and 97%. Diltiazem is given as a 5 mg bolus every 5 min until rate control is achieved or a maximal dose of 15 mg is administered, followed by an infusion of up to 15 mg/h. Esmolol, an ultra-short-acting non-selective β-blocker, has been demonstrated to be effective in controlling the ventricular response in AF. Similarly, IV metoprolol (5 mg boluses) may be used for rate control. However, β-blockers may cause hypotension particularly in patients with poor LV function. Amiodarone or digoxin may be used for rate control in patients with poor LV function. Magnesium has been shown to reduce the ventricular response in AF, with a greater effect when combined with digoxin. Magnesium may act by increasing the atrio-His interval and atrioventricular nodal refractoriness.

Digoxin and calcium channel blockers should not be given to patients who have atrial fibrillation with an anterogradely conducting accessory pathway, because blocking atrioventricular nodal conduction may provoke conduction down the accessory pathway, leading to an increase rather than decrease in the ventricular rate and hemodynamic collapse.

Pharmacological Cardioversion

A number of randomized controlled studies (RCTs) have evaluated procainamide, amiodarone, flecainide, sotalol, propafenone, and ibutilide in patients presenting to hospital with acute atrial fibrillation (non-ICU setting). In general, these studies have found the rate of conversion to be similar with the anti-arrhythmic drug as with placebo, with approximately 60% of patients spontaneously converting to sinus rhythm within 24 h.[8] The natural history of AF in acutely ill ICU patients has not been studied. However, it is likely that untreated arrhythmia will persist until the underlying medical condition which precipitated the arrhythmia has improved or resolved. The role of anti-arrhythmic agents in facilitating pharmacological cardioversion is unclear; however, it would appear that these agents have a limited role in the critically ill patient. Amiodarone is the agent most commonly used to facilitate cardioversion in the ICU. Amiodarone is not without risks, with hypotension and bradycardia being the most common adverse events, usually occurring during the loading infusion. Acute hepatotoxicity with liver function test abnormalities has been reported in 9–17% of patients. Amiodarone has also been associated with acute pulmonary toxicity presenting as ARDS. High inspired oxygen concentration and pre-existing ARDS may be risk factors for acute amiodarone pulmonary toxicity. Sleeswijk et al.[9] reported the efficacy of magnesium–amiodarone step-up scheme in critically ill patients with new-onset atrial fibrillation. A $MgSO_4$ bolus of 0.037 g/Kg over 15 minutes, was followed by a continuous infusion of 0.025 g/kg/hr (bolus of 2-3 g followed by 2g/hr in a 70 Kg patient). Intravenous amiodarone (loading dose 300 mg, followed by continuous infusion of 1,200 mg/24 h) was given to those not responding to $MgSO_4$ within 1 h. Clinical response was defined as conversion to sinus rhythm or decrease in heart rate <110 beats/min. Sixteen of the twenty-nine patients responded to $MgSO_4$ monotherapy, whereas the addition of amiodarone was required in 13 patients. Median time until conversion to sinus rhythm after $MgSO_4$ was 2 h, while the median conversion time in patients requiring amiodarone was 4 h. The 24-h conversion rate was 90%. As this approach obviates the need for anti-coagulation, it may be the preferable approach to AF in ICU patients.

Anti-coagulation

According to the most recent guidelines on anti-thrombotic therapy from the American College of Chest Physicians, anti-coagulation is not required for AF of less than 48 h.[10] This recommendation is supported by the study of Weigner and colleagues[11] who demonstrated three thromboembolic events in 357 patients (1%) with new-onset AF who converted to sinus rhythm. However, in patients in whom the arrhythmia lasts more than 48 h or its duration is uncertain, full anti-coagulation may be required. In these patients, this risk of anti-coagulation must be balanced against the risk of thromboembolic disease. The presence of structural heart disease, chronic/recurrent atrial fibrillation, and increased atrial dimensions may increase the risk of embolic events. Patients planned for pharmacological cardioversion in whom the arrhythmia has been present for more than 48 h require transesophageal echocardiography to exclude the presence of an atrial thrombus before attempting cardioversion.

■ MULTI-FOCAL ATRIAL TACHYCARDIA (MAT)

MAT has been defined as a rhythm with an atrial rate >100 beats/min, with at least three morphologically distinct P waves, irregular P–P intervals, and an isoelectric baseline between P waves. An exacerbation of COPD is the most common setting in which MAT arises. The treatment of COPD may promote the arrhythmia. A weak relationship exists between MAT and pulmonary embolism. This arrhythmia is typically an epiphenomenon of an underlying disorder and usually should not be treated. MAT is commonly transient and will often resolve after precipitating causes are reversed. MAT should be treated only if it causes hypotension, CHF, or myocardial ischemia. Calcium channel blockers, β-blockers (avoid in acute exacerbation of COPD), and magnesium have demonstrated some utility in treating this arrhythmia. Magnesium may be particularly effective and should probably be the first line of treatment (a loading dose of 2 g in 10 ml dextrose water over 5 min, followed by 10 g in 500 ml dextrose water over 5 h).

■ ATRIOVENTRICULAR NODAL RE-ENTRANT TACHYCARDIA

Atrioventricular nodal re-entrant tachycardia is usually not associated with underlying heart disease and may be precipitated by the same factors as atrial fibrillation/atrial flutter. This arrhythmia is characterized by a sudden onset and a sudden termination. The rate may range from 150 to 200 beats/min but most often it is 180–200 beats/min. In the common atrioventricular nodal re-entrant tachycardia, there is antegrade conduction over the slow AV nodal pathway and retrograde conduction over the fast pathway. As there is almost simultaneous excitation of both the atria and ventricles, the P wave occurs at the time of the QRS complex and is difficult to appreciate on the electrocardiogram. In 10% of patients, the re-entrant pathway is reversed. This tachycardia, referred to as the "uncommon atrioventricular nodal re-entrant tachycardia," is characterized by clearly visible P waves that are inverted in leads II, III, and aVF.

Management

- Vagal maneuvers are the initial treatment of choice:
  - Valsalva maneuver.
  - Muller maneuver – deep inspiration against a closed glottis.
  - Carotid sinus massage. Check that the patient has no carotid bruit or history of TIAs.
- Adenosine is the pharmacological agent of choice in patients who have failed vagal maneuvers. The usual dose is 6–12 mg by slow IV push. After termination of the tachycardia, brief periods of asystole are common:
  - Due to denervation hypersensitivity, adenosine should not be given to heart transplant recipients.
- Verapamil is also effective in terminating an atrioventricular nodal re-entrant tachycardia.
- Electrical cardioversion if the patient is hemodynamically unstable.

■ SUPRAVENTRICULAR TACHYCARDIA MEDIATED BY ACCESSORY PATHWAYS

Accessory pathways are anomalous bands of conducting tissue that form a connection between the atrium and the ventricle. When there is ante-grade accessory-pathway conduction during sinus rhythm, ventricular pre-excitation occurs. This results in the combination of a short PR interval and a delta wave, the electrocardiographic features of the Wolff–Parkinson–White (WPW) syndrome. Nearly 25% of accessory pathways are capable of only retrograde conduction (concealed bypass tracts).

The most common SVT in patients with WPW is the orthodromic atrioventricular re-entrant tachycardia; the impulse travels anterogradely over the AV node and then retrogradely through the accessory pathway. In about 10% of patients with WPW, the re-entrant circuit travels in the opposite direction (anti-dromic). This tachycardia is characterized by a wide QRS configuration (exaggeration of the delta wave).

A number of acute therapies are available for an orthodromic recipro-cating tachycardia:

- Electrical cardioversion if the patient is hemodynamically unstable.
- Adenosine is the pharmacological agent of choice (6–12 mg IV).
- Procainamide may be safely used in WPW syndrome.
- *Digoxin* and *verapamil* should not be administered as these drugs can shorten the refractory period of the bypass tract.

Atrial fibrillation and atrial flutter are frequently seen in patients with WPW syndrome because most accessory pathways have rapid conduc-tion. These patients may achieve ventricular rates that approach 300 beats/min; ventricular fibrillation may occur under such circumstances.

Adenosine, digoxin, and calcium channel blockers should *not* be given to patients who have atrial fibrillation with an accessory path-way, because blocking AV nodal conduction may provoke conduction down the accessory pathway, leading to an increase in the ventricular rate and hemodynamic collapse. The treatment of choice of these patients is procainamide.

■ SINUS BRADYCARDIA

Sinus bradycardia is not uncommon in ICU patients. This may occur due to myocardial ischemia, digoxin toxicity, sick sinus syndrome, and/or β-blockers and calcium channel blockers. The patient should be treated only if symptomatic and/or hypotensive:

- Atropine 0.5 mg repeated up to a total of 3 mg
- Isoproterenol 1–2 μg/min up to 20 μg/min

- A dopamine infusion, especially in hypotensive patients
- Pacing
  - Transvenous temporary pacemaker
  - External pacemaker (transcutaneous)

■ SICK SINUS SYNDROME

This syndrome is also known as the tachycardia–bradycardia syndrome. As the name implies, these patients have episodes of both tachycardia and bradycardia. The critically ill patient with this syndrome often requires temporary pacing in order to achieve hemodynamic stability.

■ ACCELERATED IDIOVENTRICULAR RHYTHM

This rhythm is characterized by a wide QRS complex and a regular ventricular rate, usually 60–110 beats/min. This is a benign rhythm that is usually asymptomatic and should just be observed.

■ VENTRICULAR PREMATURE COMPLEXES AND BIGEMINY

These are recognized by wide QRS complexes (>120 ms) with a bizarre configuration. Identify and treat possible precipitating factors, such as hypoxia and electrolyte disturbances. Ensure that the K^+ >4 mEq/l and that the Mg^{2+} >2 mg/dl. Treat the underlying cause and *not* the VPCs.

■ NON-SUSTAINED VENTRICULAR TACHYCARDIA

This is defined as 3 or more consecutive PVS's with a duration of up to 30s and a rate >100 beats/min. This arrhythmia is usually associated with an underlying heart disease and is associated with an increased mortality. In the ICU setting, precipitating factors should be diagnosed and treated. In the setting of acute myocardial ischemia, progressively longer runs of this arrhythmia may herald the onset of VF and should therefore be suppressed. In most other situations, unless the patient is symptomatic, this arrhythmia should just be observed.

■ SUSTAINED VENTRICULAR TACHYCARDIA

A wide QRS complex tachycardia: ectopy or aberration?

Factors Favoring Ectopy

- AV dissociation
- R or qR in V1 with taller *left* rabbit ear
- QS or RS in V6
- Bizarre frontal plane axis
- Concordant V leads
- LBBB pattern with wide R in V1

Factors Favoring SVT with Aberration

- Preceding P wave
- RBBB pattern
- Triphasic contour in V1 and V6
- Initial vector identical with that of flanking conducted beats
- qRs in V6

If there is any question of doubt, the arrhythmia should be considered to be ventricular rather than supraventricular. Adenosine may be used to differentiate between these two arrhythmias. The treatment of a ventricular tachycardia with a calcium channel blocker can result in a fatal outcome.

Sustained ventricular tachycardias usually occur in patients with severe underlying heart disease, usually ischemic heart disease. The prognosis depends largely on that of the underlying heart disease. The treatment of patients with sustained VT is dependent on the hemodynamic consequences. Cardioversion is the treatment of choice in hemodynamically compromised patients. If the patient is asymptomatic or only mildly symptomatic, a number of therapeutic options can be pursued (alone and in combination) including the following:

- Elective synchronized cardioversion.
- Procainamide is considered the drug of choice. Loading dose of 15 mg/kg at a rate of 25–50 mg/min followed by an infusion at 1–4 mg/min. Monitor levels and ECG.
- Amiodarone.
- Implantable anti-tachycardia device.

■ POLYMORPHIC VENTRICULAR TACHYCARDIA (TORSADES DE POINTES)

The hallmark of polymorphic ventricular tachycardia (PVT) is a QRS morphology that changes constantly. Torsades de pointes (translated) means "twisting of the points." Multiple leads may be required to demonstrate this phenomenon. This arrhythmia is classified as being associated with either (i) a normal QT interval or (ii) a prolonged QT interval.

Normal QT Interval

- Acute myocardial ischemia
- Hypertrophic cardiomyopathy
- Dilated cardiomyopathy

Prolonged QT Interval

- Congenital long-QT syndrome
- Acute myocardial ischemia
- Anti-arrhythmic drugs, especially class 1 agents; rarely sotalol (hypokalemia) and amiodarone
- Other drugs, including phenothiazines, tricyclic anti-depressants, erythromycin, ampicillin, and pentamidine
- Electrolyte disturbances
  - Hypokalemia
  - Hypomagnesemia
  - Hypocalcemia
- Acute intracranial pathology, such as subarachnoid hemorrhage and intracerebral bleed

Management

- Electrolyte abnormalities must be aggressively corrected, particularly potassium and magnesium deficiency.
- Magnesium sulfate (1–2 g) is usually highly successful, even in the absence of magnesium deficiency. Two grams (10 ml of 20% solution) is given IV for over 10 min, followed by 4 g for over 4–8 h as an infusion.
- Accelerating the heart rate is a simple and quick method of shortening the QT interval. Transvenous pacing is a safe and effective method of controlling this arrhythmia. As an immediate measure, transcutaneous pacing may be used while preparations are being made for electrode placement.
- An infusion of isoproterenol (2–8 μg/min) titrated to increase the heart rate above 120 beats/min is sometimes used if pacing

is not available. Isoproterenol is contraindicated in patients with an acute myocardial infarction, active ischemia, and severe hypertension.

- If the arrhythmia occurs during therapy with a type 1A agent, amiodarone may terminate the arrhythmia.
- PVT occurring in the setting of myocardial ischemia does not usually respond to anti-arrhythmic therapy. These patients usually require coronary revascularization. If the QT interval is prolonged, standard class I anti-arrhythmic agents should not be used.
- Patients with congenital long-QT syndrome are usually treated with β-blockers or phenytoin.

■ REFERENCES

1. Annane D, Sebille V, Duboc D, et al. Incidence and prognosis of sustained arrhythmias in critically ill patients. *Am J Respir Crit Care Med.* 2008;178:20–25.
2. Artucio H, Pereira M. Cardiac arrhythmias in critically ill patients: epidemiologic study. *Crit Care Med.* 1990;18:1383–1388.
3. Vieillard-Baron A, Schmitt JM, Augarde R, et al. Acute cor pulmonale in acute respiratory distress syndrome submitted to protective ventilation: incidence, clinical implications, and prognosis. *Crit Care Med.* 2001;29:1551–1555.
4. Onalan O, Crystal E, Daoulah A, et al. Meta-analysis of magnesium therapy for the acute management of rapid atrial fibrillation. *Am J Cardiol.* 2007;99:1726–1732.
5. Cagli K, Ozeke O, Ergun K, et al. Effect of low-dose amiodarone and magnesium combination on atrial fibrillation after coronary artery surgery. *J Card Surg.* 2006;21:458–464.
6. Davey MJ, Teubner D. A randomized controlled trial of magnesium sulfate, in addition to usual care, for rate control in atrial fibrillation. *Ann Emerg Med.* 2005;45:347–353.
7. Auer J, Weber T, Berent R, et al. Serum potassium level and risk of postoperative atrial fibrillation in patients undergoing cardiac surgery. *J Am Coll Cardiol.* 2004;44:938–939.
8. Galve E, Rius T, Ballester R, et al. Intravenous amiodarone in treatment of recent-onset atrial fibrillation: results of a randomized, controlled study. *J Am Coll Cardiol.* 1996;27:1079–1082.
9. Sleeswijk ME, Tulleken JE, Van NT, et al. Efficacy of magnesium–amiodarone step-up scheme in critically ill patients with new-onset atrial fibrillation: a prospective observational study. *J Intensive Care Med.* 2008;23:61–66.

10. Singer DE, Albers GW, Dalen JE, et al. Antithrombotic therapy in atrial fibrillation: American College of Chest Physicians Evidence-Based Clinical Practice Guidelines (8th Edition). *Chest.* 2008;133:546S–592S.
11. Weigner MJ, Caulfield TA, Danias PG, et al. Risk for clinical thromboembolism associated with conversion to sinus rhythm in patients with atrial fibrillation lasting less than 48 hours. *Ann Intern Med.* 1997;126:615–620.

29

Acute Decompensated Cardiac Failure

Heart failure (HF) is a serious condition affecting an estimated 2 million Americans and is a common reason for hospitalization. Acute decompensated heart failure (ADHF) refers broadly to new or worsening of signs and symptoms of HF that are progressing rapidly, whereby unscheduled medical care or hospital evaluation is necessary. The ADHERE registry is a national registry (in the United States) designed to study the characteristics, the management, and outcomes of patients (over 200,000) hospitalized with ADHF.[1] A preliminary analysis of this registry reported the mean age to be 72 years with 52% of the patients being women. The most common comorbid conditions were hypertension (73%), coronary artery disease (57%), and diabetes (44%). Evidence of mild or no impairment of systolic function was found in 46% of patients. In-hospital mortality was 4.0% and the median hospital length of stay was 4.3 days.

Patients presenting with an acute deterioration of cardiac function are often admitted to the ICU. These patients are likely to benefit from treatment. However, patients with "end-stage" cardiac failure whose condition has progressed slowly and inexorably despite maximal medical therapy are poor candidates for admission to the ICU, unless they are candidates for cardiac transplantation or have suffered from an acute medical complication. The following patients with cardiac failure may benefit from admission to an ICU:

- Worsening pulmonary edema with acute respiratory failure
- Acute myocardial ischemia
- Acute hemodynamic compromise due to arrhythmias
- Severe complicating disease, e.g., pneumonia

P.E. Marik, *Handbook of Evidence-Based Critical Care*,
DOI 10.1007/978-1-4419-5923-2_29,
© Springer Science+Business Media, LLC 2010

■ CONFIRM THE DIAGNOSIS OF CARDIAC FAILURE

In the ADHERE Registry, dyspnea occurred in about 89% of all patients presenting with cardiac failure.[2] Dyspnea on exertion was the most sensitive symptom and paroxysmal nocturnal dyspnea the most specific (positive likelihood ratio 2.6). However, many other diseases may cause symptoms that mimic cardiac failure. Dyspnea can be caused by a wide range of conditions. It may be difficult to distinguish dyspnea caused by cardiac failure from that caused by COPD; this distinction is critically important in the management of the patient with a history of cardiac failure who becomes dyspneic. Indeed, in an intriguing study which randomized patients with suspected heart failure to prehospital treatment with furosemide, morphine and nitroglycerine resulted in a higher than expected mortality in patients with asthma, chronic obstructive pulmonary disease, pneumonia, or bronchitis who were erroneously diagnosed with and treated for heart failure.[3]

ALERT

Lasix® (furosemide) is not the treatment for all patients with dyspnea.

Patients with peripheral edema may be inappropriately labeled as having heart failure when there is another cause for the edema. Physical examination is not sensitive for diagnosing heart failure. Many patients with severely impaired left ventricular function have no signs of heart failure. Marantz et al.[4] reported that 20% of patients with EF less than 40% had no clinical features of heart failure, and only 42% of patients with left ventricular EFs of less than 30% had dyspnea on exertion.

■ EVALUATION OF THE PATIENT WITH CARDIAC FAILURE

B-Type Natriuretic Peptides

Brain natriuretic peptide (BNP) and N-terminal pro-brain natriuretic peptide (NT-proBNP) are useful biomarkers to assist in the diagnosis of heart failure. BNP belongs to the natriuretic peptide family, which also includes atrial natriuretic peptide, C-type natriuretic peptide, and urodilatin. Although present in the human brain, BNP is mainly synthesized and secreted by ventricular myocardium. Myocardial wall stress is the most important stimulus for increased synthesis and secretion of BNP.

It is released into the circulation as a pro-hormone and cleaved into the biologically active 32-amino-acid BNP and the biologically inactive 76-amino-acid NT-proBNP. The half-life of BNP is 20 min, whereas the half-life of NT-proBNP is 120 min, which explains why NT-proBNP serum values are approximately six times higher than BNP values, even though both molecules are released in equimolar proportions.[5,6]

In a large number of studies it has been consistently found that BNP and NT-proBNP are elevated in patients with heart failure, and values were found to be related to disease severity as assessed by New York Heart Association (NYHA) functional class, left ventricular systolic ejection fraction, and left ventricular diastolic function.[5,6] In the Breath Not Properly (BNP) trial, 1,586 patients presenting to the emergency department with shortness of breath were investigated.[7] The main finding of this study was that BNP testing provided high test accuracy for the detection of heart failure, being superior to clinical judgment. At a cutoff value of 100 pg/ml, BNP had a very high negative predictive value, thus making it especially applicable as a rule-out test for heart failure in this setting. Thus, the particular strength of these markers is their ability to rule out the diagnosis of heart failure. In general, heart failure is unlikely at BNP values <100 pg/ml and is very likely at BNP values >500 pg/ml.

Independent of their diagnostic value, several large-scale studies have convincingly shown that BNP and NT-proBNP provide strong prognostic information for an unfavorable outcome (death, cardiovascular death, readmission, or cardiac events) in patients with heart failure or asymptomatic left ventricular dysfunction.[8]

It should be appreciated that acute right ventricular failure, as occurs with acute pulmonary embolism and acute cor pulmonale (ARDS, etc.), will result in increased BNP and NT-PROBNP levels.[9,10] BNP levels therefore have little utility in distinguishing cardiogenic from non-cardiogenic pulmonary edema.[10]

Echocardiography

Assessment of left ventricular function is a critical step in the evaluation and management of patients with heart failure. All patients should undergo echocardiography unless this investigation or angiography has been performed recently (within the last few months). An ejection fraction of less than 45%, with or without symptoms of heart failure, is accepted as evidence of left ventricular systolic dysfunction. Substantial proportions (up to 50% in some studies) of patients with signs and symptoms of heart failure have preserved systolic function (EFs greater than 45%). The cause of heart failure in these patients is on the basis of diastolic dysfunction (see below) or valvular heart disease. This distinction is important as the management of these patients differs somewhat.

Quantitative assessment of left ventricular function is important as the EF is the most important predictor of the 5-year survival rate in patients with systolic heart failure.

Laboratory Testing

Laboratory testing should include serum electrolytes and a complete blood count. In the ADHERE registry, a serum urea nitrogen (BUN) of greater than 43 mg/dl was the single best predictor of in-hospital mortality, with a systolic blood pressure of less than 115 mmHg being second and a creatinine of greater than 2.75 mg/dl being third.[2] Hyponatremia in a patient with cardiac failure is a sign of failing circulatory homeostasis and is associated with longer length of stay and higher in-hospital and early postdischarge mortality.[11] Anemia is also a poor prognostic marker.[12]

ALERT

A high BUN is a poor prognostic marker in cardiac failure; this is often a consequence of over-diuresis.

■ HEMODYNAMIC MONITORING

Invasive hemodynamic monitoring in cardiac failure has come under close scrutiny, and its value has been questioned, especially after the results of the ESCAPE trial.[13] In this study, patients were randomized to routine care or treatment guided by a PAC. In-hospital adverse events were more common among patients in the PAC group; however, there were no significant differences in 30-day mortality or clinical outcomes or adverse events at 6 months between the two groups of patients. This study, in keeping with the general critical care literature, has demonstrated the PAC to be of limited clinical utility.

■ PRECIPITATING FACTORS

It is important to determine the precipitating factor(s) that have led to a deterioration of cardiac function. The most important include the following:

- Myocardial ischemia
- Poorly controlled hypertension

- Arrhythmias, particularly atrial arrhythmias
- Poor compliance with medication
- Drug reactions/side effects
- Fluid overload due to deterioration of renal function
- Anemia
- Intercurrent illness, particularly infections
- Excessive diuresis

■ TREATMENT

The treatment of ADHF involves relief of symptoms and treatment of pulmonary edema, hemodynamic stabilization, management of comorbidities and precipitating factors, and the initiation of long-term therapy.

Acute Phase

While the management and outcome of patients with chronic systolic heart failure has improved in recent years largely due to interventions based on well conducted RCTs, the management of ADHF remains problematic with few evidence-based interventions available. Indeed, emerging data suggest that the "conventional" therapeutic interventions for ADHF including morphine, high-dose furosemide, and inotropic agents may be harmful.

Oxygen

Patients require supplemental oxygen; this should be guided by pulse oximetry. Strong evidence supports the use of NIPPV to treat acute cardiogenic pulmonary edema (see Chapter 15). Positive-pressure ventilation is "good for the left ventricle"; it reduces the work of breathing, reduces preload, and reduces LV afterload. Both CPAP and BiPAP lower intubation and mortality rates compared to conventional therapy with oxygen.[14,15] However, CPAP should be considered as the first-line intervention as it is as efficacious as BiPAP and CPAP is cheaper and easier to implement in clinical practice.[14,15]

Morphine

Morphine sulfate has long been used to treat ADHF on the basis that it is a potent venodilator with additional anxiolytic properties. However, data from the ADHERE registry suggest that the use of morphine is associated with an increased risk for intubation and is an independent predictor of mortality (OR 4.84).[16] Based on these data, morphine should be avoided in patients with ADHF.

Diuretics

Diuretics have been the mainstay for the treatment of ADHF for the past four decades; indeed these drugs (particularly furosemide) are still widely used and recommended for this indication.[17] The ADHERE study reported that 89% of patients presented with symptoms of volume over-load and that 88% received intravenous diuretics. However, although patients are volume overloaded with features of "congestion," there are little data to support the use of loop diuretics; indeed high-dose furosemide is associated with worse outcomes. It is important to note that loop diuretics are associated with a *fall in GFR* (see Chapters 8 and 42); this further compromises renal function in patients with cardiac fail-ure. High-dose diuretics have a number of adverse effects in patients with heart failure which include the following:

- Activation of the renin–angiotensin system
- Increased AVP
- Increased heart rate
- Increased norepinephrine levels
- *Decreased* GFR
- Increased SVR

Diuretics are appropriate therapy in patients with symptomatic cardio-genic pulmonary edema. However, it is important to realize that patients with failing hearts (chronic) are able to tolerate high pulmonary venous pressures without developing pulmonary edema. Patients with severe chronic left heart failure frequently lack pulmonary rales on examination or alveolar edema on chest X-ray despite high pulmonary venous pressure (and features of pulmonary venous hypertension on chest X-ray); these patients may have pulmonary venous pressures >30 mmHg. This obser-vation is explained by reduced pulmonary microvascular permeability as well as increased lymphatic flow in these patients.

It is widely (although incorrectly) believed that diuresis improves car-diac function in patients with congestive cardiac failure. It has been postulated that diuretic-induced changes in preload increase ventricular performance by two mechanisms: either by shifting the ventricle to a "more optimal position on the descending limb on the Starling curve" or by reducing left ventricular size and thereby reducing systolic wall stress (afterload) by the Laplace effect. However, it has been clearly demon-strated that in the physiological range, there is *no* descending limb of the left ventricular stroke volume–pressure curve (Frank–Starling curve) in the mammalian heart (this includes humans). Furthermore, there is currently no evidence to support the contention that diuresis increases stroke volume or cardiac output in patients with congestive cardiac failure. Braunwald and colleagues[18] demonstrated an average fall in cardiac output of 20% following diuresis in patients with impaired cardiac function both at rest and during exercise.

It should therefore be no surprise that the use of high-dose loop diuretics in patients with ADHF has been associated with adverse outcomes. Data from the ADHERE registry demonstrated that patients treated with IV diuretics had longer lengths of stay and higher in-hospital mortality rates when compared to non-IV, diuretic-treated patients, even after adjustment for confounding factors.[19] In an intriguing study, Cotter et al. randomized 110 patients with cardiogenic pulmonary edema to either high-dose nitrates or high-dose furosemide (80 mg IV every 15 min until improvement) after receiving an initial 40 mg dose of furosemide.[20] Mechanical ventilation was required in 7 (13%) patients in the nitrate group and 21 (40%) patients in the furosemide group ($p = 0.0041$). Myocardial infarction occurred in 9 (17%) and 19 (37%) patients ($p = 0.047$) and death in 1 and 3 patients ($p = 0.61$), respectively. One or more of these end points occurred in 13 (25%) and 24 (46%) patients, respectively ($p = 0.041$). Worsening renal function during hospitalization is a powerful independent prognostic factor for adverse outcomes. Metra and colleagues[21] demonstrated that the daily furosemide dose was an independent predictor of worsening renal function, which itself was a predictor of death and rehospitalization. The initial daily dose of furosemide was 82 mg in the group whose renal function remained stable as compared to 160 mg in those with worsening renal function.

Based on these data, patients with ADHF should receive no more than 40–80 mg furosemide per day and this dose should be reduced in patients with worsening renal function.

ALERT

Furosemide is the Devil's Medicine and should be used with utmost caution.

Vasodilators

Nitroglycerin is the most commonly used vasodilator in the setting of acute heart failure; however, it should be used with caution in hypotensive patients. Nitroglycerin's effects are mediated through the relaxation of vascular smooth muscle; it reduces preload and afterload. Nitroglycerin increases cardiac output, decreases systemic vascular resistance, and improves microcirculating perfusion.[22] Nitroglycerin can be given orally, topically, or intravenously as long as blood pressure is maintained. This is one of the few agents which has been shown to improve outcome in ADHF,[20] and it is likely that this agent is underutilized for the treatment of this condition The IV route is recommended in patients admitted to the ICU. The dosing of nitroglycerin is often suboptimal and may need to reach doses of about 160 μg/min to achieve measurable decreases in pulmonary capillary wedge pressure. Headache is a common adverse effect but is generally ameliorated with acetaminophen.

Due to its toxicity, nitroprusside is best avoided (see Chapter 25). While ACE inhibitors and ARBs play a central role in the management of "compensated heart failure," they are best avoided in ADHF as they may adversely affect renal function.

Nesiritide is identical to the endogenous BNP produced by the body. It acts as a vasodilator (arterial and venous) and antagonizes the renin–angiotensin–aldosterone and sympathetic nervous systems. Nesiritide is given as a 2 mg/kg bolus, followed by an infusion of 0.01 mg/kg/min. Pooled analyses have raised concerns about the safety of this agent, with the drug being linked to worsening renal function and increased mortality.[18,23] Nesiritide cannot be recommended in patients with ADHF based on the current data.

Inotropic Agents

Dobutamine may have a role in patients with acute left ventricular failure due to myocardial ischemia. In this setting, dobutamine may recruit hibernating myocardium and improve cardiac function. The role of dobutamine in patients with chronic heart failure is unclear. Chronic heart failure is characterized by sympathetic hyperactivation and β-receptor downregulation. Short-term infusions or continuous β-stimulant therapies have not been demonstrated to be beneficial in these patients.[24] This therapy is associated with an increased frequency of ventricular arrhythmias, which may increase mortality. β-Blockers have been demonstrated to improve outcome in patients with compensated heart failure (see below); it therefore appears counterintuitive that β-stimulant therapy would have a role in ADHF.

Milrinone acts by inhibiting the phosphodiesterase III isoenzyme, which leads to increased cyclic adenosine monophosphate (cAMP) and enhanced inotropy. It differs from dobutamine, because it elevates cAMP by preventing its degradation as opposed to dobutamine, which increases cAMP production. In the OPTIME-CHF study, the use of milrinone in patients with an ischemic cardiomyopathy was associated with an increase in the composite of death or rehospitalization (42% vs. 36% for placebo, $p = 0.01$).[25] Furthermore, in the ESCAPE heart failure trial, the use of an inotrope was associated with an increased risk of death, RR of 2.14 (95% CI 1.10–4.15).[26] These data suggest that both dobutamine and milrinone have a limited role in the management of patients with ADHF.

Management of Atrial Fibrillation (AF)

AF may occur in up to 50% of patients with severe heart failure. If AF causes sudden severe worsening of heart failure, immediate cardioversion may be necessary. However, most patients can be stabilized by using amiodarone or digoxin to control heart rate. Approximately 60% of patients with acute AF (less than 1 week) will spontaneously revert back to sinus rhythm. A randomized placebo-controlled study demonstrated that the rate of conversion of acute AF to sinus rhythm was similar in a group of patients treated with amiodarone compared to the group receiving placebo.[27] It had previously been assumed that the prognosis of patients with heart failure and AF was improved if these patients were converted to sinus rhythm. However, a recent RCT demonstrated that a strategy of rhythm control does not reduce the rate of death or cardiovascular complications as compared to a rate-control strategy.[28]

Management of Hypertension

Reduction of blood pressure may in itself have a beneficial effect on the signs and symptoms of heart failure. Hypertension is a relative concept in patients with heart failure. Although a blood pressure of 135/85 mmHg may be acceptable for a patient with a normal EF, that same blood pressure may be harmful for patients with left ventricular systolic dysfunction. Intravenous nicardipine, clevidipine, or fenoldopam (see Chapter 25) followed by treatment with an oral ACE inhibitor, ARBs, or amlodipine is recommended for blood pressure control in these patients.

Anti-coagulation

Routine anti-coagulation is not recommended. Patients with a history of systemic or pulmonary embolism, recent atrial fibrillation, or mobile left ventricular thrombi should be anti-coagulated aiming to achieve a prothrombin time ratio of 1.2–1.8 times control (INR 2.0–3.0).

Anemia and Treatment with EPO

Anemia is a recognized poor prognostic indicator in cardiac failure.[12] Multiple factors contribute to the anemia of heart failure including decreased erythropoietin production due to kidney injury, ACE inhibitors, increased levels of pro-inflammatory mediators as well as iron deficiency. This, however, does not mean that blood transfusion improves outcome (see Chapter 51). Blood transfusion (a single unit at a time) should be considered only in highly symptomatic patients with a hemoglobin level below 7–8 g/dl. Recombinant erythropoietin (EPO) or darbepoetin should be strongly considered in these patients. In addition to stimulating erythropoiesis and increasing the hemoglobin concentration, EPO has a number of other beneficial effects that may be particularly important in patients with heart failure. Animal studies have shown that EPO appears to directly improve LV function. EPO can induce myocardial neovascularization and prevent myocardial cell apoptosis, myocardial fibrosis, and oxidative stress secondary to myocardial infarction, CHF, or ischemic injury.

Silverberg et al.[29] randomized 32 patients with moderate-to-severe CHF who had LVEF <40% and whose Hb levels were persistently between 10.0 and 11.5 g/dl to receive subcutaneous EPO and IV iron to increase the level of Hb to at least 12.5 g% or no specific therapy. Over a mean of 8.2±2.6 months, the patients who received EPO received less therapy for heart failure and spent fewer days in hospital compared to the control group. Furthermore, NYHA class and LVEF improved in the EPO patients, while these end points worsened in the control patients. In a similar double-blind, placebo-controlled study in 38 anemic patients with CHF, these authors demonstrated favorable effects on NYHA, BNP, oxygen utilization during maximal exercise, exercise endurance and distance walked, serum creatinine and creatinine clearance, and hospitalization over a 4-month double-blind period.[30]

Treatment of ADHF: Summary

- CPAP + oxygen.
- Furosemide 40–80 mg initially (on presentation) and then 40 mg daily. Stop if BUN increases.
- Intravenous nitroglycerin, titrate up to 160 μg/min (hold/stop for hypotension).
- EPO if Hb less than 12 g/dl.
- Treat complications.
- *No* morphine, nitroprusside, nesiritide, or inotropic agents.
- Anti-coagulation for chronic AF.

■ LONG-TERM MANAGEMENT

Once the patients' condition has stabilized (i.e., resolution of features of pulmonary edema and the patient is normotensive with stable renal function), chronic therapy can be reinstated or initiated. At this point it is important to determine if the patient has predominantly systolic (low EF) or diastolic (normal EF) heart failure, as this has some impact on the long-term therapeutic plan. While a considerable number of large RCTs have evaluated the utility of various interventions in patients with systolic heart failure, the optimal management of patients with diastolic heart failure is somewhat less clear.

Diuretics do not improve heart function and they should be used with great caution in the chronic phase of heart failure (both systolic and diastolic) and only in the lowest dose to control symptoms of congestion (pulmonary edema). Patient's nutritional status should be optimized (with iron and vitamin supplementation) and comorbidities aggressively treated. Erythropoietin should be strongly considered in patients with anemia.

■ SYSTOLIC HEART FAILURE

ACE Inhibitors

ACE inhibitors have been shown to decrease mortality and hospitalizations in patients with systolic heart failure.[31] It is recommended that all patients with systolic heart failure be on an ACE inhibitor before hospital discharge unless there is a contraindication.[17]

ACE inhibitors are contraindicated in patients with moderate to severe aortic stenosis, bilateral renal artery stenosis, hypertrophic obstructive cardiomyopathy, and pericardial tamponade. Oliguria and serum creatinine levels above 3 mg/dl are also contraindications to the use of ACE inhibitors. In addition, ACE inhibitors should be avoided in patients whose renal function has acutely declined. ACE inhibitors should not be started (or be discontinued) in patients with a serum potassium greater than 5.5 mEq/l. ACE inhibitors should be used very cautiously in patients with poorly controlled angina, as ACE inhibitors may cause an increase in angina in these patients.

Mild azotemia may occur when ACE inhibitors are started; this is usually well tolerated. A rapid rise in the serum creatinine should prompt a consideration of bilateral renal artery stenosis. Patients should be started on low doses and titrated up to target levels. Even lower than target doses have been shown to decrease mortality, although higher doses are more cost effective.

ARBs block the angiotensin II receptors, thereby reducing LV remodeling, arterial vasoconstriction, and renal damage. They seem to have a more favorable adverse effect profile with less cough and angioedema; they are reserved for patients who are intolerant of ACE inhibitors.

β-Blockers

β-Blocker therapy is effective in reducing sympathetic nervous system activity, symptoms, and mortality in patients who have HF. The hyperadrenergic state of HF, as measured by increases in norepinephrine levels, leads to myocardial hypertrophy, increases in afterload, coronary vasoconstriction, and mortality. Both carvedilol and long-acting metoprolol have been shown to reduce mortality in heart failure.[32,33]

Aldactone

The aldosterone receptor antagonist Aldactone (12.5–50 mg daily) when used in conjunction with an ACE inhibitor has been demonstrated to reduce the risk of death from progressive heart failure and sudden death from cardiac causes in patients with severe heart failure.[34] The drug is well tolerated with few side effects. It has been suggested that the beneficial effect of Aldactone may be mediated by preventing myocardial and vascular fibrosis associated with increased circulating levels of aldosterone. Aldactone should therefore be added to the regimen of an ACE inhibitor in patients with severe heart failure due to left ventricular systolic dysfunction. The serum potassium level should be closely monitored and the dose reduced (or stopped) should hyperkalemia develop.

Digoxin

Digoxin inhibits the Na^+/K^+-ATPase of the myocardial cellular membrane and has been used for years to control ventricular response in atrial fibrillation. Digoxin has a very narrow therapeutic index and unless the patient is dosed precisely and the serum levels monitored, the patient is likely to suffer significant toxicity. A serum level greater than 1.2 ng/ml offers very little therapeutic advantage but increases the risk of toxicity. The patient's age, weight, and renal function must be taken into account when dosing (loading and maintenance) the patient. Because digoxin does not improve survival in patients with heart failure, this drug has a limited role in heart failure patients in sinus rhythm.[35]

Calcium Channel-Blocking Drugs

First-generation calcium channel-blocking drugs such as verapamil, diltiazem, and nifedipine should be avoided in patients with left ventricular systolic dysfunction as these agents have been demonstrated to increase morbidity and mortality. The PRAISE study demonstrated that amlodipine does not adversely affect the natural history of chronic heart failure.[36] This drug should be considered second-line therapy for the management of hypertension or angina in patients with left ventricular dysfunction.

Implantable Defibrillators

Ventricular arrhythmias in patients with congestive heart failure are associated with increased rates of overall mortality and sudden death. However, attempts at suppressing ventricular arrhythmias with anti-arrhythmic agents have not been demonstrated to improve survival. The MADIT study demonstrated that in patients with prior myocardial infarction who have an EF less than 35%, a documented episode of asymptomatic VT and inducible non-suppressible VT (EPS studies), that prophylactic therapy with an implantable defibrillator leads to improved survival as compared to conventional therapy.[37] The AVID study demonstrated that an implantable cardioverter–defibrillator resulted in lower mortality than did anti-arrhythmic drug therapy among patients resuscitated from ventricular fibrillation or symptomatic, sustained ventricular tachycardia with hemodynamic compromise.[38]

Cardiac Resynchronization

Atrial-synchronized biventricular pacing (cardiac resynchronization therapy, CRT) has proven to be an effective treatment in symptomatic patients with reduced left ventricular ejection fraction and electromechanical dyssynchrony. A meta-analysis of six studies showed that CRT reduced all-cause mortality by 28% and new hospitalizations for worsening HF by 37%.[39] The COMPANION trial suggested that the benefits of biventricular pacing and ICDs are additive in patients with LV systolic failure.[40]

Evaluation of Patients for Revascularization

Coronary artery disease is currently the most common cause of heart failure in the United States, and some heart failure patients may benefit from revascularization. Patients with a history of angina or AMI should undergo physiological testing for ischemia, followed by coronary artery angiography if ischemic regions are detected. Patients with heart failure who have significant angina (exercise limiting, occurring at rest, and recurrent episodes of pulmonary edema) should undergo coronary arteriography as the initial test for operable coronary lesions.

Mechanical Support Devices

The optimal management strategy for patients with ADHF has been limited to the use of various pharmacological agents. However, with technological advances in mechanical devices, non-pharmacological approaches are now available to supplement pharmacological manage-ment. In general, these devices can be used to support those patients with acute left ventricular failure (i.e., shock) and/or those patients with ADHF.[41]

Intra-aortic balloon pump counterpulsation (IABP) is the oldest tech-nology in current use for mechanical circulatory support; its development dates back to the 1950s. The physiological theory behind aortic counter-pulsation is that balloon inflation during ventricular diastole augments antegrade coronary perfusion and balloon deflation during ventricu-lar systole decreases aortic impedance, which decreases resistance to ejection. These effects result in decreased myocardial wall stress and increased cardiac output; myocardial oxygen consumption may fall by >50% and stroke volume may increase by as much as 30%.[42] In most settings, IABP counterpulsation is used as a bridge to more definitive therapies such as coronary bypass surgery, transplantation, or placement of a ventricular assist device (VAD).

VADs are mechanical blood pumps that serve to either augment or replace the function of either the left or the right ventricle. They are currently used for three purposes:

- A bridge to myocardial recovery in acute ventricular failure (i.e., postcardiotomy or shock complicating myocarditis or myocardial infarction)
- A bridge to heart transplantation in chronic ventricular failure
- As permanent therapy for end-stage chronic heart failure, also known as destination therapy

Most currently available devices are surgically implanted and require cardiopulmonary bypass to implant. Percutaneous assist devices are in development, and one is commercially available (e.g., TandemHeart). The TandemHeart device is a left atrial to femoral arterial bypass sys-tem that can be inserted percutaneously and is able to provide active flow via a centrifugal pump independent of native heart rhythm.[43]

■ MANAGEMENT OF PATIENTS WITH HEART FAILURE WITH PRESERVED EJECTION FRACTION

Many patients with features of cardiac failure have a preserved ejection fraction (>40%); this syndrome is referred to as diastolic heart failure or most recently "heart failure with normal ejection fraction" (HFnEF). The ADHERE registry demonstrated that up to 46% of patients with ADHF had preserved systolic function.[1] In patients with HFnEF, the left ventricle has increased diastolic stiffness (reduced compliance) and is unable to fill adequately at normal diastolic pressures.[44] This condition results in reduced end-diastolic volume and elevated end-diastolic pressures. The reduced left ventricular filling leads to decreased stroke volume and symptoms of low cardiac output, whereas the increased filling pressure leads to symptoms of pulmonary congestion.

Hypertension is the commonest cause of diastolic dysfunction which can develop even in the absence of left ventricular hypertrophy. Left ventricular compliance decreases with aging; this syndrome is therefore very common in the elderly hypertensive patients. Diabetes results in a cardiomyopathy characterized by the presence of cardiac hypertrophy and myocardial stiffness. Myocardial fibrosis and collagen deposition are the primary structural changes observed in diabetic cardiomyopathy. Both hypertension and diabetes may coexist in many patients with HFnEF. The results of large recent study found that 96% of patients with HFnEF had hypertension and 37% had diabetes.[45] The prognosis of HFnEF is almost as poor as the prognosis of heart failure with reduced EF. After a first hospitalization for heart failure, HFnEF patients have a 5-year survival rate of only 43%.[46]

In patients with features of HFnEF, it is important to exclude other diagnoses, including the following:

- Primary valvular disease
- Restrictive cardiomyopathies
    - Amyloidosis
    - Sarcoidosis
    - Hemochromatosis
- Pericardial constriction
- Chronic pulmonary disease with right heart failure
- Heart failure associated with high output state
    - Anemia
    - Thyrotoxicosis
    - AV fistula
- Atrial myxoma

In contrast to the treatment of HF in patients with reduced EF, few clinical trials are available to guide the management of patients with HFnEF.

Although controlled studies have been performed with digitalis, ACE inhibitors, ARBs, β-blockers, and calcium channel blockers in patients with HFnEF, for the most part, these trials have been small or have produced inconclusive results. The use of β-blockers and rate-slowing calcium channel blockers is advocated in HFnEF on the premise that they decrease blood pressure and afterload and prolong the diastolic filling period. However, these drugs can have a direct detrimental effect on LV relaxation and negative chronotropic properties. Therefore, the final balance between all these effects determines the clinical response in a given patient. In the OPIMIZE-HF study, β-blockers did not significantly influence the mortality and rehospitalization risk for patients with LVnEF.[47] Diuretics are required in the presence of signs of volume overload, but caution is needed to avoid a precipitous drop in LV stroke volume. ACE inhibitors and ARBs (and potentially statins) that can lead to regression of not only LV mass but also interstitial fibrosis can be beneficial, in part through their favorable effect on LV stiffness. The CHARM study, the largest study to date in patients with HFnEF, demonstrated that candesartan (an ARB) had a moderate impact in preventing admissions for CHF.[48] These data suggest that an ACE inhibitor or an ARB together with risk factor modification (glucose and cholesterol control, weight loss, smoking cessation, etc.) is the preferred approach to the management of patients with HFnEF.

■ CLINICAL PEARLS

- Heart failure is unlikely with BNP values <100 pg/ml and is very likely with BNP values >500 pg/ml.
- Anemia and an increased BUN are poor prognostic features in patients with heart failure.
- It is important to differentiate heart failure with preserved EF (HFnEF) from heart failure with reduced EF (HFrEF).
- High-dose diuretics are independent predictors for the development of renal failure and *death. Beware.*

■ REFERENCES

1. Adams KF Jr., Fonarow GC, Emerman CL, et al. Characteristics and outcomes of patients hospitalized for heart failure in the United States: rationale, design, and preliminary observations from the first 100,000 cases in the Acute Decompensated Heart Failure National Registry (ADHERE). *Am Heart J.* 2005;149:209–216.
2. Fonarow GC. The Acute Decompensated Heart Failure National Registry (ADHERE): opportunities to improve care of patients hospitalized with

acute decompensated heart failure. *Rev Cardiovasc Med.* 2003;4(Suppl 7):S21–S30.

3. Wuerz RC, Meador SA. Effects of prehospital medications on mortality and length of stay in congestive heart failure. *Ann Emerg Med.* 1992;21:669–674.

4. Marantz PR, Tobin JN, Wassertheil-Smoller S, et al. The relationship between left ventricular systolic function and congestive heart failure diagnosed by clinical criteria. *Circulation.* 1988;77:607–612.

5. Levin ER, Gardner DG, Samson WK. Natriuretic peptides. *N Engl J Med.* 1998;339:321–328.

6. Weber M, Hamm C. Role of B-type natriuretic peptide (BNP) and NT-proBNP in clinical routine. *Heart.* 2006;92:843–849.

7. Maisel AS, Krishnaswamy P, Nowak RM, et al. Rapid measurement of B-type natriuretic peptide in the emergency diagnosis of heart failure. *N Engl J Med.* 2002;347:161–167.

8. Anand IS, Fisher LD, Chiang YT, et al. Changes in brain natriuretic peptide and norepinephrine over time and mortality and morbidity in the Valsartan Heart Failure Trial (Val-HeFT). *Circulation.* 2003;107:1278–1283.

9. Cavallazzi R, Nair A, Vasu T, et al. Natriuretic peptides in acute pulmonary embolism: a systematic review. *Intensive Care Med.* 2008;34:2147–2156.

10. Levitt JE, Vinayak AG, Gehlbach BK, et al. Diagnostic utility of B-type natriuretic peptide in critically ill patients with pulmonary edema: a prospective cohort study. *Crit Care.* 2008;12:R3.

11. Gheorghiade M, Abraham WT, Albert NM, et al. Relationship between admission serum sodium concentration and clinical outcomes in patients hospitalized for heart failure: an analysis from the OPTIMIZE-HF registry. *Eur Heart J.* 2007;28:980–988.

12. Groenveld HF, Januzzi JL, Damman K, et al. Anemia and mortality in heart failure patients a systematic review and meta-analysis. *J Am Coll Cardiol* 2008;52:818–827.

13. Binanay C, Califf RM, Hasselblad V, et al. Evaluation study of congestive heart failure and pulmonary artery catheterization effectiveness: the ESCAPE trial. *JAMA.* 2005;294:1625–1633.

14. Winck JC, Azevedo LF, Costa-Pereira A, et al. Efficacy and safety of non-invasive ventilation in the treatment of acute cardiogenic pulmonary edema – a systematic review and meta-analysis. *Crit Care.* 2006;10:R69.

15. Ho KM, Wong K. A comparison of continuous and bi-level positive airway pressure non-invasive ventilation in patients with acute cardiogenic pulmonary oedema: a meta-analysis. *Crit Care.* 2006;10:R49.

16. Peacock WF, Hollander JE, Diercks DB, et al. Morphine and outcomes in acute decompensated heart failure: an ADHERE analysis. *Emerg Med J.* 2008;25:205–209.

17. Hunt SA, Abraham WT, Chin MH, et al. ACC/AHA 2005 guideline update for the diagnosis and management of chronic heart failure in the adult: a report of the American College of Cardiology/American Heart Association Task Force on Practice Guidelines. *Circulation*. 2005;112:e154–e235.

18. Stampfer M, Epstein SE, Beiser GD, et al. Hemodynamic effects of diuresis at rest and during intense upright exercise in patients with impaired cardiac function. *Circulation*. 1968;37:900–911.

19. Emerman CL, Marco TD, Costanzo MR, et al. Impact of intravenous diuretics on the outcomes of patients hospitalized with acute decompensated heart failure: insights from the ADHERE registry. *J Card Fail*. 2009;10:S116.

20. Cotter G, Metzkor E, Kaluski E, et al. Randomised trial of high-dose isosorbide dinitrate plus low-dose furosemide versus high-dose furosemide plus low-dose isosorbide dinitrate in severe pulmonary oedema. *Lancet*. 1998;351:389–393.

21. Metra M, Nodari S, Parrinello G, et al. Worsening renal function in patients hospitalised for acute heart failure: clinical implications and prognostic significance. *Eur J Heart Fail*. 2008;10:188–195.

22. den Uil CA, Caliskan K, Lagrand WK, et al. Dose-dependent benefits of nitroglycerin on microcirculation of patients with severe heart failure. *Intensive Care Med*. 2009;35:1893–1899.

23. Sackner-Bernstein JD, Kowalski M, Fox M, et al. Short-term risk of death after treatment with nesiritide for decompensated heart failure. A pooled analysis of randomized controlled trials. *JAMA*. 2005;293:1900–1905.

24. Leier CV. Positive inotropic therapy: an update and new agents. *Curr Probl Cardiol*. 1996;21:521–581.

25. Felker GM, Benza RL, Chandler AB, et al. Heart failure etiology and response to milrinone in decompensated heart failure: results from the OPTIME-CHF study. *J Am Coll Cardiol*. 2003;41:997–1003.

26. Elkayam U, Tasissa G, Binanay C, et al. Use and impact of inotropes and vasodilator therapy in hospitalized patients with severe heart failure. *Am Heart J*. 2007;153:98–104.

27. Galve E, Rius T, Ballester R, et al. Intravenous amiodarone in treatment of recent-onset atrial fibrillation: results of a randomized, controlled study. *J Am Coll Cardiol*. 1996;27:1079–1082.

28. Roy D, Talajic M, Nattel S, et al. Rhythm control versus rate control for atrial fibrillation and heart failure. *N Engl J Med*. 2008;358:2667–2677.

29. Silverberg DS, Wexler D, Sheps D, et al. The effect of correction of mild anemia in severe, resistant congestive heart failure using subcutaneous erythropoietin and intravenous iron: a randomized controlled study. *J Am Coll Cardiol*. 2001;37:1775–1780.

30. Palazzuoli A, Silverberg D, Iovine F, et al. Erythropoietin improves anemia exercise tolerance and renal function and reduces B-type natriuretic peptide and hospitalization in patients with heart failure and anemia. *Am Heart J*. 2006;152:e9-1096–e15-1096.

31. Effect of enalapril on survival in patients with reduced left ventricular ejection fractions and congestive heart failure. The SOLVD Investigators. *N Engl J Med.* 1991;325:293–302.

32. Packer M, Bristow MR, Cohn JN, et al. The effect of carvedilol on morbidity and mortality in patients with chronic heart failure. US Carvedilol Heart Failure Study Group. *N Engl J Med.* 1996;334:1349–1355.

33. Effect of metoprolol CR/XL in chronic heart failure: Metoprolol CR/XL Randomised Intervention Trial in Congestive Heart Failure (MERIT-HF). *Lancet.* 1999;353:2001–2007.

34. Pitt B, Zannad F, Remme WJ, et al. The effect of spironolactone on morbidity and mortality in patients with severe heart failure. Randomized Aldactone Evaluation Study Investigators. *N Engl J Med.* 1999;341:709–717.

35. The effect of digoxin on mortality and morbidity in patients with heart failure. The Digitalis Investigation Group. *N Engl J Med.* 1997;336:525–533.

36. O'Connor CM, Carson PE, Miller AB, et al. Effect of amlodipine on mode of death among patients with advanced heart failure in the PRAISE trial. Prospective Randomized Amlodipine Survival Evaluation. *Am J Cardiol.* 1998;82:881–887.

37. Moss AJ, Hall WJ, Cannom DS, et al. Improved survival with an implanted defibrillator in patients with coronary disease at high risk for ventricular arrhythmia. Multicenter Automatic Defibrillator Implantation Trial Investigators. *N Engl J Med.* 1996;335:1933–1940.

38. An international randomized trial comparing four thrombolytic strategies for acute myocardial infarction. The GUSTO investigators. *N Engl J Med.* 1993;329:673–682.

39. Rossi A, Rossi G, Piacenti M, et al. The current role of cardiac resynchronization therapy in reducing mortality and hospitalization in heart failure patients: a meta-analysis from clinical trials. *Heart Vessels.* 2008;23:217–223.

40. Bristow MR, Saxon LA, Boehmer J, et al. Cardiac-resynchronization therapy with or without an implantable defibrillator in advanced chronic heart failure. *N Engl J Med.* 2004;350:2140–2150.

41. Kale P, Fang JC. Devices in acute heart failure. *Crit Care Med.* 2008;36:S121–S128.

42. Schreuder JJ, Maisano F, Donelli A, et al. Beat-to-beat effects of intraaortic balloon pump timing on left ventricular performance in patients with low ejection fraction. *Ann Thorac Surg.* 2005;79:872–880.

43. Burkhoff D, Cohen H, Brunckhorst C, et al. A randomized multicenter clinical study to evaluate the safety and efficacy of the TandemHeart percutaneous ventricular assist device versus conventional therapy with intraaortic balloon pumping for treatment of cardiogenic shock. *Am Heart J.* 2006;152:469–468.

44. Zile MR, Baicu CF, Gaasch WH. Diastolic heart failure – abnormalities in active relaxation and passive stiffness of the left ventricle. *N Engl J Med.* 2004;350:1953–1959.

45. Lam CS, Roger VL, Rodeheffer RJ. Cardiac structure and ventricular–vascular function in persons with heart failure and preserved ejection fraction from Olmsted County, Minnesota. *Circulation*. 2007;115:1982–1990.
46. Tribouilloy C, Rusinaru D, Mahjoub H. Prognosis of heart failure with preserved ejection fraction: a 5-year prospective population-based study. *Eur Heart J*. 2008;29:339–347.
47. Hernandez AF, Hammill BG, O'Connor CM, et al. Clinical effectiveness of beta-blockers in heart failure: findings from the OPTIMIZE-HF (Organized Program to Initiate Lifesaving Treatment in Hospitalized Patients with Heart Failure) Registry. *J Am Coll Cardiol*. 2009;53:184–192.
48. Yusuf S, Pfeffer MA, Swedberg K, et al. Effects of candesartan in patients with chronic heart failure and preserved left-ventricular ejection fraction: the CHARM-Preserved Trial. *Lancet*. 2003;362:777–781.

30

Takotsubo Cardiomyopathy

Takotsubo cardiomyopathy also known as apical ballooning syndrome (ABS) is a unique reversible cardiomyopathy that is frequently precipitated by a stressful event and has a clinical presentation that is often indistinguishable from an acute myocardial infarction. This distinct cardiac syndrome was originally described in Japan in 1990 and named after the "octopus trapping pot," which has a round bottom and a narrow neck, which closely resembles the left ventriculogram during systole in these patients.[1] Approximately 90% of all reported cases have been in women. The mean age has ranged from 58 to 75 years, with <3% of the patients being <50 years.[2,3] The reason for the female predominance is unknown but raises the question as to whether withdrawal from estrogens contributes to the pathogenesis.

■ STRESSORS REPORTED TO TRIGGER TAKOTSUBO CARDIOMYOPATHY

- Emotional stress[2,4]
  - Death or severe illness or injury of a family member, a friend, or a pet
  - Receiving bad news – diagnosis of a major illness, daughter's divorce, spouse leaving for war
  - Severe argument
  - Public speaking
  - Involvement with legal proceedings
  - Financial loss – business, gambling

P.E. Marik, *Handbook of Evidence-Based Critical Care*,
DOI 10.1007/978-1-4419-5923-2_30,
© Springer Science+Business Media, LLC 2010

- Car accident
- Surprise party
- Move to a new residence
- Physical stress
  - Non-cardiac surgery or procedure – cholecystectomy, hysterectomy
  - Severe illness – asthma or COPD exacerbation, acute cholecystitis, pseudomembranous colitis
  - Severe pain – fracture, renal colic, pneumothorax, pulmonary embolism
  - Recovery from general anesthesia
  - Cocaine use
  - Opiate withdrawal
  - Stress test – dobutamine stress echo, exercise sestamibi
  - Thyrotoxicosis

This condition probably accounts for 1–2% of all cases of suspected acute myocardial infarction. Takotsubo cardiomyopathy occurs predominantly in postmenopausal women soon after the exposure to sudden, unexpected emotional or physical stress. In Takotsubo cardiomyopathy, left ventricular dysfunction, which can be remarkably depressed, recovers within a few weeks. Although the left ventricular dysfunction is transient, there is no evidence of obstructive epicardial coronary disease.

The most frequent clinical symptoms of Takotsubo cardiomyopathy on admission are chest pain and dyspnea, resembling acute myocardial infarction. The classic presentation is that of a postmenopausal woman presenting with chest pain or dyspnea that is temporally related to emotional or physical stress, with positive cardiac biomarkers or an abnormal electrocardiogram.[2] Takotsubo cardiomyopathy should also be considered in the differential diagnosis of inpatients, including those in the ICU, who develop an acute reduction in left ventricular systolic function in association with the following features:

- Hemodynamic compromise.
- Pulmonary edema.
- Troponin elevation.
- ECG evidence of ischemia or infarction. There may be a higher prevalence of males in the ICU population.

In general, hemodynamic compromise is unusual, but mild-to-moderate congestive heart failure is frequent. Transient ST elevation may be present on the electrocardiogram, and a small rise in cardiac troponins is invariable. When anterior ST elevation is present, the magnitude of ST shift is usually less in Takotsubo cardiomyopathy than that seen in a STEMI. Diffuse T-wave inversion and a prolonged QTc interval are typical findings (see Figure 30-1). The T-wave inversion and QTc interval

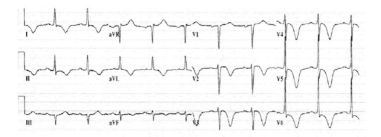

Figure 30-1. ECG demonstrating diffuse T-wave inversion and QTc prolongation. Reproduced from Ref. 4 with permission from Elsevier.

prolongationtypically resolve over 3–4 months but may occur as early as 4–6 weeks and, in some cases, be present beyond 1 year. Arrhythmias resulting from QT prolongation are commonly observed. Typically, there is hypokinesis or akinesis of the mid and apical segments of the left ventricle with sparing of the basal systolic function (see Figure 30-2).

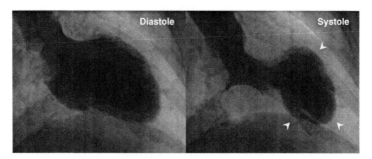

Figure 30-2. Diastolic and systolic freeze frames from a left ventriculogram of a patient with classic ABS illustrating hyperdynamic basal contraction but akinesis of the mid and apical segments (*arrows*). Reproduced from Ref. 4 with permission from Elsevier.

■ MAYO CLINIC CRITERIA FOR TAKOTSUBO CARDIOMYOPATHY

- Transient hypokinesis, akinesis, or dyskinesis of the left ventricular mid segments with or without apical involvement; the regional wall

motion abnormalities extend beyond a single epicardial vascular distribution; a stressful trigger is often, but not always, present.[4]
• Absence of obstructive coronary disease or angiographic evidence of acute plaque rupture.
• New electrocardiographic abnormalities (either ST segment elevation and/or T-wave inversion) or modest elevation in cardiac troponin.
• Absence of the following:
  – Pheochromocytoma.
  – Myocarditis.

Patients with Takotsubo cardiomyopathy on admission have high levels of serum catecholamines and of plasma brain natriuretic peptide (BNP). The myocardial histological changes in Takotsubo cardiomyopathy strikingly resemble those seen in catecholamine cardiotoxicity in both animals and humans. These changes, which differ from those in ischemic cardiac necrosis, include contraction band necrosis, neutrophil infiltration, and fibrosis.

The optimal management of Takotsubo cardiomyopathy has not been established, but supportive therapy invariably leads to spontaneous recovery. Patients have been treated with both β-blockers and ACE inhibitors.[2] Given the findings in animal models, treatment with a combined α- and β-blocker seems rational.[3] Treatment with a catecholamine as a cardiotonic appears contraindicated.

It is important to exclude dynamic left ventricular outflow tract obstruction with echocardiography in patients with severe heart failure or hypotension. Dynamic outflow obstruction occurs in up to 20% of patients. β-Blockers have been demonstrated to reverse the obstruction presumably by reducing the hypercontractility of the base of the left ventricle and increasing cardiac filling.[5]

■ REFERENCES

1. Kurisu S, Sato H, Kawagoe T, et al. Tako-tsubo-like left ventricular dysfunction with ST-segment elevation: a novel cardiac syndrome mimicking acute myocardial infarction. *Am Heart J.* 2002;143:448–455.
2. Regnante RA, Zuzek RW, Weinsier SB, et al. Clinical characteristics and four-year outcomes of patients in the Rhode Island Takotsubo Cardiomyopathy Registry. *Am J Cardiol.* 2009;103:1015–1019.
3. Akashi YJ, Goldstein DS, Barbaro G, et al. Takotsubo cardiomyopathy: a new form of acute, reversible heart failure. *Circulation.* 2008;118: 2754–2762.
4. Prasad A, Lerman A, Rihal CS. Apical ballooning syndrome (Tako-Tsubo or stress cardiomyopathy): a mimic of acute myocardial infarction. *Am Heart J.* 2008;155:408–417.

5. Yoshioka T, Hashimoto A, Tsuchihashi K, et al. Clinical implications of midventricular obstruction and intravenous propranolol use in transient left ventricular apical ballooning (Tako-tsubo cardiomyopathy). *Am Heart J.* 2008;155:526–527.

Part IV

Gastrointestinal

31

Nutrition

During the last decade, the seemingly simple task of feeding critically ill patients has become exceedingly complex with much controversy. While many consider nutrition support "an afterthought," current evidence suggests that in critically ill patients the approach to nutritional support directly impacts patient outcome. In reality, the approach is simple:

- Route – enteral nutrition (EN)
  - PO (first choice)
  - OG tube (second choice)
  - Postpyloric feeding tube (third choice)
- When
  - Within 24 h
- Quantity
  - Day 1: 10–15 kcal/kg/day
  - Day 2–4: 15–20 kcal/kg/day
  - Day ≥5: 20–25 kcal/kg/day
- Composition
  - Omega-3 fatty acids
  - High-quality protein
  - Low glycemic index
  - Soluble fiber

ALERT

The two commandments of nutrition support are the following:

- "If the bowel works, use it" (and if it does not work, make it work).
- "There is no disease process that benefits from starvation."

P.E. Marik, *Handbook of Evidence-Based Critical Care*,
DOI 10.1007/978-1-4419-5923-2_31,
© Springer Science+Business Media, LLC 2010

■ THE MYTHS OF NUTRITIONAL SUPPORT

- PN is safe.[1]
- EN contraindicated with vasopressors.
- EN contraindicated with mechanical ventilation.
- EN contraindicated with "gastroparesis" and "poor b/s."
- Starvation is "okay."
- The concept of "bowel rest" is as absurd as "cardiac rest:"
  - Starvation injures the bowel.

The results of a number of RCTs (and meta-analyses of these trials) have established the following principles on which to base nutritional support in critically ill patients[2]:

- There are no data that parenteral nutrition (PN) is of any benefit to critically ill patients. The available evidence suggests that PN increases complications and mortality rates. PN should therefore be limited to patients who after 5–7 days of starvation are unable to tolerate even small volumes of enteral nutrition. This includes patients with proximal fistula, bowel obstruction, and short gut syndrome.[3] This concept is best illustrated in patients who have severe pancreatitis in whom PN as compared to EN is associated with more septic complications, a longer LOS, and a higher mortality.[4]
- Early enteral nutrition (within 24 h of admission to the ICU) has been shown to reduce complications and improve the outcome of critically ill patients when compared to delayed enteral nutrition.[5,6] No studies demonstrate an advantage to delaying nutritional support in seriously ill patients.
- Overfeeding patients is associated with significant complications including hyperglycemia, hepatic steatosis with hepatic dysfunction, elevated BUN, and excessive CO_2 production.
- There are no data to suggest that accurately measuring resting energy expenditure (REE) to determine nutritional requirements improves outcome. Measurement of REE may be appropriate in morbidly obese patients.
- Enteral nutritional formulas high in omega-3 fatty acids have been shown to improve the outcome of patients with sepsis and ARDS.[7,8] This topic is, however, likely to become more controversial with the "negative" ARDSNet EDEN-Omega Study (see http://www.ardsnet.org/front).
- Enteral nutritional formulas with added arginine, glutamine, omega-3 FA, and anti-oxidants reduce complications and LOS when used in the perioperative period (in non-septic patients).[9]
- Enteral nutritional feeding formulas of low osmolarity and enriched with fiber (non-digestible plant cell wall constituents) reduce the risk of diarrhea and improve feeding tolerance (see Chapter 38).

The composition of commonly prescribed commercially available enteral formulas available in the United States are listed in Table 31-1.

Recent studies have shown that dietary fatty acids can reduce the severity of inflammatory injury by altering the availability of arachidonic acid in tissue phospholipids. Animal and clinical studies have shown that nutritional intervention with dietary fish oil-containing eicosapentaenoic acid (an omega-3 fatty acid) can favorably modulate pro-inflammatory eicosanoid production from arachidonic acid. Similarly, γ-linolenic acid suppresses leukotriene biosynthesis and is further metabolized to the monoenoic prostaglandins, such as prostaglandin E1. Prostaglandin E1 is a potent vasodilator of pulmonary and systemic circulation and inhibits platelet aggregation, neutrophil chemotaxis, and oxygen radical release. In patients with sepsis and ARDS, an enteral nutritional formula high in omega-3 FA has been demonstrated to decrease BAL neutrophil count, improve oxygenation, increase the number of ventilator-free days, reduce ICU LOS, and reduce mortality.[7,8] The benefits of omega-3 fatty acid supplementation in critically ill patients will need to be re-evaluated once the data from the ARDSNet EDEN-Omega Study become available. While a large body of experimental and clinical data support the use of omega-3 fatty acids in modulating inflammation, the clinical benefits and the cost effectiveness of this approach are likely to be more controversial.

Nevertheless, an enteral formula with high-quality protein, omega-3 fatty acids, anti-oxidants, and soluble fiber (prebiotic) with a low osmolarity and a low glycemic index would appear to be the "ideal" enteral formulation for critically ill ICU patients.

The absence of bowel sounds does not mean that the bowel is not working. Bowel sounds result from air moving through the small intestine. The presence of bowel sounds requires gastric emptying and gastric air. Many seriously ill patients have gastroparesis and are being treated with nasogastric suctioning. These patients have little movement of air from the stomach to the small intestine and therefore have decreased bowel sounds. Furthermore, to declare the absence of bowel sounds, one should listen for 2–4 min in each of the four quadrants (total of 10–16 min). Few clinicians listen for more than a few seconds. In addition, the quantity of bowel sounds (or volume of flatus) does not directly correlate with gut motility. Thus, bowel sounds are a poor indicator of small intestine function. The presence of bowel sounds is a better indicator of active gastric emptying.

ALERT

In the ICU patient population, neither the presence nor the absence of bowel sounds nor evidence of the passage of flatus or stool is required for the initiation of enteral feeding.

Table 31-1. Composition of common enteral formulas.

Category	Osmolite 1.2 Standard without Fiber	Jevity 1.2 Standard with Fiber	Oxepa High N-3 IMD	Fibersource HN Standard with Fiber	Novasource Renal Fluid Elect restricted	Replete with Fiber High protein with Fiber	Crucial[a] Semi-elem. IMD	Peptamen AF Semi-elem. IMD, H-Pr
kcal/ml	1.2	1.2	1.5	1.2	2.0	1.0	1.5	1.2
Sodium (mEq/l)	58	58	57	52	70	38	51	35
Potassium (mEq/l)	46	47	50	51	28	38	48	41
Osmolarity	360	450	535	490	700	310	490	390
CHO (g/l, cal%)	158/53	169/52	105/28	160/53	200/40	113/45	135/36	107/36
Protein (g/l, cal%)	56/18	55/18	63/17	53/18	74/15	62/25	94/25	75/25
Fat (g/l, cal%)	39/29	39/29	94/55	39/29	100/45	34/30	68/39	55/39
Source lipid	Canola oil, MCT oil	Canola oil, MCT oil	Canola oil, fish oil, MCT oil	Canola oil, MCT oil	Sunflower oil, corn oil, MCT oil	Canola oil, MCT oil	MCT oil, fish soy oil	MCT oil, fish soy oil
$n-6:n-3$	6.3:1	6.3:1	1.7:1	2.7:1	–	2.3:1	1.5:1	1.8:1
Dietary fiber (g/l)	0	18	0	10	0	14	0	5.2
Manufacturer	Abbott	Abbott	Abbott	Nestle	Nestle	Nestle	Nestle	Nestle

IMD, immunomodulating diet; H-Pr, high protein.
[a] Arginine, 15 g/l.

Gastric feeding is delivered using nasogastric tubes or gastrostomy tubes. Larger bore nasogastric tubes are preferred when feeding the stomach. Nasogastric tubes are generally easily placed; the oral route is preferred in intubated patients due to the lower risk of sinusitis (see Chapter 13). Confirmation of gastric location must be confirmed prior to feeding (aspiration of gastric contents and X-ray confirmation). Most critically ill patients can be fed gastrically via an OG tube. This is the preferred route, as gastric intubation is easier to achieve, the tube rarely clogs, it allows for the administration of oral medications, and for the monitoring of gastric residual volumes. Most importantly, however, gastric feeding protects the gastric mucosa from stress ulceration negating the need for stress ulcer prophylaxis, (see Chapter 32). In patients with delayed gastric emptying, IV erythromycin (70–100 mg q 8–12 h) and/or metoclopramide is recommended.[10,11] In patients who fail gastric feeding despite these measures, postpyloric, small-bore feeding tubes are recommenced.

Numerous techniques have been described for placement of small bowel-feeding tubes, including fluoroscopic or endoscopic methods, the use of magnets and ECG electrodes, and the bedside "cork-screw" method. These techniques are cumbersome, impractical, and have a high failure rate. Recently, a novel method (electromagnetic guidance system) of nasojejunal feeding tube placement at the bedside has been introduced (Corpak, VIASYS Medical Systems, Wheeling, IL). In our hands, we have a 90% success rate at postpyloric placement with an average procedure time (nose to distal duodenum) of 5 min (unpublished data).[12] It has been suggested the postpyloric feeding results in fewer compilations than does gastric feeding. However, two meta-analyses found no difference in the rate of aspiration pneumonia and mortality with gastric as compared to postpyloric feeding.[13,14] For the reasons outlined above, we prefer gastric feeding as our primary mode of enteral access; only when this approach fails would we recommend placement of a distal "postpyloric" feeding tube.

One of the most feared complications of enteral feeding is aspiration of enteral formula with resultant hypoxia and/or pneumonia. Thus, in an attempt to minimize the risk for aspiration, many clinicians monitor gastric residual volumes (GRVs). The presumption is that GRV measurements are accurate and useful markers for the risk of aspiration and pneumonia. Frequently, enteral feeding is interrupted when the GRV exceeds 150 ml. There is however no data to support this practice. High GRVs (i.e., >400 ml) do not necessarily predict aspiration, and low GRVs (i.e., <100 ml) are no guarantee that aspiration will not occur. Interrupting enteral nutrition when the GRV exceeds 100 ml has not been shown to decrease the incidence of aspiration. Nonetheless, GRV measurements are routinely measured in most ICUs to monitor "tolerance" to enteral nutrition. McClave and colleagues[15] randomized critically ill ventilated patients to two management strategies using a GRV >200 or >400 ml to withhold feeding. In this study, there was no relationship between GRV and aspiration or regurgitation. In addition, there was no correlation between aspiration/regurgitation and pneumonia. Pinilla et al.[16] demonstrated a reduction in "feeding intolerance," improved enteral nutrition provision, and reduced time to reach the goal rate in patients in whom a gastric residual volume threshold of 250 ml as opposed to 150 ml was used. There was no statistical difference between the two protocols with regard to emesis.

ALERT

There is a poor relationship between the gastric residual volume and the risk of aspiration. *Do not* hold tube feeds unless the gastric residual volume >400 ml and/or the patient shows signs of intolerance (distended abdomen, vomiting).

■ THE "FEED" PROTOCOL (*FEED EARLY ENTERALLY IN D*-STOMACH)

- Place OG tube on admission to ICU.
- Initiate tube feeds immediately at 20 ml/hr.[a,b,c]
- Check residuals every 6 h.
- Increase to 40 ml/hr after 12 h.
- Increase to 60 ml/hr after 24 h.
- Increase to 70–80 ml/hr after 3–4 days.
- If residuals >400 ml or nausea/vomiting/abdominal distension:
  - Empty the stomach.
  - Give prokinetic agent (erythromycin).
  - Restart at half previous rate.
  - If Pt remains intolerant, place a small bowel-feeding tube.

---

[a] Assumes 1 kcal/ml formula and average IBW.

[b] In shocked patients, stabilize with fluids and pressors before initiating feeds (within 12 h of ICU admission).

[c] In patients in whom extubation is expected within 24 h of ICU admission, feeding can be delayed until after extubation.

In patients at high risk for aspiration (i.e., severe multiple trauma and history of gastroparesis), it may be prudent to place a small bowel-feeding tube on admission to the ICU. The head of the bed should be elevated to 30° in all patients to decrease the risk of aspiration. Additional routine measures should be taken to reduce the risk of aspiration and VAP (see Chapter 17).

Note:

- Propofol emulsion contains approximately 0.1 g of fat (1.1 kcal) for every milliliter. An infusion of propofol may therefore provide a significant caloric load. In patients receiving high-dose propofol infusions, the enteral feeds need to be adjusted to take into account the added caloric load. A low-fat enteral formulation, such as Vivonex, may be used.
- Making the patient nil per os surrounding the time of diagnostic tests or procedures should be minimized to prevent inadequate delivery of nutrients and prolonged periods of ileus. Ileus may be propagated by nil per os status.

ALERT

When tube feeds are suddenly discontinued, the patient should be placed on a D5 or a D10 solution (to prevent hypoglycemia) and the blood glucose monitored closely (particularly when the patient is on an insulin protocol).

■ NUTRITION IN SPECIFIC DISEASE STATES

Liver failure (see Chapter 33)
Pancreatitis (see Chapter 37)
Renal failure (see Chapter 44)

■ OBESITY

In the critically ill obese patient, permissive underfeeding or hypocaloric feeding with EN is recommended. For all classes of obesity where BMI is >30, the goal of the EN regimen should not exceed 60–70% of target energy requirements or 11–14 kcal/kg actual body weight/day (or 22–25 kcal/kg ideal body weight/day). Protein should be provided in a range ≥2.0 g/kg ideal body weight/day for class I and class II patients (BMI

30–40) and ≥ 2.5 g/kg ideal body weight/day for class III patients (BMI >40).[2]

■ PARENTERAL NUTRITION

PN is associated with significant complications, including an increased incidence of infections (particularly, catheter-associated septicemia and fungemia); metabolic disturbances such as hyperglycemia, hypophosphatemia, hypokalemia, and trace element deficiency; atrophy of the gastrointestinal mucosa, predisposing to bacterial translocation; and immune suppression. TPN frequently causes hepatic dysfunction which results in both biochemical and histological changes in the liver.

■ THE REFEEDING SYNDROME

Protein-calorie malnutrition may exist in up to 50% of hospitalized patients. Feeding malnourished patients, particularly after a period of starvation, may result in severe metabolic disturbances, most notably hypophosphatemia. Hypophosphatemia developing after initiating parenteral or enteral nutrition has been termed the refeeding syndrome. In addition to hypophosphatemia, changes in potassium, magnesium, and glucose metabolism occur during refeeding. Although classically described in cachectic patients after prolonged starvation, this syndrome has been reported to occur commonly in poorly nourished ICU patients who have been starved for as short as 48 h.

The commercially available tube feed preparations contain between 50 and 60 mg/dl of phosphorus (the recommended daily allowance). However, in patients with high metabolic demands and phosphorus-depleted patients, these formulas may not meet the requirements necessary to accommodate the massive transcellular shifts and possible whole-body depletion of phosphorus found in these patients.

■ REFERENCES

1. Elke G, Schadler D, Engel C, et al. Current practice in nutritional support and its association with mortality in septic patients – Results from a national prospective multicenter study. *Crit Care Med.* 2008;36:1762–1767.
2. Martindale RG, McClave SA, Vanek VW, et al. Guidelines for the provision and assessment of nutrition support therapy in the adult critically

ill patient: Society of Critical Care Medicine and American Society for Parenteral and Enteral Nutrition: Executive Summary. *Crit Care Med.* 2009;37:1757–1761.

3. Marik PE, Pinsky MR. Death by total parenteral nutrition. *Intensive Care Med.* 2003;29:867–869.

4. Marik PE. What is the best way to feed patients with pancreatitis? *Curr Opin Crit Care.* 2009;15:131–138.

5. Marik PE, Zaloga GP. Early enteral nutrition in acutely ill patients: a systematic review. *Crit Care Med.* 2001;29:2264–2270.

6. Artinian V, Krayem H, DiGiovine B. Effects of early enteral feeding on the outcome of critically ill mechanically ventilated medical patients. *Chest.* 2006;129:960–967.

7. Pontes-Arruda A, DeMichele S, Srth A, et al. The use of an inflammation modulating diet in patients with acute lung injury or acute respiratory distress syndrome: a Meta-analysis evaluation of outcome data. *JPEN.* 2008;32(6):596–605.

8. Marik PE, Zaloga GP. Immunonutrition in critically ill patients: a systematic review and analysis of the literature. *Intensive Care Med.* 2008;34:1980–1990.

9. Marik PE, Zaloga GP. Immunonutrition in high risk surgical patients: A systematic review and analysis of the literature. *JPEN.* 2010; (in press).

10. Nguyen NQ, Chapman MJ, Fraser RJ, et al. Erythromycin is more effective than metoclopramide in the treatment of feed intolerance in critical illness. *Crit Care Med.* 2007;35:483–489.

11. Ritz MA, Chapman MJ, Fraser RJ, et al. Erythromycin dose of 70 mg accelerates gastric emptying as effectively as 200 mg in the critically ill. *Intensive Care Med.* 2005;31:949–954.

12. Gray R, Tynan C, Reed L, et al. Bedside electromagnetic-guided feeding tube placement: an improvement over traditional placement technique? *Nutr Clin Pract.* 2007;22:436–444.

13. Ho KM, Dobb GJ, Webb SA. A comparison of early gastric and post-pyloric feeding in critically ill patients: a meta-analysis. *Intensive Care Med.* 2006;32:639–649.

14. Marik PE, Zaloga G. Gastric vs. Post-Pyloric Feeding? A systematic Review. *Crit Care.* 2003;7:R46–R51.

15. McClave SA, Lukan JK, Stefater JA, et al. Poor validity of residual volumes as a marker for risk of aspiration in critically ill patients. *Crit Care Med.* 2005;33:324–330.

16. Pinilla JC, Samphire J, Arnold C, et al. Comparison of gastrointestinal tolerance to two enteral feeding protocols in critically ill patients: a prospective, randomized controlled trial. *JPEN.* 2001;25:81–86.

32

Stress Ulcer Prophylaxis

In 1969, Skillman and colleagues reported a clinical syndrome of lethal stress ulceration in 7 of 150 (5%) consecutive ICU patients. These patients had in common respiratory failure, hypotension, and sepsis.[1] Pathological examination demonstrated multiple superficial ulcers which were confined to the gastric fundus. Following this report, these authors performed a randomized controlled study in which 100 critically ill ICU patients at risk of "stress ulceration" were randomized to either antacid prophylaxis (titrated to keep the gastric pH above 3.5) or no prophylaxis.[2] Two of 51 (4%) treated patients had gastrointestinal bleeding (GIB) as compared to 12 of 49 (25%) control patients (p <0.005). Subsequent studies confirmed this finding and two meta-analyses published by Cook and colleagues[3,4] demonstrated that both histamine-2 receptor blockers (H2RBs) and sucralfate decreased the risk of bleeding from stress ulceration when compared to placebo. Stress ulcer prophylaxis (SUP) is regarded as the standard of care in patients admitted to the ICU and this intervention is currently endorsed by many professional bodies.[5,6] The universal use of SUP has been reinforced with the adoption of "ventilator bundles." Currently the Joint Commission and the Institute for Healthcare Improvement recommend universal stress ulcer prophylaxis as a core "quality" measure for mechanically ventilated patients.[7] Estimates indicate that approximately 90% of critically ill patients admitted to the ICU receive some form of stress ulcer prophylaxis. Furthermore, although proton pump inhibitors (PPIs) have never been demonstrated to reduce the rate of bleeding from stress ulceration, these agents have assumed a pre-eminent role for the prevention of this condition.[8,9]

Stress ulcers are superficial erosions in the gastric mucosa that are common in patients with acute, life-threatening diseases. These lesions are usually shallow and well demarcated, primarily involving the superficial layers of the gastric epithelium.[10] Endoscopic studies have shown

P.E. Marik, *Handbook of Evidence-Based Critical Care*,
DOI 10.1007/978-1-4419-5923-2_32,
© Springer Science+Business Media, LLC 2010

that nearly all critically ill patients develop upper gastrointestinal erosions after critical illness or major surgery. Gastric erosions are present
in 10–25% of patients on admission to the ICU and in up to 90% of
patients by the third ICU day.[11,12] Although gastric erosions are common
in critically ill patients, they are usually clinically silent. The reported
frequencies of clinically significant GIB vary from about 0.6 to 2% in
the absence of SUP and was 1.5% in the large, prospective multi-center
cohort study conducted by Cook and colleagues.[13] In the study by Cook
and colleagues, the independent risk factors of GIB were respiratory failure requiring mechanical ventilation for more than 48 h (OR 15.6) and a
coagulopathy (OR 4.3).[13]

The pathogenesis of stress ulceration remains poorly understood.
Various factors and mechanisms, alone or in combination, are probably responsible for the lesions. Despite the multi-factorial mechanisms
proposed as contributing to the development of stress-related gastrointestinal erosions, the presence of luminal gastric acid appears essential.
However, the majority of patients with stress ulceration have normal acid
secretion. Alterations in mucosal blood flow, the mucus layer, protein
synthesis, bicarbonate and prostaglandin secretion, and epithelial cell
renewal have been postulated to alter the gastric mucosal barrier leading to the back diffusion of acid leading to mucosal damage. In addition,
alterations in endothelin-1 and serotonin production as well as infection
with *Helicobacter pylori* may play a role in the development of stress
ulceration.

■ **DOES SUP REDUCE GI BLEEDING?**

During the early years of critical care, stress-related GIB was an important cause of morbidity and mortality. During the past 2 decades, the rate
of stress-related GIB has declined probably due to improved resuscitation and early enteral feeding of critically ill patients. To be useful, SUP
should affect clinical outcome. No clinical trial of stress ulcer prophylaxis
has demonstrated a reduction in mortality or length of stay. Surprisingly
the effect of SUP on the risk of bleeding is unclear. Cook and colleagues
performed a meta-analysis of 10 studies which randomized patients to
receive a H2RA or placebo. The authors reported that H2RAs reduced
the risk of clinically significant bleeding (OR 0.44; 95% CI 0.22–0.88),
with a trend toward an increased risk of nosocomial pneumonia (OR 0.25;
95% CI 0.78–2.0) with no effect on mortality.[4] It should be pointed out
that these studies were performed in the 1980s when early enteral nutrition was not encouraged and many patients received parenteral nutrition
(see below). Messori and colleagues[14] performed a more recent meta-
analysis of studies that compared ranitidine with placebo in ICU patients.

These authors concluded that "ranitidine is ineffective in the prevention of gastrointestinal bleeding in patients in the ICU and might increase the risk of pneumonia."

Zandstra and Stoutenbeek[15] reported that 1 of 183 patients (0.6%) receiving prolonged mechanical ventilation without any SUP developed stress ulcer-related bleeding. Erstad and colleagues[16] conducted a prospective study on 543 patients and reported that clinically significant GIB rates were similar for those patients with ineffective SUP and those with appropriate SUP. Faisy and colleagues[17] compared the rate of clinically significant GIB during two sequential time periods. During the first phase, all patients ($n = 736$) received SUP, while SUP was withheld during the second period ($n = 737$). Although the patients during the second phase of the study were sicker (higher SAPS II score), the rate of overt (1.9% vs. 1.6%) and clinically significant bleeding (1.4% vs. 1.1%) as well as the use of blood products was similar between the two time periods. More recently, Kantorova and colleagues[9] performed a randomized, placebo-controlled study in critically ill patients at high risk for stress-related GIB (mechanical ventilation >48 h and coagulopathy) in which they compared three SUP regimens (omeprazole, famotidine, and sucralfate) with placebo. The overall bleeding rate was 1% with no significant difference between treatment groups (placebo 1%). Gastric pH and bacterial colonization were significantly greater in the patients who received acid-suppressive therapy with a trend toward a higher incidence of VAP in these patients.

These data suggest that the rate of clinically significant bleeding from stress ulceration in critically ill ICU patients is currently very low and that SUP does not alter this risk or the natural history of this disease.

■ ENTERAL NUTRITION AND STRESS ULCER PROPHYLAXIS

It has been suggested that patients receiving enteral alimentation have a lower incidence of stress ulceration than do unfed patients.[18] In animal models, enteral alimentation has been demonstrated to protect the gastric mucosa from stress-related gastric mucosal damage.[19,20] It has been suggested that enteral nutrients buffer acid and may act as a direct source of mucosal energy, induce the secretion of cytoprotective prostaglandins, and improve mucosal blood flow.[19,20] Furthermore, mucosal immunity may be supported via stimulation of the gut-associated lymphoid tissue.

Bonten and colleagues[21] demonstrated that continuous enteral nutrition was more likely to raise gastric pH to >3.5 than patients receiving H2RAs or PPIs. Two rat studies have evaluated the role of enteral nutrition in preventing stress ulceration.[22,23] The results of both trials showed that continuous intragastric administration of elemental formulas significantly reduced the occurrence of macroscopic mucosal lesions compared with intragastric administration of an antacid or intravenous administration of cimetidine. In a retrospective analysis, Raff and colleagues[24] demonstrated that early (within 12 h post-trauma) enteral nutrition was at least as effective as H2RAs and/or antacids as stress ulcer prophylaxis in a cohort of 526 severely burned patients. Pingleton and Hadzima[18] reported a similar finding in 43 ventilated patients. A review of the "historical" randomized controlled trials that studied the effectiveness of acid-suppressive therapy in reducing the risk of bleeding demonstrates that SUP was beneficial only in those patients who were NPO (received no gastric feeding). However, in those studies in which patients were fed enterally, the risk of bleeding was equivalent in the treatment and placebo groups.[9,25–27] It is unclear whether post-pyloric alimentation protects against stress ulceration. While reflux of enteral nutrition into the stomach is common with post-pyloric feeding, gastric pH is significantly lower in patients fed intra-duodenally as compared to intragastrically.[28,29] However, in animal models both routes of nutrition are equally efficacious in preventing stress ulceration. While definitive data are lacking, SUP should probably be administered to patients receiving post- pyloric nutritional support who are at high risk for stress ulceration (i.e., coagulopathic patients receiving mechanical ventilation).

These data suggest that in those patients receiving intragastric enteral nutrition, SUP is not required and indeed may increase the risk of complications (see below). As early enteral nutrition (as opposed to delayed enteral nutrition or parenteral nutrition) has been demonstrated to reduce the morbidity and the mortality of critically ill patients,[30,31] intragastric nutrition should be initiated within 24 h of admission to the ICU unless an absolute contraindication exists (bowel obstruction, short gut syndrome).

■ COMPLICATIONS ASSOCIATED WITH ACID-SUPPRESSIVE THERAPY

It would appear to be no accident of natural selection that the gastric mucosa of mammalian species secretes acid. Acid plays an important role in protein digestion but more importantly sterilizes the upper gastrointestinal tract. Acid-suppressive therapy is associated with increased colonization of the upper gastrointestinal tract with potentially pathogenic organism. This may be of critical importance in ICU patients where protocols of oral and enteric decontamination (with non-absorbable antibiotics/anti-microbials) have been demonstrated to reduce the incidence of ventilator-associated pneumonia (VAP).[32,33] As an extension of these observations, acid-suppressive therapy has been demonstrated to increase the gastric colonization and the risk of VAP.[9,14] In a large prospective pharmacoepidemiological cohort study involving non-ICU hospitalized patients, Herzig and colleagues[34] demonstrated that acid-suppressive medication was associated with a 30% increased odds ratio of hospital-acquired pneumonia. In a subset analysis, these authors demonstrated that this risk was related to the use of PPIs and not H2RB. Furthermore, the use of gastric-suppressive therapy together with the use of broad-spectrum antibiotics has been associated with an increased risk of *Clostridium difficile* infection.[35–37] Gastric acidity may be important in destroying ingested *C. difficile* spores, while broad-spectrum antibiotics reduce colonization resistance. PPIs have been shown to significantly raise gastric pH compared with H2RAs, which may result in a greater risk of *C. difficile* and pneumonia. Dial and colleagues demonstrated that PPIs doubled the risk of hospitalized patients developing *C. difficile* colitis, whereas H2RAs did not increase this risk.[36] These authors subsequently demonstrated that the use of both PPIs and H2RAs increased the risk of community-acquired *C. difficile*; however the risk was greater with PPIs.[38] The rapid increase in the incidence of *C. difficile* colitis in hospitalized patients may be causally related to the exploding use of PPIs.

■ COMPLICATIONS ASSOCIATED WITH SPECIFIC DRUGS

H2 Receptor Antagonists (H2RAs)

H2RAs are widely used for SUP. They decrease gastric acid secretion through a reversible, competitive inhibition of histamine-stimulated acid secretion. H2RAs have a wide therapeutic index; however, adverse reactions occur on average in 7% of hospitalized patients.[39] Drug interactions can occur with H2RAs, particularly cimetidine. Ben-Joseph and colleagues demonstrated that the failure to reduce the dose of H2RAs in patients with renal dysfunction doubled the likelihood of the patients experiencing an adverse drug reaction.[40] Those reactions of most concern in critically ill patients include altered mental status, neutropenia, and thrombocytopenia. H2RAs may rarely cause a sinus bradycardia with rapid infusion. The central nervous system reactions include confusion, delirium, disorientation, hallucinations, and obtundation. These reactions have been reported to occur in 2–3% of hospitalized patients.[41] While an altered mental status and cognition is a common problem in ICU patients, treatment with H2RAs is associated with a significant increase in central nervous system dysfunction, having been reported in up to 80% of patients.[41–43]. Considering the frequency of this reaction, the advanced age of most ICU patients, and the enormous concerns with ICU-related delirium, these agents are therefore best avoided.

Proton Pump Inhibitors (PPIs)

PPIs are substituted benzimidazoles that inhibit gastric secretion in a dose-dependent manner. They are the most potent anti-secretory agents available and can elevate or maintain intragastric pH above 6, which is necessary to maintain clotting in patients at risk for rebleeding and for ulcer healing (from peptic ulcer disease). PPIs irreversibly inhibit the final step in acid production (the transport of H^+ by the proton pump H^+/K^+ ATPase) providing long-lasting suppression of acid secretion. In addition, because PPIs are activated in the acidic compartments of parietal cells, they only inhibit secreting proton pumps. PPIs have the potential for drug interactions. PPIs are metabolized by hepatic cytochrome (CYP450) isoenzymes and therefore may interfere with the elimination of other drugs cleared by this route. Of the available PPIs, omeprazole has the highest potential for drug interaction, while pantoprazole has the lowest (low affinity for CYP enzymes). Omeprazole interferes with the metabolism of cyclosporine, diazepam, phenytoin, Coumadin, and several anti-psychotic drugs. Clopidogrel is an anti-platelet drug that is commonly used following acute coronary syndromes. Clopidogrel is a prodrug whose bioactivation is mediated by hepatic cytochrome P450 isoenzymes.[44] As these enzymes are inhibited by PPIs, patients taking clopidogrel together with a PPI have been reported to have a higher incidence of cardiac events than those taking clopidogrel alone.[45–47]

Sucralfate

Sucralfate is a basic non-absorbable aluminum salt of saccharose octasulfate. It is physiochemically an antacid, but it does not lead to significant pH increase. Its mechanism of protection is believed to be multi-factorial. Sucralfate forms a protective barrier on the surface of the gastric mucosa; it stimulates the secretion of mucous, bicarbonate, prostaglandins, and epidermal growth factor as well as improves mucosal blood flow. Since sucralfate is not systemically absorbed, it may decrease the absorption of other concomitantly administered oral medications including ciprofloxacin, phenytoin, digoxin, and levothyroxine. To minimize these interactions, it is recommended that these drugs be administered 2 h before sucralfate. Sucralfate may also interact with enteral feeding, resulting in clotted feeding tubes and bezoars. Furthermore, its "pharmacodynamic activity" requires an empty stomach; therefore the use of sucralfate necessitates the interruption of tube feeding. Sucralfate should not be administrated through duodenal or jejunostomy feeding tubes because the medication would bypass its site of action. Toxic levels of aluminum have been reported in critically ill patients requiring continuous venovenous hemofiltration who were receiving sucralfate.[48] As this drug appears to be less effective than acid-suppressive therapy in preventing bleeding from stress ulceration and as its administration requires the interruption of tube feeds, it would appear that this agent has a limited role in the ICU.[49]

■ EVIDENCE-BASED APPROACH TO STRESS ULCER PROPHYLAXIS

An analysis of best available evidence suggests that SUP should not be routinely used in the ICU. ICU patients who can be fed gastrically within 24 h of ICU admission do not routinely require SUP. SUP may be indicated in gastrically fed patients who are mechanically ventilated and have a severe coagulopathy or DIC. SUP should also be considered in patients with a history of upper gastrointestinal bleeding. Ventilated ICU patients receiving postpyloric feeding may require SUP. SUP is required in mechanically ventilated patients who are not receiving enteral nutrition (this should be a very rare occurrence). In those patients in whom SUP is required, a PPI would appear to be the drug of choice.

■ CLINICAL PEARLS

- Stress ulcer prophylaxis is not routinely required in the ICU.
- The use of PPIs may increase the risk of *C. difficile* colitis and VAP.
- H2RA may increase the risk of delirium.

■ REFERENCES

1. Skillman JJ, Bushnell LS, Goldman H, et al. Respiratory failure, hypotension, sepsis and jaundice: a clinical syndrome associated with lethal haemorrhage from acute stress ulceration of the stomach. *Am J Surg*. 1969;117:523–530.
2. Hastings PR, Skillman JJ, Bushnell LS, et al. Antacid titration in the prevention of acute gastrointestinal bleeding: a controlled, randomized trial in 100 critically ill patients. *N Engl J Med*. 1978;298:1041–1045.
3. Cook DJ, Witt LG, Cook RJ, et al. Stress ulcer prophylaxis in the critically ill: a meta-analysis. *Am J Med*. 1991;1991:519–527.
4. Cook DJ, Reeve BK, Guyatt GH, et al. Stress ulcer prophylaxis in critically ill patients. Resolving discordant meta-analyses. *JAMA*. 1996;275:308–314.

5. Dellinger RP, Levy MM, Carlet JM, et al. Surviving sepsis Campaign: international guidelines for management of severe sepsis and septic shock. *Crit Care Med.* 2008;36:296–327.
6. American Society of Hospital Pharmacists therapeutic guidelines on stress ulcer prophylaxis. *Am J Health System Pharm.* 1999;56:347–379.
7. Quality Measures Compendium. Division of Quality, Evaluation and Health Outcomes, Centers for Medicare and Medicaid Services. Available at http://www.cms.hhs.gov/MedicaidSCHIPQualPrac/Downloads/pmfinalaugust06.pdf 2. 2007. Accessed March 13, 2009.
8. Jung R, MacLaren R. Proton-pump inhibitors for stress ulcer prophylaxis in critically ill patients. *Ann Pharmacother.* 2002;36:1929–1937.
9. Kantorova I, Svoboda P, Scheer P, et al. Stress ulcer prophylaxis in critically ill patients: a randomized controlled trial. *Hepatogastroenterology.* 2004;51:757–761.
10. Fisher RL, Pipkin GA, Wood JR. Stress-related mucosal disease. Pathophysiology, prevention and treatment. *Crit Care Clin.* 1995;11:323–345.
11. Eddleston JM, Pearson RC, Holland J, et al. Prospective endoscopic study of stress erosions and ulcers in critically ill adult patients treated with either sucralfate or placebo. *Crit Care Med.* 1994;22:1949–1954.
12. Martin LF. Stress ulcers are common after aortic surgery. Endoscopic evaluation of prophylactic therapy. *Am Surg.* 1994;60:169–174.
13. Cook DJ, Fuller HD, Guyatt GH, et al. Risk factors for gastrointestinal bleeding in critically ill patients. Canadian Critical Care Trials Group. *N Engl J Med.* 1994;330:377–381.
14. Messori A, Trippoli S, Vaiani M, et al. Bleeding and pneumonia in intensive care patients given ranitidine and sucralfate for prevention of stress ulcer: meta-analysis of randomised controlled trials. *BMJ.* 2000;321:1103–1106.
15. Zandstra DF, Stoutenbeek CP. The virtual absence of stress-ulceration related bleeding in ICU patients receiving prolonged mechanical ventilation without any prophylaxis. A prospective cohort study. *Intensive Care Med.* 1994;20:335–340.
16. Erstad BL, Camamo JM, Miller MJ, et al. Impacting cost and appropriateness of stress ulcer prophylaxis at a university medical center. *Crit Care Med.* 1997;25:1678–1684.
17. Faisy C, Guerot E, Diehl JL, et al. Clinically significant gastrointestinal bleeding in critically ill patients with and without stress-ulcer prophylaxis. *Intensive Care Med.* 2003;29:1306–1313.
18. Pingleton SK, Hadzima SK. Enteral alimentation and gastrointestinal bleeding in mechanically ventilated patients. *Crit Care Med.* 1983;11:13–16.
19. Ephgrave KS, Kleiman-Wexler RL, Adair CG. Enteral nutrients prevent stress ulceration and increase intragastric volume. *Crit Care Med.* 1990;18:621–624.

20. Shorr LD, Sirinek KR, Page CP, et al. The role of glucose in preventing stress gastric mucosal injury. *J Surg Res*. 1984;36:384–388.
21. Bonten MJ, Gaillard CA, van Tiel FH, et al. Continuous enteral feeding counteracts preventive measures for gastric colonization in intensive care unit patients. *Crit Care Med*. 1994;22:939–944.
22. Mabogunje OA, Andrassy RJ, Isaacs H Jr, et al. The role of a defined formula diet in the prevention of stress-induced gastric mucosal injury in the rat. *J Pediatr Surg*. 1981;16:1036–1039.
23. Lally KP, Andrassy RJ, Foster JE, et al. Evaluation of various nutritional supplements in the prevention of stress-induced gastric ulcers in the rat. *Surg Gynecol Obstet*. 1984;158:124–128.
24. Raff T, Germann G, Hartmann B. The value of early enteral nutrition in the prophylaxis of stress ulceration in the severely burned patient. *Burns*. 1997;23:313–318.
25. Cheadle WG, Vitale GC, Mackie CR, et al. Prophylactic postoperative nasogastric decompression. A prospective study of its requirement and the influence of cimetidine in 200 patients. *Ann Surg*. 1985;202: 361–366.
26. Ben-Menachem T, Fogel R, Patel RV, et al. Prophylaxis for stress-related gastric hemorrhage in the medical intensive care unit. A randomized, controlled, single-blind study. *Ann Intern Med*. 1994;121: 568–575.
27. Apte NM, Karnad DR, Medhekar TP, et al. Gastric colonization and pneumonia in intubated critically ill patients receiving stress ulcer prophylaxis: a randomized, controlled trial. *Crit Care Med*. 1992;20: 590–593.
28. MacLaren R, Jarvis CL, Fish DN. Use of enteral nutrition for stress ulcer prophylaxis. *Ann Pharmacother*. 2001;35:1614–1623.
29. Valentine RJ, Turner WW, Borman K, et al. Does nasoenteral feeding afford adequate gastroduodenal stress prophylaxis? *Crit Care Med*. 1986;14:599–601.
30. Artinian V, Krayem H, DiGiovine B. Effects of early enteral feeding on the outcome of critically ill mechanically ventilated medical patients. *Chest*. 2006;129:960–967.
31. Marik PE, Pinsky MR. Death by total parenteral nutrition. *Intensive Care Med*. 2003;29:867–869.
32. de Smet AM, Kluytmans JA, Cooper BS, et al. Decontamination of the digestive tract and oropharynx in ICU patients. *N Engl J Med*. 2009;360(1):20–31.
33. Chan EY, Ruest A, O'Meade M, et al. Oral decontamination for prevention of pneumonia in mechanically ventilated adults: systemic review and meta-analysis. *Br Med J*. 2007;-doi:10.1136/bmj.39136.528160.BE.
34. Herzig SJ, Howell MD, Ngo LH, et al. Acid-suppressive medication use and the risk for hospital-acquired pneumonia. *JAMA*. 2009;301: 2120–2128.

35. Cunningham R, Dale B, Undy B, et al. Proton pump inhibitors as a risk factor for *Clostridium difficile* diarrhoea. *J Hosp Infect.* 2003;54: 243–245.
36. Dial S, Alrasadi K, Manoukian C, et al. Risk of *Clostridium difficile* diarrhea among hospital inpatients prescribed proton pump inhibitors: cohort and case-control studies. *CMAJ.* 2004;171:33–38.
37. Louie TJ, Meddings J. *Clostridium difficile* infection in hospitals: risk factors and responses. *CMAJ.* 2004;171:45–46.
38. Dial S, Delaney JA, Barkun AN et al. Use of gastric acid-suppressive agents and the risk of community-acquired *Clostridium difficile*-associated disease. *JAMA.* 2005;294:2989–2995.
39. Segal R, Russell WL, Oh T, et al. Use of i.v. cimetidine, ranitidine, and famotidine in 40 hospitals. *Am J Hosp Pharm.* 1993;50:2077–2081.
40. Ben-Joseph R, Segal R, Russell WL. Risk for adverse events among patients receiving intravenous histamine-2-receptor antagonists. *Ann Pharmacother.* 1993;27:1532–1537.
41. Cantu TG, Korek JS. Central nervous system reactions to histamine-2 receptor blockers. *Ann Intern Med.* 1991;114:1027–1034.
42. Cerra FB, Schentag JJ, McMillen M, et al. Mental status, the intensive care unit and cimetidine. *Ann Surg.* 1982;196:565–570.
43. Welage LS, Wing PE, Schentag JJ, et al. An evaluation of intra-venous famotidine (F) versus cimetidine (C) therapy in the critically ill. *Gastroenterology.* 1988;94:A491.
44. Kim KA, Park PW, Hong SJ, et al. The effect of CYP2C19 polymorphism on the pharmacokinetics and pharmacodynamics of clopidogrel: a possible mechanism for clopidogrel resistance. *Clin Pharmacol Ther.* 2008;84:236–242.
45. Li XQ, Andersson TB, Ahlstrom M, et al. Comparison of inhibitory effects of the proton pump-inhibiting drugs omeprazole, esomeprazole, lansoprazole, pantoprazole, and rabeprazole on human cytochrome P450 activities. *Drug Metab Dispos.* 2004;32:821–827.
46. Ho PM, Maddox TM, Wang L, et al. Risk of adverse outcomes associated with concomitant use of clopidogrel and proton pump inhibitors following acute coronary syndrome. *JAMA.* 2009;301:937–944.
47. Juurlink DN, Gomes T, Ko DT, et al. A population-based study of the drug interaction between proton pump inhibitors and clopidogrel. *CMAJ.* 2009;180:713–718.
48. Mulla H, Peek G, Upton D, et al. Plasma aluminum levels during sucralfate prophylaxis for stress ulceration in critically ill patients on continuous venovenous hemofiltration: a randomized, controlled trial. *Crit Care Med.* 2001;29:267–271.
49. Cook D, Guyatt G, Marshall J, et al. A comparison of sucralfate and ranitidine for the prevention of upper gastrointestinal bleeding in patients requiring mechanical ventilation. *N Engl J Med.* 1998;338:791–797.

33

Chronic Liver Failure

Chronic liver failure (CLF) and cirrhosis accounted for more than 26,000 deaths and more than half a million hospitalizations in the United States in 2004, making liver disease the 12th leading cause of death.[1] The Child–Turcotte–Pugh (CTP) scoring system classifies CLF into three categories based on severity (Table 33-1). A total CTP score of 5–6 is Child's class A, well-compensated disease; a CTP score of 7–9 is Child's class B, in which there is significant functional compromise; and a CTP score of 10–15 is Child's class C, advanced decompensated disease.[2] The model for end-stage liver disease (MELD) score provides another classification of the severity of chronic liver failure based on the readily obtainable laboratory values of serum creatinine, total bilirubin, and prothrombin time, expressed as the international normalized ratio.[2,3]

Cirrhosis is defined histologically as an advanced form of progressive hepatic fibrosis with distortion of the hepatic architecture and regenerative nodule formation. It may be due to a variety of causes. The major clinical consequences of cirrhosis are impaired hepatocyte function, an increased intrahepatic resistance (portal hypertension), and the development of hepatocellular carcinoma. The general circulatory abnormalities in cirrhosis (splanchnic vasodilation, systemic vasoconstriction and hypoperfusion of the kidneys, water and salt retention, and increased cardiac output) are intimately linked to the hepatic vascular alterations and resulting portal hypertension. The clinical picture of chronic liver disease is frequently dominated by the complications of portal hypertension. In addition, infectious complications are common and associated with worsening of hepatocyte function and portal hypertension.

P.E. Marik, *Handbook of Evidence-Based Critical Care*,
DOI 10.1007/978-1-4419-5923-2_33,
© Springer Science+Business Media, LLC 2010

Table 33-1. The Child–Turcotte–Pugh (CTP) scoring system.

Parameter	1	2	3
Ascites	Absent	Easily controlled	Poorly controlled
Bilirubin (mg/dl)	<2	2–3	>3
Albumin (g/dl)	>3.5	2.8–3.5	<2.8
INR	<1.7	1.7–2.3	>2.3
Encephalopathy	None	Grade 1–2	Grade 3–4

■ CAUSES OF CIRRHOSIS

- Viral/infectious
  - Hepatitis B
  - Hepatitis C
  - Schistosomiasis
- Metabolic
  - Alcohol
  - Toxins, medications
- Hereditary hemochromatosis
- Wilson's disease
- Non-alcoholic steatohepatitis
- Autoimmune hepatitis
- Cholestatic
  - Primary biliary cirrhosis
  - Primary sclerosing cholangitis
  - Secondary biliary cirrhosis
- Vascular
  - Right heart failure
  - Budd–Chiari syndrome
- α-1-Anti-trypsin deficiency
- Sarcoidosis
- Cystic fibrosis

Cirrhosis represents a clinical spectrum, ranging from asymptomatic liver disease to hepatic decompensation. Manifestations of hepatic decompensation include the following:

- Variceal bleeding (see Chapter 36)
- Ascites with spontaneous bacterial peritonitis
- Hepatic encephalopathy
- Hepatorenal syndrome
- Hepatopulmonary syndrome
- Portopulmonary hypertension
- Hepatocellular carcinoma
- Hepatoadrenal syndrome

> **ALERT**
>
> The liver never fails in isolation. . ..
> it takes each and every organ system down with it!

■ METABOLIC/HEMATOLOGIC DERANGEMENTS IN CIRRHOSIS

- Hyperglycemia (portal to systemic shunting)
- Hypoglycemia (hepatocyte failure)
- Hypoalbuminemia
- Decreased synthesis of clotting factors. . .prolonged INR
- Decreased production of AT, protein S and C. . . thrombotic risk
- Increased ammonia
- Cholestasis
  - Impaired absorption of fat and fat soluble vitamins
- Anemia
  - Microcytic from iron deficiency
  - Macrocytic folate and B12 deficiency
- Hyponatremia (Na <135 mmol/l)
  - An independent predictor of mortality[4]
  - From increased ADH due to decreased effective circulating volume
- Thrombocytopenia
  - Hypersplenism
  - Alcohol
  - Marrow suppression
- "Low-level" DIC
- Renal dysfunction
- Impaired immunity

■ SPONTANEOUS BACTERIAL PERITONITIS

Spontaneous bacterial peritonitis (SBP) is seen in up to 30% of patients with ascites. Patients who have SBP present with fever, diffuse abdominal pain or tenderness, altered mental status, leukocytosis, or worsening renal function. Approximately 15% of patients do not have any signs or symptoms of SBP. The diagnostic test of choice is abdominal paracentesis. An ascitic fluid neutrophil count higher than 250/mm^3 in the absence of a known or a suspected intra-abdominal surgical source of infection, such as a perforated peptic ulcer or an abscess, is diagnostic of SBP. Fluid cultures are positive in approximately half of the cases. Almost all cases of SBP are secondary to a single microorganism, with *Escherichia coli* and *Klebsiella pneumoniae* accounting for approximately half of the cases and gram-positive bacteria accounting for one-third.[5] Treatment consists of a 5-day course of a third-generation cephalosporin, such as intravenous cefotaxime/ceftriaxone, and usually results in an excellent clinical response with resolution of SBP. For patients unable to take a cephalosporin, intravenous ciprofloxacin, followed by oral administration, is recommended.[5] SBP is associated with the development of hepatorenal syndrome in about 30% of patients. The risk can be decreased by intravenous albumin infusion at a dose of 1.5 mg/kg at the time of SBP diagnosis and 1.0 mg/kg after 48 h.[6]

Primary prophylaxis, defined as antibiotic treatment of patients without prior SBP, has been suggested in patients with chronic liver failure and ascites who fulfill the following criteria:

• Ascitic fluid protein concentration lower than 1 g/dl,
• Serum bilirubin level higher than 3.2 mg/dl, and
• Platelet count higher than 98,000/mm^3, as these patients have a threefold increased risk of developing SBP within 1 year.

A recent RCT demonstrated that primary prophylaxis with norfloxacin significantly reduced the 1-year risk of developing SBP when compared with placebo (7% vs. 61%; p <0.001).[7] Following an initial episode of SBP, 1-year recurrence rate is 55%, 1-year survival is less than 50%, and antibiotic prophylaxis with fluoroquinolones is recommended. Amoxicillin–clavulanate and trimethoprim–sulfamethoxazole are acceptable alternatives in those unable to tolerate quinolones.

■ HEPATIC ENCEPHALOPATHY

Hepatic encephalopathy has a wide range of clinical manifestations, from impaired memory and diminished attention to confusion and coma. Many factors have been implicated in its pathogenesis, including derangements in neurotransmitter pathways, cerebral blood flow modulation, and systemic inflammatory responses. The ammonia hypothesis states that impaired hepatic breakdown of ammonia results in multiple neurotoxic effects, including altering the transit of amino acids, water, and electrolytes across the neuronal membrane and propagating astrocyte swelling and cerebral edema. Contrary to "classic teaching," Ong and colleagues[8] found a good correlation between the serum ammonia levels and the severity of hepatic encephalopathy. Furthermore, there was no significant difference between venous and arterial ammonia levels.

Acute worsening of hepatic encephalopathy should prompt an evaluation for reversible causes, such as gastrointestinal bleeding, hypovolemia, hypoglycemia, hypokalemic metabolic alkalosis, infection, constipation, hypoxia, or excessive use of sedatives.

The treatment of hepatic encephalopathy is with non-absorbable disaccharides (such as lactulose) to lower ammonia levels. The starting dose of lactulose is commonly 30 g twice a day, titrated to two to three soft stools per day. The addition of non-absorbable antibiotics such as rifaximin may further decrease intestinal ammonia production. Previously, aggressive protein restriction was recommended; however, this is now believed to worsen the nutritional status of patients and decreases overall survival.[9] Guidelines published by the European Society for Clinical Nutrition and Metabolism (ESPEN) recommended that patients with cirrhosis should have an energy intake of 35–40 kcal/kg body weight per day and a protein intake of 1.2–1.5 g/kg body weight per day.[10]

Zinc deficiency impairs the activity of urea cycle enzymes and glutamine synthetase. Zinc deficiency has been implicated in the pathogenesis of hepatic encephalopathy as diminished serum zinc levels and their inverse correlation with blood ammonia levels have been reported.[11] Zinc supplementation in the treatment of hepatic encephalopathy is based on a small number of controlled studies that provided inconsistent results regarding efficacy, types, and doses of zinc used, and duration of therapy.

Grading of Mental Status

- Grade 0
  - No signs or symptoms
- Grade 1
  - Trivial lack of awareness, euphoria or anxiety, shortened attention span impaired performance of addition
- Grade 2
  - Lethargy or apathy, minimal disorientation for time or place, subtle personality change, inappropriate behavior, impaired performance of subtraction
- Grade 3
  - Somnolence to semi-stupor but responsive to verbal stimuli, confusion, gross disorientation
- Grade 4 Coma (unresponsive to verbal or noxious stimuli)

■ HEPATORENAL SYNDROME

Hepatorenal syndrome (HRES) is a functional form of renal failure that occurs in patients with end-stage liver disease. The pathophysiological hallmark of HRS is vasoconstriction of the renal circulation. The mechanism of the vasoconstriction is incompletely understood; it may be multi-factorial, involving disturbances in the circulatory function and activity of the systemic and renal vasoactive mechanisms. In 1996 the International Ascites Club (IAC) established major and minor diagnostic criteria for the diagnosis of HRS.[12] HRS was further classified as type 1 and type 2 according to the rate of decline of renal function. Type 1 was arbitrarily defined as a 100% increase in serum creatinine reaching a value of greater than 1.5 mg/dl in less than 2 weeks. Patients who had a slower decline in renal function were deemed to have type 2 HRS.

Patients with type 1 HRS have a very poor prognosis compared to patients with type 2 HRS. The median survival time for type 1 HRS has been reported to be 14 days. The only effective medical therapy currently available for the management of HRS is the administration of vasoconstrictors together with volume expansion with albumin. Volume expansion with albumin and vasopressin analogues (ornipressin and terlipressin), norepinephrine, and somatostatin has been used with variable success.[13,14] Liver transplantation is considered the treatment of choice for patients with cirrhosis and type 1 HRS because it "allows for both the liver disease and associated renal failure to be cured."

HRS is a frequent complication over overdiuresis, particularly in the setting of a contrast study or a therapeutic paracentesis. Patients who undergo a contrast study and/or paracentesis require fluid loading (with albumin).

ALERT

LASIX is NOT a volume expander; its use may lead to a fatal outcome in patients with cirrhosis.

■ HEPATOADRENAL SYNDROME

Sepsis and end-stage liver disease have a number of pathophysiological mechanisms in common (endotoxemia, increased levels of proinflammatory mediators, decreased levels of HDL), and it is therefore not surprising that adrenal insufficiency is common in patients with end-stage liver disease.[15] Tsai and colleagues[16] performed a corticotrophin stimulation test in 101 patients with cirrhosis and sepsis. In this study, 51.4% of the patients were diagnosed with adrenal insufficiency;

survival at 90 days was 15.3% in these patients compared to 63.2% in those patients with normal adrenal function. Fernandez and coauthors[17] compared the survival of patients with cirrhosis and sepsis who underwent adrenal function testing in which patients with adrenal insufficiency were treated with hydrocortisone (Group 1) to a control group (Group 2) that did not undergo a cosyntropin testing and were not treated with corticosteroids. The incidence of adrenal failure was 68% in Group 1; the hospital survival was 64% in Group 1 as compared to 32% in Group 2 ($p = 0.003$). These data suggest that adrenal dysfunction is common in critically ill patients with end-stage liver disease and that treatment with corticosteroids may improve outcome.

■ PULMONARY CONSEQUENCES OF PORTAL HYPERTENSION

Two distinct pulmonary vascular disorders can occur in cirrhosis: hepatopulmonary syndrome (HPS) and portopulmonary hypertension (POPH). Both can coexist in the same patient. Portopulmonary hypertension is seen in 0.5–5% of patients with cirrhosis and/or portal hypertension and presents in similar ways to patients with pulmonary hypertension from other causes. Diagnosis is established by echocardiography and right heart catheterization. Recent case reports and series have demonstrated improvement of pulmonary hypertension with oral sildenafil.[18]

HPS is defined as a defect in arterial oxygenation induced by intrapulmonary vascular dilatations. This entity is seen in 8–17% of patients with cirrhosis, and median survival is 11 months. Liver transplantation resolves HPS in the majority of patients.

■ INFECTION AND CIRRHOSIS

Cirrhotic patients have several abnormalities which increase the susceptibility to bacterial infection; these include deficiency of bactericidal and opsonic activities, impaired monocyte function, depressed phagocytic activity, defective chemotaxis, and low levels of serum complement. A National Hospital Discharge Survey demonstrated that hospitalized cirrhotics are more likely to develop sepsis (RR 2.6) and to die from sepsis (RR 2.0) than are hospitalized non-cirrhotics.[19] Fifteen to thirty-five percent of cirrhotics develop nosocomial infection, with infection accounting for 30–50% of deaths in patients with cirrhosis.

- Usual infections
  - SBP
  - Pneumonia
  - Gram-negative bacteremia
  - UTI
- Common pathogens
  - *E. coli*
  - *Staphylococcus aureus*
  - *Enterococcus faecalis*
  - *Streptococcus pneumoniae*
  - *Pseudomonas aeruginosa*
- Diagnosis of infection is difficult in patients with cirrhosis
  - Reduced WBC due to hypersplenism
  - Tachycardia and hyperdynamic circulation
  - Hyperventilation due to hepatic encephalopathy
  - Blunted febrile response
  - Cirrhosis itself results in low-grade fever
- In patients with cirrhosis infections
  - Further impair systemic and splanchnic hemodynamics
  - Impair coagulation
  - Worsen liver function
  - May trigger variceal bleeding

■ SUPPORTIVE CARE OF THE HOSPITALIZED CIRRHOTIC

- Do not replace clotting factors or platelets unless bleeding (see Chapters 52 and 53).
- Feed with a 1 g/kg protein diet.
- SCDs for DVT prophylaxis.
- Exclude infection; culture blood, ascitic fluid.
- Prophylactic antibiotics in high-risk patients.
- Do not diurese; give 25% albumin.
- Paracentesis in patients with tense ascites (replace albumin).
- Avoid nephrotoxic drugs.
- Lactulose for regular stool.
- Rifaximin 200 mg PO q 8 hourly to decrease ammonia production by GI flora.
- Monitor venous ammonia.
- ACTH stimulation test in all; replace with hydrocortisone if AI (see Chapter 40).
- Avoid sedatives (haloperidol and dexmedetomidine are okay).

- Ultrasound + Doppler to exclude portal/splenic vein thrombosis and hepatocellular carcinoma.
- α-Fetoprotein level.

■ REFERENCES

1. Minino AM, Heron MP, Smith BL. Deaths: preliminary data for 2004. *Natl Vital Stat Rep*. 2006;54:1–49.
2. Pugh RN, Murray-Lyon IM, Dawson JL, et al. Transection of the oesophagus for bleeding oesophageal varices. *Br J Surg*. 1973;60:646–649.
3. Durand F, Valla D, Durand F, et al. Assessment of the prognosis of cirrhosis: Child–Pugh versus MELD. *J Hepatol*. 2005;42(Suppl):S100–S107.
4. Angeli P, Wong F, Watson H, et al. Hyponatremia in cirrhosis: results of a patient population survey. *Hepatology*. 2006;44:1535–1542.
5. Arora G, Keeffe EB. Management of chronic liver failure until liver transplantation. *Med Clin North Am*. 2008;92:839–860.
6. Sort P, Navasa M, Arroyo V, et al. Effect of intravenous albumin on renal impairment and mortality in patients with cirrhosis and spontaneous bacterial peritonitis. *N Engl J Med*. 1999;341:403–409.
7. Fernandez J, Navasa M, Planas R, et al. Primary prophylaxis of spontaneous bacterial peritonitis delays hepatorenal syndrome and improves survival in cirrhosis [see comment]. *Gastroenterology*. 2007;133: 818–824.
8. Ong JP, Aggarwal A, Krieger D, et al. Correlation between ammonia levels and the severity of hepatic encephalopathy. *Am J Med*. 2003;114:188–193.
9. Cordoba J, Lopez-Hellin J, Planas M, et al. Normal protein diet for episodic hepatic encephalopathy: results of a randomized study. *J Hepatol*. 2004;41:38–43.
10. Plauth M, Cabre E, Riggio O, et al. ESPEN guidelines on enteral nutrition: liver disease. *Clin Nutr*. 2006;25:285–294.
11. Reding P, Duchateau J, Bataille C. Oral zinc supplementation improves hepatic encephalopathy. Results of a randomised controlled trial. *Lancet*. 1984;2:493–495.
12. Arroyo V, Gines P, Gerbes AL, et al. Definition and diagnostic criteria of refractory ascites and hepatorenal syndrome in cirrhosis. International Ascites Club. *Hepatology*. 1996;23:164–176.
13. Saner FH, Fruhauf NR, Schafers RF, et al. Terlipressin plus hydroxyethyl starch infusion: an effective treatment for hepatorenal syndrome. *Eur J Gastroenterol Hepatol*. 2003;15:925–927.
14. Duvoux C, Zanditenas D, Hezode C, et al. Effects of noradrenalin and albumin in patients with type I hepatorenal syndrome: a pilot study. *Hepatology*. 2002;36:374–380.

15. Marik PE, Gayowski T, Starzl TE, et al. The hepatoadrenal syndrome: a common yet unrecognized clinical condition. *Crit Care Med.* 2005;33:1254–1259.
16. Tsai MH, Peng YS, Chen YC, et al. Adrenal insufficiency in patients with cirrhosis, severe sepsis and septic shock. *Hepatology.* 2006;43: 673–681.
17. Fernandez J, Escorsell A, Zabalza M, et al. Adrenal insufficiency in patients with cirrhosis and septic shock: effect of treatment with hydrocortisone on survival. *Hepatology.* 2006;44:1288–1295.
18. Reichenberger F, Voswinckel R, Steveling E, et al. Sildenafil treatment for portopulmonary hypertension. *Eur Respir J.* 2006;28:563–567.
19. Foreman MG, Mannino DM, Moss M. Cirrhosis as a risk factor for sepsis and death: analysis of the National Hospital Discharge Survey. *Chest.* 2003;124:1016–1020.

34

Alcoholic Hepatitis

Alcoholic hepatitis is observed in approximately 20% of heavy drinkers and about 50% of heavy drinkers who are admitted to an acute-care hospital. Alcoholic hepatitis is a serious disease, with a 28-day mortality of 35% in high-risk patients (Maddrey's discriminant function $\geq$32).[1] Alcoholic hepatitis is a clinical syndrome of jaundice and liver failure that generally occurs after decades of heavy alcohol use (mean intake, approximately 100 g/day).[2] Not uncommonly, the patient will have ceased alcohol consumption several weeks before the onset of symptoms. The cardinal sign of alcoholic hepatitis is the rapid onset of jaundice. Other common signs and symptoms include fever, ascites, and proximal muscle loss. Patients with severe alcoholic hepatitis may have encephalopathy. Typically, the liver is enlarged and tender. Histology of the liver reveals hepatocellular injury characterized by ballooned (swollen) hepatocytes that often contain amorphous eosinophilic inclusion bodies called Mallory bodies (also called alcoholic hyaline) surrounded by neutrophils. The presence in hepatocytes of large fat globules, also known as steatosis, is common in alcoholic hepatitis. While the pathophysiology of alcoholic hepatitis is complex and incompletely understood, the prevailing theory postulates that ethanol promotes the translocation of lipopolysaccharide (LPS) from the lumen of the small and large intestines to the portal vein, where it travels to the liver. LPS activates Kupffer cells in the liver. TNF-α, produced by Kupffer cells, appears to play a pivotal role in the genesis of alcoholic hepatitis.

Laboratory studies characteristically reveal the following:

- Increased AST (but usually <300 IU)
- AST:ALT >2
- Increased WBC with neutrophilia
- Increased bilirubin (usually >5 mg/dl)

P.E. Marik, *Handbook of Evidence-Based Critical Care*, DOI 10.1007/978-1-4419-5923-2_34, © Springer Science+Business Media, LLC 2010

- Increased INR
- Increased creatinine

A variety of scoring systems have been developed to assess the severity of alcoholic hepatitis and to guide treatment. Maddrey's discriminant function (mDF) and the Glasgow alcoholic hepatitis score (GAHS) help the clinician decide whether corticosteroids should be initiated (Table 34-1). These scoring systems share common elements, such as the serum bilirubin level and prothrombin time (or INR).

Table 34-1. Glasgow alcohol hepatitis score.[3]

Score	1	2	3
Age	<50	>50	–
WCC	<15	≥25	–
BUN (mg/dl)	<14	≥14	–
INR	<1.5	1.5–2.0	>2.0
Bilirubin	<7.3	7.3–14.7	>14.7

Maddrey's discriminant function is calculated as [4.6 × (patient's prothrombin time – control prothrombin time, in seconds)] + serum bilirubin level (mg/dl).

■ MANAGEMENT

- Enteral feeding is recommended as the patients are frequently malnourished. A daily protein intake of 1.5 g/kg of body weight is recommended, even among patients with hepatic encephalopathy.[4]
- Patients may develop alcohol withdrawal syndrome. While benzodiazepines are usually recommended, dexmedetomidine may be particularly useful in this situation (see Chapter 60).
- Valproic acid and divalproex sodium (Depakote) are useful alternatives to consider in this situation.
- Corticosteroid therapy abrogates the inflammatory process. However, the use of these agents has been controversial.[5] An individual patient meta-analysis demonstrated that corticosteroids reduce mortality in patients with an mDF ≥32.[1] More recently, Forrest et al.[6] demonstrated that in patients with an mDF >32, only those with a GAHS ≥9 benefit from corticosteroids. Prednisolone at a dosage of 40 mg/day for 28 days is usually recommended. A prompt decline in serum bilirubin indicates a favorable response to therapy. Patients who do not exhibit a reduction in serum bilirubin within 1 week are considered non-responders and have a 6-month mortality rate of 50% or higher.

- One randomized controlled trial showed that pentoxifylline (400 mg q 8 h), a phosphodiesterase inhibitor which modulates TNF-α transcription, reduced short-term mortality among patients with alcoholic hepatitis.[7] The survival benefit of pentoxifylline appears to be related to a significant reduction in the development of the hepatorenal syndrome.
- Direct TNF-α inhibitors have not been demonstrated to improve outcome.[8]

■ REFERENCES

1. Mathurin P, Mendenhall CL, Carithers RL Jr, et al. Corticosteroids improve short-term survival in patients with severe alcoholic hepatitis (AH): individual data analysis of the last three randomized placebo controlled double blind trials of corticosteroids in severe AH. *J Hepatol.* 2002;36:480–487.
2. Lucey MR, Mathurin P, Morgan TR. Alcoholic hepatitis. *N Engl J Med.* 2009;360:2758–2769.
3. Forrest EH, Evans CD, Stewart S, et al. Analysis of factors predictive of mortality in alcoholic hepatitis and derivation and validation of the Glasgow alcoholic hepatitis score. *Gut.* 2005;54:1174–1179.
4. Cabre E, Rodriguez-Iglesias P, Caballeria J, et al. Short- and long-term outcome of severe alcohol-induced hepatitis treated with steroids or enteral nutrition: a multicenter randomized trial. *Hepatology.* 2000;32:36–42.
5. Rambaldi A, Saconato HH, Christensen E, et al. Systematic review: glucocorticosteroids for alcoholic hepatitis – a Cochrane Hepato-Biliary Group systematic review with meta-analyses and trial sequential analyses of randomized clinical trials. *Aliment Pharmacol Ther.* 2008;27:1167–1178.
6. Forrest EH, Morris AJ, Stewart S, et al. The Glasgow alcoholic hepatitis score identifies patients who may benefit from corticosteroids. *Gut.* 2007;56:1743–1746.
7. Akriviadis E, Botla R, Briggs W, et al. Pentoxifylline improves short-term survival in severe acute alcoholic hepatitis: a double-blind, placebo-controlled trial. *Gastroenterology.* 2000;119:1637–1648.
8. Boetticher NC, Peine CJ, Kwo P, et al. A randomized, double-blinded, placebo-controlled multicenter trial of etanercept in the treatment of alcoholic hepatitis. *Gastroenterology.* 2008;135:19531960.

35

Fulminant Hepatic Failure

Fulminant hepatic failure (FHF) also known as acute liver failure is defined as the development of impaired hepatic synthetic function with coagulopathy and the development of hepatic encephalopathy in the absence of underlying liver disease within a time period of 2–3 months. This condition is uncommon but not rare, affecting approximately 2,000 cases annually in the United States with a mortality ranging 50–90% despite intensive care therapy.[1]

The clinical picture of chronic liver disease is frequently dominated by the complication of portal hypertension. On the other hand, the clinical picture of acute/fulminant hepatic failure is dominated by hepatocyte failure. Cerebral edema leading to intracranial hypertension (IH) complicates approximately 50–80% of patients with severe FHF (grade III or IV coma) in whom it is the leading cause of death.[2] Recovery of functional liver mass in acute liver injury occurs more readily than in the chronic setting because of the lack of long-standing fibrosis and portal hypertension, and the host's overall better nutritional status. Therefore, if the individual can be supported throughout the acute event, and the inciting injury is removed or ameliorated, recovery will follow the rapid regeneration of liver cells. For those in whom spontaneous recovery is not possible, liver transplant may be life saving.

■ CAUSES OF FULMINANT HEPATIC FAILURE

- Viral Hepatitis
  - Hepatitis B, C, and E, and rarely A and D infections

P.E. Marik, *Handbook of Evidence-Based Critical Care*,
DOI 10.1007/978-1-4419-5923-2_35,
© Springer Science+Business Media, LLC 2010

- CMV infection
- Viral hemorrhagic fevers
- Drugs and toxins
  - Acetaminophen (see   Chapter 59)
  - Alcohol
  - Isoniazid
  - Valproic acid
  - Phenytoin
  - Amanita phalloides
  - Carbon tetrachloride
  - Methylenedioxymethamphetamine ("ecstasy")
- Miscellaneous
  - Fatty liver of pregnancy
  - Reye's syndrome
  - Wilson's disease
  - Autoimmune chronic active hepatitis
  - Budd–Chiari syndrome (especially in patients with underlying hepatic disease

■ WORKUP OF PATIENTS PRESENTING WITH FHF

Blood and Urine Testing

- Complete blood cell count with platelets
- Electrolytes BUN and creatinine
- International normalized ratio (INR)
- Liver panel
- Blood lactate
- Ammonia
- Blood gas with pH
- HIV testing (rapid)
- Hepatitis A, B, C, E (all markers)
- Cytomegalovirus (CMV) PCR and Ab
- Herpes simplex virus (HSV) PCR and Ab
- Epstein–Barr virus Ab
- Autoimmune markers
  - Anti-nuclear antibody
  - Anti-smooth muscle antibody
  - Anti-liver kidney microsomal antibody
- Metabolic markers
  - Uric acid
  - Serum copper and urine copper
- Hypercoagulable markers
  - Lupus anti-coagulant

- – Factor 5 Leiden
- Toxicology screen and drug panel
  - – Acetaminophen
  - – Opiates
  - – Barbiturates
  - – Cocaine
  - – Alcohol
- Pregnancy testing (females)
- Urine electrolytes and osmolarity
- Blood cultures
- Urine cultures

Imaging and Other Testing

- Chest radiograph
- Abdominal ultrasound with Doppler study of the liver
- ECG
- Echocardiogram with estimation of pulmonary artery pressures

■ CEREBRAL EDEMA IN FHF

Currently the mechanisms which produce cerebral edema and IH in the setting of FHF are multi-factorial in etiology and are only partially understood. Possible contributing mechanisms include cytotoxicity due to the osmotic effects of ammonia, glutamine, and other amino acids, and pro-inflammatory cytokines. Cerebral hyperemia and vasogenic edema occur due to the disruption of blood–brain barrier with rapid accumulation of low molecular substances. Dysfunction of the sodium–potassium ATPase pump with loss of autoregulation of cerebral blood flow has been implicated as a cause of hyperemia. As encephalopathy progresses, there is gradual cerebral vasodilation due to the loss of cerebral autoregulation resulting in increased cerebral blood volume and edema. Finally, in the preterminal phase, there is a marked reduction in cerebral blood flow due to cerebral edema with ultimate cerebral herniation.

Clinical signs of IH include systemic hypertension, bradycardia, pupillary abnormalities, decerebrate posturing, epileptiform activity, and brainstem respiratory patterns. These are however late signs and usually indicate impending herniation. An ammonia level higher than 200 μg/dl in stage III and IV encephalopathy is a strong predictor of brain herniation.[3] Though high ICP often results in death in patients with FHF, it is not clear how to identify those patients at risk and how to monitor them. Computed tomogram brain scanning often fails to demonstrate cerebral edema in patients with elevated ICP. The use of ICP monitoring in patients with FHF is controversial. There is no evidence that ICP monitoring improves outcome (due to lack of data). In addition, both intraparenchymal and intraventricular monitoring devices are contraindicated as these patients are usually severely coagulopathic. Furthermore, epidural devices are less accurate and many centers no longer use these devices. Consequently, in many centers, the ICP is not monitored. Nevertheless, the US Acute Liver Failure Study Group has endorsed the use of ICP monitors in patients with FHF who are at high risk for IH.[4]

Transcranial Doppler is a valuable non-invasive technique which measures systolic flow velocity of the middle cerebral artery. Cerebral blood flow measured with transcranial Doppler appears to correlate fairly well with more direct measures of flow such as xenon and A–V oxygen content trends.[5] Normal systolic velocity is <120 cm/s. Attenuation of the diastolic flow signal may be a sign of intracranial hypertension and diminished effective cerebral perfusion. In addition, the diastolic waveform may indicate early or late signs of elevated ICP as diastolic flow begins to attenuate. A pulsatility index (systolic velocity – diastolic velocity/systolic velocity) >1.6 is a poor prognostic sign.

■ MANAGEMENT OF INCREASED ICP

Optimal management of IH and FHF begins with the recognition that a patient with acute liver disease may die suddenly and are therefore best cared for in an ICU with expertise in the management of liver failure (also see Chapter 49). Since the transportation of patients with advanced levels of coma is hazardous and the disease often worsens rapidly, transfer to a liver transplantation center should be considered at the time of admission of any patient with altered mentation. Increase in ICP often occurs in conjunction with the multiple organ dysfunction syndrome.

Assisted ventilation must be instituted in all patients with grade III and IV coma. In general, sedation of any kind should be avoided in early stages of coma. Patient's head must be positioned at a 30° upright angle to improve jugular venous outflow and to optimize cerebral perfusion pressure. Coughing, gagging, agitation, fever, seizures, arterial hypertension, frequent head turning, and endotracheal suctioning are all associated with surges in ICP and are best avoided. Although neuromuscular blockade may be needed if patients are particularly difficult to ventilate or if severe hypoxia exists, they are best avoided.

Propofol is the sedative agent of choice in patients with FHF. Propofol permits a faster return to wakefulness and is a useful agent for neurological evaluation in patients with FHF. Liver failure does not influence propofol pharmacokinetics. Propofol has additional properties that may be beneficial in patients with FHF including a decrease in cerebral metabolic rate, decrease in ICP, potentiation of GABAminergic inhibition, inhibition of NMDA glutamate receptors, and voltage-dependent calcium channels and prevention of lipid peroxidation.[6] Propofol decreases intracranial pressure (ICP) in patients with either normal or increased ICP.

There are no randomized controlled clinical trials which have evaluated lactulose or non-absorbable antibiotics in patients with FHF. However, considering the central role that ammonia is postulated to play in the pathophysiology of FHF, it may be prudent to "detoxify" the gastrointestinal tract with one of these agents.

Moderate induced hypothermia (32–33°C) has been shown to delay the onset of encephalopathy and control cerebral edema in several studies.[7] Several mechanisms have been proposed by which induced hypothermia reduces cerebral edema in patients with FHF. Hypothermia reduces cerebral ammonia levels by decreased brain ammonia uptake, decreases production of ammonia in situ, and improves ammonia clearance in the brain by stimulation of glutamine synthesis.[8] Induced hypothermia should be considered in patients with grade III and IV coma (see Chapter 58). Mannitol and hypertonic saline have a role in patients with evidence of severely raised ICP.

The US Acute Liver Failure Study Group conducted an RCT in which patients with FHF not due to acetaminophen were randomized to *N*-acetylcysteine (NAC) or placebo.[9] Spontaneous survival amongst patients stratified by grade of encephalopathy is shown in Table 35-1.

Table 35-1. Spontaneous survival of patients with FHF (not due to acetaminophen) randomized to NAC or placebo.

Grade at Admission	Placebo	NAC	p-Value
1–2	17/56 (30%)	30/58 (52%)	0.021
3–4	8/36 (22%)	2/23 (9%)	0.177
Total	25/92 (27%)	32/81 (45%)	0.09

The primary outcome of the trial, overall survival rate (i.e., spontaneous survival + survival after OLT), was 61 of 92 patients (67%) in the placebo group and 57 of 81 patients (70%) in the NAC group ($p = 0.57$). Although, the outcome of the trial was considered "negative," considering the safety profile of NAC and greater spontaneous survival in the patients who received NAC, the administration of NAC should be considered for FHF patients (at least in those with mild-to-moderate hepatic encephalopathy)

■ SUPPORTIVE MEASURES

- Monitor blood glucose; 5–10% D/W to prevent hypoglycemia.
- Monitor neurological status very closely.
- Monitor volume status, urine output.
- Exclude/treat sepsis.
- Routine cultures and infection surveillance.
- Prophylactic antibiotics are generally not recommended.
- Enteral feeding should be commenced within 24 h of ICU admission and should provide 20–25 kcal/kg/day for the initial phase of the illness and 25–30 kcal/kg/day during recovery. Protein (1 g/kg/day) is recommended. In patients considered to be at high risk for IH or in whom circulating ammonia is approaching or above 150 mmol/l, this protein load may be reduced (to 0.5 g/kg/day) for periods of 1–2 days only.
- Vitamin K 10 mg intravenously given as a single dose.
- Prophylactic transfusions to normalize coagulation profile are not recommended. FFP/fibrinogen for active bleeding only. Unnecessary correction of coagulopathy will remove one of the most important parameters for determining patient prognosis and further complicate the already difficult decision-making process around transplantation listing.
- Monitor INR and lactate closely, at least every 8 h.
- N-Acetylcysteine should be considered.
- Extracorporeal liver-assist devices (ELADs) hold promise for temporary hepatic support.

■ INDICATIONS FOR LIVER TRANSPLANTATION

The uncertainty as to whether a patient will recover with conservative management or require transplantation has been the subject of many different reports and case series; however, the Kings College Criteria remain the current standard for clinicians.[10] These criteria are used to predict death in patients presenting with ALF in the setting of acetaminophen and other causes of ALF. Despite these criteria, the decision as to when to "list" a patient with FHF is extremely difficult. In the authors' experience, the trend in both the INR and the serum lactate are very useful in assisting with this decision.

■ KINGS CRITERIA

Acetaminophen-Induced Acute Liver Failure (ALF)

- Hepatic encephalopathy coma grades 3–4

- Arterial pH <7.3
- Prothrombin time (PT) greater than 100 s
- Serum creatinine greater than 3.4 mg/dl

Non-acetaminophen-Induced ALF

- PT of greater than 100 s or three of the following five criteria:
  - Age less than 10 years or greater than 40 years
  - ALF caused by non-A, non-B, non-C, hepatitis, halothane hepatitis, or idiosyncratic drug reactions
  - Jaundice present more than 1 week before the onset of encephalopathy
  - PT >50 s
  - Serum bilirubin greater than 17.5 mg/dl

■ REFERENCES

1. Hoofnagle JH, Carithers RL Jr, Shapiro C, et al. Fulminant hepatic failure: summary of a workshop. *Hepatology.* 1995;21:240–252.
2. Ostapowicz G, Fontana RJ, Schiodt FV, et al. Results of a prospective study of acute liver failure at 17 tertiary care centers in the United States. *Ann Intern Med.* 2002;137:947–954.
3. Clemmesen JO, Larsen FS, Kondrup J, et al. Cerebral herniation in patients with acute liver failure is correlated with arterial ammonia concentration. *Hepatology.* 1999;29:648–653.
4. Stravitz RT, Kramer AH, Davern T, et al. Intensive care of patients with acute liver failure: recommendations of the US Acute Liver Failure Study Group. *Crit Care Med.* 2007;35:2498–2508.
5. Strauss GI, Moller K, Holm S, et al. Transcranial Doppler sonography and internal jugular bulb saturation during hyperventilation in patients with fulminant hepatic failure. *Liver Transpl.* 2001;7:352–358.
6. Marik PE. Propofol: therapeutic indications and side effects. *Curr Pharm Design.* 2004;10:3639–3649.
7. Stravitz RT, Larsen FS. Therapeutic hypothermia for acute liver failure. *Crit Care Med.* 2009;37:S258–S264.
8. Chatauret N, Rose C, Butterworth RF. Mild hypothermia in the prevention of brain edema in acute liver failure: mechanisms and clinical prospects. *Metab Brain Dis.* 2002;17:445–451.
9. Lee WM, Rossaro L, Fontana RJ. Intravenous N-acetylcysteine improves survival in early stage non-acetaminophen acute liver failure [abstract]. *Hepatology.* 2007;46:268A.
10. O'Grady JG, Alexander GJ, Hayllar KM, et al. Early indicators of prognosis in fulminant hepatic failure. *Gastroenterology.* 1989;97:439–445.

36

GI Bleeding

■ INITIAL ASSESSMENT

- The urgency with which GI bleeding is managed is dictated by the rate of bleeding:
  - The patient with trace heme-positive stools and without severe anemia can be managed as an outpatient.
  - Visible blood requires hospitalization and inpatient evaluation.
  - Persistent bleeding or rebleed with hemodynamic instability necessitates ICU admission.
  - Massive bleeding is defined as loss of 30% or more of estimated blood volume or bleeding requiring blood transfusion of 6 or more units/24 h.
- Hemodynamic assessment (see Table 36-1):
  - Blood pressure, pulse, postural changes, and assessment of peripheral perfusion.
- The presence of comorbid disease must be determined, especially CAD and cardiac failure.
- Estimating blood loss. This can be estimated by measuring the return from an NG tube.
- An approximate estimate of blood loss can also be made by the hemodynamic response to a 2-L crystalloid fluid challenge:
  - If BP returns to normal and stabilizes, blood loss of 15–30% has occurred.
  - If BP rises but falls again, blood volume loses of 30–40% has occurred.
  - If BP continues to fall, blood volume loss of >40% has probably occurred.
- History and examination: Attempt to localize most likely source of bleeding:

P.E. Marik, *Handbook of Evidence-Based Critical Care*,
DOI 10.1007/978-1-4419-5923-2_36,
© Springer Science+Business Media, LLC 2010

Table 36-1. Correlation between physical signs and severity of UGIB.

Physical Sign	Mild	Moderate	Severe
Blood loss	<1 l	1–2 l	>2 l
Blood pressure	Normal	N-borderline low	Hypotensive
Orthostasis	No	Possible	Likely
Tachycardia	None–mild	Moderate	Severe
Skin	Warm, perfused	Diaphoretic	Cool, clammy
Urine output	Normal	Diminished	Poor
Sensorium	Alert/anxious	Anxious	Confused/drowsy

- Use of NSAID, alcohol, anti-platelet drugs, and anti-coagulants.
- History of GERD, chronic epigastric pain, renal failure, weight loss, vomiting before bleeding, etc.
- Previous history of bleeding
- The presence of melena indicates upper GI bleeding.
- Hematemesis indicates upper GI bleeding.
- When small amounts of bright red blood are passed per rectum, the lower GI tract can be assumed to be the source.
- In patients with large-volume maroon stools, NG tube aspiration should be performed to exclude upper GI hemorrhage. It should be noted that in about 15% of patients with upper gastrointestinal bleeding, NG aspirate will fail to obtain blood or "coffee ground" material.

- Nasogastric aspiration with saline lavage is beneficial to detect the presence of intragastric blood, to determine the type of gross bleeding, to clear the gastric field for endoscopic visualization, and to prevent aspiration of gastric contents. NG tube placement is essential to monitor ongoing bleeding and to decompress the stomach.
- Concerns that placement of a nasogastric tube may induce bleeding in patients with coagulopathies are outweighed by the benefits of the information obtained.
- Laboratory tests:
    - Serum chemistries (incl. BUN and creatinine), CBC, coagulation profile (PT, PTT, INR), liver function tests.
    - Cardiac enzymes (troponins) and ECG.

■ INITIAL RESUSCITATION

- Establish two large bore IV lines or a large bore central line.
- Insert NG tube and aspiration (by hand).

- Volume expansion with crystalloids (LR preferred, see Chapter 8).
- Monitor BP, pulse, and urine output.
- Cross match blood. Blood products are the most efficient volume expanders and should be infused as soon as possible in patients with significant bleeds. Transfusion requirements are determined by multiple factors, including patient age, presence of comorbidities, cardiovascular status, baseline hematocrit, and tempo of the bleeding, along with the current hematocrit level. RBCs are transfused in patients who have significant blood loss, continuing active bleeding, and those who manifest cardiac, renal, or cerebral ischemia (regardless of HCT). The rate of blood transfusion is determined by the severity of the hypovolemia, by the tempo of the bleeding, and by the presence of cardiac, renal, or cerebrovascular comorbidities. Generally RBSs should be transfused to maintain a hemoglobin concentration between 8 and 10 g/dl (see Chapter 51):
  - It is important to note that it takes up to 72 h for the hematocrit to reach its nadir after a single episode of bleeding (assuming no other intervention). Therefore, a normal hemoglobin (on admission) does not exclude significant bleeding. Blood transfusion should not be withheld from actively bleeding patients, based on their hemoglobin/hematocrit. Conversely a falling hematocrit does not imply continued bleeding but rather may represent equilibration of fluid between the intravascular and the extracellular extravascular compartment.
  - Patients who have variceal bleeding should be transfused to a hematocrit of 25–27 (Hb 8–9 g/dl) to avoid exacerbating the bleeding by increasing the portal pressure. In a small RCT, 25 cirrhotic patients who were transfused aggressively with transfusion of at least 2 units of PRBs had a significantly higher risk for rebleeding than did 25 similar cirrhotic patients who were transfused conservatively with transfusion only for shock or a hemoglobin <8.[1]
- In patients with active bleeding, fresh frozen plasma should be given if the INR >1.4. Platelet transfusion is indicated if the platelet count is <50,000/mm^3. In addition, FFP should be given after 6 units of RBCs and platelets after 10 units (see Chapters 52 and 53).
- Airway protection. The risk of aspiration is especially high in patients with massive bleeding or those who have an altered mental status. Endotracheal intubation is recommended in these patients. In addition, endotracheal intubation facilitates endoscopy. It may be advisable to place an NG tube prior to intubation in an attempt to empty the stomach and reduce the risk of aspiration during endotracheal intubation.
- In patients with severe upper GI bleeding and clinical evidence or a history of advanced liver disease, or a history of previous

variceal bleeding, an octreotide infusion should be commenced prior to endoscopy (see treatment of variceal hemorrhage below)

- In patients with presumed UGIB, proton pump inhibitor (PPI) therapy is recommended before EGD. The rationale for PPI therapy is that the most common causes of UGIB, including ulcers, gastritis, duodenitis, and hemorrhagic reflux esophagitis, are medically treated with acid-suppressive therapy. PPI therapy is also useful, however, for hemostasis of lesions that are not caused by acid and are not in other circumstances treated by PPI therapy, probably because neutralization of intraluminal gastric acid promotes hemostasis by stabilizing blood clots. Experimental data have shown that gastric acid impairs clot formation, promotes platelet disaggregation, and favors fibrinolysis.
- Intravenous erythromycin (70–100 mg), through its effect as a motilin receptor agonist, has been shown to promote gastric motility and substantially improve visualization of the gastric mucosa on initial endoscopy.
- All patients who have acute GIB require gastroenterology consultation.
- Surgical consultation is recommended for patients who have ongoing active bleeding, massive bleeding, recurrent bleeding, bleeding associated with significant abdominal pain, acute lower gastrointestinal bleeding, and abdominal findings suggestive of an acute abdomen.

■ TRIAGE OF PATIENTS: WHO TO ADMIT TO THE ICU?

At the time of triage the following criteria can stratify patients into a high-risk group (high risk of rebleeding, requiring surgery, and dying):

- A systolic blood pressure of <100 mmHg on admission;
- Severe comorbid disease;
- Evidence of active, ongoing GI hemorrhage at the time of triage;
- INR >1.4.

The rate of rebleeding is approximately 3% in the low-risk group as compared to 25% in the high-risk group. Patients in the low-risk group do not require admission to an ICU and can be adequately managed on a general medical floor.

■ UPPER GI BLEEDING (UGIB)

Upper gastrointestinal bleeding (UGIB) is a common, potentially life-threatening condition responsible for more than 300,000 hospital admissions and about 30,000 deaths per annum in the United States. Accurate patient evaluation and appropriate early management before esophagogastroduodenoscopy (EGD) are critical to decrease the morbidity and mortality.[2]

UGIB is defined as bleeding proximal to the ligament of Treitz to differentiate it from lower gastrointestinal bleeding involving the colon and middle gastrointestinal bleeding involving the small intestine distal to the ligament of Treitz. It has a mortality of 7–10%.[2] The mortality has decreased only minimally during the last 30 years despite the introduction of endoscopic therapy that reduces the rate of rebleeding. This observation has been attributed to the increasing percentage of UGIB occurring in the elderly who have a much worse prognosis than other patients because of their frequent use of anti-platelet medications or anti-coagulants and their frequent comorbid conditions.

The major causes of UGIB include the following:

- Peptic ulcer disease
- Esophageal and gastric varices
- Hemorrhagic gastritis
- Esophagitis
- Mallory–Weiss tear
- Upper GI malignancy
- Dieulafoy lesion

Helicobacter pylori and the use of NSAIDs are the predominant cause of PUD in the United States accounting for approximately 50 and 25% of cases, respectively.[3]

■ FURTHER MANAGEMENT OF UPPER GI BLEEDING

Early upper gastrointestinal endoscopy is the cornerstone of management of upper gastrointestinal bleeding. Endoscopy within 12–24 h of presentation is generally recommended. EGD is the prime diagnostic and therapeutic tool for UGIB.[4]

Early endoscopy serves three vital roles:

- Diagnosis:
  - It accurately delineates the bleeding site and determines the specific cause. EGD is 90–95% diagnostic for acute UGIB.

- Treatment:
  - *Non-variceal bleeding*. Endoscopic therapy has been shown to improve outcomes in patients with non-variceal bleeding. The endoscopic methods of controlling bleeding include thermal coagulation of a bleeding vessel, injection of a bleeding site with epinephrine or a sclerosing agent, and laser therapy to produce tissue coagulation. Endoscopic therapy has been shown to be of benefit to patients with actively bleeding lesions or lesions that have a protuberance in the ulcer crater (i.e., a visible vessel) seen on endoscopy. The rate of rebleeding in patients with active bleeding or non-bleeding visible vessel is reduced by about 50% with endoscopic therapy.[5] However, in about 20% of such patients, bleeding recurs.
  - *Variceal bleeding*. Endoscopic sclerotherapy and/or band ligation is the method of choice in controlling active variceal hemorrhage.
- Risk stratification:
  - Establishing an endoscopic diagnosis of the lesion and associated stigmata greatly enhances the ability to predict outcomes (i.e., the risk of rebleeding).
  - The endoscopic appearance of a bleeding ulcer can be used to predict the likelihood of recurrent bleeding on the basis of the Forrest classification, which ranges from IA to III. High-risk lesions include those characterized by active spurting of blood (grade IA) or oozing blood (grade IB), a non-bleeding visible vessel described as a pigmented protuberance (grade IIA), and an adherent clot (grade IIB). Low-risk lesions include flat, pigmented spots (grade IIC), and clean-base ulcers (grade III).[5]

■ FURTHER MANAGEMENT OF BLEEDING PEPTIC ULCERS

- A meta-analyses showed that the use of PPIs significantly decreased the risk of ulcer rebleeding (odds ratio 0.40; 95% CI 0.24–0.67), the need for urgent surgery (odds ratio 0.50; 95% CI 0.33–0.76), and the risk of death (odds ratio 0.53; 95% CI 0.31–0.91).[6]
- A pooled analysis of 16 RCTs that enrolled more than 3,800 patients suggested that an intravenous bolus loading followed by a continuous infusion of a PPI is more effective than bolus dosing alone in decreasing the rates of rebleeding and the need for surgery.[7] Based on these data, an intravenous bolus followed by a continuous infusion of a PPI for 72 h after endoscopic hemostasis is recommended.

- Planned, second-look endoscopy that is performed within 24 h after initial endoscopic therapy is not recommended.[5]
- For most patients with evidence of persistent ulcer bleeding or rebleeding, a second attempt at endoscopic hemostasis is often effective, may result in fewer complications than surgery, and is the recommended management approach.[4,8]
- Angiography with transcatheter embolization provides a non-operative option for patients in whom a site of acute bleeding has not been identified or controlled by endoscopy. Transcatheter embolization has been shown to significantly reduce mortality in patients with UGIB, although uncommon complications include bowel ischemia, secondary duodenal stenosis, and gastric, hepatic, and splenic infarction. In most institutions, radiological intervention is reserved for patients in whom endoscopic therapy has failed, especially if such patients are high-risk surgical candidates.
- Patients should be tested and treated for *H. pylori* infection.
- Evaluation for any ongoing need for a non-steroidal anti-inflammatory or anti-platelet agent and, if such treatment is indicated, appropriate coadministration of a gastroprotective agent are important.

■ FURTHER MANAGEMENT OF ESOPHAGEAL VARICES

- In patients with variceal hemorrhage, there remains a 40% chance of recurrent variceal bleeding within 72 h and a 60% chance within 10 days if no additional treatment is pursued.
- Octreotide 50 μg bolus followed by an infusion of at a rate of 50 μg/h has been demonstrated to reduce the risk of early rebleeding.
- Endoscopic banding in combination with an octreotide infusion is more effective than endoscopic therapy alone for controlling bleeding and reducing the incidence of rebleeding.
- There is a close association between infection and variceal bleeding (see Chapter 33). A complete microbiological workup, including blood cultures and diagnostic paracentesis, when appropriate should be performed. Furthermore, antibiotic prophylaxis has been demonstrated to reduce the risk of infections in patients with variceal bleeding and to improve short-term survival.[9] Prophylaxis with a third-generation cephalosporin, quinolone, or amoxicillin–clavulanic acid is recommended.
- Paracentesis significantly decreases variceal pressure and tension.[10] This suggests that ascites removal can be useful in the treatment of variceal bleeding in cirrhotic patients.

- There is a small chance that placement of a feeding tube/NG tube after variceal banding may dislodge the bands and or cause bleeding. This should therefore be delayed for 48–72 h.
- Balloon tamponade with a Minnesota or Sengstaken–Blakemore tube can be lifesaving in the presence of severe ongoing bleeding when carried out by experienced staff. However, placement by inexperienced staff is associated with an increased risk of death largely due to esophageal perforation and pulmonary aspiration.
- TIPPS (transjugular intrahepatic portosystemic shunt) is a radiological intervention that creates a portosystemic tract through the liver parenchyma, through which an 8–12-mm expandable metal stent is inserted. TIPPS has become the treatment of choice as rescue therapy in the 10–20% of patients with variceal hemorrhage unresponsive to endoscopic management. TIPPS has largely replaced emergency surgical shunting. The main limitations of TIPPS are the development of encephalopathy in about 20% of patients and progressive development of shunt insufficiency (thrombosis).
- Gastric varices are the source of bleeding in 10–36% of patients with variceal hemorrhage. Unless the gastric varices are located on the proximal lesser curve, they are not amenable to endoscopic ligation and for this reason, early TIPPS is generally recommended.
- Non-selective β-blockers (nadolol or propranolol) reduce the risk of rebleeding. A combination of endoscopic treatment together with β-blockers reduces overall and variceal rebleeding more than either therapy alone.[11]
- The role of TIPPS in preventing recurrent bleeding is unclear with studies showing discordant results with no clear survival benefit.

■ MANAGEMENT OF PATIENTS WITH LOWER GI BLEEDING

Angiodysplasia and diverticular disease of the right colon account for the vast majority of episodes of acute lower GI bleeding. The spontaneous remission rate, even with massive bleeding, is approximately 80%. In patients with ongoing lower GI bleeding, a radionuclide bleeding scan is indicated. There are two types of bleeding scan. The first is a technetium-labeled sulfur colloid scan, which although very sensitive can only detect bleeding that occurs during the 1–2 h following injection of the isotope. Alternatively, a technetium-labeled ("tagged") red blood cell bleeding scan can detect bleeding sites for up to 24 h after the cessation of bleeding. If the result of either type of bleeding scan is positive, angiography should then be performed.

Selective mesenteric angiography detects arterial bleeding that occurs at a rate of 0.5 ml/min or faster. It can be both diagnostic and therapeutic. When active bleeding is seen selective, arterial infusion of vasopressin arrests the hemorrhage in 90% of patients; adding sterile, absorbable gelatin powder further increases the efficacy of vasopressin. If bleeding continues and no source has been found, surgical intervention is warranted. Surgical intervention is also recommended in patients with recurrent diverticular bleeding.

■ REFERENCES

1. Blair SD, Janvrin SB, McCollum CN, et al. Effect of early blood transfusion on gastrointestinal haemorrhage. *Br J Surg*. 1986;73:783–785.
2. Cappell MS, Friedel D. Initial management of acute upper gastrointestinal bleeding: from initial evaluation up to gastrointestinal endoscopy. *Med Clin North Am*. 2008;92:491–509.
3. Kurata JH, Nogawa AN. Meta-analysis of risk factors for peptic ulcer. Nonsteroidal antiinflammatory drugs, *Helicobacter pylori*, and smoking. *J Clin Gastroenterol*. 1997;24:2–17.
4. Barkun A, Sabbah S, Enns R, et al. The Canadian Registry on Nonvariceal Upper Gastrointestinal Bleeding and Endoscopy (RUGBE): endoscopic hemostasis and proton pump inhibition are associated with improved outcomes in a real-life setting. *Am J Gastroenterol*. 2004;99:1238–1246.
5. Gralnek IM, Barkun AN, Bardou M. Management of acute bleeding from a peptic ulcer. *N Engl J Med*. 2008;359:928–937.
6. Bardou M, Toubouti Y, Benhaberou-Brun D, et al. Meta-analysis: proton-pump inhibition in high-risk patients with acute peptic ulcer bleeding. *Aliment Pharmacol Ther*. 2005;21:677–686.
7. Morgan D. Intravenous proton pump inhibitors in the critical care setting. *Crit Care Med*. 2002;30:S369–S372.
8. Lau JY, Sung JJ, Lam YH, et al. Endoscopic retreatment compared with surgery in patients with recurrent bleeding after initial endoscopic control of bleeding ulcers. *N Engl J Med*. 1999;340:751–756.
9. Soares-Weiser K, Brezis M, Tur-Kaspa R, et al. Antibiotic prophylaxis of bacterial infections in cirrhotic inpatients: a meta-analysis of randomized controlled trials. *Scand J Gastroenterol*. 2003;38:193–200.
10. Kravetz D, Romero G, Argonz J, et al. Total volume paracentesis decreases variceal pressure, size, and variceal wall tension in cirrhotic patients. *Hepatology*. 1997;25:59–62.
11. Gonzalez R, Zamora J, Gomez-Camarero J, et al. Meta-analysis: combination endoscopic and drug therapy to prevent variceal rebleeding in cirrhosis. *Ann Intern Med*. 2008;149:109–122.

37

Pancreatitis

Acute pancreatitis is a common disease that causes significant morbidity and mortality. More than 300,000 patients are admitted per year for pancreatitis and about 20,000 patients die from this disease per year in the United States.[1] In developed countries, obstruction of the common bile duct by stones (38%) and alcohol abuse (36%) are the most frequent causes of acute pancreatitis. Gallstone-induced pancreatitis is caused by duct obstruction of gallstone migration. Obstruction is localized in the bile duct, the pancreatic duct, or both. Other well-established causes of acute pancreatitis include the following:

- Hypertriglyceridemia
- Post-ERCP
- Drug induced
- Autoimmune
- Genetic
- Abdominal trauma
- Postoperative
- Ischemia
- Infections
- Hypercalcemia and hyperparathyroidism
- Posterior penetrating ulcer
- Scorpion venom

Abdominal pain is the cardinal symptom. It occurs in about 95% of cases. Typically it is generalized to the upper abdomen, but it may be more localized to the right upper quadrant, epigastric area, or, occasionally, left upper quadrant. The pain typically occurs acutely, without a prodrome, and rapidly reaches maximum intensity. It tends to be moderate to severe in intensity and tends to last for several days. The pain typically is boring and deep because of the retroperitoneal location of the pancreas. About 90% of patients have nausea and vomiting, which can be

P.E. Marik, *Handbook of Evidence-Based Critical Care*,
DOI 10.1007/978-1-4419-5923-2_37,
© Springer Science+Business Media, LLC 2010

severe and unremitting. The severity of the physical findings depends on the severity of the attack. Mild disease presents with only mild abdominal tenderness. Severe disease presents with severe abdominal tenderness and guarding, generally localized to the upper abdomen. Rebound tenderness is unusual.

■ DIAGNOSIS

- Leukocytosis is common because of a systemic inflammatory response.
- Mild hyperglycemia is common because of decreased insulin secretion and increased glucagon levels.
- The serum lipase level is the primary diagnostic marker for acute pancreatitis because of its high sensitivity and specificity. Serum lipase is more than 90% sensitive for acute pancreatitis.[2] The serum lipase level rises early in pancreatitis and remains elevated for several days.
- Serum amylase concentrations exceeding three times the normal upper limit support the diagnosis of acute pancreatitis. However, the serum amylase is within the normal range on admission in up to 20% of the patients.
- In a meta-analysis, a serum ALT level higher than 150 IU/l had a positive predictive value of 95% in diagnosing acute gallstone pancreatitis.[3]
- Any patient who has unexplained, severe abdominal pain should undergo supine and upright chest and abdominal radiographs. Abdominal radiographs are performed mainly to exclude alternative abdominal diseases, such as gastrointestinal perforation.
- Abdominal ultrasonography is the primary imaging study for abdominal pain associated with jaundice and for excluding gallstones as the cause of acute pancreatitis. It has the advantages of low cost, ready availability, and easy portability for bedside application in very sick patients. It is thus ubiquitous in the evaluation of pancreatitis. When adequately visualized, an inflamed pancreas is recognized as hypoechoic and enlarged because of parenchymal edema. The pancreas is visualized inadequately in 30% of cases.
- Patients who present with severe pancreatitis or who present initially with mild-to-moderate pancreatitis that does not improve after several days of supportive therapy should undergo abdominal CT imaging. A CT scan *with contrast* is now standard for the diagnosis and workup of suspected severe pancreatitis. Patients should receive both intravenous and oral contrast. Intravenous contrast is, however, contraindicated in the presence of renal insufficiency.

Furthermore, patients must be "fully" volume resuscitated prior to receiving contrast:

- Improvements in the contrast bolus techniques allow one to image the perfusion of the pancreatic parenchyma with accuracy. Areas of necrosis with diminished or no enhancement upon contrast bolus are detected with an accuracy of 87% (see CT grading system below).
- Except in cases of initial diagnostic uncertainty, it is advisable to wait for 1–2 days to obtain the initial scan. Before this point, pancreatic necrosis may not be apparent, and in addition, the delay allows the patient to receive initial aggressive fluid resuscitation, thus reducing the risk of contrast-induced nephropathy.

■ RISK STRATIFICATION

Most episodes of acute pancreatitis are mild and self-limiting, needing only brief hospitalization. However, 20% of patients develop severe disease with local and extrapancreatic complications characterized by early development and persistence of hypovolemia and multiple organ dysfunction. Risk stratification plays a key role in the management of patients with acute pancreatitis. Although amylase and lipase remain the standard for diagnosis, they are poor predictors of severity. A number of scoring systems have been developed to assess the severity of pancreatitis. The Ranson criteria is the first scoring system to be developed and remains commonly employed today. More recently, the APACHE II scoring system and the Imrie score have been used to predict severity. The Balthazar computed tomography grading system is widely used in patients who have undergone CT scanning. Severe acute pancreatitis as defined by the Atlanta Symposium includes a Ranson score ≥3, APACHE II score ≥8, organ failure, and/or local complications (necrosis, abscess, or pseudocyst).[4]

Ranson's Criteria

- At presentation
  - Age older than 55 years
  - Blood glucose level greater than 200 mg/dl
  - White blood cell count greater than 16,000/mm³
  - Lactate dehydrogenase level greater than 350 IU/l
  - Alanine aminotransferase level greater than 250 U/l
- Forty-eight hours after presentation
  - Hematocrit 10% decrease
  - Serum calcium less than 8 mg/dl
  - Base deficit greater than 4 mEq/l

- Blood urea nitrogen increase greater than 5 mg/dl
- Fluid sequestration greater than 6 l
- PaO$_2$ less than 60 mmHg

Glasgow (Imrie) Severity Scoring System

- Age >55 years
- White cell count >15 × 10^9/l
- PaO$_2$ <60 mmHg
- Serum lactate dehydrogenase >600 units/l
- Serum aspartate aminotransferase >200 units/l
- Serum albumin <3.2 g/dl
- Serum calcium <8.2 mg/dl
- Serum glucose >180 mg/dl
- Serum BUN >45 mg/dl

Balthazar CT Grading System

- A: Normal
- B: Gland enlargement, small intrapancreatic fluid collections
- C: Peripancreatic inflammation, >30% pancreatic necrosis
- D: Single extrahepatic fluid collection, 30–50% pancreatic necrosis
- E: Extensive extrapancreatic fluid collections, >50% pancreatic necrosis

■ COMPLICATIONS

- Renal dysfunction/failure.
- Pulmonary complications:
  - ARDS.
  - Pleural effusion.
  - Atelectasis.
  - Pneumonia.
- Abdominal:
  - Pancreatic necrosis is the most severe local complication because it is frequently associated with pancreatic infection. Infection of pancreatic necrosis develops during the second or the third week in 40–70% of patients.
  - Pancreatic abscess consists of a circumscribed collection of pus that arises around a restricted area of pancreatic necrosis.
  - Pseudocyst is a collection of pancreatic fluid enclosed by a wall of granulation tissue that results from pancreatic duct leakage.
  - Intraperitoneal hemorrhage.
  - Splenic vein thrombosis (causing left-sided portal hypertension).
  - Obstructive jaundice.

- Other:
  - DIC/coagulopathy.
  - Upper GI bleeding.
  - Hypocalcemia.
  - Hyperglycemia.
  - Hypertriglyceridemia.

ALERT

Enteral nutrition is the "treatment of choice" in patients with pancreatitis.

■ MANAGEMENT

- In mild forms of disease, besides the etiological treatment (mostly for gallstone-induced pancreatitis), therapy is supportive and includes fluid resuscitation, analgesia, oxygen administration, and anti-emetics.
- Early fluid resuscitation to correct fluid losses in the third space and maintain an adequate intravascular volume is an important component of the management of patients with severe pancreatitis (see Chapter 8).
- Respiratory, cardiovascular, and renal function must be closely monitored.
- Morphine traditionally has been disfavored for acute pancreatitis because it increases the sphincter of Oddi pressure. Meperidine (50–100 mg every 4–6 h) has been the traditional opiate regimen of choice because it does not raise the sphincter pressure. Caution should be used with this agent as its active metabolite normeperidine accumulates with renal dysfunction and can cause seizures. Fentanyl is a useful alternative in this situation.
- Nasogastric tube aspiration traditionally was used to prevent pancreatic stimulation induced by gastric distension and acid secretion. Multiple clinical trials, however, have demonstrated no benefit from nasogastric aspiration (see feeding below).[5]
- Prophylactic antibiotics have previously been recommended to reduce the risk of pancreatic infection.[6] However, recent meta-analyses have failed to demonstrate a benefit from prophylactic antibiotics.[7,8] Recent guidelines issued by the American College of Gastroenterology do not recommend antibiotic prophylaxis to prevent pancreatic infection.[9]

- Peritoneal lavage to remove toxic necrotic compounds is no longer recommended for severe pancreatitis. In a meta-analysis of eight RCTs involving a total of 333 patients, peritoneal lavage did not reduce morbidity or mortality.[10]
- Adrenal insufficiency (CIRCI) has been reported to occur in up to 35% of patients with severe pancreatitis.[11] Cosyntropin stimulation test and treatment with hydrocortisones are recommended in those patients with adrenal insufficiency (see Chapter 40).
- To discriminate between sterile and infected pancreatic necrosis in patients who continue to deteriorate, ultrasound- or CT-guided fine-needle aspirations of pancreatic tissues should be performed. When infection is proven or in the presence of abscesses, targeted antibiotic therapy is warranted.
- Most patients with gallstone-induced pancreatitis present with mild disease and quickly recover after early resuscitation. ERCP is indicated for clearance of bile duct stones in patients with severe pancreatitis, in those with cholangitis, in those who are poor candidates for cholecystectomy, in those postcholecystectomy, and in those with strong evidence of persistent biliary obstruction.[9]
- Probiotics should be avoided in patients with pancreatitis (see Chapter 38).[12]
- Patients with acute pancreatitis have traditionally been treated with "bowel rest"; this included NG suction and NPO. Patients with mild pancreatitis were started on oral feeds once the pain had subsided, while patients with severe pancreatitis were treated with parenteral nutrition until the disease process resolved. There is, however, no scientific data to support this approach to the management of patients with acute pancreatitis. Both experimental and clinical data strongly support the concept that enteral nutrition started within 24 h of admission to hospital reduces complications (primarily pancreatic infection), length of hospital stay, and mortality in patients with acute pancreatitis.[13,14] Enteral nutrition should begin within 24 h after admission and following the initial period of volume resuscitation and control of nausea and pain. Patients with mild pancreatitis can take a low fatty diet by mouth, while patients with severe pancreatitis should receive enteral tube feeds. Clinical trials suggest that both gastric and jejunal tube feeding are well tolerated in patients with severe pancreatitis. However, post-pyloric feeding is generally recommended. While there are limited data as to the optimal type of tube feed, a semi-elemental formula with omega-3 fatty acids and soluble fiber is recommended (see Chapter 31). Parenteral nutrition is associated with increased complications and mortality and should be avoided in patients with acute pancreatitis.

- Nasojejunal enteral nutrition with prebiotic fiber supplementation has been demonstrated to improve hospital stay, duration of nutrition therapy, acute-phase response, and overall complications in patients with severe pancreatitis when compared to standard enteral nutrition.[15]

■ CLINICAL PEARLS

- Patients with pancreatitis should be risk stratified into a mild and severe group.
- Patients with severe pancreatitis require a dynamic CT scan to determine the presence of local complication, the extent of necrosis, and to guide pancreatic aspiration.
- Enteral nutrition is the treatment of choice for patients with pancreatitis.
- Prophylactic antibiotics are not recommended.

■ REFERENCES

1. Sandler RS, Everhart JE, Donowitz M, et al. The burden of selected digestive diseases in the United States. *Gastroenterology.* 2002;122:1500–1511.
2. Smith RC, Southwell-Keely J, Chesher D. Should serum pancreatic lipase replace serum amylase as a biomarker of acute pancreatitis? *ANZ J Surg.* 2005;75:399404.
3. Tenner S, Dubner H, Steinberg W. Predicting gallstone pancreatitis with laboratory parameters: a meta-analysis. *Am J Gastroenterol.* 1994;89:1863–1866.
4. Bollen TL, van Santvoort HC, Besselink MG, et al. The Atlanta classification of acute pancreatitis revisited. *Br J Surg.* 2008;95:6–21.
5. Sarr MG, Sanfey H, Cameron JL. Prospective, randomized trial of nasogastric suction in patients with acute pancreatitis. *Surgery.* 1986;100:500–504.
6. Golub R, Siddiqi F, Pohl D. Role of antibiotics in acute pancreatitis: a meta-analysis. *J Gastrointest Surg.* 1998;2:496–503.
7. Jafri NS, Mahid SS, Idstein SR, et al. Antibiotic prophylaxis is not protective in severe acute pancreatitis: a systematic review and meta-analysis. *Am J Surg.* 2009;197:806–813.
8. Mazaki T, Ishii Y, Takayama T. Meta-analysis of prophylactic antibiotic use in acute necrotizing pancreatitis. *Br J Surg.* 2006;93:674–684.
9. Banks PA, Freeman ML. Practice guidelines in acute pancreatitis. *Am J Gastroenterol.* 2006;101:2379–2400.

10. Platell C, Cooper D, Hall JC. A meta-analysis of peritoneal lavage for acute pancreatitis. *J Gastroenterol Hepatol.* 2001;16:689–693.
11. Peng YS, Wu CS, Chen YC, et al. Critical illness-related corticosteroid insufficiency in patients with severe acute biliary pancreatitis: a prospective study. *Crit Care.* 2009;13:R123.
12. Besselink MG, van Santvoort HC, Buskins E, et al. Probiotic prophylaxis in predicted severe acute pancreatitis: a randomised, double-blind, placebo-controlled trial. *Lancet.* 2008;371:651–659.
13. Marik PE. What is the best way to feed patients with pancreatitis? *Curr Opin Crit Care.* 2009;15:131–138.
14. Petrov MS, van Santvoort HC, Besselink MG, et al. Enteral nutrition and the risk of mortality and infectious complications in patients with severe acute pancreatitis: a meta-analysis of randomized trials. *Arch Surg.* 2008;143:1111–1117.
15. Karakan T, Ergun M, Dogan I, et al. Comparison of early enteral nutrition in severe acute pancreatitis with prebiotic fiber supplementation versus standard enteral solution: a prospective randomized double-blind study. *World J Gastroenterol.* 2007;13:2733–2737.

38

Diarrhea and Constipation

■ DIARRHEA

Diarrhea is a common problem in the ICU.[1] Diarrhea is best defined as ≥3 loose stools per day.[2,3] The incidence of diarrhea in the ICU varies widely according to the definition used.[1] However, approximately 20–30% of ICU patients will develop clinically relevant diarrhea.[4,5] In the ICU, diarrhea is best classified as infectious or non-infectious, based on the different therapeutic approaches. Multiple risk factors contribute to the causation of both infectious and non-infectious diarrhea.

The risk factors for "non-infectious" diarrhea include previous/concurrent antibiotic use, hypoalbuminemia, change in tube-feeding formula, high-volume tube feeds, intermittent bolus tube feeds (as compared to a continuous infusion), high osmolarity tube feeds, ICU/hospital LOS, previous starvation (NPO), and medications (containing sorbitol).[4–8] The use of third-generation cephalosporins has been strongly associated with both "non-infectious" diarrhea and *Clostridium difficile* colitis.[4,9–11]

Infectious Diarrhea

Clostridium difficile is the primary cause of infectious nosocomial diarrhea in developed countries (see Chapter 13). Risk factors include broad-spectrum antibiotics, acid-suppressive therapy, and direct/indirect contact with infected/colonized patients (see Chapter 32). *Clostridium difficile* must be excluded in all ICU patients who develop diarrhea; stool should be sent for culture and for *C. difficile* toxins (at least two

P.E. Marik, *Handbook of Evidence-Based Critical Care*,
DOI 10.1007/978-1-4419-5923-2_38,
© Springer Science+Business Media, LLC 2010

specimens). In addition, *Pseudomonas aeruginosa* has been reported to be a cause of outbreaks of diarrhea associated with the use of antibiotics in ICU patients.[4] Other enteric pathogens that can cause diarrhea include salmonella, *C. perfringens* type A, and *Staphylococcus aureus*.[9] Although *Candida* species have been considered culprit pathogens associated with infectious diarrhea, there is no convincing data to support this association.[12]

"Non-Infectious" Diarrhea

Antibiotic-Associated Diarrhea (AAD)

Bartlett defines AAD as diarrhea of unknown etiology that occurs in patients who are receiving antibiotics; in 10–20% of these cases, *C. difficile* infection is found.[9,10] The pathophysiological explanation for AAD is that antibiotics reduce the concentration of anaerobic bacteria normally present in the intestine; this decreases carbohydrate (dietary fiber) fermentation and causes an osmotic diarrhea (see below).[9]

Enteral Feeding-Associated Diarrhea

Enteral feeding is frequently "blamed" as the cause of diarrhea resulting in the interruption of tube feeds. However, many studies have found no association between the risk of nosocomial diarrhea and enteral tube feeds.[4,7] Interestingly, in a recent meta-analysis comparing the complications of parenteral and enteral nutrition, enteral feeding was not found to increase the risk of diarrhea.[13] Furthermore, many experimental and clinical studies have demonstrated that, in comparison with parenteral nutrition, enteral nutrition can actually reduce the incidence of diarrhea due to better preservation of the gastrointestinal mucosal structure and function.[1]

Energy-dense formulae have a high osmolality, resulting in significant fluid shifts into the stomach and the proximal small bowel. The resulting excessive intraluminal volume may accelerate small intestinal transit, resulting in a greater fluid load in the large bowel and subsequent diarrhea. In addition, high enteral feed volumes and bolus feeding increase the risk of diarrhea.[5]

Management of "Non-infectious" Diarrhea

- A continuous infusion of a low-osmolarity enteral formula is preferred. If patients develop diarrhea on one of these formulas, *do not stop* the feed, rather reduce the rate.

- Dietary fibers are carbohydrates that cannot be digested by endogenous digestive enzymes and undergo fermentation by the colonic bacteria. Short-chain fatty acids, products of carbohydrate fermentation in the colon, play an important role in salt and water absorption in the colon. Furthermore, short-chain fatty acids, such as butyrate, are an important fuel for colonocytes. Consequently, dietary fibers have been added to enteral nutrition formulas to normalize bowel function. Experimental studies have shown that enteral feeding with fiber results in better colonic mucosal trophicity and in a lower rate of bacterial translocation than does enteral feeding without fiber.[14] The clinical use of dietary fiber in patients receiving tube feed is controversial, with contradictory findings.[15–18] However, a recent meta-analysis which included hospitalized patients receiving enteral nutrition demonstrated that the incidence of diarrhea was reduced with fiber administration (OR 0.68, 95% CI 0.48–0.96).[19] This effect was attenuated when ICU patients were analyzed as a distinct group. Meta-regression showed a more pronounced effect when the baseline incidence of diarrhea was high:
  - Soluble fibers are a better substrate for colonic bacterial fermentation than are insoluble fiber. However, until recently, water-soluble fiber supplements were used rarely in enteral formulas because of their high viscosity.
  - Recently, new fiber-processing techniques have been used to produce highly water-soluble and low-viscosity dietary fibers for use in enteral formulas. A multi-fiber-enriched enteral formula and/or the enteral administration of a fiber mixture should be considered in patients with diarrhea.[19,20]
- The use of opioids including loperamide can induce a paralytic ileus. These drugs are best avoided. However, they can be considered as a "last resort" in patients in whom an infectious diarrhea has been excluded.

The Use of Probiotics and Prebiotics

- The gut flora is profoundly disturbed during critical illness and this can profoundly alter gut function. Ingestion of specific fiber-fermenting lactic acid bacteria (probiotics) and fermentable fiber (prebiotics) is known to reduce intestinal colonization with potentially pathogenic gram-negative bacteria, to reduce bacterial translocation, to reduce pro-inflammatory cytokine induction, and to upregulate immune function The use of probiotics and prebiotics is however controversial[21]:
  - Two meta-analyses demonstrated that probiotics significantly reduced the risk of AAD (RR 0.43, 95% CI 0.31, 0.58, $p<0.001$)

and were beneficial in patients with *C. difficile* colitis (RR 0.59, 95% CI 0.41, 0.85, $p = 0.005$).[22,23]

- The Dutch Acute Pancreatitis Study randomized 298 patients with severe pancreatitis to receive a probiotic preparation (containing multiple species of *Lactobacilli* and *Bifidobacterium*) or placebo administered enterally twice daily for 28 days.[24] There was no difference in the rate of infection complications between groups; however, the group of patients receiving the probiotic had a significantly higher incidence of multi-system organ failure and a higher mortality (16% vs. 6%, $p = 0.01$). Nine patients in the probiotic group developed non-occlusive mesenteric ischemia, while none of the patients in the placebo group developed this complication. The cause of the increased occurrence of bowel ischemia in the probiotic group is unclear.

- A meta-analysis which evaluated the use of probiotics alone in critically ill patients (10 studies) reported a reduction in infections but no effect on mortality, ICU, or hospital length of stay.[25] The author concluded that because of methodological bias it was not *clear that probiotics are beneficial (and they may even be harmful) in the critically ill patient group.*

- *Saccharomyces boulardii* (a live fungus) is frequently used in critically ill patients to treat diarrhea and is the only yeast probiotic that has been proved to be effective. *Saccharomyces fungemia* has been described in ICU patients being treated with this agent.[26]

• Due to the uncertainty on the benefits and risks associated with probiotics in critically ill patients, it is difficult to justify the use of these agents until we can obtain more conclusive data.

■ CONSTIPATION

Constipation has been defined as the lack of a bowel movement for three consecutive days. The reported incidence of constipation in ICU patients varies between 20 and 80%.[27,28] Risk of constipation is increased in critically ill patients due to immobility and inability to act or respond to the urge to defecate, which can result in abdominal distension, vomiting, restlessness, gut obstruction, and perforation. Activation of opioid receptors, particularly μ-receptors within the gastrointestinal tract, contributes to the pathophysiology of ileus with opioid use.

The ideal pharmacological regimen for the prophylaxis and treatment of constipation has yet to be determined for critically ill patients. Stool softeners are unlikely to be effective in the critically ill patient. Bulk laxatives such as psyllium, methylcellulose, and polycarbophil may not be an appropriate choice for critically ill patients who need immediate relief from constipation. Moreover, these laxatives must be administered with adequate amounts of fluid, which may not be possible in these patients. Bulk laxatives should be avoided in patients who require fluid restriction, are confined to bed, or have strictures or partial obstructions. The use of fiber-based laxatives may result in fecal impaction without adequate fluid intake and may further complicate existing fecal impaction. Two commonly used stimulant laxatives in the United States are senna and bisacodyl, which work by increasing intestinal motility and secretions. Onset of action is within hours, and the major adverse effect is abdominal cramps. Patanwala et al.[27] reported that the use of stimulant (senna and bisacodyl) or osmotic laxatives (lactulose) were effective in treating constipation in ICU patients.

■ CLINICAL PEARLS

- Do not stop tube feeds in patients who develop diarrhea; exclude *C. difficile* infection and look for reversible factors.
- Stimulant laxatives should be used in patients who fail to have a bowel movement for 2–3 days.

■ REFERENCES

1. Wiesen P, Van GA, Preiser JC. Diarrhoea in the critically ill. *Curr Opin Crit Care*. 2006;12:149–154.
2. Whelan K, Judd PA, Preedy VR, et al. Enteral feeding: the effect on faecal output, the faecal microflora and SCFA concentrations. *Proc Nutr Soc*. 2004;63:105–113.
3. Manatsathit S, Dupont HL, Farthing M, et al. Guideline for the management of acute diarrhea in adults. *J Gastroenterol Hepatol*. 2002;17(Suppl):S54–S71.
4. Marcon AP, Gamba MA, Vianna LA. Nosocomial diarrhea in the intensive care unit. *Braz J Infect Dis*. 2006;10:384–389.
5. Barrett JS, Shepherd SJ, Gibson PR. Strategies to manage gastrointestinal symptoms complicating enteral feeding. *JPEN*. 2009;33:21–26.
6. Shimoni Z, Averbuch Y, Shir E, et al. The addition of fiber and the use of continuous infusion decrease the incidence of diarrhea in elderly tube-fed patients in medical wards of a general regional hospital: a controlled clinical trial. *J Clin Gastroenterol*. 2007;41:901–905.
7. Edes TE, Walk BE, Austin JL. Diarrhea in tube-fed patients: feeding formula not necessarily the cause. *Am J Med*. 1990;88:91–93.
8. Smith CE, Marien L, Brogdon C, et al. Diarrhea associated with tube feeding in mechanically ventilated critically ill patients. *Nurs Res*. 1990;39:148–152.

9. Bartlett JG. Clinical practice. Antibiotic-associated diarrhea. *N Engl J Med.* 2002;346:334–339.
10. Wistrom J, Norrby SR, Myhre EB, et al. Frequency of antibiotic-associated diarrhoea in 2,462 antibiotic-treated hospitalized patients: a prospective study. *J Antimicrob Chemother.* 2001;47:43–50.
11. Schwaber MJ, Simhon A, Block C, et al. Factors associated with nosocomial diarrhea and *Clostridium difficile*-associated disease on the adult wards of an urban tertiary care hospital. *Eur J Clin Microbiol Infect Dis.* 2000;19:9–15.
12. Krause R, Reisinger EC. Candida and antibiotic-associated diarrhoea. *Clin Microbiol Infect.* 2005;11:1–2.
13. Gramlich L, Kichian K, Pinilla J, et al. Does enteral nutrition compared to parenteral nutrition result in better outcomes in critically ill adult patients? A systematic review of the literature. *Nutrition.* 2004;20: 843–848.
14. Nakamura T, Hasebe M, Yamakawa M, et al. Effect of dietary fiber on bowel mucosal integrity and bacterial translocation in burned rats. *J Nutr Sci Vitaminol.* 1997;43:445–454.
15. Dobb GJ, Towler SC. Diarrhoea during enteral feeding in the critically ill: a comparison of feeds with and without fibre. *Intensive Care Med.* 1990;16:252–255.
16. Yang G, Wu XT, Zhou Y, et al. Application of dietary fiber in clinical enteral nutrition: a meta-analysis of randomized controlled trials. *World J Gastroenterol.* 2005;11:3935–3938.
17. Rushdi TA, Pichard C, Khater YH. Control of diarrhea by fiber-enriched diet in ICU patients on enteral nutrition: a prospective randomized controlled trial. *Clin Nutr.* 2004;23:1344–1352.
18. Schultz AA, Ashby-Hughes B, Taylor R, et al. Effects of pectin on diarrhea in critically ill tube-fed patients receiving antibiotics. *Am J Crit Care.* 2000;9:403–411.
19. Elia M, Engfer MB, Green CJ, et al. Systematic review and meta-analysis: the clinical and physiological effects of fibre-containing enteral formulae. *Aliment Pharmacol Ther.* 2008;27:120–145.
20. Schneider SM, Girard-Pipau F, Anty R, et al. Effects of total enteral nutrition supplemented with a multi-fibre mix on faecal short-chain fatty acids and microbiota. *Clin Nutr.* 2006;25:82–90.
21. Morrow LE, Kollef MH. Probiotics in the intensive care unit: why controversies and confusion abound. *Crit Care.* 2008;12:160.
22. Sazawal S, Hiremath G, Dhingra U, et al. Efficacy of probiotics in prevention of acute diarrhoea: a meta-analysis of masked, randomised, placebo-controlled trials. *Lancet Infect Dis.* 2006;6:374–382.
23. McFarland LV. Meta-analysis of probiotics for the prevention of antibiotic associated diarrhea and the treatment of *Clostridium difficile* disease. *Am J Gastroenterol.* 2006;101:812–822.

24. Besselink MG, van Santvoort HC, Buskins E, et al. Probiotic prophy-
    laxis in predicted severe acute pancreatitis: a randomised, double-blind,
    placebo-controlled trial. *Lancet*. 2008;371:651–659.
25. Koretz RL. Probiotics, critical illness, and methodologic bias. *Nutr Clin
    Pract*. 2009;24:45–49.
26. Nikolaos L, Dimitrios V, Hellen M, et al. *Saccharomyces boulardii* fun-
    gaemia in an intensive care unit patient treated with caspofungin. *Crit
    Care*. 2008;12:414-(doi:10.1186/cc6843).
27. Patanwala AE, Abarca J, Huckleberry Y, et al. Pharmacologic man-
    agement of constipation in the critically ill patient. *Pharmacotherapy*.
    2006;26:896902.
28. Mostafa SM, Bhandari S, Ritchie G, et al. Constipation and its implica-
    tions in the critically ill patient. *Br J Anaesth*. 2003;91:815–819.

Part V

Metabolic

39

Stress Hyperglycemia and Glycemic Control

Stress hyperglycemia is common in critically ill and injured patients and is a component of the "fight-and-flight" response. Until recently, stress hyperglycemia was considered a beneficial adaptive response, with the raised blood glucose providing a ready source of fuel for the brain, skeletal muscle, heart, and other vital organs at a time of increased metabolic demand. However, retrospective studies in patients undergoing cardiac surgery suggested that perioperative hyperglycemia was associated with an increased risk of postoperative infections and increased mortality.[1–3] Furthermore, these studies suggested that control of blood glucose reduced these complications. Following the first *Leuven Intensive Insulin Therapy Trial* in 2001, "tight glucose control" became regarded as the standard of care in all ICU patients around the world.[4]

Prior to 2001, stress hyperglycemia was defined as a plasma glucose level above 180–200 mg/dl. However, following the *Leuven Intensive Insulin Therapy Trial*, the American College of Endocrinology, the American Diabetes Association, and other authorities suggested that stress hyperglycemia be considered in any critically ill patient with a blood glucose level in excess of 110 mg/dl.[5] In the *Leuven Intensive Insulin Therapy Trial*, 12% of patients had a baseline blood glucose level above 200 mg/dl on the day following ICU admission. However, 74.5% of patients had a baseline blood glucose level above 110 mg/dl, with 97.5% having a recorded blood glucose level above 110 mg/dl sometime during their ICU stay.[4]

P.E. Marik, *Handbook of Evidence-Based Critical Care*,
DOI 10.1007/978-1-4419-5923-2_39,
© Springer Science+Business Media, LLC 2010

■ RISK FACTORS OF HYPERGLYCEMIA

- Activation of the stress response
  - Hypotension
  - Hypoxia
  - Sepsis
  - Trauma
  - Surgery
  - Burns
  - Myocardial infarction, etc.
- Intravenous glucose (especially TPN)
- Glucocorticoids
- Exogenous catecholamines
- Enteral formula high in glucose (high glucose load)

■ PATHOPHYSIOLOGY

Activation of the stress response with the production of

- glucagon
- epinephrine
- cortisol
- growth hormone
- pro-inflammatory cytokines including
  - interleukin-1 (IL-1)
  - IL-6
  - tumor necrosis factor-α (TNF-α)

results in increased gluconeogenesis, glycogenolysis, and insulin resistance. Increased hepatic gluconeogenesis appears central to the pathogenesis of stress hypoglycemia.

Both acute and chronic hyperglycemia have been demonstrated to have adverse effects, most notably the following:

- Increases oxidative injury
- Potentiates the pro-inflammatory response
- Promotes clotting
- Causes abnormal vascular reactivity
- Impairs leukocyte and mononuclear cell immune responsiveness

■ DIAGNOSIS

Most ICUs in the world (and in the United States in particular) use bedside capillary blood glucose measurements to monitor blood glucose levels. However, multiple studies have shown that these devices are inaccurate and tend to overestimate "true" plasma glucose levels.[6,7] A number of factors may lead to inaccurate capillary blood glucose measurements, including

- poor peripheral perfusion (shock)
- peripheral edema
- use of vasopressors
- low hemoglobin
- single-channel "glucometers"
- poor technique

Using bedside capillary blood glucose measurements to manage insulin infusions is likely to lead to an unacceptably high rate of hypoglycemia. It is therefore suggested that arterial/venous rather than capillary blood be used for the bedside "measurement" of blood glucose and that these values be correlated with the blood glucose measured at the central laboratory (at least 12 hourly).

■ TREATMENT

In 2001, van den Berghe and coworkers[4] published a "landmark study" (the *Leuven Intensive Insulin Therapy Trial*) in which they demonstrated that tight glycemic control using intensive insulin therapy improved the outcome of critically ill surgical patients. Following this study, tight glycemic control was rapidly adopted as the standard of care for ICUs throughout the world and endorsed by the *Institute for Health Care Improvement* and other national organizations in the United States. In 2006, van den Berghe and colleagues[8] repeated this study design in medical ICU patients. Although failing to reproduce the improvement in survival in the entire set of patients, this study demonstrated a reduction in morbidity in the patients randomized to the tight glycemic group with a reduction in mortality in the subset of patients with an ICU stay of 3 days or more. Following this study, two multi-center randomized European studies were prematurely discontinued due to an alarmingly high rate of hypoglycemia in the "tight glycemic control" arm with no mortality benefit.[9,10] Two additional single-center randomized studies showed a trend toward a higher mortality in the "tight glycemic" arm.[11,12] Recently, "NICE-SUGAR," a large (6,022 patients) multi-center

RCT was published which was unable to confirm the findings of van den Berghe et al.[13] Indeed, this study demonstrated a 2.6% absolute increase in 90-day mortality in patients randomized to tight glucose control ($p = 0.02$). Summary data of these five studies (excluding the van den Berghe studies) demonstrate that intensive insulin therapy is associated with an increased risk of death (OR 0.89; 95% CI 0.81–0.99, $p = 0.04$). The most likely explanation for the disparate findings between the van den Berge studies and the subsequent studies lies with the high rate of use of parenteral nutrition (PN) in the van den Berghe studies (87%). This explanation is supported by both experimental and clinical studies which have demonstrated that excessive parenteral glucose may lead to severe hyperglycemia and that the parenteral glucose load may be an independent predictor of organ failure and death.

■ COMPLICATIONS

Tight glycemic control is associated with significant hazards. Severe hypoglycemia occurs in up to 18% of treated patients, with these patients being at an increased risk of death. Hypoglycemia is particularly hazardous in ICU patients who are frequently intubated and sedated and therefore unable to respond appropriately (masked hypoglycemia). Using cerebral microdialysis in patients following severe brain injury, Oddo and colleagues[14] demonstrated that tight glycemic control is associated with a greater risk of brain energy crisis and death. These data suggest that tight glycemic control may result in neuroglycopenia at the time of increased cerebral metabolic demand.

■ WHAT TO DO NOW!

The results of the NICE-SUGAR study as well as the additional four randomized controlled studies which have attempted to replicate the van den Berghe studies clearly demonstrate that tight glycemic control (70–110 mg/dl) has no role in the management of general ICU patients. However, the role of tight glycemic control in patients undergoing cardiac surgery remains unclear. In these patients, it is likely that both pre- and postoperative optimization of blood glucose may improve outcome; however, the optimal blood glucose target is unknown (probably between 100 and 140 mg/dl). In all other ICU patients, it appears reasonable to maintain the blood glucose concentration between 140 and 180 mg/dl. The optimal method of achieving this goal is unclear; however, a number of options are available, which are as follows:

- In the control arm of the NICE-SUGAR study, an insulin infusion was administered if the blood glucose level exceeded 180 mg/dl and insulin administration was reduced and then discontinued if the blood glucose level dropped below 144 mg/dl.
- In patients receiving enteral tube feeds, we suggest a 6-hourly, subcutaneous, regular insulin sliding scale when the blood glucose exceeds 160 mg/dl, followed by twice daily NPH/intermediate-acting insulin (together with the regular insulin sliding scale). We limit NPH to a maximum of 20 units 12 hourly. If this approach does not adequately control blood glucose (<200 mg/dl), we would then switch to an insulin infusion:
    - Although the use of "sliding scales" in hospitalized patients (who are eating) is considered "a relic from the past" (and reactive rather than proactive), this approach does have some utility in ICU patients who are receiving continuous tube feeds.[15] Although the absorption of subcutaneous insulin may be impaired in the critically ill, absorption may be adequate to control blood glucose.

ALERT

- Avoid long-acting insulins in the ICU (glargine, etc.).
- Avoid oral hypoglycemic agents in the ICU (these agents can be restarted on discharge from the ICU).

■ ADDITIONAL TREATMENT

General Measures

- Avoid TPN at all costs.
- Limit the amount of intravenous dextrose.
- Use a low-carbohydrate enteral formula.
- Avoid high-dose corticosteroids.

■ CLINICAL PEARLS

- Hypoglycemia is much worse than hyperglycemia in ICU patients.
- Tight glycemic control increases mortality in ICU patients:
    - The number needed to harm (NNH) is 38!!
- Insulin should be used only when the blood glucose exceeds 160–180 mg/dl.
- Limit the intravenous glucose load (i.e., *No* TPN).

■ REFERENCES

1. Furnary AP, Wu Y. Clinical effects of hyperglycemia in the cardiac surgery population: the Portland Diabetic Project. *Endoc Pract.* 2006;12(Suppl) 3:22–26.
2. Furnary AP, Wu Y. Eliminating the diabetic disadvantage: the Portland diabetic project. *Semin Thorac Cardiovasc Surg.* 2006;18:302–308.
3. Zerr KJ, Furnary AP, Grunkemeier GL, et al. Glucose control lowers the risk of wound infection in diabetics after open heart operations. *Ann Thorac Surg.* 1997;63:356–361.
4. van den Berghe G, Wouters P, Weekers F, et al. Intensive insulin therapy in critically ill patients. *N Engl J Med.* 2001;345:1359–1367.
5. Garber AJ, Moghissi ES, Bransome ED Jr, et al. American College of Endocrinology position statement on inpatient diabetes and metabolic control. *Endoc Pract.* 2004;10:77–82.
6. Critchell C, Savarese V, Callahan A, et al. Accuracy of bedside capillary blood glucose measurements in critically ill patients. *Intensive Care Med.* 2007;33:2079–2084.
7. Kanji S, Buffie J, Hutton B, et al. Reliability of point-of-care testing for glucose measurement in critically ill adults. *Crit Care Med.* 2005;33:2778–2785.
8. van den Berghe G, Wilmer A, Hermans G, et al. Intensive insulin therapy in the medical ICU. *N Engl J Med.* 2006;354:449–461.
9. Devos P, Preiser JC, Melot C. Impact of tight glucose control by intensive insulin therapy on ICU mortality and the rate of hypoglycaemia: final results of glucotrol [European society of Intensive Care Medicine 20th Annual Congress abstract 0735]. *Intensive Care Med.* 2007;33 (suppl 2):S189.
10. Brunkhorst FM, Engel C, Bloos F, et al. Intensive insulin therapy and pentastarch resuscitation in severe sepsis. *N Engl J Med.* 2008;358: 125–139.
11. De La Rosa GD, Donado JH, Restrepo AH, et al. Strict glycemic control in patients hospitalized in a mixed medical and surgical intensive care unit: a randomized clinical trial. *Crit Care.* 2008;12:R120.
12. Arabi Y, Dabbagh OC, Tamim HM, et al. Intensive versus conventional insulin therapy: A randomized controlled trial in medical and surgical critically ill patients. *Crit Care Med.* 2008;36:3190–3197.
13. Finfer S, Chittock DR, Su SY, et al. Intensive versus conventional glucose control in critically ill patients. The NICE-Sugar Study Investigators. *N Engl J Med.* 2009;360:1283–1297.
14. Oddo M, Schmidt M, Carrera E, et al. Impact of tight glycemic control on cerebral glucose metabolism after severe brain injury: a microdialysis study. *Crit Care Med.* 2008;36:33233–33238.
15. Umpierrez GE, Palacio A, Smiley D. Sliding scale insulin use: myth or insanity? *Am J Med.* 2007;120:563–567.

40

Adrenal Insufficiency and CIRCI

The stress system receives and integrates a diversity of cognitive, emotional, neurosensory, and peripheral somatic signals that are directed to the central nervous system through distinct pathways. The stress response is normally adaptive and time limited and improves the chances of the individual for survival. The stress response is mediated largely by activation of the hypothalamic–pituitary–adrenal (HPA) axis with the release of cortisol. In general, there is a graded cortisol response to the degree of stress, such as the type of surgery. Cortisol levels also correlate with the severity of injury, the Glasgow Coma Scale, and the APACHE score. Cortisol effects the transcription of thousands of genes in every cell of the body. In addition, the cortisol–glucocorticoid receptor complex effects cellular function by non-transcriptional mechanisms. Cortisol has several important physiological actions on metabolism, cardiovascular function, and the immune system. Cortisol increases the synthesis of catecholamines and catecholamine receptors, which are partially responsible for its positive inotropic effects. In addition, cortisol has potent anti-inflammatory actions including the reduction in number and function of various immune cells, such as T and B lymphocytes, monocytes, neutrophils, and eosinophils at sites of inflammation. Cortisol is the most important inhibitor of the transcription of pro-inflammatory mediators (inhibits NF-κB and AP-1 by multiple mechanisms).[1]

There is increasing evidence that in many critically ill patients, activation of the HPA axis and the release of cortisol are impaired. The reported incidence varies widely (0–77%) depending upon the population of patients studied and the diagnostic criteria used to diagnose adrenal insufficiency (AI).[2] However, the overall incidence of adrenal insufficiency in critically ill medical patients approximates 10–20%, with

P.E. Marik, *Handbook of Evidence-Based Critical Care*,
DOI 10.1007/978-1-4419-5923-2_40,
© Springer Science+Business Media, LLC 2010

an incidence as high as 60% in patients with septic shock.[2] The major sequela of adrenal insufficiency in the critically ill is on the systemic inflammatory response (excessive inflammation) and the cardiovascular function (hypotension).

Until recently, the exaggerated pro-inflammatory response that characterizes patients with systemic inflammation has focused on the suppression of the HPA axis and "adrenal failure." However, experimental and clinical data suggest that corticosteroid tissue resistance may also play an important role. This complex syndrome is referred to as "critical illness-related corticosteroid insufficiency (CIRCI)."[1,3] CIRCI is defined as inadequate cellular corticosteroid activity for the severity of the patient's illness, i.e. CIRCI may be due to acute adrenal insufficiency, corticosteroid tissue resistance, or both. The mechanisms leading to dysfunction of the HPA axis and tissue glucocorticoid resistance during critical illness are complex and poorly understood.[1] CIRCI manifests with insufficient corticosteroid-mediated downregulation of inflammatory transcription factors.

CIRCI is most common in patients with severe sepsis (septic shock) and patients with ARDS. In addition, patients with liver disease have a high incidence of AI (hepatoadrenal syndrome). CIRCI should also be considered in patients with pancreatitis. A subset of critically ill patients may suffer structural damage to the adrenal gland from either hemorrhage or infarction and this may result in long-term adrenal dysfunction. Furthermore, a number of drugs are associated with adrenal failure. However, most patients with AI (and CIRCI) develop reversible dysfunction of the HPA system; this is probably initiated by inflammatory mediators, may be self-perpetuating, and follows the same time course of the immune deregulation in patients with sepsis and SIRS.[1]

■ CAUSES OF ADRENAL INSUFFICIENCY/CIRCI

Reversible Dysfunction of HPA Axis

- Sepsis/SIRS
- Pancreatitis
- Drugs
  - Corticosteroids (secondary AI)
  - Ketoconazole (primary AI)
  - *Etomidate* (primary AI)
  - Megesterol acetate (secondary AI)
  - Rifampin (increased cortisol metabolism)
  - Phenytoin (increased cortisol metabolism)
  - Metyrapone (primary AI)
  - Mitotane (primary AI)
- Hypothermia

Primary Adrenal Insufficiency

- Autoimmune adrenalitis
- HIV infection
  - HART therapy
  - HIV virus
  - CMV
- Metastatic carcinoma
  - Lung
  - Breast
  - Kidney
- Systemic fungal infection
  - Histoplasmosis
  - Cryptococcus
  - Blastomycosis
- Tuberculosis
- Adrenal hemorrhage/infarction
  - DIC
  - Meningococcemia
  - Anti-coagulation
  - Anti-phospholipid syndrome
  - HIT
  - Trauma

Glucocorticoid Tissue Resistance

- Sepsis
- SIRS
  - ARDS
  - Trauma
  - Burns
  - Pancreatitis
  - Liver failure
  - Postcardiac surgery
  - HELLP syndrome (see Chapter 54)

■ CLINICAL FEATURES OF ADRENAL INSUFFICIENCY/CIRCI

Patients with chronic adrenal insufficiency (Addison's disease) usually present with the following:

- Weakness
- Weight loss

- Anorexia and lethargy
- Nausea, vomiting, and abdominal pain

Clinical signs include the following:

- Orthostatic hypotension
- Hyperpigmentation (primary adrenal insufficiency).

Laboratory testing may demonstrate the following:

- Hyponatremia
- Hyperkalemia
- Hypoglycemia
- Normocytic anemia

This presentation contrasts with the features of CIRCI. The clinical manifestations of CIRCI are consequent upon an exaggerated pro-inflammatory immune response and include the following:

- Hypotension refractory to fluids and requiring vasopressors is a common manifestation of CIRCI:
  - CIRCI should therefore be considered in all ICU patients requiring vasopressor support.
- An excessive systemic inflammatory response:
  - ALI/ARDS.
  - Trauma.
  - Burns.
  - Pancreatitis.
  - Liver failure.
  - Postcardiac surgery.
  - HELLP syndrome (see Chapter 54).

Laboratory assessment may demonstrate the following:

- Eosinophilia.
- Hypoglycemia.
- Hyponatremia and hyperkalemia are uncommon.

■ DIAGNOSIS OF ADRENAL INSUFFICIENCY/CIRCI

At the current time, there are no clinically useful tests to assess the cellular actions of cortisol; the accurate clinical diagnosis of CIRCI therefore remains somewhat elusive. Furthermore, while the diagnosis of AI in the critically ill is fraught with difficulties, at this time this diagnosis is best made by[1]

- a random (stress) cortisol of less than 10 μg/dl or
- a delta cortisol of less than 9 μg/dl after a 250 μg ACTH stimulation test.

From a mechanistic and practical standpoint, it may be useful to divide CIRCI into two subgroups[4]:

Type I: Characterized by a random (stress) cortisol <10 μg/dl
Type II: Characterized by a random cortisol ≥10 μg/dl and a delta cortisol less than 9 μg/dl

Type II CIRCI is typically associated with high levels of pro-inflammatory mediators (notably IL-6 and IL-10), high CRP levels, and high ACTH levels. These patients may have both ACTH and tissue glucocorticoid resistance.[4]

Type I CIRCI is associated with low levels of pro-inflammatory mediators and "normal" stress ACTH levels; these patients may have impaired cortisol production (adrenal insufficiency). Future studies should distinguish between these two subtypes, as this may have prognostic and therapeutic implications.

■ TREATMENT OF ADRENAL INSUFFICIENCY/CIRCI

Who to Treat with Steroids?

The use of stress doses of corticosteroids (200–300 mg hydrocortisone/day) in critically ill ICU patients is controversial with little consensus in the literature. Hopefully, ongoing clinical trial will help resolve this issue. However, corticosteroids should be considered in the treatment of patients with septic shock who have responded poorly to fluids and vasopressors (requiring >0.05–0.1 μg/kg/min of norepinephrine or equivalent) and patients with ARDS who show progressive disease after 48 h of supportive care. Adrenal testing is not required in these patients. Two recent meta-analyses support the use of low-dose (stress doses) corticosteroids in these patients with a very favorable risk/benefit profile.[5,6] Additional ICU patients who meet the diagnostic criteria for CIRCI (as defined above) *and* who have hemodynamic instability or evidence of an excessive inflammatory response should also be treated with corticosteroids (liver failure, pancreatitis, etc.). Corticosteroids have also proven beneficial in patients with the HELLP syndrome (see Chapter 54) and in preventing atrial fibrillation (and limiting SIRS) in patients undergoing cardiopulmonary bypass surgery.[1]

The suggested treatment approach is outlined below. Corticosteroids should never be stopped abruptly; this will lead to a "rebound" of inflammatory mediators with an increased likelihood of hypotension and/or rebound inflammation (lung injury). A continuous infusion of glucocorticoid may be associated with better (smoother) glycemic control.[7] Since blood glucose variability has been demonstrated to have prognostic implications,[8,9] a continuous infusion of a glucocorticoid may have additional benefits.

■ MEDICATION (DRUGS) FOR ADRENAL INSUFFICIENCY/CIRCI

- Hydrocortisone 50 mg IV q 6 h or a 100 mg bolus followed by a continuous infusion at 10 mg/hr for at least 7 days, and ideally for 10–14 days. Patients should be vasopressor and ventilator-"free" before taper.
- Hydrocortisone taper:
  – Hydrocortisone 50 mg IV q 8 h for 3–4 days.
  – Hydrocortisone 50 mg IV/PO q 12 h for 3–4 days.
  – Hydrocortisone 50 mg IV/p.o. daily for 3–4 days.
  – Reinstitution of full-dose hydrocortisone with recurrence of shock or worsening oxygenation.
- Hydrocortisone and methylprednisolone are considered interchangeable.
- Dexamethasone should be avoided; it lacks mineralocorticoid activity. Dexamethasone has a long half-life and suppresses the HPA axis; it should therefore *not* be used pending an ACTH stimulation test.

■ ADDITIONAL TREATMENT

General Measures

- Active infection surveillance is required in all patients receiving corticosteroids with a low threshold for performing blood cultures, mini-BAL, and other appropriate cultures.
- Blood glucose should be monitored closely and hyperglycemia managed by reducing the glycemic load and treating with insulin as appropriate.
- Clinicians should monitor CPKs and muscle strength and avoid neuromuscular blocking agents (at all costs).

■ CLINICAL PEARLS

- CIRCI is best defined as inadequate cellular corticosteroid activity for the severity of the patient's illness; this includes AI, glucocorticoid tissue resistance, or both.
- Consider treatment with corticosteroids in patients with septic shock, ARDS, and patients with hemodynamic instability as well as patients with pancreatitis, liver failure, and HELLP syndrome.
- Hydrocortisone in a dose of 200 mg daily (50 mg q 6 h or as a continuous infusion at 10 mg/h) is suggested.
- Monitor response to corticosteroids and taper the drug slowly.

■ REFERENCES

1. Marik PE. Critical illness related corticosteroid insufficiency. *Chest.* 2009;135:181–193.
2. Annane D, Maxime V, Ibrahim F, et al. Diagnosis of adrenal insufficiency in severe sepsis and septic shock. *Am J Respir Crit Care Med.* 2006;174:1319–1326.
3. Marik PE, Pastores SM, Annane D, et al. Recommendations for the diagnosis and management of corticosteroid insufficiency in critically ill adult patients: consensus statements from an international task force by the American College of Critical Care Medicine. *Crit Care Med.* 2008;36:1937–1949.
4. Kwon YS, Suh GY, Jeon K, et al. Cytokine levels and dysfunction in the hypothalamus–pituitary–adrenal axis in critically-ill patients. (in press).
5. Tang BM, Craig JC, Eslick GD, et al. Use of corticosteroids in acute lung injury and acute respiratory distress syndrome: a systematic review and meta-analysis. *Crit Care Med.* 2009;37:1595–1603.
6. Annane D, Bellissant E, Bollaert PE, et al. Corticosteroids in the treatment of severe sepsis and septic shock in adults: a systematic review. *JAMA.* 2009;301:2349–2361.
7. Loisa P, Parviainen I, Tenhunen J, et al. Effect of mode of hydrocortisone administration on glycemic control in patients with septic shock: a prospective randomized trial. *Crit Care.* 2007;11:R21 (doi:10.1186/cc5696).
8. Egi M, Bellomo R, Stachowski E, et al. Variability of blood glucose concentration and short-term mortality in critically ill patients. *Anesthesiol.* 2006;105:244–252.
9. Dossett LA, Cao H, Mowery NT, et al. Blood glucose variability is associated with mortality in the surgical intensive care unit. *Am Surg.* 2008;74:679–685.

41

Hypo- and Hypercalcemia

Calcium is a critical intracellular messenger and regulator of cell function. Calcium is essential for excitation–contraction coupling in muscle, neurotransmission, cell division, hormonal release, phagocytosis, chemotaxis, and numerous other activities. Although these functions are usually beneficial, calcium also regulates processes that can injure and kill cells such as digestive enzyme activation, cytokine release, free radical production, inhibition of ATP synthesis, and vasoconstriction. Thus, calcium is truly a double-edged sword.

Calcium circulates in the blood in three fractions:

- A protein-bound fraction (primarily albumin)
- A chelated fraction
- An ionized fraction

It is the ionized fraction that is physiologically active and homeostatically regulated. Most critically ill patients have low concentrations of albumin and will have low total calcium concentrations in the blood. However, the ionized calcium fraction may be elevated, normal, or decreased. Thus, it is important to assess circulating calcium concentrations by ionized calcium measurement.

Circulating concentrations of ionized calcium are primarily maintained within a narrow range by the combined actions of parathyroid hormone and vitamin D. These hormones increase gastrointestinal absorption of calcium, decrease urinary loss of calcium, and increase calcium mobilization from bone. It is important to realize that dietary calcium is not required to maintain normal circulating calcium concentrations,

P.E. Marik, *Handbook of Evidence-Based Critical Care*,
DOI 10.1007/978-1-4419-5923-2_41,
© Springer Science+Business Media, LLC 2010

because adequate calcium can be mobilized from bone. When interpreting concentrations of parathyroid hormone or calcitriol, it is important to consider the concentrations of ionized calcium. Normally, concentrations of these hormones should be high during hypocalcemia and decreased during hypercalcemia. Failure of parathyroid hormone to increase during ionized hypocalcemia suggests parathyroid gland suppression or insufficiency. On the other hand, elevated concentrations of parathyroid hormone in the context of ionized hypercalcemia suggest hyperparathyroidism. Normal ionized calcium concentrations in the context of elevated parathyroid hormone concentrations suggest that parathyroid hormone is appropriately compensating for some other factor that is lowering the ionized calcium concentration (such as a chelator).

■ HYPOCALCEMIA

Hypocalcemia is a common electrolyte abnormality in critically ill patients. Depending on the definition used and population studied, hypocalcemia is reported to occur in 12–88% of critically ill patients. Generally the incidence and the degree of hypocalcemia correlate with disease severity and mortality.[1]

Hypocalcemia is best defined as an ionized calcium <4.65 mg/dl (1.16 mmol/l). Ionized calcium should be measured to confirm hypocalcemia in patients with low total serum calcium. Measuring magnesium, creatinine, phosphate, vitamin D levels, amylase, lipase, and CPK will help determine the etiology of hypocalcemia. Serum intact PTH is the most valuable test as an inappropriately normal or low level in the face of hypocalcemia confirms hypoparathyroidism.

Decreased circulating concentrations of ionized calcium are common in critically ill patients with sepsis. Patients with pancreatitis, burns, and multiple trauma are also predisposed to ionized hypocalcemia. Hypocalcemia secondary to blood transfusion is usually transient and often not clinically significant unless >5 units of packed red blood cells are given.

The cause of ionized hypocalcemia in critically ill patients is frequently multi-factorial.[2,3] Many critically ill patients (especially those with infection) have suppressed or inappropriately low parathyroid hormone concentrations in the context of ionized hypocalcemia. Hypomagnesemia contributes to hypoparathyroidism in some of these patients. It has also been suggested that elevated intracellular calcium or magnesium concentrations during sepsis suppress the parathyroid glands. Elevated concentrations of intracellular divalent cations may occur despite decreased circulating concentrations of the ions. Another proposed mechanism for hypocalcemia is suppression of the parathyroid glands via the direct or the indirect effects of circulating mediators such as cytokines.

In addition, ionized hypocalcemia may result from the lack of activated vitamin D (calcitriol). Vitamin D deficiency is reported to be extremely common in critically ill patients.[4] In the study by Lee et al., hypovitaminosis D was associated with adverse outcomes independent of hypocalcaemia, however vitamin D supplementation was not protective. The cause of the hypovitaminosis D is postulated to be due to lack of exposure to sunlight as well as alterations in vitamin D and parathyroid metabolism.

Elevated concentrations of intracellular calcium have been linked to cell dysfunction and death during sepsis and ischemia.[5,6] It has been hypothesized that hypocalcemia may be a protective mechanism in critical illness. Thus, parathyroid gland suppression, secondary to the release of various inflammatory mediators, may have evolved to be protective during these states. If this premise is correct, one would hypothesize that administration of calcium would be detrimental during ischemia and sepsis. Indeed, this appears to be the case. Calcium administration increases cellular injury during ischemia. Calcium administration increases mortality in animals administered endotoxin as shown by Malcolm et al.[7] and after cecal ligation and puncture as shown by Zaloga et al.[8] It is noteworthy that in these studies although intravenous calcium increased blood pressure, mortality increased. Furthermore, calcium antagonists appear to be beneficial during sepsis. Experimental studies have demonstrated that verapamil, nifedipine, and diltiazem decrease the production of pro-inflammatory mediators, increase IL-10 (anti-inflammatory mediator), improve the hemodynamic profile, and reduce the mortality in lipopolysaccharide-induced septic shock.[9–13] Todd and Mollitt[5] demonstrated that sepsis increased RBC intracellular calcium and that this effect could be partly ameliorated by calcium channel blockade.

Should Hypocalcemia Be Corrected in Critically Ill Patients?

This is controversial as hypocalcemia may be an adaptive response to severe stress. Furthermore, there are inadequate data currently available to make strong recommendations with regard to treatment of this common electrolyte disorder in the critically ill.[14] Most recommendations are therefore based on expert opinion.[1,15,16] While hypocalcemia may decrease cardiac contractility[17] and while intravenous calcium chloride has been demonstrated to increase the blood pressure and cardiac function,[18] the effect of this intervention on patient outcome is unknown.[14] It is plausible that intravenous calcium has short-term beneficial hemodynamic effects which are outweighed by the longer term effects on immune and cell function. Consequently most experts suggest that symptomatic hypocalcemia (tetany, etc) warrants treatment; however, "asymptomatic" hypocalcemia should not be treated until the serum-ionized calcium is <3.2 mg/dl (0.8 mmol/l).[1,15,16]

ALERT

These data suggest that hypocalcemia may have a protective effect in acute critical illness. Treatment of hypocalcemia may be akin to treating stress hyperglycemia; it normalizes the numbers but increases mortality! *We should not mess with that which we do not understand.*

However, similar to stress hyperglycemia, treatment of hypocalcemia may be indicated when severe or in chronically critically ill patients.

Treatment

- Correct hypomagnesemia.
- Treat hyperphosphatemia.
- Intravenous calcium gluconate is indicated for acutely symptomatic patients and following an acute fall in serum calcium. One to two grams (90–180 mg of elemental calcium) is injected in 50 ml of 5% dextrose slowly over 10–20 min with EKG monitoring. Rapid injection may precipitate cardiac arrest in systole.
- Treatment with IV calcium is contraindicated in concomitant hyperphosphatemia for fear of precipitation of the calcium–phosphate product.
- As vitamin D has pleiotropic effects on immunity, endothelial and mucosal function, and glucose metabolism, replacement with 1,25-dihydroxyvitamin D may have a role in critically ill patients, particularly the chronically critically ill (see Chapter 7).

■ HYPERCALCEMIA

Hypercalcemia is defined as an increase in serum calcium >1 mg/ml above the normal range (8.5–10.2 mg/dl or 2.2–2.5 mmol/l):

- – Mild hypercalcemia 10.2–11.9 mg/dl
- – Moderate hypercalcemia 12–13.9 mg/dl
- – Severe hypercalcemia ≥14 mg/dl

The most common cause of asymptomatic hypercalcemia in an outpatient setting is primary hyperparathyroidism. The most common cause of inpatient hypercalcemia is malignancy.[19,20] Twenty to thirty percent of patients with cancer have hypercalcemia at some point in the course of their disease. Primary hyperparathyroidism can coexist with cancer in up to 15% of cases.

The most common cancers associated with hypercalcemia are the following:

- Breast
- Squamous-cell cancer (head and neck, esophagus, cervix, or lung)
- Renal
- Ovarian/endometrial
- HTLV-associated lymphoma
- Multiple myeloma
- Lymphoma

Malignancy-associated hypercalcemia results from any of four mechanisms:

- Local osteolytic hypercalcemia from increased osteoclastic resorption of bone surrounding malignant cells in the bone marrow
- Humoral hypercalcemia of malignancy (HHM) caused by secretion of parathyroid hormone-related protein (PTHrP) from the cancer cells
- Secretion of the active form of vitamin D
- Ectopic secretion of PTH which is very rare

In chronically critically ill patients, bone hyperabsorption is an important cause of hypercalcemia (see Chapter 7). Other less common causes include the following:

- Tertiary hyperparathyroidism – from autonomous parathyroid glands in end-stage renal disease
- Chronic granulomatous disease from increased production of active vitamin D
- Drug induced
  - Vitamin D intoxication
  - Lithium
  - Thiazide diuretics
  - Vitamin A toxicity
  - Theophylline
- Hyperthyroidism
- TPN

Hypercalcemia must be confirmed by ionized calcium measurements. Intact PTH levels help aid in the diagnosis, with high levels indicating primary hyperparathyroidism and low levels indicating other causes. Plasma 1,25-dihydroxyvitamin D levels may be useful in sarcoidosis or other granulomatous disorders.

An EKG may show shortened QTc from shortening of the myocardial action potential and there have been reports of ST segment elevation and arrhythmias though uncommon.

Treatment

- Rehydration and calciuresis:
  - Normal saline 200–500 ml/h.
  - Guided clinically by volume status and evidence of fluid overload and cardiovascular status.
  - Use of loop diuretics is controversial and should not be used until volume resuscitation is complete.
- Intravenous bisphosphonates:
  - Block osteoclastic bone resorption.
  - Superior to all other modes of treatment.
  - Pamidronate 60–90 mg IV over 2 h in 50–200 ml of saline or 5% dextrose in water.
  - Zoledronate 4 mg IV over 15 min in 50 ml saline or 5% dextrose in water.
  - Both drugs are associated with renal failure, flu-like symptoms, chills, and fever.
  - A response is noted in 2–4 days with the nadir in serum calcium occurring in 4–7 days.
  - Lasts for 1–3 weeks.

Second Line

- Glucocorticoids:
  - In lymphomas with elevated levels of active vitamin D.
  - Prednisone (60 mg) for 10 days.
- Calcitonin:
  - Maximal response occurs in 12–24 h.
  - Reductions in serum calcium are small and transient (1 mg/dl).
  - Can cause flushing and nausea.
- Mithramycin:
  - Effective but limited by adverse effects like thrombocytopenia, anemia, leucopenia, hepatitis, and renal failure.
- Gallium nitrate:
  - Body surface area (100–200 mg/m^2) given IV continuously over 24 h for 5 days.
  - Can cause renal failure.

Additional Therapies

- Hemodialysis:
  - In patients with acute or chronic renal failure who cannot be hydrated safely and in whom bisphosphonates may not be safe.
  - The dialysate contains little or no calcium.
  - Especially when the GFR is <10–20 ml/min.
- New therapies:
  - Receptor activator of nuclear factor-κB ligand (RANKL) is involved in osteoclast-mediated bone resorption in cancer.
  - Osteoprotegerin and antibodies against RANKL and PTHrP.

■ CLINICAL PEARLS

- Hypocalcemia should not be treated unless the serum-ionized calcium is <3.2 mg/dl (0.8 mmol/l).
- The most common cause of hypercalcemia in the hospitalized setting is malignancy.
- First-line treatment of hypercalcemia includes vigorous hydration.

■ REFERENCES

1. Zivin JR, Gooley T, Zager RA, et al. Hypocalcemia: a pervasive metabolic abnormality in the critically ill. *Am J Kidney Dis.* 2001;37:689–698.
2. Lind L, Carlstedt F, Rastad J, et al. Hypocalcemia and parathyroid hormone secretion in critically ill patients. *Crit Care Med.* 2000;28:93–99.
3. Zaloga GP, Chernow B. The multifactorial basis for hypocalcemia during sepsis. Studies of the parathyroid hormone–vitamin D axis. *Ann Intern Med.* 1987;107:36–41.
4. Lee P, Eisman JA, Center JR. Vitamin D deficiency in critically ill patients. *N Engl J Med.* 2009;360:1912–1913.
5. Todd JC, III, Mollitt DL. Effect of sepsis on erythrocyte intracellular calcium homeostasis. *Crit Care Med.* 1995;23:459–465.
6. Sayeed MM, Zhu M, Maitra SR, et al. Alterations in cellular calcium and magnesium during circulatory/septic shock. *Magnesium.* 1989;8:179–189.
7. Malcolm DS, Zaloga GP, Holaday JW. Calcium administration increases the mortality of endotoxic shock in rats. *Crit Care Med.* 1989;17:900–903.
8. Zaloga GP, Sager A, Black KW, et al. Low dose calcium administration increases mortality during septic peritonitis in rats. *Circ Shock.* 1992;37:226–229.

9. Cuschieri J, Gourlay D, Garcia I, et al. Slow channel calcium inhibition blocks proinflammatory gene signaling and reduces macrophage responsiveness. *J Trauma*. 2002;52:434–442.

10. Lee HC, Hardman JM, Lum BK. Effects of nicardipine in rats subjected to endotoxic shock. *Gen Pharmacol*. 1992;23:71–74.

11. Szabo C, Hasko G, Nemeth ZH, et al. Calcium entry blockers increase interleukin-10 production in endotoxemia. *Shock*. 1997;7:304–307.

12. Sirmagul B, Kilic FS, Tunc O, et al. Effects of verapamil and nifedipine on different parameters in lipopolysaccharide-induced septic shock. *Heart Vessels*. 2006;21:162–168.

13. Mustafa SB, Olson MS. Effects of calcium channel antagonists on LPS-induced hepatic iNOS expression. *Am J Physiol*. 1999;277:G351–G360.

14. Forsythe RM, Wessel CB, Billiar TR, et al. Parenteral calcium for intensive care unit patients. *Cochrane Database Syst Rev*. 2008;CD006163.

15. Carlstedt F, Lind L. Hypocalcemic syndromes. *Crit Care Clin*. 2001;17:139–153.

16. Zaloga GP. Hypocalcemia in critically ill patients. *Crit Care Med*. 1992;20:251–262.

17. Lang RM, Fellner SK, Neumann A, et al. Left ventricular contractility varies directly with blood ionized calcium. *Ann Intern Med*. 1988;108:524–529.

18. Vincent JL, Bredas P, Jankowski S, et al. Correction of hypocalcaemia in the critically ill: what is the haemodynamic benefit? *Intensive Care Med*. 1995;21:838–841.

19. Ariyan CE, Sosa JA. Assessment and management of patients with abnormal calcium. *Crit Care Med*. 2004;32:S146-S154.

20. Stewart AF. Clinical practice. Hypercalcemia associated with cancer. *N Engl J Med*. 2005;352:373–379.

42

Electrolyte Disturbances

■ SODIUM AND WATER

Rules of the Game

Sodium balance determines volume status. Water balance determines tonicity, i.e., Na^+ concentration:

- Volume overload, increased total body sodium (regardless of serum Na concentration).
- Euvolemia, normal total body sodium (regardless of serum Na concentration).
- Volume depletion, decreased total body sodium (regardless of serum Na concentration).
- Hyponatremia, relative water excess.
- Hypernatremia, relative water deficit.
- In volume depleted patients, volume should be corrected prior to correction of tonicity, i.e., patients should initially be volume resuscitated with lactated ringer's solution or normal saline regardless of serum sodium concentration (see Chapter 8).
- Hyponatremic dehydration; volume replacement with 0.9% NaCl.
- Hypertonic dehydration; volume replacement with lactated Ringer's solution, then change to 0.45% NaCl.

■ HYPONATREMIA

Assessment of volume status (fluid overloaded, euvolemia or dehydration) is central to the evaluation and management of patients with hyponatremia (see Figure 42-1). Further diagnostic workup includes

P.E. Marik, *Handbook of Evidence-Based Critical Care*,
DOI 10.1007/978-1-4419-5923-2_42,
© Springer Science+Business Media, LLC 2010

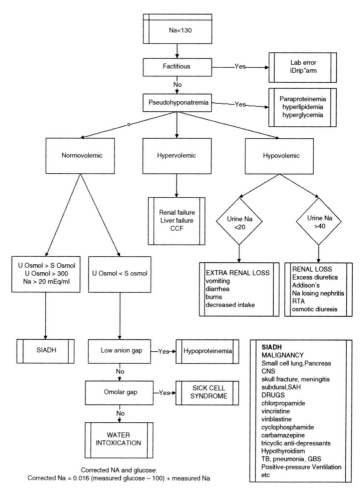

Figure 42-1. Hyponatremia diagnostic algorithm.

urine and serum electrolytes and osmolarity, thyroid function tests, lipid profile, and serum cortisol (and possibly ACTH stimulation test).

Most patients with hyponatremia are asymptomatic and have a plasma sodium concentration above 120 mEq/l. In these patients there is no urgency in correcting the serum sodium concentration and treatment should occur over a number of days. Treatment typically consists of iso-tonic saline if the patient has true volume depletion or water restriction in the syndrome of inappropriate ADH secretion (SIADH). More aggressive therapy is indicated in those patients who have symptomatic or severe hyponatremia (plasma sodium concentration below 110 mEq/l). In this setting, hypertonic saline can be given initially to raise the plasma sodium concentration (to ~120 mEq/l), although the rate at which this occurs must be carefully monitored to minimize the risk of central demyelinating lesions (see below). Hyponatremia in the setting of effective intravascu-lar volume depletion and edema (congestive cardiac failure and cirrhosis) results from the release of ADH in response to "hypovolemia" and carries a poor prognosis. Such patients require volume expansion with albumin and attempts to correct the underlying hemodynamic derangement. The role of ADH antagonists in these patients is unclear.[1,2]

The treatment of hyponatremia requires either the addition of sodium or the removal of water. When excess water rather than sodium deficit is the main mechanism of hyponatremia, removal of water alone is indi-cated. Water removal may be difficult, however, but sodium addition is easy. Net water removal can be achieved by the removal of sodium and water with a loop diuretic administered simultaneously with sodium in the form of hypertonic saline. The administration of hypertonic saline alone will also induce sodium and water diuresis, resulting in net loss of water, but the urine concentration is less predictable in this situation.

The optimal rate of correction of hyponatremia varies with the clini-cal state of the patient. Acute symptomatic hyponatremia (less than 48 h) results in cerebral edema due to water movement into the brain. In con-trast, chronic hyponatremia allows time for cerebral adaption to occur, resulting in the return of brain volume toward normal and usually causes no neurological symptoms. Rapid initial correction of hyponatremia is warranted in symptomatic patients, but overly rapid correction can be deleterious (osmotic demyelinating syndrome), particularly in patients with chronic hyponatremia.[3]

In general the sodium concentration should initially be corrected to a level of 120 mEq/l. The rate at which this correction should occur will depend on the presence of symptoms and the rate at which the disorder occurred. Alcoholic patients are particularly prone to cerebral demyelinolysis. In asymptomatic patients the plasma sodium concentra-tion should be raised at a maximal rate of below 0.5 mEq/l/h and more importantly, less than 10 mEq/l in the first day and less than 18 mEq/l over the first two days; a more rapid elevation can increase the risk of osmotic demyelination.[4]

More rapid correction is indicated in patients with symptomatic hyponatremia who present with seizures or other severe neurologi-cal manifestations; these findings are primarily due to cerebral edema induced by acute hyponatremia. In this setting, the plasma sodium concentration can be raised at an initial rate of 1.5–2 mEq/l/h for the first 3–4 h, since the risk of persistent severe hyponatremia is greater than the possible danger of overly rapid correction. Despite the more rapid initial rate of correction with symptomatic hyponatremia, the total increase in the plasma sodium concentration over the first 24 h should not exceed 10–12 mEq/l, the same limit noted with asymptomatic patients.

Hyponatremia occurring after transurethral resection of the bladder or prostate is one setting in which even more rapid correction may be warranted. The dilutional fall in plasma sodium concentration induced by absorption of non-electrolyte irrigation fluids occurs over a very short period of time, before significant cerebral adaption has begun.

The amount of Na^+ required to raise the plasma Na^+ concentration to a safe level (120 mEq/l) can be calculated from the following formula:

$$Na^+ \text{ deficit} = 0.6 \times \text{lean body weight(kg)} \times (120 - \text{plasma[Na +]}),$$
$$\text{substitute } 0.6 \text{ for } 0.5 \text{ in women}$$

Since 3% saline contains ~500 mEq/l, the total amount of this solution (in liters) required to increase the serum sodium to 120 mEq/l can be calculated as follows:

$$\text{Total volume of 3\% saline (liters)} = Na^+ \text{ deficit}/500$$

When 3% saline is used, the initial rate is usually between 50 and 100 ml/h; the serum sodium should be checked after 2 h and then 2 hourly until the sodium has stabilized.

An alternative (and perhaps safer) approach in euvolemic hyponatremic patients is to use a 0.9% saline infusion together with furosemide to increase the free water loss.

■ HYPERNATREMIA

Hypernatremia is not uncommon in ICU patients primarily due to excessive resuscitation with 0.9 NaCl ([Na+] 154 mEq/l). Hypernatremia may also occur in dehydrated patients in whom thirst is impaired (e.g., bed ridden or altered mental status). The treatment of the former is free water (e.g., 200 ml water orally q 4–6 h). In hypertonic dehydration, volume status should be corrected first (lactated Ringer's solution) followed by correction of tonicity (0.45% saline and/or free water). Rapid correction of hypernatremia can induce cerebral edema, seizures, permanent neurological damage, and death. To minimize these risks, the plasma Na^+ concentration should be corrected slowly. The maximum rate at which the plasma Na^+ should be corrected is 0.5 mEq/l/h or 12 mEq/l/day, a rate equivalent to that of hyponatremia. The water deficit can be calculated using the following formula:

Water deficit $= 0.5 \times (([Na+]/140) - 1)$, substitute 0.5 with 0.4 in women

■ HYPOKALEMIA

Only a small fraction of the total body K^+ is extracellular. Therefore, serum K^+ levels do not accurately reflect the total body K^+. The degree of K^+ deficit is dependent on the duration of the precipitating cause (time for equilibration) and the serum K^+ level. In patients with chronic hypokalemia, 1 mEq fall in serum K^+ is approximately equal to a 200 mEq total body deficit. In critically ill ICU patients, it is generally recommended to keep the serum $[K^+] \geq 4.0$ mEq/l. In patients with severe hypokalemia ($K <3.0$ mEq/l), both p.o. and IV potassium is recommended.

IV Replacement Therapy of KCl

- No more than 20 mEq/h should be given: central line infusion
  - 20 mEq in 50 ml over 1 h
  - 40 mEq in 100 ml over 2 h
- Peripheral line infusion
  - 10 mEq in 100 ml over 1 h
  - 20 mEq in 200 ml over 2 h

■ HYPERKALEMIA

Acute hyperkalemia is usually the result of renal failure. Hyperkalemia may also occur with overzealous potassium replacement and in patients receiving ACE inhibitors and potassium-sparing diuretics. Factors such as the duration of hyperkalemia, the plasma Ca^{2+} concentration, and the acid–base balance modify the toxicity of hyperkalemia. However, a $K^+ >6.5$ mEq/l or hyperkalemia associated with ECG changes should be regarded as life-threatening requiring immediate treatment.

Clinical features usually occur when the $K^+ >6.5$ mEq/l and include the following:

- Weakness
- Paresthesia
- Ileus

- Paralysis
- Cardiac arrest

ECG changes include the following:

- Peaked T waves
- Flattened P
- Prolonged PR interval
- Widening of the QRS complex
- Sine wave leading to ventricular fibrillation or asystole

The rate of progression of the ECG changes is not predictable and patients may progress from minor ECG changes to dangerous conduction disturbances or arrhythmias within minutes. The ECG changes are exacerbated by coexisting hyponatremia, hypocalcemia, hypermagnesemia, and acidosis.

Patients should be treated when the K^+ is greater than 5.5 mEq/l; urgent treatment is required when the K^+ >6.5 mEq/l. The goals of treatment are to

- protect the heart from the effects of K^+ by antagonizing the effect on cardiac conduction (calcium);
- shift the K^+ from the extracellular to the intracellular compartment;
- reduce the total body potassium.

Life-threatening arrhythmia may occur at any time during therapy; hence, continuous ECG monitoring is required. Patients with a serum K^+ >6.5 mEq/l and/or significant ECG changes should be treated immediately with calcium gluconate, followed by a glucose/insulin infusion and then an iron exchange resin.

■ HYPOPHOSPHATEMIA

Phosphorus is an essential component of phospholipid and nucleic acids, and plays an essential role in energy metabolism. Only about 1% of the total body phosphorus is extracellular, with the major phosphate store being in bone and the intracellular compartment. The normal range of serum phosphorus concentration in the serum is between 2.2 and 4.4 mg/dl, of which about 55% is in an ionized form that is physiologically active. The serum phosphate concentration is a poor indicator of the total body phosphorus and rapid shifts of phosphate between the extracellular and the intracellular compartments only confound this situation. Interpretation of the serum phosphate is further complicated by a normal diurnal variation, which may be as large as 0.5 mg/dl. However, hypophosphatemia may cause severe life-threatening complications, particularly in patients with depleted phosphate stores.

Causes of Severe Hypophosphatemia

- Alcohol abuse and withdrawal
- Refeeding after starvation
- Respiratory alkalosis
- Malabsorption
- Oral phosphate binders
- TPN
- Severe burns
- Therapy of diabetic ketoacidosis

There is a poor correlation between serum phosphate levels and symptoms. Although hypophosphatemia becomes life threatening when the serum levels are less than 1 mg/dl, symptoms may develop when the serum phosphate is less than 2 mg/dl.

Manifestations include the following:

- Myocardial depression
- Weakness, rhabdomyolysis, and respiratory failure
- Confusion, stupor, coma, and seizures
- Hemolysis, platelet dysfunction, and leukocyte dysfunction

Management of Hypophosphatemia

Therapy is usually empirical and phosphate level must be closely followed to prevent hyperphosphatemia. It has been recommended that patients with severe hypophosphatemia (serum phosphate level less than 1 mg/dl) be given an infusion of phosphate at a rate of 6 mg/kg/h (or 0.1 mM phosphate/kg in 500 ml 0.45 NS over 6 h), with serum levels being checked every 6 h and discontinued when the serum phosphate level exceeds 2 mg/dl. Thereafter the patients should receive oral phosphate to replace the intracellular stores. Phosphate solutions should be used with extreme caution in patients with renal failure. Charron et al. demonstrated that a potassium phosphate solution may be given at a faster rate in patients with severe hypophosphatemia if the serum potassium is less than 4 mEq/l; these authors reported using an infusion of 30 mmol in 40 ml/NS over 2 h and 45 mmol/l in 100 ml/NS given over 3 h.[5]

Patients with mild-to-moderate hypophosphatemia (serum phosphate between 1.0 and 2.2 mg/dl) should receive oral supplementation (1 g Neutra-Phos/day) unless diarrhea precludes using this route of supplementation.

■ HYPOMAGNESEMIA

Magnesium in the fourth most abundant cation in the body and the second most prevalent intracellular cation. Approximately 53% of total Mg stores are in bone, 27% in muscle, 19% in soft tissues, 0.5% in erythrocytes, and 0.3% in serum. Serum Mg is 67% ionized, 19% protein bound, and 14% complexed. Standard clinical determinations of serum total Mg reflect all three forms. Of note, protein-bound and complexed Mg are unavailable for most biochemical processes. Since serum contains only 0.3% of total body Mg stores, serum total Mg measurements poorly reflect total body status. Serum total Mg concentrations normally average 1.7–2.3 mg/dl.

Mg^{2+} is essential for the function of important enzymes, including those related to the transfer of phosphate groups, all reactions that require ATP, for the replication and transcription of DNA, as well as cellular energy metabolism, membrane stabilization, nerve conduction, and calcium channel function. Magnesium plays an essential role in the function of the cell membrane sodium–potassium ATPase pump. Hypomagnesemia is reported to be common in ICU patients ($\sim$60%) and an important prognostic marker. The causes of "hypomagnesemia" include the following:

- Alcoholism and alcohol withdrawal
- Emesis
- Diarrhea
- Nasogastric suction
- Parenteral nutrition
- Refeeding syndrome
- Diabetes
- Drugs
  - Loop diuretics
  - Aminoglycosides
  - Amphotericin B
  - *Cis*-platinum
  - Cyclosporin

The reported manifestations of hypomagnesemia include the following:

- Hypokalemia and hypocalcemia
- Lethargy, confusion, coma, seizures, ataxia, nystagmus
- Prolonged PR and QT interval on ECG
- Atrial and ventricular arrhythmias

Assessing Mg status in the critically ill beyond serum total Mg levels is difficult. As for calcium, normal total Mg levels may coexist with ionized hypomagnesemia and vice versa. A major advance in evaluating Mg deficiency is the ability to measure Mg^{2+}. The incidence of ionized hypo-magnesemia in ICU patients has been reported to be between 14–18%.[6] The clinical significance of this finding is unclear. Serum total Mg levels are not correlated with serum Mg^{2+} in the critically ill because of accompanying variations in plasma protein concentrations, acid–base balance, metabolic derangements, and drugs that affect Mg balance.[7]

Management of Hypomagnesemia

Most episodes of hypomagnesemia in intensive care are asymptomatic. In theory, symptoms and signs occur when the serum total Mg concentrations fall below 1.2 mg/dl. In light of the above information the value of routinely measuring the serum magnesium is in question. However, it is probably prudent to measure the serum magnesium level in patients at risk of magnesium deficiency and to treat those who have severe hypomagnesemia (<1.2 mg/dl). Treatment of hypomagnesemia (aiming for a serum magnesium level of ∼2.5 mg/dl) may be particularly important in patients with arrhythmias and those with seizures. Magnesium should be replaced cautiously in patients with renal impairment. The recommended dose is 2 g $MgSO_4$ over 10 min intravenously, followed either by an infusion at 0.5 g/h for 6 h or by a 1 g bolus hourly for 4 h, followed by a repeat serum magnesium level. In renal failure the dose should be halved.

■ REFERENCES

1. Finley JJ, Konstam MA, Udelson JE. Arginine vasopressin antagonists for the treatment of heart failure and hyponatremia. *Circulation.* 2008;118:410–421.
2. Decaux G, Soupart A, Vassart G. Non-peptide arginine–vasopressin antagonists: the vaptans. *Lancet.* 2008;371:1624–1632.
3. Pirzada NA, Ali II. Central pontine myelinolysis. *Mayo Clin Proc.* 2001;76:559–562.
4. Patel GP, Balk RA. Recognition and treatment of hyponatremia in acutely ill hospitalized patients. *Am J Med.* 2007;29:211–229.
5. Charron T, Bernard F, Skrobik Y, et al. Intravenous phosphate in the intensive care unit: more aggressive repletion regimens for moderate and severe hypophosphatemia. *Intensive Care Med.* 2003;29:1273–1278.
6. Soliman HM, Mercan D, Lobo SS, et al. Development of ionized hypomagnesemia is associated with higher mortality rates. *Crit Care Med.* 2003;31:1082–1087.
7. Escuela MP, Guerra M, Anon JM, et al. Total and ionized serum magnesium in critically ill patients. *Intensive Care Med.* 2005;31:151–156.

43

Acid–Base Disturbances

■ AN APPROACH TO ARTERIAL BLOOD GAS ANALYSIS

Step 1: Is there an acid–base disorder?
Look at the $PaCO_2$ and the HCO_3 to determine whether they are in the normal range (see Table 43-1). If abnormal, go to step 2; if normal, go to step 5.

Step 2: Is the patient acidemic or alkalemic?
Look at the pH. Is the pH normal (i.e., pH between 7.35 and 7.45) or is the pH on the acidemic or the alkalemic side of 7.40?.

Step 3: What is the primary acid–base disorder? (Table 43-2).
From an analysis of the pH, $PaCO_2$ and HCO_3, determine the primary defect:

- If the pH is decreased, the patient has an acidemia, which may be either a
    - metabolic acidosis – characterized by a low HCO_3
    - respiratory acidosis – characterized by an increased PCO_2
- If the pH is increased, the patient has an alkalemia, which may be either
    - metabolic alkalosis – characterized by an increase in plasma HCO_3
    - respiratory alkalosis – characterized by a decreased PCO_2

Step 4: Expected compensatory response.
Determine whether the compensatory response is of the magnitude expected (see Tables 43-3 and 43-4), i.e., is there a secondary (uncompensated) acid–base disturbance?

Step 5: How to recognize mixed acid–base disorders?

P.E. Marik, *Handbook of Evidence-Based Critical Care*,
DOI 10.1007/978-1-4419-5923-2_43,
© Springer Science+Business Media, LLC 2010

Table 43-1. Normal acid–base values.

	Mean	1 SD	2 SD
PaCO$_2$ (mmHg)	40	38–42	35–45
pH	7.4	7.38–7.42	7.35–7.45
HCO$_3$	24	23–25	22–26

Table 43-2. Acid–base disorders.

Acid–Base Disorder	Criteria
Respiratory failure/respiratory acidosis	PaCO$_2$ >45 mmHg
Respiratory alkalosis	PaCO$_2$ <35 mmHg
Acute respiratory failure	PaCO$_2$ >45 mmHg; pH <7.35
Chronic respiratory failure	PaCO$_2$ >45 mmHg; pH 7.36–7.44
Acute respiratory alkalosis	PaCO$_2$ <35 mmHg; pH >7.45
Chronic respiratory alkalosis	PaCO$_2$ <35 mmHg; pH 7.36–7.44
Acidemia	pH <7.35
Alkalemia	pH >7.45
Acidosis	HCO$_3$ <22 mEq/l
Alkalosis	HCO$_3$ >26 mEq/l

Table 43-3. Traditional acid–base definitions.

		pH	PaCO$_2$	HCO$_3$	BE
Respiratory acidosis	Uncompensated	↓	↑	N	N
	Partly compensated	↓	↑	↑	↑
	Compensated	N	↑	↑	↑
Respiratory alkalosis	Uncompensated	↑	↓	N	N
	Partly compensated	↑	↓	↓	↓
	Compensated	N	↓	↓	↓
Metabolic acidosis	Uncompensated	↓	N	↓	↓
	Partly compensated	↓	↓	↓	↓
	Compensated	N	↓	↓	↓
Metabolic alkalosis	Uncompensated	↑	N	↑	↑
	Partly compensated	↑	↑	↑	↑
	Compensated	N	↑	↑	↑

Acid–base disorders may present as two or three coexisting disorders. It is possible for a patient to have an acid–base disorder with a normal pH, PCO$_2$, and HCO$_3$, the only clue to an acid–base disorder being an increased anion gap:

$$\text{Anion gap} = [Na] - ([Cl] + [HCO_3]), \text{ normal } 12 \pm 2 \text{ mEq/l}$$

Table 43-4. Compensation for acid–base disorders.

Primary Disorder	Primary Change	Compensatory Change	Expected Compensation
Metabolic acidosis	$\downarrow HCO_3$	$\downarrow PaCO_2$	$\Delta PaCO_2 = 1.0\ \Delta HCO_3$
Metabolic alkalosis	$\uparrow HCO_3$	$\uparrow PaCO_2$	$\Delta PaCO_2 = 0.7\ \Delta HCO_3$
Respiratory acidosis	$\uparrow PaCO_2$	$\uparrow HCO_3$	Acute: $\Delta HCO_3 = 0.1\ \Delta PaCO_2$ $\Delta pH \sim \Delta PaCO_2 \times 0.01$ Chronic: $\Delta HCO_3 = 0.35\ \Delta PaCO_2$ $\Delta pH \sim \Delta PaCO_2 \times 0.003$
Respiratory alkalosis	$\downarrow PaCO_2$	$\downarrow HCO_3$	Acute: $\Delta HCO_3 = 0.2\ \Delta PaCO_2$ $\Delta pH \sim \Delta PaCO_2 \times 0.01$ Chronic: $\Delta HCO_3 = 0.5\ \Delta PaCO_2$ $\Delta pH \sim \Delta PaCO_2 \times 0.002$

- Calculate the plasma anion gap; if it is increased by >5 mEq/l, the patient most likely has a metabolic acidosis.
- Compare the fall in plasma HCO_3 $(25 - HCO_3)$ with the increase in the plasma anion gap; these should be of similar magnitude. If there is a gross discrepancy (5 mEq/l), there is a mixed disturbance present:
    - Increase in AG > fall in HCO_3 suggests that a component of the metabolic acidosis is due to HCO_3 loss.
    - Increase in AG < fall in HCO_3 suggests coexistent metabolic alkalosis.

Step 6: Calculate the osmolar gap (in patients with an unexplained AG metabolic acidosis):

$$\text{Estimated serum osmolality} = 2 \times Na + glucose/18 + BUN/2.8,$$
$$\text{normal} \approx 290\ mOsm/kg\ H_2O$$

$$\text{Osmolal gap} = Osm\ (measured) - Osm\ (calculated), \text{normal} < 10$$

Causes of an increased osmolal gap (see Table 43-5):

- Ethylene glycol

- Alcohol (ethanol)
- Methanol
- Isopropyl alcohol (causes neither an anion gap nor an acidosis)
- Mannitol
- Sorbitol
- Paraldehyde
- Acetone

Table 43-5. Osmolal gap and lethal intoxications.

Substance	Mol. Wt	Lethal Level (mg/dl)	Osmolal Gap at this Level
Ethanol	46	350	80
Ethylene glycol	62	21	4
Isopropyl alcohol	60	340	60
Methanol	32	80	27
Acetone	58	55	10

■ METABOLIC ACIDOSIS

The manifestations of metabolic acidosis are largely dependent on the underlying cause and the rapidity with which the condition developed. An acute severe metabolic acidosis results in myocardial depression with decreased cardiac output, decreased blood pressure, and decreased hepatic and renal blood flow. Re-entrant arrhythmia and a reduction in the ventricular fibrillation threshold can occur. Brain metabolism becomes impaired with progressive obtundation and coma.

See Figure 43-1 for an approach to the diagnosis of metabolic acidosis. Metabolic acidosis in the critically ill patient is an ominous sign and warrants an aggressive approach to the diagnosis and management of the cause(s) of the disorder. In almost all circumstances the treatment of a metabolic acidosis involves the treatment of the underlying disorder. Except in specific circumstances (outlined below), there is no scientific evidence to support treating a metabolic or a respiratory acidosis with sodium bicarbonate.[1] Furthermore, it is the intracellular pH which is of importance in determining cellular function. The intracellular buffering system is much more effective in restoring pH to normal than are the extracellular buffers. Consequently, patients have tolerated a pH as low as 7.0 during sustained hypercapnia without obvious adverse effects. Paradoxically, sodium bicarbonate can decrease intracellular pH (in circumstances where CO_2 elimination is fixed).

There are no data to support the use of bicarbonate in patients with lactic acidosis.[1,2] The prognosis is related to the underlying disorder causing

METABOLIC ACIDOSIS

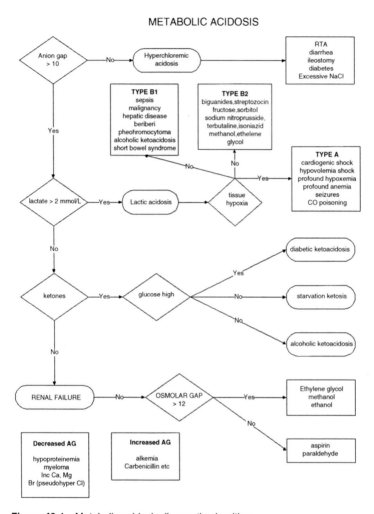

Figure 43-1. Metabolic acidosis diagnostic algorithm.

the acidosis. The infusion of bicarbonate can lead to a variety of problems in patients with acidosis, including fluid overload, a postrecovery metabolic alkalosis, and hypernatremia. Furthermore, studies in both animals and humans suggest that alkali therapy may only transiently raise the plasma bicarbonate concentration. This finding appears to be related in part to the carbon dioxide generated as the administered bicarbonate buffers excess hydrogen ions. Unless the minute ventilation is increased (in ventilated patients), CO_2 elimination will not be increased; this will paradoxically worsen the intracellular acidosis.

Indications for Bicarbonate Therapy

In hyperchloremic acidosis (e.g., that produced by severe diarrhea, fistula, etc.), endogenous regeneration of bicarbonate cannot occur (as bicarbonate has been lost rather than buffered). Therefore, even if the cause of the acidosis can be reversed, exogenous alkali is often required for prompt attenuation of severe acidemia. Bicarbonate therapy is therefore indicated in patients with severe hyperchloremic acidosis in which the pH is less than 7.2; these are predominantly patients with severe diarrhea, high-output fistulas, and renal tubular acidosis. In order to prevent sodium overload, we suggest that 2×50 ml ampoules of $NaHCO_3$ (each containing 50 mmol of $NaHCO_3$) be added to 1 l of 5% D/W and infused at a rate of 100–200 ml/h.

Methanol and ethylene glycol intoxication can produce a severe, acute, high-anion-gap metabolic acidosis caused by the accumulation of toxic metabolites. Large amounts of alkali are often required to control the severe acidemia (see Chapter 59).

Bicarbonate and Ketoacidosis

Bicarbonate is frequently administered to "correct the acidosis" in patients with diabetic ketoacidosis. However, paradoxically, bicarbonate has been demonstrated to increase ketone production. Studies have demonstrated an increase in acetoacetate levels during alkali administration, followed by an increase in 3-hydroxybutyrate levels after its completion. In pediatric patients, treatment with bicarbonate has been demonstrated to prolong hospitalization.[3] In addition, bicarbonate may decrease CSF pH as increased CO_2 produced by buffering acid crosses the blood–brain barrier, combines H_2O, and regenerates H^+. It is generally believed that adjunctive bicarbonate is unnecessary and potentially disadvantageous in severe DKA.

D-Lactic Acidosis

Certain bacteria in the GI tract may convert carbohydrate into organic acids. The two factors that make this possible are slow GI transit (blind loops, obstruction) and change of the normal flora (usually with antibiotic therapy). The most prevalent organic acid is D-lactic acid. Since humans metabolize this isomer more slowly than L-lactate and production rates can be very rapid, life-threatening acidosis can be produced. This usual laboratory test for lactate is specific for the L-lactate isomer. Therefore, to confirm the diagnosis, the plasma D-lactate must be measured.

■ METABOLIC ALKALOSIS

Metabolic acidosis (MA) is a common acid–base disturbance in ICU patients, characterized by an elevated serum pH (>7.45) secondary to plasma bicarbonate (HCO_3-) retention. The MA is usually the result of several therapeutic interventions in the critically ill patient. Nasogastric drainage, diuretic-induced intravascular volume depletion, hypokalemia, and the use of corticosteroids are common causes of MA in these patients. In addition, the citrate in transfused blood is metabolized to bicarbonate which may compound the MA. Overventilation in patients with type 2 respiratory failure may result in a posthypercapnic MA. In many patients, the events that generated the MA may not be present at the time of diagnosis.

MA may have adverse effects on cardiovascular, pulmonary, and metabolic function. It can decrease cardiac output, depress central ventilation, shift the oxyhemoglobin saturation curve to the left, worsen hypokalemia and hypophosphatemia, and negatively affect the ability to wean patients from mechanical ventilation. Increasing serum pH has been shown to correlate with ICU mortality. Correction of MA has been shown to increase minute ventilation, increase arterial oxygen tension and mixed venous oxygen tension, and decrease oxygen consumption. It is therefore important to correct MA in all critically ill patients.

The first therapeutic maneuver in patients with MA is to replace any fluid (with normal saline) and electrolyte deficits. Aggressive potassium supplementation is warranted to achieve a K^+ >4.5 mEq/l. If these interventions fail, ammonium chloride, hydrochloric acid, or arginine hydrochloride may be given. The disadvantage of these solutions is that they are difficult to use and require the administration of a large volume of hypotonic fluid. Extravasation of hydrochloric acid may result in severe tissue necrosis, mandating administration through a well-functioning central line. Acetazolamide is a carbonic anhydrase inhibitor that promotes the renal excretion of bicarbonate and has been demonstrated to be very effective in treating an MA in ICU patients. A single dose of 500 mg is recommended. The onset of action is within 1.5 h with a duration of approximately 24 h.[4,5] Repeat doses may be required as necessary.

■ CLINICAL PEARLS

- NaHCO$_3$ is basically a useless therapy.
- Correct the volume deficit and potassium (first) in patients with a metabolic alkalosis.

■ REFERENCES

1. Aschner JL, Poland RL. Sodium bicarbonate: basically useless therapy. *Pediatrics*. 2008;122:831–835.
2. Boyd JH, Walley KR. Is there a role for sodium bicarbonate in treating lactic acidosis from shock. *Curr Opin Crit Care*. 2008;14:379–383.
3. Green SM, Rothrock SG, Ho JD, et al. Failure of adjunctive bicarbonate to improve outcome in severe pediatric diabetic ketoacidosis. *Ann Emerg Med*. 1998;31:41–48.
4. Marik PE, Kussman BD, Lipman J, et al. Acetazolamide in the treatment of metabolic alkalosis in critically ill patients. *Heart Lung*. 1991;20:455–459.
5. Mazur JE, Devlin JW, Peters MJ, et al. Single versus multiple doses of acetazolamide for metabolic alkalosis in critically ill medical patients: a randomized, double-blind trial. *Crit Care Med*. 1999;27:1257–1261.

44

Acute Renal Failure

Acute renal failure (ARF) is a common problem in the ICU. Even modest degrees of ARF not resulting in dialysis treatment increase the risk of death approximately fivefold.[1] The mortality of patients who require dialysis has remained in excess of 50% despite improvements in renal replacement therapy and aggressive supportive care. It is therefore essential that all efforts be made to avoid this complication, i.e., aggressive (early) fluid resuscitation and avoidance of potentially nephrotoxic drugs (especially aminoglycosides and contrast media). The therapeutic intervention of choice in patients with oliguria is fluid resuscitation and not furosemide/Lasix™ (see Chapter 8).

While low-dose dopamine increases renal blood flow and urine output in patients with normal renal function, dopamine does not improve renal function, reduce the need for dialysis, or alter the course of ARF in critically ill patients.[2] In addition, studies have demonstrated that furosemide is of no value in modifying azotemia, reducing the need for dialysis, altering the time to recovery of renal function, reducing hospital stay, or impacting survival in established ARF.[3-5] Indeed, diuretics have been reported to be associated with a significant increase in the risk of death and non-recovery of renal function.[6] A recent meta-analysis concluded that furosemide was not associated with any significant clinical benefit but perhaps was associated with an increased risk of harm.[7] Diuretics in any form (bolus, continuous infusion, topical) have no role in the management/prevention of acute renal failure (the only exceptions are patients with hypercalcemia/tumor lysis as part of a forced diuresis protocol). Optimization of intravascular volume, cardiac output, and mean arterial pressure remains the cornerstone of both the prevention and the treatment of ARF. No pharmacological intervention has yet been demonstrated to alter the natural history of this condition. In patients who remain oliguric/anuric after adequate fluid resuscitation, it is important to exclude

P.E. Marik, *Handbook of Evidence-Based Critical Care*,
DOI 10.1007/978-1-4419-5923-2_44,
© Springer Science+Business Media, LLC 2010

urinary tract obstruction (and urinary catheter obstruction), as this is an immediately reversible cause of acute renal failure.

■ PRERENAL AZOTEMIA

Patients with prerenal azotemia (urinary Na <40 mEq/l) and increased serum BUN/creatinine ratio should receive aggressive fluid resuscitation. Glomerular filtration is highly dependent on renal blood flow and renal perfusion pressure. When both/either falls, the kidney autoregulates to maintain GFR. However, when the mean arterial pressure (MAP) falls below 60 mmHg, the filtration pressure drops close to 0. It is therefore essential that all patients with prerenal azotemia be adequately fluid resuscitated to achieve an adequate MAP (>80 mmHg) and cardiac index (CI >3.0 l/min/m^2). In the elderly and in patients with diseases affecting the integrity of the afferent arterioles, lesser degrees of hypotension may cause a decline in renal function and oliguria. In patients with compromised renal function, nephrotoxic drugs (particularly aminoglycosides and contract agents) should be avoided.

■ CONTRAST AGENTS AND THE KIDNEY

Contrast-induced nephropathy, defined as an increase in serum creatinine greater than 25% (or >0.5 mg/dl) within 3 days of intravascular contrast administration in the absence of an alternative cause, is the third most common cause of ARF in hospitalized patients.[8,9] Contrast-induced nephropathy develops in up to 10% of patients with normal renal function. However, the incidence may be as high as 25% in high-risk patients, namely those with

- pre-existing renal dysfunction, especially diabetic nephropathy
- congestive heart failure
- dehydration
- multiple myeloma
- concomitant drugs
  - angiotensin-converting enzyme inhibitors
  - non-steroidal anti-inflammatory drugs

All attempts should be made to avoid iodinated contrast agents in patients with prerenal azotemia and in patients with acute renal insults. In all patients receiving intravenous contrast agents, vigorous prehydration is required. There is evidence that low-osmolality contrast agents lower the risk of nephrotoxicity in patients with elevated serum creatinine concentrations (>1.5 mg/dl).[10]

Prevention of Contrast-Induced ARF

- Effective interventions[11-13]
  - Volume expansion with saline solutions
  - Avoidance of high-osmolar contrast agents
  - Minimization of volume of contrast media
  - Discontinue NSAIDS, diuretics, etc.
  - N-Acetylcysteine
- Potentially effective interventions [11]
  - Theophylline
- Ineffective or potentially harmful interventions[11,14]
  - Dopamine
  - Fenoldopam
  - Atrial natriuretic peptide
  - Diuretics
  - Mannitol

Acetylcysteine and vigorous prehydration should be considered in all patients at high risk of contrast-induced nephrotoxicity. Acetylcysteine should be given as 600 or 1,200 mg PO (or IV) twice daily the day before and the day of the procedure.[12,13]

In patients with acute renal failure in whom the use of contrast agents is essential, dialysis immediately after the contrast procedure may limit additional renal compromise (contrast agents are dialyzable). However, postprocedure dialysis is not required in patients on chronic hemodialysis who receive an intravenous contrast agent unless the patient becomes volume overloaded.

Extreme caution should be exercised when using contrast agents in patients with cirrhosis. These patients have a diminished intravascular volume which is frequently exacerbated by the use of diuretics. Contrast-induced renal failure is a devastating complication in these patients. Should contrast be required, all cirrhotic patients should be vigorously volume resuscitated (5% albumin) and given acetylcysteine.

■ AMINOGLYCOSIDES AND THE KIDNEY

Aminoglycoside antibiotics are reported to be the most common cause of drug-induced nephrotoxicity in hospitalized patients. It is probable that between 5 and 15% of patients treated with an aminoglycoside will develop clinically significant nephrotoxicity. The risk factors of aminoglycoside nephrotoxicity include the following:

- More than 10 days of treatment
- A second course of aminoglycosides within 3 months of the first course
- Underlying renal dysfunction
- Advanced age
- Multiple daily dosing schedule
- Hypokalemia and hypomagnesemia
- Concurrent administration of nephrotoxic agents, especially
  - Vancomycin
  - Amphotericin B
  - Cyclosporine

In patients with renal dysfunction, the half-life of aminoglycosides is increased, resulting is serum levels being elevated for a prolonged period of time. This enhances the renal uptake of the drug with increased nephrotoxicity. Aminoglycoside antibiotics should therefore be avoided in patients with significant renal dysfunction.

■ "COMMON" NEPHROTOXIC AGENTS

- Interstitial nephritis
  - β-Lactams (esp. ampicillin)
  - Quinolones
  - NSAIDS
  - Rifampicin
  - Sulphonamides
  - Acyclovir
  - Vancomycin
  - Cisplatin
  - Cimetidine
  - Allopurinol
  - Omeprazole and lansoprazole
- Tubular cell toxicity
  - Aminoglycosides
  - Amphotericin B
  - Anti-retrovirals
  - Cisplatin
- Crystal nephropathy
  - Foscarnet
  - Ganciclovir
- Altered intraglomerular hemodynamics
  - Cyclosporine
  - Tacrolimus
  - NSAIDS
  - ACE inhibitors

■ MANAGEMENT OF ESTABLISHED ACUTE RENAL FAILURE

Acute renal failure is a reversible process in the majority of cases requiring careful fluid and electrolyte management and adjustment of drug dosages according to the level of the glomerular filtration rate. Multiple pharmacological agents including dopamine, fenoldopam, loop diuretics, atrial natriuretic peptide, insulin growth factor-1, and thyroxine have proven beneficial for the treatment of ARF in animal models. However, similar success has not been observed in human studies.[15] Indeed, once the patient has established acute renal failure, no intervention or therapy has been demonstrated to hasten the recovery of renal function. However, further kidney insults should be rigorously avoided as this will delay renal recovery.

■ WHEN TO INITIATE RENAL REPLACEMENT THERAPY (RRT)

The "classic" criteria for initiating renal replacement therapy include the following:

- Hyperkalemia (K >6.5 mmol/l)
- Progressive acidosis with pH <7.20
- Fluid overload with pulmonary edema
- Pericardial effusion
- Uremic symptoms, i.e., nausea, vomiting, altered mental status, asterixis
- Increase of serum creatinine >2 mg/dl/day

These recommendations were formulated for patients with chronic renal failure. However, most intensivists (and critical-care nephrologists) contend that there is no reason to wait for significant physiological derangements (hyperkalemia, severe acidosis, fluid overload, uremic complication) to develop in the already physiologically fragile, critically ill patient before initiating RRT. The early initiation of RRT facilitates early nutritional support, simplifies fluid management, and may prevent complications. However, there are no solid data to support this strategy and a review of the literature does not allow recommendations regarding the optimal indications for or timing of renal replacement therapy.[16]

Mode of Renal Replacement Therapy

Continuous renal replacement therapies (CRRTs) have been developed to enable the critically ill patient with acute renal failure to be treated more effectively. Acute renal failure in the critically ill patient almost always develops in the setting of shock, sepsis, major surgery, and/or major trauma, and is invariably associated with multi-organ dysfunction and/or failure. In addition, these patients usually have hemodynamic and respiratory abnormalities that make conventional intermittent hemodialysis both technically difficult and fraught with many complications. The patients' fluid, electrolyte, and acid–base status fluctuate widely within a 24 hour period; intermittent dialysis is not suited to these changing circumstances. Continuous renal replacement therapies were developed with the aim of providing a more physiological method of renal replacement therapy, i.e., to function more like a normal kidney. Over the last 2 decades, CRRT has undergone a remarkable revolution, the major aspects of which include the introduction of countercurrent dialysate flow, the use of double lumen venous access, and the development of modular, portable CVVHD machines.

Advantages of CRRT Therapy

- Hemodynamically well tolerated
- Minimal change in plasma osmolarity
- Better control of azotemia, electrolytes and acid–base balance
- Very effective in removing fluid
- Technically simple
- Membrane capable of removing cytokines in septic patients
- Better membrane biocompatibility

From a conceptual standpoint, it seems logical that the use of CRRT with its gradual fluid and solute removal would be superior to the rapid volume and solute flux associated with IHD in the critically ill patient with hemodynamic instability. However, clinical trials have not demonstrated outcome benefits associated with CRRT.[16–19] Based on the current data, IHD and CRRT appear to lead to similar clinical outcomes for patients with ARF.

Dosing of RRT

Until recently, the optimal dosing of IHD and CRRT in the ICU was unclear with data suggesting that more aggressive RRT (daily IHD or CVVHD at an ultrafiltration rate of at least 35 ml/kg/h) was associated with improved renal recovery.[16,20] The VA/NIH Acute Renal Failure Trial Network randomized 1,124 patients with ARF to receive intensive or less intensive RRT.[21] Hemodynamically stable patients underwent intermittent HD (six vs. three times per week) and hemodynamically unstable patients underwent CVVHD (35 vs. 20 ml/kg/h). There was no difference in clinical outcomes between the two groups of patients.

■ CLINICAL PEARLS

- Optimization of preload and cardiac output (and avoidance of nephrotoxic agents) is the treatment of choice in patients with prerenal azotemia.
- Lasix/furosemide is the "Devil's medicine" and should be avoided in patients with prerenal azotemia and ARF.
- RRT should be initiated in patients with hyperkalemia, progressive acidosis, or volume overload.
- Thrice weekly IHD is indicated in hemodynamically stable patients and low-intensity CVVHD in hemodynamically unstable patients.

■ REFERENCES

1. Levy EM, Viscoli CM, Horwitz RI. The effect of acute renal failure on mortality. A cohort analysis. *JAMA*. 1996;275:1489–1494.
2. Australian and New Zealand Intensive Care Society (ANZICS) Clinical Trials Group. Low dose dopamine in patients with early renal dysfunction: a placebo-controlled trial. *Lancet*. 2000;356:2139–2143.
3. Brown CB, Ogg CS, Cameron JS. High dose furosemide in acute renal failure: a controlled trial. *Clin Nephrol*. 1981;15:90–96.
4. Lucas CE, Zito JG, Carter KM, et al. Questionable value of furosemide in preventing renal failure. *Surgery*. 1977;82:341–320.
5. Kleinknecht D, Ganeval D, Gonzalez-Duque LA, et al. Furosemide in acute oliguric renal failure. A controlled trial. *Nephron*. 1976;17:51–58.
6. Mehta RL, Pascual MT, Soroko S, et al. Diuretics, mortality, and non-recovery of renal function in acute renal failure. *JAMA*. 2002;288: 2547–2553.
7. Ho KM, Sheridan DJ. Meta-analysis of furosemide to prevent or treat acute renal failure. *BMJ*. 2006;333:420.
8. Morcos SK, Thomsen HS, Webb JA. Contrast-media-induced nephrotoxicity: a consensus report. Contrast Media Safety Committee, European Society of Urogenital Radiology (ESUR). *Eur Radiol*. 1999;9: 1602–1613.

9. Thomsen HS, Morcos SK. Contrast-medium-induced nephropathy: is there a new consensus? A review of published guidelines. *Eur Radiol.* 2006;16:1835–1840.

10. Barrett BJ, Carlisle EJ. Metaanalysis of the relative nephrotoxicity of high- and low-osmolality iodinated contrast media. *Radiology.* 1993;188:171–178.

11. Kelly AM, Dwamena B, Cronin P, et al. Meta-analysis: effectiveness of drugs for preventing contrast-induced nephropathy. *Ann Intern Med.* 2008;148:284–294.

12. Marenzi G, Assanelli E, Marana I, et al. N-acetylcysteine and contrast-induced nephropathy in primary angioplasty. *N Engl J Med.* 2006;354:2773–2782.

13. Tepel M, van der Giet M, Schwarzfeld C, et al. Prevention of radiographic-contrast-agent-induced reductions in renal function by acetylcysteine. *N Engl J Med.* 2000;343:180–184.

14. Solomon R, Werner C, Mann D, et al. Effects of saline, mannitol, and furosemide to prevent acute decreases in renal function induced by radiocontrast agents. *N Engl J Med.* 1994;331:1416–1420.

15. Weisbord SD, Palevsky PM. Acute renal failure in the intensive care unit. *Semin Respir Crit Care Med.* 2006;27:262–273.

16. Pannu N, Klarenbach S, Wiebe N, et al. Renal replacement therapy in patients with acute renal failure: a systematic review. *JAMA.* 2008;299:793–805.

17. Mehta RL, McDonald B, Gabbai FB, et al. A randomized clinical trial of continuous versus intermittent dialysis for acute renal failure. *Kidney Int.* 2001;60:1154–1163.

18. Augustine JJ, Sandy D, Seifert TH, et al. A randomized controlled trial comparing intermittent with continuous dialysis in patients with ARF. *Am J Kidney Dis.* 2004;44:1000–1007.

19. Tonelli M, Manns B, Feller-Kopman D. Acute renal failure in the intensive care unit: a systematic review of the impact of dialytic modality on mortality and renal recovery. *Am J Kidney Dis.* 2002;40:875–885.

20. Ronco C, Bellomo R, Homel P, et al. Effects of different doses in continuous veno-venous haemofiltration on outcomes of acute renal failure: a prospective randomised trial. *Lancet.* 2000;356:26–30.

21. Palevsky PM, Zhang JH, O'Connor TZ, et al. Intensity of renal support in critically ill patients with acute kidney injury. *N Engl J Med.* 2008;359:7–20.

45

Rhabdomyolysis

Rhabdomyolysis means destruction or disintegration of striated muscle. This syndrome is characterized by muscle breakdown and necrosis resulting in the leakage of the intracellular muscle constituents into the circulation and the extracellular fluid. Rhabdomyolysis ranges from an asymptomatic illness with elevation in the creatine kinase (CK) to a life-threatening condition associated with extreme elevations in CK, electrolyte imbalances, acute renal failure (ARF), and disseminated intravascular coagulation (DIC).[1] The cause of rhabdomyolysis is usually easily identified; however, in some instances, the etiology is elusive. Muscular trauma is the most common cause of rhabdomyolysis. Less common causes include muscle enzyme deficiencies, electrolyte abnormalities, infectious causes, drugs, toxins, and endocrinopathies. Rhabdomyolysis is commonly associated with myoglobinuria, and if this is sufficiently severe, it can result in ARF. Weakness, myalgia, and tea-colored urine are the main clinical manifestations. The most sensitive laboratory finding of muscle injury is the CPK; a level greater than 5,000 U/l indicates serious muscle injury in the absence of myocardial or brain infarction. The management of patients with rhabdomyolysis includes advanced life support (airway, breathing, and circulation) followed by measures to preserve renal function. The latter includes vigorous hydration. The use of alkalizing agents and osmotic diuretics, while commonly used, remains of unproven benefit.

■ EPIDEMIOLOGY

About 10–40% of patients with rhabdomyolysis develop acute renal failure.[1] Indeed, it has been suggested by some authors that rhabdomyolysis

P.E. Marik, *Handbook of Evidence-Based Critical Care*,
DOI 10.1007/978-1-4419-5923-2_45,
© Springer Science+Business Media, LLC 2010

from all causes leads to 5–25% of cases of ARF. Recent clinical series of patients developing acute renal failure report mortality rates of 7–80%. Patients with severe injury who develop rhabdomyolysis-induced renal failure have a mortality of approximately 20%. Mortality is higher in patients with multi-organ dysfunction syndrome. Rhabdomyolysis occurs in up to 85% of patients with traumatic injuries.

■ ETIOLOGY

There are multiple causes of rhabdomyolysis, which can be classified as physical and non-physical causes.[1]

Physical Causes

- Trauma and compression
  - Crush injuries
  - Motor vehicle accidents
  - Confinement/incapacitation without changing position
  - Prolonged surgery without changing position
- Vessel occlusion
  - Embolism/in vitro thrombosis
  - Vessel clamping during surgery
  - Compartment syndrome
- Excessive muscle activity
  - Delirium tremens
  - Seizures
  - Overexertion (marathon running)
  - Tetanus
- Electrical current
  - Cardioversion
  - High-voltage electrical injury
  - Lightning
- Hyperthermia
  - Exercise
  - Malignant hyperthermia
  - Serotonin syndrome
  - Neuroleptic malignant syndrome
  - Sepsis

Non-physical Causes

- Inborn errors of metabolism
- Drugs and toxins
  - Cocaine
  - Ethanol
  - Heroin
  - Insect and snake venoms
  - Statins
  - Fibrates
  - Anti-depressants
  - Benzodiazepines
- Infections
  - *Legionella*
  - Streptococcal (necrotizing fasciitis)
  - Coxsackie
  - Herpes virus
  - Influenza A and B
  - Epstein–Barr
  - Adenovirus
  - HIV
  - Cytomegalovirus
- Electrolyte imbalances
  - Hyperosmotic conditions
  - Hypernatremia
  - Hypocalcemia
  - Hyponatremia
  - Hypokalemia
  - Hypophosphatemia

The major causes of rhabdomyolysis in patients admitted to the emergency department of an urban population in the United States are cocaine, exercise, and immobilization. In the United States, rhabdomyolysis is commonly diagnosed in intoxicated patients subjected to prolonged muscle compression as they lay motionless, in elderly patients following a fall or stroke, and in patients with seizure disorders. Trauma and crush injuries following motor vehicle accidents and collapse of buildings are other common causes of rhabdomyolysis. All trauma patients should be screened for rhabdomyolysis.[2] Acute alcohol-induced rhabdomyolysis can occur after binge drinking or a sustained period of alcohol abuse, and is associated with pain and swelling of muscles, particularly the quadriceps. Rhabdomyolysis has rarely been reported when a surgical procedure is performed in an improper position or following the prolonged use of a tourniquet. Myoglobinemia and myoglobinuria and a mild elevation of CPK may occur after strenuous physical exertion. However, when physical exertion is extreme, it can cause myolysis with severe rhabdomyolysis; this is especially likely to occur when strenuous exercise is performed under condition of high temperature and humidity. Hypokalemia increases the risk of rhabdomyolysis during strenuous exercise. Athletes who abuse diuretics are therefore at a high risk of developing rhabdomyolysis during strenuous exercise. Medications and recreational drugs are important causes of rhabdomyolysis. Drug-induced rhabdomyolysis encompasses a large group of substances that can affect muscles by different mechanisms.

Statins (3-hydroxy-3-methylglutaryl coenzyme A reductase inhibitors) are an important cause of myositis and rhabdomyolysis.[3,4] Risk factors for the development of a statin-induced myopathy include the following:

- High dosages
- Increasing age
- Female sex
- Renal and hepatic insufficiency
- Diabetes mellitus
- Concomitant therapy with drugs such as
    - fibrates
    - cyclosporine
    - azole anti-fungals
    - macrolide antibiotics
    - warfarin
    - digoxin

Individual statins may differ in their risk of inducing rhabdomyolysis with some patients developing this syndrome when switching from one statin to another. Other patients develop rhabdomyolysis when exposed to any statin. It is probable that genetic factors play a role in the pathogenesis of this syndrome.[5]

■ PATHOPHYSIOLOGY

Muscle injury, regardless of mechanism, results in a cascade of events that leads to leakage of extracellular calcium ions into the intracellular space.[6] The excess of calcium causes a pathological interaction of actin and myosin and activates cellular proteases with muscle destruction and fiber necrosis. The final common effector pathway is thought to be an increase in free cytosolic ionized calcium, which may start a cascade of effects leading to major cell permeability and capillary leak. With muscle injury, large quantities of potassium, phosphate, myoglobin, CK, and urate leak into the circulation. Myoglobin in the renal glomerular filtrate can precipitate and cause renal tubular obstruction, leading to renal damage.

Mechanisms of Acute Renal Failure in Rhabdomyolysis Patients

It has been suggested that there are two crucial factors in the development of myoglobinuric acute renal failure; these include hypovolemia/dehydration and aciduria.[6] Three main mechanisms influence heme protein toxicity: renal vasoconstriction with diminished renal circulation, intraluminal cast formation, and direct heme protein-induced cytotoxicity. In the absence of hypovolemia and aciduria, heme proteins have minimal nephrotoxic effects; however, when these conditions are present, heme proteins can induce renal dysfunction by a variety of mechanisms.[7] Released heme proteins produce a synergistic effect on renal vasoconstriction initiated through hypovolemia and activation of the cytokine cascade. Pigmented casts are a characteristic of rhabdomyolysis-associated acute renal failure. These are a result of the interaction of Tamm–Horsfall protein with myoglobin, which is enhanced at a low pH.

■ CLINICAL MANIFESTATIONS

There is a wide variation in the clinical presentation of rhabdomyolysis. The "classic" triad of symptoms includes muscle pain, weakness and dark urine. The most frequently involved muscle groups are the calves and lower back. The muscles can be tender and swollen, and there can be skin changes indicating pressure necrosis. However, these classic features are seen in less than 10% of patients. Some patients experience severe excruciating pain. The calf pain may erroneously result in a workup for deep venous thrombosis and the back pain can mimic renal colic. Similarly, involvement of the chest musculature can present with "anginal"-type chest pain. Over 50% of the patients may not complain of muscle pain or weakness. The initial clinical sign of rhabdomyolysis may be the appearance of discolored urine. Urine can range from pink-tinged, to cola colored, to dark black.

Severe hyperkalemia occurs secondary to massive muscle breakdown, causing cardiac dysrhythmias and possibly cardiac arrest. Hepatic dysfunction occurs in 25% of patients with rhabdomyolysis.[8] Proteases released from injured muscle cause hepatic injury. Acute renal failure and diffuse intravascular coagulation are late complications, developing 12–72 h after the acute insult.

Laboratory Findings

Although history and physical examination can provide clues, the diagnosis of rhabdomyolysis is confirmed by laboratory studies. CK levels are the most sensitive indicator of myocyte injury in rhabdomyolysis. Normal CK enzyme levels are 45–260 U/l. In rhabdomyolysis, CK rises within 12 h of the onset of muscle injury, peaks in 1–3 days, and declines 3–5 days after cessation of muscle injury. The peak CK level may be predictive of the development of renal failure. Abnormal CK levels are commonly seen in injured ICU patients, and a level of 5,000 U/l or greater is related to renal failure.[2,9] The half-life of CK is 1.5 days and so it remains elevated longer than serum myoglobin levels.

Both ARF and the increased release of creatinine from skeletal muscle increase the serum concentrations of urea nitrogen and creatinine. However, the creatinine is elevated to a greater extent than the blood urea nitrogen (BUN), narrowing the normal 10:1 ratio of urea nitrogen to creatinine to 6:1 or less. Other findings include hyperkalemia, hypocalcemia, hyperphosphatemia, hyperuricemia, and elevated levels of other muscle enzymes like lactate dehydrogenase, aldolase, aminotransferases, and carbonic anhydrase III.

■ MANAGEMENT

The treatment of rhabdomyolysis includes initial stabilization and resuscitation of the patient while concomitantly attempting to preserve renal function. Retrospective analysis seems to show that early aggressive fluid replacement with saline is beneficial in minimizing the occurrence of renal failure. The longer it takes for rehydration to be initiated, the more likely it is that renal failure will develop.[10] Forced diuresis, when started within 6 h of admission, has been reported to minimize the risk of acute renal failure.[11] Mannitol and bicarbonate are commonly employed following the initial resuscitation with saline.[12,13] It has been suggested that mannitol may be protective due to the associated diuresis which minimizes intratubular heme pigment deposition and mannitol may act as a free radical scavenger, thereby minimizing cell injury. Furosemide and other loop diuretics have been advocated for use in patients with myoglobinuric renal impairment in an attempt to initiate diuresis and convert anuric to oliguric renal failure.

Alkalinization of the urine has been suggested to minimize renal damage after rhabdomyolysis. After resuscitation and restoration of normal renal perfusion, the kidneys clear a large acid load resulting in an acidic urine. It has been postulated that these patients may be unable to alkaline their urine without the administration of bicarbonate, and this increases the risk of tubular cast development and renal injury. However, others have argued that large volume infusion of crystalloid alone creates a solute diuresis sufficient to alkalinize the urine.[14] Furthermore, large doses of bicarbonate may worsen the degree of hypocalcemia, especially if hypovolemia is corrected.

While mannitol and bicarbonate are considered the standard of care in preventing acute renal failure, there is little clinical evidence to support the use of these agents. While randomized controlled trials are lacking, the available evidence suggests that mannitol and bicarbonate have no benefit over and above aggressive fluid resuscitation alone.[15] In a retrospective study of 24 patients, Homsi et al. demonstrated that volume expansion with saline alone prevented progression to renal failure and that the addition of mannitol and bicarbonate had no additional benefit.[16] Using their Trauma Registry and intensive care unit database, Brown and colleagues[2] reviewed the case records of 1,771 trauma patients with increased CK levels. Overall 217 patients (12%) developed renal failure, with 97 requiring dialysis. In this study, peak CK >5,000 U/l was associated with an increased risk of developing renal failure. Of the 382 patients with CK >5,000 U/l, 154 patients (40%) received mannitol and bicarbonate, whereas 228 patients did not. There was no significant difference in the incidence of renal failure (22% vs. 18%), of dialysis (7% vs. 6%), or of mortality (15% vs. 18%) between the two groups. Based on these data it would appear that mannitol and bicarbonate have little additional benefit over aggressive volume replacement with saline alone.

Dialysis

Despite optimal treatment, some patients will develop acute renal failure; severe acidosis and hyperkalemia can also be present. These patients will require renal replacement therapy to correct fluid and electrolyte abnormalities. Daily hemodialysis or continuous hemofiltration may be required initially to remove urea and potassium that are released from damaged muscles. Normalization of potassium is the priority, because hyperkalemic cardiac arrest is a life-threatening early complication. The removal of myoglobin by plasma exchange has not shown benefit.

A unique management issue in rhabdomyolysis-induced acute renal failure is the development of hypercalcemia during the recovery phase in 20–30% of patients. To minimize this complication, the administration of calcium should be avoided during the renal failure phase, unless the patient has symptomatic hypocalcemia or severe hyperkalemia.

■ CLINICAL PEARLS

- Rhabdomyolysis should be considered in all trauma patients as well as patients found unconscious.

- A CPK >5,000 is predictive of renal injury.
- Vigorous fluid resuscitation is the most effective method of limiting renal dysfunction in patients with rhabdomyolysis.

■ REFERENCES

1. Huerta-Alardin AL, Varon J, Marik PE. Bench-to-bedside review: rhabdomyolysis – an overview for clinicians. *Crit Care*. 2005;9:158–169.
2. Brown CV, Rhee P, Chan L, et al. Preventing renal failure in patients with rhabdomyolysis: do bicarbonate and mannitol make a difference? *J Trauma*. 2004;56:1191–1196.
3. Antons KA, Williams CD, Baker SK, et al. Clinical perspectives of statin-induced rhabdomyolysis. *Am J Med*. 2006;119:400–409.
4. Thompson PD, Clarkson P, Karas RH. Statin-associated myopathy. *JAMA*. 2003;289:1681–1690.
5. The Search Collaborative Group. SLCO1B1 variants and statin-induced myopathy- A genomewide study. *N Engl J Med*. 2008;359:789–799.
6. Knochel JP. Mechanisms of rhabdomyolysis. *Curr Opin Rheumatol*. 1993;5:725–731.
7. Zager RA. Studies of mechanisms and protective maneuvers in myoglobinuric acute renal injury. *Lab Invest*. 1989;60:619–629.
8. Akmal M, Massry SG. Reversible hepatic dysfunction associated with rhabdomyolysis. *Am J Nephrol*. 1990;10:49–52.
9. Sharp LS, Rozycki GS, Feliciano DV. Rhabdomyolysis and secondary renal failure in critically ill surgical patients. *Am J Surg*. 2004;188:801–806.
10. Odeh M. The role of reperfusion-induced injury in the pathogenesis of the crush syndrome. *N Engl J Med*. 1991;324:1417–1422.
11. Zager RA. Rhabdomyolysis and myohemoglobinuric acute renal failure. *Kidney Int*. 1996;49:314–326.
12. Ron D, Taitelman U, Michaelson M, et al. Prevention of acute renal failure in traumatic rhabdomyolysis. *Arch Intern Med*. 1984;144:277–280.
13. Gunal AI, Celiker H, Dogukan A, et al. Early and vigorous fluid resuscitation prevents acute renal failure in the crush victims of catastrophic earthquakes. *J Am Soc Nephrol*. 2004;15:1862–1867.
14. Knottenbelt JD. Traumatic rhabdomyolysis from severe beating – experience of volume diuresis in 200 patients. *J Trauma*. 1994;37:214–219.
15. Conger JD. Interventions in clinical acute renal failure: what are the data? *Am J Kidney Dis*. 1995;26:565–576.
16. Homsi E, Barreiro MF, Orlando JM, et al. Prophylaxis of acute renal failure in patients with rhabdomyolysis. *Ren Fail*. 1997;19:283–288.

Part VI

Central Nervous System

46

Ischemic Strokes and Intracerebral Hemorrhage

Stroke causes 9% of all deaths worldwide and is the second most common cause of death after ischemic heart disease. In over 75% of cases the stroke is ischemic in nature. However, unlike acute myocardial infarction, therapeutic interventions which attempt to limit infarct size have been of limited success. Indeed, apart from thrombolytic therapy in a highly selected group of patients (probably less than 5% of "stroke" patients) and aspirin, no therapeutic intervention has been demonstrated to impact on the course of this illness. Considering these data, the rationale for admitting patients to an ICU needs to be evaluated. In addition, aspects of medical care which maximize the potential for recovery and limit complications need to be explored. In most instances, such treatment is best provided by specialized "low-technology" stroke units.

■ STROKE ICUs, MEDICAL ICUs, OR STROKE UNITS

Stroke intensive care units were abandoned in the 1970 s after it was demonstrated that such units had very little impact on the outcome of patients following a stroke. The situation is not much different today; for the overwhelming majority of patients suffering a stroke, acute medical interventions in an ICU have not been established to improve outcome, and in fact, certain interventions may be harmful. Admission to and aggressive management in an ICU may only serve to prolong the dying

P.E. Marik, *Handbook of Evidence-Based Critical Care*,
DOI 10.1007/978-1-4419-5923-2_46,
© Springer Science+Business Media, LLC 2010

process of a patient who has suffered a catastrophic neurological event. Burtin and colleagues[1] evaluated 199 stroke patients who underwent mechanical ventilation in an ICU. The 1-year survival rate was just 8%. Berrouschot et al.[2] reported a 3-month mortality of 79% in patients admitted to an ICU following a space-occupying ("malignant") middle cerebral artery infarction despite aggressive medical care.

A small group of patients who suffer a stroke may benefit from admission to the ICU if they develop a reversible/treatable medical complication. Endotracheal intubation should be reserved for patients with reversible respiratory failure or comatose patients who are likely to have a good prognosis for a functional recovery. Burtin and colleagues have demonstrated that patients with an absent gag reflex on admission to hospital will almost always die from their stroke.[1] Although intubation and hyperventilation are routine, though heroic measures in patients after severe stroke, their efficacy in reducing mortality and improving functional recovery has never been established. In fact, hyperventilation with induced hypocarbia may reduce perfusion to the penumbral brain regions and increase infarct size. Furthermore, it is arguable that endotracheal intubation and mechanical ventilation will reduce the risk of atelectasis and pneumonia in patients with an impaired level of consciousness when compared to good nursing and respiratory care without endotracheal intubation.

■ PROFILES PREDICTIVE OF FUTILITY AFTER A DEVASTATING STROKE

- Aneurysmal SAH[3]
  - Persistent coma after attempts to lower ICP
  - Massive intraventricular hemorrhage with hydrocephalus
  - Presence of delayed global edema on CT
- Lobar intracerebral hemorrhage
  - Coma with extensor posturing and absent pontomesencephalic reflexes
  - Coma with septum pellucidum shift >6 mm on CT
- Ganglionic intracerebral hemorrhage
  - Coma with hydrocephalus and hematoma size >60 cm^3
- Pontine hemorrhage
  - Coma with hyperthermia and tachycardia
  - Coma with acute hydrocephalus and hemorrhage extension into the thalamus
- Cerebellar hemorrhage
  - Absent corneal reflexes
  - Absent oculocephalic response with hydrocephalus

- Hemispheric ischemic infarction
  - Clinical deterioration with coma and loss of pontomesencephalic reflexes
  - Shift of pineal gland >4 mm on CT scan performed within 48 h
- Cerebellar ischemic infarction
  - Persistent coma after decompressive surgery

The failure of specific interventions to improve the outcome of patients suffering a stroke should not imply that physicians should adopt a fatalistic approach when managing these patients. A number of well-conducted clinical trials have demonstrated that the mortality and functional recovery of patients following a stroke is significantly improved when these patients are cared for in a specialized stroke unit as compared to a general medical ward. These units provide specialized nursing care and a well-organized multi-disciplinary rehabilitation program. Stroke unit care reduces the medical complications in stroke patients and allows for earlier and more intense rehabilitation. The Stroke Council of the American Heart Association (AHA) recommends "rapid transfer of a patient to a hospital that has a specialized stroke care unit."[4]

■ ACUTE ISCHEMIC STROKES

Ischemic stokes may be conveniently classified as follows:

- Large vessel atherosclerotic
- Cardioembolic
- Small artery (lacuna)
- Stroke of other identified cause (e.g., vasculitis)
- Stroke of undetermined cause

At present, no intervention with putative neuroprotective actions has been established as effective in improving outcomes after stroke and therefore none currently can be recommended.[4] Similarly hemodilution, volume expansion, vasodilators, and induced hypertension cannot be recommended.

Thrombolytic Therapy

The National Institute of Neurological Disorders and Stroke (NINDS) rt-PA Stroke Trial demonstrated that rt-PA given to patients within 3 h of the onset of stroke resulted in an 11–13% absolute increase in the chance of minimum or no disability at 3 months.[5] Studies with a longer time window for enrollment have demonstrated a higher mortality in the treatment group, largely due to an increased incidence of intracerebral hemorrhage. In the European Cooperative Acute Stroke Study (ECASS), patients with moderate to severe acute ischemic strokes were randomized (<6 h) to placebo or rt-PA. Patients with infarction involving more than one-third of the middle cerebral artery territory on CT scan were excluded. At 30 days, there was a higher mortality in the rt-PA group (17.9% vs. 12.7%).[6] Large parenchymal hemorrhages were increased threefold in the rt-PA group. The lack of benefit of in the rt-PA group was ascribed to inappropriate CT scan interpretation in the haste of emergency management of the stroke patients (109 of the 620 randomized patients were not appropriate). In the second European Cooperative Acute Stroke Study (ECASS II), no benefit for rt-PA was demonstrated; furthermore, treatment differences were similar whether patients were treated within 3 h or 3–6 h.[7]

More recently ECASS III reported the results of a study in which alteplase (0.9 mg/kg) or placebo was administered between 3 and 4.5 h after the onset of acute ischemic stroke.[8] Patients with severe stroke were excluded from this trial. Although mortality did not differ between groups, more patients have a favorable outcome with alteplase than with placebo (52.4% vs. 45.2%; OR 1.34; 95% CI 1.02–1.76, $p = 0.04$).

These data demonstrate that the benefits of thrombolytic therapy decrease with time, while the risks (intracranial bleeding) increase with time; time is therefore of the essence. Thrombolytic therapy is best administered at regional centers that have experience with this therapy and where the timely evaluation and initiation of therapy can be instituted; selected patients may benefit when the window of treatment is extended up to 4.5 h.

The most recent guidelines from the Stroke Council of the American Heart Association suggest the following inclusion and exclusion criteria for thrombolytic therapy[4]:

- Diagnosis of ischemic stroke causing measurable neurological deficit.
- The neurological signs should not be clearing spontaneously.
- The neurological signs should not be minor or isolated.
- Caution should be exercised in treating patients with major deficits.
- The symptoms of stroke should not be suggestive of subarachnoid hemorrhage.
- Onset of symptoms <3 h before beginning treatment (this can now be extended up to 4.5 h in selected patients).
- No head trauma or stroke in previous 3 months.
- No myocardial infarction in previous 3 months.
- No GIT or urinary tract hemorrhage in previous 21 days.

- No major surgery in previous 14 days.
- No history of previous intracranial hemorrhage.
- Blood pressure not elevated (SBP <185 mmHg or DBP <110 mmHg).
- Not taking an oral anti-coagulant or if anti-coagulant being taken, INR <1.5
- If receiving heparin in previous 48 h, aPTT must be normal.
- Platelet count >100,000.
- No seizure.
- CT does not show multi-lobar infarction (hypodensity >one-third of the cerebral hemisphere.
- The patient or family members understand the potential risks and benefits from treatment.

The role of intra-arterial thrombolysis in patients with ischemic stroke is unclear. This treatment modality is however an option in selected patients who have had a major stoke of <4 h duration due to occlusion of the MCA and who are not otherwise candidates for intravenous rt-PA (recent surgery, etc.).[4] Treatment requires the patient to be at an experienced stroke center with immediate access to cerebral angiography and qualified interventionists.

Treatment of Acute Ischemic Stroke with Intravenous rt-PA

- Infuse 0.9 mg/kg (maximum dose 90 mg) over 60 min with 10% of the dose given as a bolus over 1 min.[4]
- Admit the patient to an ICU or a stroke unit for monitoring.
- Perform neurological assessments every 15 min during the infusion and every 30 min thereafter for the next 6 h, then hourly until 24 h after treatment.
- If the patient develops severe headache, acute hypertension, nausea, or vomiting, discontinue the infusion (if rt-PA being administered) and obtain emergency CT scan.
- Measure blood pressure every 15 min for the first 2 h and subsequently every 30 min for the next 6 h, then hourly until 24 h after treatment.
- Increase the frequency of BP measurements if SBP >180 mmHg or if DBP >105 mmHg; administer anti-hypertensive medication to maintain BP below these levels (see Chapter 25).
- Delay placement of NG tubes, CVCs, bladder catheters, or intra-arterial catheters.
- Obtain a follow-up CT scan at 24 h before starting anti-coagulants or anti-platelet drugs.

Anti-platelet Therapy and Anti-coagulation

The International Stroke Trial (IST) randomized (using a factorial design) over 19,000 patients within 48 h of an acute ischemic stroke to 14 days of treatment with placebo, heparin (5,000 or 12,500 U q 12 h), or aspirin 300 mg daily.[9] Aspirin resulted in a 1.1% absolute reduction in recurrent ischemic strokes at 14 days; both heparin regimens had no effect on outcome. Additional studies have demonstrated that heparin, low molecular weight heparin, and heparinoids do not improve outcome following a stroke.[10,11] The current AHA/American Stroke Association (ASA) guidelines do not recommend urgent anti-coagulation for patients with moderate to severe strokes because of an increased risk of serious intracranial hemorrhage. Nor do they recommend anti-coagulant therapy following rt-PA.[4] However, these guidelines recommend treatment with aspirin (initial dose of 325 mg) within 24–48 after stroke onset.

Anti-coagulation in Cardioembolic Stroke

Hemorrhage into the infarct occurs in about 30% of cases of all embolic infarcts; it may however, require 3 or 4 days or longer to become apparent on the CT scan. However, magnetic resonance imaging has demonstrated that by 3 weeks, hemorrhagic conversion occurs in up to 70% of patients. Hemorrhage ranges from the usual cortical petechial to confluent hematomas. In non-anti-coagulated patients, infarct volume seems to be the only independent predictor of hemorrhagic conversion.

Chronic anti-coagulant therapy has been demonstrated to reduce the risk of recurrent embolization in patients who have suffered an embolic stroke. Approximately 80% of patients who have suffered a cerebral embolic stroke will suffer a subsequent embolic stroke without anti-coagulation. In the "ORG 19172" study, only 2 of 123 patients with cardioembolic strokes treated with placebo (i.e., received no heparin) suffered a recurrent ischemic event during the study period.[10] In the IST trial, recurrent ischemic stroke (during the study period) occurred in 4.9% of patients with cardioembolic stoke randomized to receive placebo compared to 2.8% who received heparin.[9] However, hemorrhagic transformation occurred in 2.1% of patients receiving heparin compared to 0.4% receiving placebo. Based on these data it may be prudent to delay anti-coagulation for 10–14 days, particularly in patients with large cerebral infarcts and hypertensive patients. The role of transesophageal echocardiography (TEE) in these patients is unclear. However, it may be prudent to perform TEE in patients at high risk of early recurrent embolization and to commence anti-coagulation earlier if clot is visualized within the cardiac cambers and CT scan does not show evidence of hemorrhagic transformation. The HAEST study compared LMWH and aspirin in 449 patients with an acute ischemic stroke and atrial fibrillation.[12] In this study, the frequency of recurrent ischemic stroke during the first 14 days was 8.5% in the LMWH group and 7.5% in the aspirin group. There was no difference in the rate of ICH between the treatment groups. These data suggest that patients with embolic stroke and atrial fibrillation should receive aspirin during the acute phase of the stroke with the initiation of chronic oral anti-coagulation between 10 and 14 days.

Decompressive Surgery

Hemispheric decompression in young patients with malignant middle cerebral artery territory infarction and space-occupying brain edema has been demonstrated to improve outcome. An individual patient meta-analysis demonstrated a marked improvement in neurological recovery and survival with decompressive craniectomy.[13] This combination occurs in about 1–10% of patients with supratentorial hemispheric infarcts and usually arises between 2 and 5 days after stroke.

Treatment of Hyperglycemia

Both animal and human data suggest that postinfarction hyperglycemia increases neuronal damage with an increase in infarct size. These data suggest that hyperglycemia should be treated, with careful monitoring of the serum glucose (hypoglycemia may extend infarct size). The optimal target blood glucose level in this group of patients is yet to be determined; however, a level between 110 and 140 mg/dl appears reasonable (see Chapter 39). Results of clinical trials in critically ill patients suggest improved outcome with early enteral nutrition. Prevention of hyperglycemia once feeding is initiated is important.

Treatment of Fever

Fever has been shown to worsen the prognosis in acute stroke. It is therefore reasonable to treat fever in stroke patients with anti-pyretics.[14] The goal should be to keep patients normothermic. In animal models of focal cerebral ischemia, hypothermia significantly reduces infarct size and improves outcome;[15] however, the role of induced hypothermia in patients with ischemic stroke has yet to be determined.

Treatment of Poststroke Hypertension

The vast majority of patients with cerebral ischemia present with acutely elevated BP regardless of the sub-type of infarct or pre-existing hypertension.[16,17] The BP elevation spontaneously decreases over time. The elevated BP is not a manifestation of a hypertensive emergency but rather a protective physiologic response to maintain cerebral perfusion pressure to the vascular territory affected by ischemia. Lowering the BP in patients with ischemic strokes may reduce cerebral blood flow, which because of impaired autoregulation may result in further ischemic injury. The common practice of "normalizing" the BP following a cerebrovascular accident is potentially dangerous. When a proximal arterial obstruction results in a mild stroke, a fall in BP may result in further infarction involving the entire territory of that artery. It should be noted that the Intravenous Nimodipine West European Trial of intravenous nimodipine for acute stroke was stopped because of increased neurological deterioration in the treatment group, which the investigators attributed to the effects of hypotension.[18,19] A meta-analysis evaluating the use of oral or intravenous calcium channel blockers initiated at 6 h–5 days after symptom onset in acute ischemic stroke patients found that intravenous administration, higher doses, and administration within 12 h of symptom onset were associated with an increased risk of poor outcomes.[20] The increased risk of poor outcomes is probably limited to patients treated very aggressively or to specific anti-hypertensive agents. The Acute Candesartan Cilexetil Evaluation in Stroke Survivors (ACCESS) trial initiated treatment with either the angiotensin receptor-1 blocker (ARB) candesartan or placebo in patients with ischemic stroke and a BP measurement >200/100 mmHg 6–24 h after admission or >180/105 mmHg at 24–36 h.[21] Both the cumulative 12-month mortality rate (2.9% vs. 7.2%) and the incidence of vascular events (9.8% vs. 18.7%) were lower in the candesartan-treated group; however, the primary outcome of disability measured by Barthel index at 3 months was not different between the two treatment groups. The mechanism(s) by which the ARB exerted its beneficial effects is unclear, as the blood pressure profiles were nearly identical in the treatment and placebo groups. Additional studies are required to confirm the benefit of ARBs in patients with ischemic stroke.

The management of high BP in acute ischemic stroke is highly controversial because of a lack of reliable evidence from randomized, controlled trials. The current recommendations regarding BP management in acute ischemic stroke are based on two observations: (1) BP reduction is associated with an increased risk of neurological deterioration and worse outcome in patients with ischemic stroke in some studies, although a causal relationship has not been demonstrated conclusively and (2) the benefit of acute BP lowering (unlike chronic treatment) in patients with ischemic stroke remains unclear. There may be a reduction of cardiovascular events with early institution of angiotensin receptor antagonists; however, the benefit is not conclusively related to BP reduction. Therefore, in the absence of definitive benefit, both the ASA and the European Stroke Initiative are consistent in not recommending routine lowering of BP unless it repeatedly exceeds 200–220 mmHg systolic or 120 mmHg diastolic in the acute period.[4,22] In these patients the aim is to reduce the pressure by not more than 10–15% in the first 24 h. While the drug of choice is unclear, a short-acting intravenous agent is currently recommended, i.e., labetalol, nicardipine, or clevidipine (see Chapter 25). These patients may benefit from weaning to an ARB.

Both the ASA and the European Stroke Initiative guidelines recommend the reduction of BP according to the eligibility thresholds for inclusion in the NINDS rt-PA efficacy trial before thrombolytics are administered. Anti-hypertensive therapy is therefore required for SBP >185 mmHg or DBP >110 mmHg with a targeted SBP of 180 mmHg and a DBP of 105 mmHg.

Supportive Medical Therapy

- General measures are aimed at maintaining an adequate cerebral perfusion pressure and preventing complications.
- Maintain euvolemia; hypovolemia will compromise cardiac output and cerebral perfusion, thereby extending the size of the infarct. Avoid hypotonic solutions which will increase cerebral edema. Stroke patients may develop the "cerebral salt-wasting syndrome," which requires aggressive volume replacement.
- Bed rest with elevation of the head to 20–35°.
- Laxatives.
- DVT prophylaxis (stockings/pneumatic boots/LMWH).
- Mild sedation/anxiolysis for agitated patients. In patients who require deeper sedation/hypnosis (for example, to facilitate mechanical ventilation), propofol is a useful agent. This drug decreases ICP (and CBF proportionately) and allows frequent neurological assessment due to its short duration of action.
- Regular chest physiotherapy and physical therapy.
- Speech and swallowing assessment. The ability of the patient to swallow should be assessed as abnormalities of swallowing occur in up to 40% of patients. In patients with swallowing dysfunction, enteral feeding should be achieved using a small bore feeding nasoenteric tube. In the majority of patients, swallowing function will recover in 7–10 days. Occasionally prolonged supportive feeding may be required, necessitating placement of a gastrostomy/gastrojejunostomy (see Chapter 20).
- Fever should be treated with acetaminophen.

- Corticosteroids have no role in the management of cerebral edema and increased intracranial pressure after stroke.
- The frequency of seizures during the acute period after stroke is reported to be between 4 and 43%. Recurrent seizures occur in approximately 20–80% of cases. There are no data concerning the value of prophylactic administration of anti-convulsants after ischemic stroke. Until such data become available, stroke patients who are seizure free should not receive anti-convulsant drugs.

■ INTRACEREBRAL HEMORRHAGES

Approximately 15% of all strokes are hemorrhagic. The mortality rate in the first 30 days after ICH is 35–50% with more than half of the deaths occurring in the first 2 days. Clot volume is the most powerful predictor of outcome. Other important variables are baseline neurological status and intraventricular hemorrhage volume. Although previously thought to be rare, recurrence or extension of ICH recently has been shown to be a relatively common occurrence affecting as many as one-third of patients in the early period after ICH. The principles of management of intracerebral hemorrhage are similar to those of acute ischemic stokes, with a few exceptions.

A urine toxic screen should be obtained as part of the initial evaluation in ICH patients, particularly the young and the normotensive; substances implicated in the causation of ICH include cocaine, amphetamines, methylphenidate, Talwin–pyribenzamine, phencyclidine, and phenylpropanolamine.

Two randomized trials showed no benefit on regional blood flow, neurological improvement, mortality, and functional outcomes from the regular use of intravenous mannitol boluses.[23,24] Those patients with ICH while receiving anti-coagulant therapy should have emergent correction of the abnormal coagulation parameters to prevent further enlargement of the hematoma (see Chapter 52). In patients with ICH and mechanical heart valves, temporary interruption of anti-coagulation therapy seems safe in patients without previous evidence of systemic embolization. For most patients at risk of cardioembolic stroke, discontinuation of anti-coagulation for 1–2 weeks should be sufficient to observe the evolution of a parenchymal hematoma (or to clip or coil a ruptured aneurysm, or to evacuate an acute subdural hematoma). Seizure prophylaxis with anti-convulsants is generally recommended for patients with lobar hematomas. A phase II study demonstrated an improvement in neurological outcome and mortality in patients with an ICH treated with activated recombinant factor VII (fVIIa).[25] However, a large phase III trial (FAST) was unable to reproduce these findings.[26]

To facilitate early and effective clearance of blood in the ventricles, recent efforts have focused on intraventricular use of thrombolytic drugs in patients who have intraventricular hemorrhage in association with spontaneous intracerebral hemorrhage.[27] Furthermore, observational studies have shown encouraging results for endoscopic removal of intraventricular hemorrhage.[28]

Blood Pressure Control

The acute hypertensive response in intracerebral hemorrhage is characterized by its high prevalence, self-limiting nature, and prognostic significance. In an analysis of 45,330 patients with intracerebral hemorrhage, 75% had systolic blood pressure greater than 140 mmHg and 20% greater than 180 mmHg at presentation.[29] The high blood pressure might be secondary to uncontrolled chronic hypertension, with disruption of central autonomic pathways by intracerebral hemorrhage. High blood pressure is associated with hematoma enlargement and poor outcome; however, an exact cause and effect relation is unproven.

The current ASA Stroke Council guidelines recommend that "until ongoing clinical trials of blood pressure intervention for intracerebral hemorrhage are completed, physicians must manage blood pressure on the basis of the present incomplete evidence..." by maintaining systolic blood pressure less than 180 mmHg in the acute period with short half-life intravenous anti-hypertensive drugs.[30]

Recent data suggest a greater therapeutic benefit with more aggressive lowering of blood pressure. The Antihypertensive Treatment of Acute Cerebral Hemorrhage (ATACH) trial and the Intensive Blood Pressure Reduction in Acute Cerebral Hemorrhage (INTERACT) trial reported that aggressive reduction of blood pressure to less than 140 mmHg probably decreases the rate of substantial hematoma enlargement without increasing adverse events.[31,32] Because the effect on clinical outcome has not been fully assessed, the more conservative targets set in the ASA Stroke Council and the EUSI guidelines should be followed.[30,33] Great caution is advised about lowering blood pressure too aggressively without concomitant management of cerebral perfusion pressure.

Surgical Interventions

Routine surgical interventions include placing an ICP monitor in patients who have large hemorrhages or performing a ventriculostomy in patients who display evidence of obstructive hydrocephalus. Urgent surgical decompression is indicated in patients with cerebellar hematomas greater than 3 cm in diameter or with brain-stem compression. Open craniotomy and decompression of cortical or lobar hemorrhages have been associated with a higher mortality over medical therapy.[34] The ASA Stroke Council and the EUSI guidelines do not recommend routine evacuation of supratentorial hemorrhage by standard craniotomy within 96 h of the ictus.[30,33] Both guidelines recommend surgery for patients presenting with lobar hemorrhage within 1 cm of the surface, particularly for those with good neurological status who are deteriorating clinically. The role of stereotactic approaches to clot evacuation is yet to be determined.

■ SUBDURAL HEMATOMA

The collection of fresh blood under the dura mater is referred to as an acute subdural hematoma. Data from the Traumatic Coma Data Bank indicate that 21% of all severely injured patients have subdural hematomas. Subdural hematoma is usually caused by injury to an artery or a vein within or over the brain surface. The clinical presentation includes a wide spectrum of neurological findings secondary to either mass effect or direct brain injury. On CT scan the lesion is seen as a hyperdense extraaxial collection that is crescent shaped. Patients presenting with acute neurological deficits and a CT scan demonstrating an acute subdural hematoma should undergo emergent surgery. Surgical intervention may not be required for patients with small lesions less than 3 mm thick on CT scan or those who present with neurological signs after a significant delay.

■ EPIDURAL HEMATOMA

Like subdural hematoma, epidural hematomas are most commonly associated with head trauma, especially in association with skull fractures. They are rarely seen in adults over the age of 60 years, because after this age the dura adheres tightly to the inner table of the calvarium. The most common locations are temporal and frontal. When identified the most common source is the middle meningeal artery. The primary therapy for an acute epidural hematoma is surgery, usually urgently. Mannitol, furosemide, and hyperventilation are used when patients deteriorate clinically from an awake state to one of decreased arousal or agitation.

■ CLINICAL PEARLS

- Patients with a stroke are best managed in a dedicated stroke unit.
- Thrombolytic therapy should be considered in patients presenting with 4.5 h of the onset of an ischemic stroke.
- As a general rule, patients who have suffered a massive stroke do not "benefit" from intubation, mechanical ventilation, and treatment in an ICU.
- Patients with an ischemic stroke and a systolic BP >200 or >180 mmHg after a hemorrhagic stroke require cautious lowering of their blood pressure with a short-acting intravenous antihypertensive agent. These patients should be managed in an ICU with meticulous attention paid to prevent excessive lowering of the BP.

■ REFERENCES

1. Burtin P, Bollaert PE, Feldmann L, et al. Prognosis of stroke patients undergoing mechanical ventilation. *Intensive Care Med.* 1994;20:32–36.
2. Berrouschot J, Sterker M, Bettin S, et al. Mortality of space-occupying ('malignant') middle cerebral artery infarction under conservative intensive care. *Intensive Care Med.* 1998;24:620–623.
3. Wijdicks EF, Rabinstein AA. Absolutely no hope? Some ambiguity of futility of care in devastating acute stroke. *Crit Care Med.* 2004;32:2332–2342.
4. Adams HP, Del ZG, Alberts MJ, et al. Guidelines for the early management of adults with ischemic stroke: a guideline from the American Heart Association/American Stroke Association Stroke Council, Clinical Cardiology Council, Cardiovascular Radiology and Intervention Council, and the Atherosclerotic Peripheral Vascular Disease and Quality of Care Outcomes in Research Interdisciplinary Working Groups: the American Academy of Neurology affirms the value of this guideline as an educational tool for neurologists. *Stroke.* 2007;38:1655–1711.
5. NINDS rtPA Stroke Study Group. Tissue plasminogen activator for acute ischemic stroke. *N Engl J Med.* 1995;333:1581–1587.
6. Hacke W, Kaste M, Fieschi C, et al. Intravenous thrombolysis with recombinant tissue plasminogen activator for acute hemispheric stroke. The European Cooperative Acute Stroke Study (ECASS). *JAMA.* 1995;274:1017–1025.
7. Hacke W, Kaste M, Fieschi C, et al. Randomised double-blind placebo-controlled trial of thrombolytic therapy with intravenous

alteplase in acute ischaemic stroke (ECASS II). Second European–Australasian Acute Stroke Study Investigators. *Lancet.* 1998;352: 1245–1251.

8. Hacke W, Kaste M, Bluhmki E, et al. Thrombolysis with alteplase 3 to 4.5 hours after acute ischemic stroke. *N Engl J Med.* 2008;359: 1317–1329.

9. International Stroke Trial Collaborative Group. The International Stroke Trial (IST): a randomised trial of aspirin, subcutaneous heparin, both, or neither among 19,435 patients with acute ischaemic stroke. *Lancet.* 1997;349:1569–1581.

10. The Publications Committee for the Trial of ORG 10172 in Acute Stroke Treatment (TOAST) Investigators. Low molecular weight heparinoid, ORG 10172 (Danaparoid), and outcome after acute ischemic stroke. A randomized controlled trial. *JAMA.* 1998;279:1265–1272.

11. Roden-Jullig A, Britton M. Effectiveness of heparin treatment for progressing ischaemic stroke: before and after study. *J Intern Med.* 2000;248:287–291.

12. Berge E, Abdelnoor M, Nakstad PH, et al. Low molecular-weight heparin versus aspirin in patients with acute ischaemic stroke and atrial fibrillation: a double-blind randomised study. HAEST Study Group. Heparin in Acute Embolic Stroke Trial. *Lancet.* 2000;355:1205–1210.

13. Vahedi K, Hofmeijer J, Juettler E, et al. Early decompressive surgery in malignant infarction of the middle cerebral artery: a pooled analysis of three randomised controlled trials. *Lancet Neurol.* 2007;6:215–222.

14. Marion DW. Controlled normothermia in neurologic intensive care. *Crit Care Med.* 2004;32:S43–S45.

15. van der Worp HB, Sena ES, Donnan GA, et al. Hypothermia in animal models of acute ischaemic stroke: a systematic review and meta-analysis. *Brain.* 2007;130:3063–3074.

16. Wallace JD, Levy LL. Blood pressure after stroke. *JAMA.* 1981;246:2177–2180.

17. Britton M, Carlsson A, de Faire U. Blood pressure course in patients with acute stroke and matched controls. *Stroke.* 1986;17:861–864.

18. Wahlgren NG, MacMohon DG, De Keyser J, et al. The Intravenous Nimodipine West European Trial (INWEST) of nimodipine in the treatment of acute ischemic stroke. *Cerebrovasc Dis.* 1994;4: 204–210.

19. Ahmed N, Nasman P, Wahlgren NG. Effect of intravenous nimodipine on blood pressure and outcome after acute stroke. *Stroke.* 2000;31: 1250–1255.

20. Horn J, Limburg M. Calcium antagonists for acute ischemic stroke. *Cochrane Database Syst Rev.* 2000;CD001928.

21. Schrader J, Luders S, Kulschewski A, et al. The ACCESS Study: evaluation of acute candesartan cilexetil therapy in stroke survivors. *Stroke.* 2003;34:1699–1703.

22. Klijn CJ, Hankey GJ, American Stroke Association and European Stroke Initiative. et al. Management of acute ischaemic stroke: new guidelines from the American Stroke Association and European Stroke Initiative. *Lancet Neurol.* 2003;2:698–701.
23. Misra UK, Kalita J, Ranjan P, et al. Mannitol in intracerebral hemorrhage: a randomized controlled study. *J Neurol Sci.* 2005;234:41–45.
24. Kalita J, Misra UK, Ranjan P, et al. Effect of mannitol on regional cerebral blood flow in patients with intracerebral hemorrhage. *J Neurol Sci.* 2004;224:19–22.
25. Mayer SA, Brun NC, Begtrup K, et al. Recombinant activated Factor VII for acute intracerebral hemorrhage. *N Engl J Med.* 2005;352:777–785.
26. Mayer SA, Brun NC, Begtrup K, et al. Efficacy and safety of recombinant activated factor VII for acute intracerebral hemorrhage. *N Engl J Med.* 2008;358:2127–2137.
27. Naff NJ, Hanley DF, Keyl PM, et al. Intraventricular thrombolysis speeds blood clot resolution: results of a pilot, prospective, randomized, double-blind, controlled trial. *Neurosurg.* 2004;54:577–583.
28. Yadav YR, Mukerji G, Shenoy R, et al. Endoscopic management of hypertensive intraventricular haemorrhage with obstructive hydrocephalus. *BMC Neurol.* 2007;7:1.
29. Qureshi AI, Ezzeddine MA, Nasar A, et al. Prevalence of elevated blood pressure in 563,704 adult patients with stroke presenting to the ED in the United States. *Am J Emerg Med.* 2007;25:32–38.
30. Broderick J, Connolly S, Feldmann E, et al. Guidelines for the management of spontaneous intracerebral hemorrhage in adults: 2007 update: a guideline from the American Heart Association/American Stroke Association Stroke Council, High Blood Pressure Research Council, and the Quality of Care and Outcomes in Research Interdisciplinary Working Group. *Stroke.* 2007;38:20012023.
31. Anderson CS, Huang Y, Wang JG, et al. Intensive blood pressure reduction in acute cerebral haemorrhage trial (INTERACT): a randomised pilot trial. *Lancet Neurol.* 2008;7:391–399.
32. Qureshi, A. I. Antihypertensive treatment of acute cerebral hemorrhage (ATACH) trial. New Orleans, LA, International Stroke Conference. 2-22-2008.
33. Steiner T, Kaste M, Forsting M, et al. Recommendations for the management of intracranial haemorrhage – part I: spontaneous intracerebral haemorrhage. The European Stroke Initiative Writing Committee and the Writing Committee for the EUSI Executive Committee. *Cerebrovasc Dis.* 2006;22:294–316.
34. Mendelow AD, Gregson BA, Fernandes HM, et al. Early surgery versus initial conservative treatment in patients with spontaneous supratentorial intracerebral haematomas in the International Surgical Trial in Intracerebral Haemorrhage (STICH): a randomised trial. *Lancet.* 2005;365:387–397.

47

Delirium

Delirium is defined in the American Psychiatric Associations Diagnostic and Statistical Manual of Mental Disorders (DSM-IV) as a disturbance of *consciousness and cognition* that develops over a short period of time (hours to days) and *fluctuates* over time.[1] Many different terms have been used to describe the syndrome of cognitive impairment in critically ill patients, including ICU psychosis, acute confusional state, ICU encephalopathy, and acute brain syndrome; however, ICU delirium is the preferred term. Delirium is a very common and serious complication in ICU patients.[2–5] McNicoll et al.[6] reported that 70.3% of elderly ICU patients developed delirium at some time during their hospitalization. Delirium in ICU patients has been demonstrated to be an independent predictor of the length of hospital stay as well as ICU and 6-month mortality rates.[2–5,7,8] In addition, delirium may be a predictor of long-term cognitive impairment in survivors of critical illness.

Delirium can be categorized into subtypes according to psychomotor behavior, and the high prevalence of hypoactive delirium in critically ill patients probably contributes to clinician's lack of recognition of delirium. Hypoactive delirium is characterized by decreased responsiveness, withdrawal, and apathy, whereas hyperactive delirium is characterized by agitation, restlessness, and emotional lability.[3] Peterson and coworkers examined delirium subtypes in a cohort of medical ICU patients; they observed that purely hyperactive delirium was rare (1.6%); in contrast, 43.5% of patients had purely hypoactive delirium and 54.1% had mixed delirium.[9]

Elderly ICU patients are particularly at risk for developing delirium. Sleep deprivation, sepsis, hypoxemia, use of physical restraints, fluid and electrolyte imbalances, and metabolic and endocrine derangements have been implicated in the causation of delirium.[10] On average, ICU patients sleep only 2 h/day, and less than 6% of their sleep is REM sleep.[11]

P.E. Marik, *Handbook of Evidence-Based Critical Care*, DOI 10.1007/978-1-4419-5923-2_47,
© Springer Science+Business Media, LLC 2010

The use of benzodiazepines for sedation appears to be a particularly important risk factor in ICU patients. Pandharipande and colleagues[12] reported that the use of lorazepam was independently associated with the development of delirium in ICU patients. Marcantonio and colleagues[13] reported that the use of meperidine and benzodiazepines were independently associated with the development of postoperative delirium in elderly patients after orthopedic surgery. Other drugs including digoxin, anti-histaminics, opiates, anti-parkinsonian medications, anti-psychotics, and anti-depressants can induce delirium. The high noise level, incessant monitor alarms, and bright lights in the ICU may contribute to the development of delirium in ICU patients. Pre-existent cognitive or functional impairment is an important risk factor for the development of delirium in hospitalized patients.

Delirium is common following major surgery in elderly patients. Postoperative delirium is associated with an increased mortality, increased incidence of medical complications, and a prolonged hospital stay.[14] Preoperative cognitive dysfunction (dementia) is a strong predictor of postoperative delirium.[15] Postoperative delirium has an onset of approximately 24 h after surgery and generally resolves within a week. Delirium was reported to occur in 33% of elderly patients undergoing coronary artery bypass surgery (CABG).[16] Due to their advanced age, delirium is common following hip fracture repair, occurring in 28–65% of patients.[17–20] Transient postoperative delirium is associated with a poor long-term functional outcome.[17,18,21] Some patents may progress into a long-term confusional state. Marcantonio et al.[18] reported that 6% of patients remained delirious 6 months after hip fracture surgery.

■ DELIRIUM ASSESSMENT

Current data suggest that delirium is frequently overlooked and under-diagnosed in ICU patients. Given the fluctuating nature of delirium, a cursory "one-time only" evaluation at the bedside in usually ineffectual and has been shown to be a poor strategy for physicians to identify delirium in acutely ill patients.[22] It is therefore important that clinicians complete frequent delirium assessments. To this end, clinicians need a scale that can be completed quickly and incorporated into their daily routine. Although there is currently a lack of evidence demonstrating that the systematic assessment and management of delirium in the ICU improves outcome, a delirium assessment tool should be incorporated into the regular bedside evaluation of ICU patients. Six delirium assessment tools have been developed for use in the ICU, with the confusion assessment method for the intensive care unit (CAM-ICU) and the intensive care delirium screening checklist (ICDSC) being the most extensively validated.[23-25] The author prefers the ICDSC due to its simplicity and ease of use; a score of 1 is given if each of the following elements is met:

- Altered level of consciousness
  - Non-responsive, poorly responsive, drowsy, or hypervigilant
- Inattention
  - Difficulty following instruction, cannot focus
- Disorientation
- Hallucinations, delusions, or psychosis
- Psychomotor agitation or retardation
  - Hyperactivity or hypoactivity
- Inappropriate speech or mood
  - Inappropriate, disorganized or incoherent speech, or inappropriate display of emotion
- Sleep–wake cycle disturbance
  - Sleeping less than 4 h or waking frequently at night
- Symptom fluctuation

A score of 4 or more is considered indicative of delirium

■ PREVENTION AND MANAGEMENT

These data suggest that prevention, early detection, and treatment of delirium should be important goals in the management of ICU patients. Establishing a sleep–wake cycle, controlling noise pollution, morning bright light therapy, reorientation, and music therapy may be useful in the prevention and treatment of delirium in the ICU.[20,26] Preoperative sleep deprivation may increase the risk of postoperative delirium.[15] Poor postoperative pain control has been associated with the development of delirium.[27] Opiates (fentanyl or morphine) should therefore not be withheld in the fear of causing delirium.

Although no placebo-controlled clinical trials have been conducted to evaluate its efficacy in ICU patients, haloperidol is recommended as the drug of choice for the treatment of delirium by the Society of Critical Care Medicine (SCCM) and the American Psychiatric Association.[28,29] Haloperidol blocks D_2 dopamine receptors, resulting in amelioration of hallucinations, delusions, and unstructured thought patterns. Patients are typically treated with 2 mg IV followed by repeated doses (doubling the previous dose) every 15–20 min while agitation persists. Once agitation subsides, scheduled doses (every 4–6 h) may be continued for a few days, followed by tapered doses for several days. The most important side effects of haloperidol are dystonia, extrapyramidal effects, laryngeal spasm, and QTc prolongation. A baseline and daily 12-lead ECG is recommended to follow the QTc interval; magnesium deficiency should be aggressively treated and other drugs which prolong the QTc interval should be used with caution. The extrapyramidal effects appear to be very uncommon in ICU patients; an alternative agent should be used if these develop. Similarly the neurolept-malignant syndrome appears to be exceedingly uncommon in these patients. Haloperidol is the "safest" anti-psychotic in patients with a seizure disorder.

Milbrandt et al.[30] reported that the use of haloperidol within 2 days of the initiation of mechanical ventilation was associated with a lower hospital mortality. The role of haloperidol in preventing delirium was not reported in this study. Kaneko and colleagues[31] administered 5 mg haloperidol (or matching placebo) intravenously at night for 5 days postoperatively in 78 geriatric patients undergoing gastrointestinal surgery. Postoperative delirium developed in 10.5% of the patients receiving haloperidol as compared to 32% in the placebo group. Haloperidol and other "atypical" anti-psychotics hold great promise for the prophylaxis of delirium in elderly patients undergoing surgery.

Skrobik et al.[32] compared oral olanzapine with oral haloperidol in treating delirium in 73 ICU patients. The mean daily dose was 6.5 mg for haloperidol and 4.5 mg for olanzapine. Both drugs were equally efficacious in controlling the features of delirium; fewer side effects were noted in the olanzapine group. Han and colleagues[33] compared oral risperidone with oral haloperidol in 28 delirious acutely ill medical patients. The starting dose was 0.5 mg twice daily for risperidone and 0.75 mg twice daily for haloperidol; these doses were adjusted daily based on the assessment of delirium. There was no difference in the efficacy or response rate between the two agents.

Reade and colleagues[34] randomized 20 patients undergoing mechanical ventilation in whom extubation was not possible because of agitated delirium to receive either haloperidol 0.5–2 mg/h or dexmedetomidine 0.2–0.7 μg/kg/h. Dexmedetomidine significantly reduced time to extubation and ICU length of stay; all dexmedetomidine patients were successfully extubated as compared to 7 of 10 haloperidol patients. This pilot study suggests that dexmedetomidine may be the drug of choice for the treatment of delirium in the ICU.

Melatonin has been suggested to reset the internal circadian rhythm and sleep–wake cycle and may have a role in the treatment and/or the prevention of delirium in ICU patients.[35] Bourne and colleagues[36] demonstrated that melatonin given at night increased the duration of sleep. Based on pharmacokinetic data, these authors recommend a dose of 2 mg.

■ CLINICAL PEARLS

- All ICU patients should be regularly screened (i.e., 8 hourly) for the presence of delirium using a validated delirium assessment tool.
- Patient orientation and preservation of the sleep–wake cycle are important to minimize the risk of delirium.
- Sedation with benzodiazepines should be avoided; benzodiazepines should not be used for the treatment of delirium.
- Dexmedetomidine is a promising drug for the prevention and treatment of delirium.

■ REFERENCES

1. American Psychiatric Association. *Diagnostic and Statistical Manual of Mental Disorders.* 4th ed. Washington DC: American Psychiatric Association; 2000.
2. Gunther ML, Jackson JC, Ely EW. The cognitive consequences of critical illness: practical recommendations for screening and assessment. *Crit Care Clin.* 2007;23:491–506.
3. Girard TD, Pandharipande PP, Ely EW. Delirium in the intensive care unit. *Crit Care.* 2008;12(Suppl 3):S3.
4. Ely EW, Shintani A, Truman B, et al. Delirium as a predictor of mortality in mechanically ventilated patients in the intensive care unit. *JAMA.* 2004;291:1753–1762.
5. Pandharipande P, Cotton BA, Shintani A, et al. Prevalence and risk factors for development of delirium in surgical and trauma intensive care unit patients. *J Trauma.* 2008;65:34–41.
6. McNicoll L, Pisani MA, Zhang Y, et al. Delirium in the intensive care unit: occurrence and clinical course in older patients. *J Am Geriatr Soc.* 2003;51:591–598.
7. Ely EW, Gautam S, Margolin R, et al. The impact of delirium in the intensive care unit on hospital length of stay. *Intensive Care Med.* 2001;27:1892–1900.
8. Lin SM, Liu CY, Wang CH, et al. The impact of delirium on the survival of mechanically ventilated patients. *Crit Care Med.* 2004;32:2254–2259.
9. Peterson JF, Pun BT, Dittus RS, et al. Delirium and its motoric subtypes: a study of 614 critically ill patients. *J Am Geriatr Soc.* 2006;54:479–484.
10. Inouye SK, Charpentier PA. Precipitating factors for delirium in hospitalized elderly persons. Predictive model and interrelationship with baseline vulnerability. *JAMA.* 1996;275:852–857.
11. Cooper AB, Thornley KS, Young GB, et al. Sleep in critically ill patients requiring mechanical ventilation. *Chest.* 2000;117:809–818.

12. Pandharipande P, Shintani A, Peterson J, et al. Lorazepam is an independent risk factor for transitioning to delirium in intensive care unit patients. *Anesthesiol.* 2006;104:21–26.
13. Marcantonio ER, Juarez G, Goldman L, et al. The relationship of postoperative delirium with psychoactive medications. *JAMA.* 1994;272: 1518–1522.
14. Parikh SS, Chung F. Postoperative delirium in the elderly. *Anesth Analg.* 1995;80:1223–1232.
15. Kaneko T, Takahashi S, Naka T, et al. Postoperative delirium following gastrointestinal surgery in elderly patients. *Surg Today.* 1997;27: 107–111.
16. Santos FS, Velasco IT, Fraguas R Jr. Risk factors for delirium in the elderly after coronary artery bypass graft surgery. *Int Psychogeriatr.* 2004;16:175–193.
17. Zakriya K, Sieber FE, Christmas C, et al. Brief postoperative delirium in hip fracture patients affects functional outcome at three months. *Anesth Analg.* 98:1798–1802.
18. Marcantonio ER, Flacker JM, Michaels M, et al. Delirium is independently associated with poor functional recovery after hip fracture. *J Am Geriatr Soc.* 2000;48:618–624.
19. Gustafson Y, Berggren D, Brannstrom B, et al. Acute confusional states in elderly patients treated for femoral neck fracture. *J Am Geriatr Soc.* 1988;36:525–530.
20. Marcantonio ER, Flacker JM, Wright RJ, et al. Reducing delirium after hip fracture: a randomized trial. *J Am Geriatr Soc.* 2001;49:516–522.
21. Olofsson B, Lundstrom M, Borssen B, et al. Delirium is associated with poor rehabilitation outcome in elderly patients treated for femoral neck fractures. *Scand J Care Sci.* 2005;19:119–127.
22. Armstrong SC, Cozza KL, Watanabe KS. The misdiagnosis of delirium. *Psychosomatics.* 1997;38:433–439.
23. Devlin JW, Fong JJ, Fraser GL, et al. Delirium assessment in the critically ill. *Intensive Care Med.* 2007;33:929–940.
24. Bergeron N, Dubois MJ, Dumont M, et al. Intensive care delirium screening checklist: evaluation of a new screening tool. *Intensive Care Med.* 2001;27:859–864.
25. Ely EW, Inouye SK, Bernard GR, et al. Delirium in mechanically ventilated patients: validity and reliability of the confusion assessment method for the intensive care unit (CAM-ICU). *JAMA.* 2001;286: 2703–2710.
26. Inouye SK, Bogardus ST Jr, Charpentier PA, et al. A multicomponent intervention to prevent delirium in hospitalized older patients. *N Engl J Med.* 1999;340:669–676.
27. Vaurio LE, Sands LP, Wang Y, et al. Postoperative delirium: the importance of pain and pain management. *Anesth Analg.* 2006;102: 1267–1273.

28. Jacobi J, Fraser GL, Coursin DB, et al. Clinical practice guidelines for the sustained use of sedatives and analgesics in the critically ill adult. *Crit Care Med.* 2002;30:119–141.

29. Practice guideline for the treatment of patients with delirium. American Psychiatric Association. *Am J Psychiatry.* 1999;156:1–20.

30. Milbrandt EB, Kersten A, Kong L, et al. Haloperidol use is associated with lower hospital mortality in mechanically ventilated patients. *Crit Care Med.* 2005;33:226–229.

31. Kaneko T, Cai J, Ishikura T, et al. Prophylactic consecutive administration of haloperidol can reduce the occurrence of postoperative delirium in gastrointestinal surgery. *Yonaga Acta Medica* 1999;42:179–184.

32. Skrobik YK, Bergeron N, Dumont M, et al. Olanzapine vs haloperidol: treating delirium in a critical care setting. *Intensive Care Med.* 2004;30:444–449.

33. Han CS, Kim YK. A double-blind trial of risperidone and haloperidol for the treatment of delirium. *Psychosomatics.* 2004;45:297–301.

34. Reade MC, O'Sullivan K, Bates S, et al. Dexmedetomidine vs. haloperidol in delirious, agitated, intubated patients: a randomised open-label trial. *Crit Care.* 2009;13:R75.

35. Hanania M, Kitain E. Melatonin for treatment and prevention of postoperative delirium. *Anesth Analg.* 2002;94:338–339.

36. Bourne RS, Mills GH, Minelli C. Melatonin therapy to improve nocturnal sleep in critically ill patients: encouraging results from a small randomised controlled trial. *Crit Care.* 2008;12:R52-doi:10.1186/cc6871.

48

Seizures and Status Epilepticus

■ SEIZURES IN THE ICU

Seizures are common neurological complications in medical and post-surgical ICU patients and commonly arise from coexisting conditions associated with critical illness. Most ICU seizures occur in patients who did not have prior seizures or neurologic pathology as part of the primary admitting diagnosis. Status epilepticus as an admitting diagnosis is much less common than seizures occurring as a complication during the course of critical illness.[1] Most seizures that occur in the ICU setting manifest as generalized tonic–clonic convulsions.

Seizures Occurring as a Complication of Critical Illness

- Hypoxia/ischemia
- Eclampsia
- Posterior reversible encephalopathy syndrome (PRESS), see Chapter 63
- Drug/substance toxicity
  - Antibiotics
    - Carbapenems, esp. imipenem
    - Penicillins
    - Cephalosporins
    - Aztreonam
    - Fluoroquinolones
    - Metronidazole

P.E. Marik, *Handbook of Evidence-Based Critical Care*,
DOI 10.1007/978-1-4419-5923-2_48,
© Springer Science+Business Media, LLC 2010

- – Anti-depressants
  - • Tricyclics
  - • Bupropion
- – Anti-psychotics
  - • Chlorpromazine
- – Immunosuppressants
  - • Tacrolimus
  - • Cyclosporine
- – Others
  - • Theophylline
  - • Cocaine
  - • Amphetamines
- • Drug/substance withdrawal
  - – Alcohol
  - – Barbiturates
  - – Benzodiazepines
  - – Opioids
- • Metabolic
  - – Hypoglycemia
  - – Hypocalcemia
  - – Hypophosphatemia
  - – Hyponatremia
  - – Renal failure

Seizures from Primary Neurological Diseases

- • Stroke
  - – Hemorrhagic
  - – Large cortical
- • Intracranial tumor
  - – Cortical primary
  - – Cortical metastatic
- • Traumatic head injury

■ MANAGEMENT

Many seizures manifest as single, self-limited episodes. Such occurrences serve to alert the ICU team that a metabolic, drug, or structural problem exists. The first step is to terminate the ictal activity followed by an evaluation as to the cause of the seizure. Neuroimaging (CT scan) is always required to exclude a structural lesion even in the context of an identifiable metabolic/drug etiology. An EEG is required in patients who do not fully regain consciousness (see status epilepticus) and in those patients whose level of consciousness is difficult to assess (due to sedation, underlying disease, etc.).

Seizure Therapy

- Acute termination of ictal activity
  - Lorazepam 0.05–0.1 mg/kg
  - Midazolam 0.05–0.2 mg/kg
- Treatment of underlying cause
  - Drug induced; consider hemodialysis if recurrent (theophylline)
  - Lorazepam for drug withdrawal
  - Alcohol (see Chapter 60)
  - INH, IV pyridoxine
  - Serotonin inhibitors (see Chapter 61)
  - Cocaine – benzodiazepine (see Chapter 59)
- Prophylaxis if risk persists (consult neurology for input)
  - Phenytoin
  - Levetiracetam
  - Gabapentin
  - Lamotrigine
  - Topiramate

Levetiracetam (Keppra) has distinct advantages over the other intravenous and oral anti-convulsants in the critically ill as it has few drug interactions and is usually well tolerated.

Management of seizures in the setting of an ischemic stroke should be no different than that of seizures from other causes. The most recent guidelines from the Stroke Council of the American Stroke Association recognize that there is no sound evidence regarding treatment options in this setting.[2] Topiramate has potential neuroprotective properties against cerebral ischemia.[3] Phenytoin, barbiturates, and benzodiazepines may in contrast have negative effects on recovery from stroke.[4]

■ STATUS EPILEPTICUS

Status epilepticus is a major medical emergency associated with significant morbidity and a mortality of up to 76% in elderly patients with refractory status epileptics.[5] This clinical entity requires prompt management. The complications of status epilepticus include cardiac dysrhythmias, derangements of metabolic and autonomic function, neurogenic pulmonary edema, hyperthermia, rhabdomyolysis, and pulmonary aspiration. Permanent neurological damage occurs with prolonged uncontrolled convulsive activity.

Status epilepticus is usually defined as continuous seizure activity lasting 30 min or as two or more discrete seizures between which consciousness is not fully regained.[6] Lowenstein, Bleck, and Macdonald have proposed that status epilepticus be defined as a continuous, generalized, convulsive seizure lasting more than 5 min or two or more seizures during which the patients do not return to baseline consciousness.[7] The rationale for this revised definition is based on the fact that a typical, generalized tonic–clonic seizure rarely lasts longer than 5 min, spontaneous termination becomes less likely in seizures lasting greater than 5 min, and the longer the seizure continues, the more difficult the seizure becomes to control with anti-epileptic drugs and the greater the degree of neuronal damage. This definition is consistent with common clinical practice in which it would be unreasonable to wait for 30 min before initiating anti-epileptic drug therapy.

Refractory status epilepticus is usually defined as seizures lasting longer than 2 h or seizures recurring at a rate of two or more episodes per hour without recovery to baseline between seizures despite treatment with conventional anti-epileptic drugs. However, from a clinical perspective it is preferable to consider refractory status epilepticus in any patient who has failed first-line therapy.

Status epilepticus may be classified by the presence of motor convulsions (convulsive status epilepticus) or their absence (non-convulsive status epilepticus). They may be further divided into status epilepticus that affects the whole brain (generalized status epilepticus) and status epilepticus that affects only part of the brain (partial status epilepticus).[6] Status epilepticus appears to be more frequent among males, blacks, and the aged.

■ ETIOLOGY

In many patients with a pre-existent seizure disorder, no obvious precipitating factor can be determined. A fall in serum levels of anti-epileptic drugs due to poor compliance with medications or due to increased clearance associated with concurrent illness has been implicated in some patients. Adult patients with a new diagnosis of epilepsy may first present in status epilepticus.

Common Causes of Status Epilepticus

- Anti-epileptic drug non-compliance
- Alcohol related
- Cerebrovascular accidents

- Drug toxicity
  - Cephalosporins
  - Carbapenems
  - Penicillins
  - Ciprofloxacin
  - Tacrolimus
  - Cyclosporine
  - Theophylline
  - Cocaine
- Central nervous system infections
  - Meningitis
  - Encephalitis
- Central nervous system tumors (primary or secondary)
- Metabolic disturbances (i.e., electrolyte abnormalities, uremia)
- Cerebrovascular accidents
- Head trauma
- Cerebral anoxia/hypoxia
- Hypoglycemia or hyperglycemia

■ PATHOPHYSIOLOGY

It is likely that ineffective recruitment of inhibitory neurons together with excessive neuronal excitation plays a role in the initiation and propagation of the electrical disturbance occurring in status epilepticus. A growing body of basic science and clinical observation supports the concept that status epilepticus becomes more difficult to control as its duration increases. It has been postulated that this may occur due to a mechanistic shift from inadequate GABAergic inhibitory receptor-mediated transmission to excessive NMDA excitatory receptor-mediated transmission. In man and experimental animals, sustained seizures cause selective neuronal loss in vulnerable regions such as the hippocampus, the cortex, and the thalamus. The degree of neuronal injury is closely related to the duration of seizures, underscoring the importance of rapid control of status epilepticus.

Complications of Generalized Status Epilepticus

- Systemic
  - Acidosis
  - Hyperthermia
  - Rhabdomyolysis
  - Renal failure

- – Arrhythmias
- – Trauma
- – Aspiration
- Neurologic
  - – Direct excitotoxic injury
  - – Epileptogenic foci
  - – Synaptic reorganization

■ DIAGNOSIS

Status epilepticus may be divided into two stages.[6] The first phase is characterized by generalized convulsive tonic–clonic seizures that are associated with an increase in autonomic activity that results in hypertension, hyperglycemia, sweating, salivation, and hyperpyrexia. During this phase, cerebral blood flow is increased due to increased cerebral metabolic demands. After approximately 30 min of seizure activity, patients enter the second phase characterized by failure of cerebral autoregulation, decreased cerebral blood flow, increased in intracranial pressure, and systemic hypotension. During this phase, electromechanical dissociation may occur in which although electrical cerebral seizure activity continues the clinical manifestations may be restricted to minor twitching.

The diagnosis of status epilepticus is straightforward in patients with witnessed generalized convulsive tonic–clonic seizures. However, status epilepticus may not be considered in patients who have progressed to the non-convulsive phase of status epilepticus and present in coma. All comatose patients should therefore be carefully examined for evidence of minor twitching which may involve the face, hands, or feet or present as nystagmoid jerking of the eyes. Towne and colleagues evaluated 236 patients with coma and no overt seizure activity. Eight percent of patients in this study were found to have non-convulsive status epilepticus by electroencephalographic monitoring.[8] An urgent EEG is therefore required in patients with unexplained coma.

■ TREATMENT

Status epilepticus is a medical emergency that requires rapid and aggressive treatment to prevent neurologic damage and systemic complications. The longer the status remains untreated, the greater the neurologic damage. In addition, the longer an episode of status continues, the more refractory to treatment it becomes and the greater the likelihood of chronic epilepsy. The management of status epilepticus involves the rapid termination of seizure activity, airway protection, measures to prevent aspiration, management of potential precipitating causes, treatment of complications, prevention of recurrent seizures, and the treatment of any underlying conditions.

General Measures

- As with any critically ill patient, the first step in the management of a patient with status epilepticus should be to ensure an adequate airway and provide respiratory support.
- The patient should be positioned so that they cannot harm themselves from the seizure activity.
- Two large gauge intravenous catheters should be inserted to allow fluid resuscitation and pharmacotherapy. Should peripheral venous access be difficult, placement of a central venous catheter is recommended.
- Despite the periods of apnea and cyanosis that occur during the tonic or the clonic phases of their seizure, most patients in status epilepticus breathe sufficiently as long as the airway remains clear. An oral airway may be required once the seizure has terminated to prevent airway obstruction. Once the seizures are controlled and if the patient is oxygenating and ventilating adequately, endotracheal intubation may not be required for "airway protection" even if the patient remains comatose.[9] However, in this situation, precautions should be taken to avoid aspiration and a nasogastric tube should be placed to ensure that the stomach is empty. Endotracheal intubation will be required in patients who continue to have seizures despite first-line therapy (see below). There is no available data as to the pharmacologic agent(s) preferred for achieving endotracheal intubation. As these patients will be comatose and already have received lorazepam, a hypnotic agent is usually not required. However, an anesthetic induction dose of propofol, midazolam, or etomidate may terminate the seizure activity and facilitate intubation. Neuromuscular blockade will be required to facilitate intubation in patients who continue to have tonic–clonic seizure activity despite these pharmacologic interventions. Rocuronium (1 mg/kg), a short acting, non-depolarizing muscle relaxant, which is devoid of significant hemodynamic effects and does not increase ICP, is the preferred agent. Succinylcholine should be avoided if possible as the patient may be hyperkalemic as a consequence of rhabdomyolysis. Prolonged neuromuscular blockade should be avoided.
- Hypoglycemia must be excluded rapidly and corrective measures instituted if serum levels of glucose are low. If prompt measurement of blood glucose levels is not possible, the patient should receive

100 mg of intravenous thiamine followed by a 50-ml bolus of 50% dextrose.

- Blood pressure, electrocardiogram, and temperature should be monitored. If the patient develops significant hyperthermia (>40°C), then passive cooling is required.
- Blood specimens should be obtained for the determination of serum chemistries.
- Continuous motor seizures may lead to muscle breakdown with the release of myoglobin into the circulation. Maintenance of adequate hydration is necessary to prevent myoglobin-induced renal failure. Forced saline diuresis should be considered in the presence of myoglobinuria or significantly elevated serum creatine kinase levels (CPK levels greater than 5,000 U/l).
- Brain imaging with a computerized tomographic scan (CT) and/or magnetic resonance imaging (MRI) as well as a lumbar puncture will be required in patients presenting with a previously undiagnosed seizure disorder once the seizure activity has been controlled. It is important to emphasize that the first priority is to control the seizures. Imaging studies should be performed only once the seizure activity has been controlled. Endotracheal intubation and neuromuscular paralysis for the sole purpose of imaging the patient may increase morbidity and is strongly discouraged.

Pharmacotherapy

Because only a small fraction of seizures go on to become status epilepticus, the probability that a given seizure will proceed to status is small at the start of the seizure and increases as the seizure duration increases. If a seizure lasts longer than 5 min, clinical experience suggests that the likelihood of spontaneous termination decreases. The goal of pharmacologic therapy is to achieve rapid and safe termination of the seizure and prevention of its recurrence without adverse effects on the cardiovascular and respiratory systems or altering the level of consciousness. Diazepam, lorazepam, midazolam, phenytoin, fosphenytoin, and phenobarbital have all been used as first-line therapy for the termination of status epilepticus. These drugs have different pharmacodynamic and pharmacokinetic properties which determine their rapidity of clinical effect, efficacy in terminating status epilepticus, and their duration of action. The benzodiazepines bind to the benzodiazepine receptor on GABA increasing GABAergic transmission, while the barbiturates act directly on the GABA receptor. The anti-seizure activity of phenytoin is complex; however, its major action appears to block the voltage-sensitive, use-dependent sodium channels.

The publication of the Veterans Administration Cooperative Trial in 1998 and the San Francisco EMS Study in 2001 allows for an evidence-based approach to the choice of the first-line agent to terminate status epilepticus.[10,11] The VA cooperative study randomized 384 patients with overt generalized status epilepticus into four treatment arms as follows:

- Lorazepam 0.1 mg/kg
- Diazepam 0.15 mg/kg, followed by 18 mg/kg of phenytoin
- Phenytoin 18 mg/kg
- Phenobarbital 15 mg/kg

Successful treatment required both clinical and EEG termination of seizures within 20 min of the start of therapy and no seizure recurrence within 60 min from the start of therapy. Patients who failed the first treatment received a second choice and if necessary, a third choice of study drug. The latter choices were not randomized, because this would have resulted in some patients receiving two loading doses of phenytoin, but the treating physician remained blinded to the treatments being given. Status epilepticus was terminated in

- patients randomized to lorazepam (64.9%),
- patients randomized to phenobarbital (58.2%),
- patients randomized to diazepam and phenytoin (55.8%), and
- patients randomized to phenytoin (43.6%; $p = 0.002$ for lorazepam vs. phenytoin).

There was no difference between arms in recurrence rates. The San Francisco EMS Study was a randomized, double-blind trial to evaluate intravenous benzodiazepine administration by paramedics for the treatment of out-of-hospital status epilepticus.[11] In this study, 205 patients were randomized to intravenous diazepam (5 mg), lorazepam (2 mg), or placebo. An identical second injection was given if needed. Status epilepticus had terminated at arrival in the emergency department in 59.1% of patients treated with lorazepam, 42.6% of patients treated with diazepam, and 21.1% of patients given placebo [odds ratio of 1.9 (95% CI 0.9–4.3) for lorazepam compared to diazepam]. The duration of the status epilepticus was shorter in the lorazepam group as compared to the diazepam group [adjusted relative hazard, 0.65 (95% CI 0.36–1.17)]. These data are supported by a double-blind study reported by Leppick in 1983 in which 78 patients with status epilepticus were randomized to receive one or two doses of either 4 mg lorazepam or 10 mg diazepam.[12] Seizures were controlled in 89% of the episodes treated with lorazepam and in 76% treated with diazepam. Although the dosages of lorazepam and diazepam differed in these three studies and phenytoin was added to diazepam in the VA study, the summed data indicate that lorazepam is significantly more effective in terminating seizures than is diazepam [odds ratio of 1.74

(95% CI 1.14–2.64), $p = 0.01$]. Furthermore, the pharmacokinetic properties of lorazepam favor it over diazepam. The anti-convulsant effect of a single dose of diazepam is very brief (20 min), whereas that of lorazepam is much longer (greater than 6 h) and the risk of respiratory depression may be greater with diazepam.[13] Although diazepam has a much longer elimination half-life, due to its high lipid solubility it is rapidly redistributed from the brain to the peripheral fat stores accounting for its shorter anti-seizure activity. Based on these data, lorazepam in a dose of 0.1 mg/kg is recommended as first-line therapy for control of status epilepticus.

Many authorities recommend 20 mg/kg phenytoin (or fosphenytoin) following the administration of lorazepam. While there are no data which demonstrate that phenytoin increases the response rate following the use of lorazepam, this agent may prevent recurrent seizures and is recommended in patients without a rapidly reversible process (e.g., the effect of subtherapeutic anti-epileptic drug concentrations).[14]

Continuous EEG monitoring is required in patients who do not recover consciousness once the convulsive seizure has aborted. In a study by DeLorenzo and colleagues, after cessation of convulsions, 48% of patients continued to have seizure activity and 14% of patients had persistent non-convulsive status epilepticus.[15]

Management of Refractory Status Epilepticus

In the VA cooperative study, 55% of patients with generalized convulsive status epilepticus failed first-line therapy. The aggregate response rate to a second first-line agent (lorazepam, diazepam, phenytoin, or phenobarbital) was 7% and 2.3% to a third first-line agent. Only 5% of patients with status epilepticus who did not respond to lorazepam and phenytoin therapy responded to phenobarbital administration These data suggest that refractory status epilepticus is much more common than is generally appreciated and that phenobarbital should not be used as a second-line (or third-line) agent in patients who have failed to respond to lorazepam. Furthermore, the limited data available suggest that the administration of further doses of lorazepam will not be useful.[12]

A variety of agents have been recommended for the treatment of refractory status epilepticus including midazolam, propofol, high-dose thiopentone or pentobarbital, intravenous levetiracetam, intravenous valproate, topiramate, tiagabine, ketamine, isoflurane, and intravenous lidocaine. Treatment guidelines are difficult as refractory status epilepticus has not been studied in a prospective clinical trial. Currently, however, a continuous intravenous infusion of midazolam or propofol together with continuous EEG monitoring is the preferred mode of treatment.[16,17] Both agents have been reported to be successful in the control of patients with refractory status epilepticus. It should, however, be pointed out that this recommendation is based on limited clinical data.[16,18] Recently, intravenous valproic acid and intravenous levetiracetam (Keppra) have become available and may have particular utility in status epilepticus both as a second-line agent and as an "add-on" to another second-line agent (midazolam or propofol).[19,20]

The goal regarding the activity on the EEG remains a matter of debate. There is no prospectively collected evidence that a burst-suppression EEG pattern is required for, or is efficacious for, the termination of status epilepticus. Many patients can achieve complete seizure control with a background of continuous slow activity and do not incur the greater risks associated with higher doses of medication required to achieve a burst-suppression pattern.

- Midazolam is given as a loading dose of 0.2 mg/kg, followed by an infusion of 0.1–2.0 mg/kg/h titrated to produce seizure suppression by continuous EEG monitoring.
- Propofol is given as a loading dose of 3–5 mg/kg, followed by an infusion of 30–100 μg/kg/min titrated to EEG seizure suppression. After 12 h of seizure suppression, the dose is gradually titrated by 50% over the next 12 h and then titrated off over the subsequent 12 h. If seizure activity should recur during the weaning period, a further loading dose of 1–3 mg/kg should be given followed by an infusion rate increased to obtain another 12 h seizure-free period.[21]
- Valproic acid is given as a loading dose of 20–40 mg/kg followed by an infusion at 5 mg/kg/h that is titrated down after 12 h of clinical and EEG seizure control. Valproic acid has a broad spectrum of activity for different seizure types and is effective in terminating status epilepticus.
- Levetiracetam (Keppra) in a dose of between 1,000 and 4,000 mg infused over 15 min has been successfully used in status epilepticus. Levetiracetam has essentially no drug–drug interactions, limited protein binding, no hepatic metabolism, and is generally well tolerated.

High-dose barbiturate therapy is associated with hemodynamic instability and immune paresis. Due to their side effects, barbiturates are reserved for those patients who fail second-line therapy. Pentobarbital in a dose of 10–15 mg/kg/h, followed by 0.5–1.0 mg/kg/h is recommended.

The Management of Non-convulsive Status Epilepticus

Non-convulsive status epilepticus constitutes approximately 20–25% of status epilepticus cases, occurring in about 8% of all comatose patients without clinical signs of seizure activity and persisting in 14% of patients after generalized convulsive status epilepticus. Some have suggested that non-convulsive status epilepticus is a benign condition which does not require aggressive therapy. However, the prognosis of non-convulsive status epilepticus depends upon the etiology and the level of consciousness, being associated with significant morbidity in those with a depressed level of consciousness. Comatose patients with non-convulsive status epilepticus following generalized convulsive status epilepticus should be treated aggressively as outlined above for refractory convulsive status epilepticus. Levetiracetam may have particular utility in these patients.[22]

Prevention of Seizure Recurrence Once Status Epilepticus Is Terminated

Once status epilepticus is controlled, attention turns to preventing its recurrence. The best regimen for an individual patient will depend on the cause of the patient's seizure and any previous history of anti-epileptic drug therapy. A patient who develops status epilepticus in the course of ethanol withdrawal may not need anti-epileptic drug therapy once the withdrawal has run its course. In contrast, patients with new, ongoing epileptogenic stimuli (e.g., encephalitis) may require high dosages of anti-epileptic drugs to control their seizures.

■ CLINICAL PEARLS

- Metabolic derangements and drug withdrawal are the commonest causes of seizures in ICU patients.
- Lorazepam at a dose of 0.1 mg/kg is recommended as first-line therapy for control of status epilepticus.
- Midazolam, propofol, valproic acid, and levetiracetam have proven efficacy as second-line therapy in status epilepticus.

■ REFERENCES

1. Bleck TP. Neurological disorders in the intensive care unit. *Semin Respir Crit Care Med*. 2006;27:201–209.
2. Adams HP, Del ZG, Alberts MJ, et al. Guidelines for the early management of adults with ischemic stroke: a guideline from the American Heart Association/American Stroke Association Stroke Council, Clinical Cardiology Council, Cardiovascular Radiology and Intervention Council, and the Atherosclerotic Peripheral Vascular Disease and Quality of Care Outcomes in Research Interdisciplinary

Working Groups: the American Academy of Neurology affirms the value of this guideline as an educational tool for neurologists. *Stroke.* 2007;38:1655–1711.
3. Leker RR, Neufeld MY. Anti-epileptic drugs as possible neuroprotectants in cerebral ischemia. *Brain Res Rev.* 2003;42:187–203.
4. Goldstein LB. Potential effects of common drugs on stroke recovery. *Arch Neurol.* 1998;55:454–456.
5. Logroscino G, Hesdorffer DC, Cascino GD, et al. Long-term mortality after a first episode of status epilepticus. *Neurology.* 2002;58: 537–541.
6. Marik PE, Varon J. The management of status epilepticus. *Chest.* 2004;126:582–591.
7. Lowenstein DH, Bleck T, Macdonald RL. It's time to revise the definition of status epilepticus. *Epilepsia.* 1999;40:120–122.
8. Towne AR, Waterhouse EJ, Boggs JG, et al. Prevalence of nonconvulsive status epilepticus in comatose patients. *Neurology.* 2000;54:340–345.
9. Coplin WM, Pierson DJ, Cooley KD, et al. Implications of extubation delay in brain-injured patients meeting standard weaning criteria. *Am J Respir Crit Care Med.* 2000;161:1530–1536.
10. Treiman DM, Meyers PD, Walton NY. A comparison of four treatments for generalized convulsive status epilepticus. Veterans Affairs Status Epilepticus Cooperative Study Group. *N Engl J Med.* 1998;339:792–798.
11. Alldredge BK, Gelb AM, Isaacs SM, et al. A comparison of lorazepam, diazepam, and placebo for the treatment of out-of-hospital status epilepticus. *N Engl J Med.* 2001;345:631–637.
12. Leppik IE, Derivan AT, Homan RW, et al. Double-blind study of lorazepam and diazepam in status epilepticus. *JAMA.* 1983;249: 1452–1454.
13. Mitchell WG. Status epilepticus and acute repetitive seizures in children, adolescents, and young adults: etiology, outcome, and treatment. *Epilepsia.* 1996;37(Suppl 1):S74–S80.
14. Lowenstein DH, Alldredge BK. Status epilepticus. *N Engl J Med.* 1998;338:970–976.
15. DeLorenzo RJ, Waterhouse EJ, Towne AR, et al. Persistent nonconvulsive status epilepticus after the control of convulsive status epilepticus. *Epilepsia.* 1998;39:833–840.
16. Claassen J, Hirsch LJ, Emerson RG, et al. Treatment of refractory status epilepticus with pentobarbital, propofol, or midazolam: a systematic review. *Epilepsia.* 2002;43:146–153.
17. Mayer SA, Claassen J, Lokin J, et al. Refractory status epilepticus: frequency, risk factors, and impact on outcome. *Arch Neurol.* 2002;59: 205–210.
18. Ulvi H, Yoldas T, Mungen B, et al. Continuous infusion of midazolam in the treatment of refractory generalized convulsive status epilepticus. *Neurol Sci.* 2002;23:177–182.

19. Selvitelli M, Drislane FW. Recent developments in the diagnosis and treatment of status epilepticus. *Curr Neurol Neurosc Rep.* 2007;7: 529–535.
20. Uges JW, van Huizen MD, Engelsman J, et al. Safety and pharmacokinetics of intravenous levetiracetam infusion as add-on in status epilepticus. *Epilepsia.* 2009;50:415–421.
21. Stecker MM, Kramer TH, Raps EC, et al. Treatment of refractory status epilepticus with propofol: clinical and pharmacokinetic findings. *Epilepsia.* 1998;39:18–26.
22. Rupprecht S, Franke K, Fitzek S, et al. Levetiracetam as a treatment option in non-convulsive status epilepticus. *Epilepsy Res.* 2007;73: 238–244.

49

Management of Raised ICP

Increased intracranial pressure (ICP) may occur in patients who have cerebral hemorrhage, cerebral infarction with associated edema, primary or metastatic brain tumors, encephalitis, global anoxic or ischemic brain injury, or traumatic brain injury (TBI). Most of the information concerning raised ICP is derived from studies on TBI; it is unclear if this information can be extrapolated to other clinical situations.

Cerebral blood flow (CBF) in humans averages about 50 ml/100 gm brain tissue/min. Irreversible neuronal damage occurs if CBF drops below 18 ml/100 gm/min for a prolonged period of time. Cerebral blood flow is equal to the cerebral perfusion pressure (CPP), which is defined as the difference between the mean arterial blood pressure (MAP) and the intracranial pressure (ICP) divided by the cerebral vascular resistance (CVR). Because the CBF is difficult to measure clinically, the CPP is used as a guide to assessing the adequacy of cerebral perfusion.

Both the ICP and the MAP need to be measured to determine the CPP. The normal ICP is between 0 and 10 mmHg. While earlier studies and recommendations centered on the importance of ICP per se, current evidence emphasizes the importance of the CPP. The guidelines proposed by the Brain Trauma Foundation recommend that the CPP should be maintained at a minimum of 70 mmHg in the brain-injured patient, although the exact target number and methodology for achieving that target remain controversial. A higher threshold may be required in patients with chronic hypertension.[1] These guidelines use 20 mmHg as the threshold for intracranial hypertension. A lower target CPP (50–60 mmHg) may be adequate in patients with cerebral edema associated with fulminant hepatic failure (see Chapter 35). The target CPP in other situations is unclear; however, a CPP as low as 50 mmHg may be adequate

P.E. Marik, *Handbook of Evidence-Based Critical Care*,
DOI 10.1007/978-1-4419-5923-2_49,
© Springer Science+Business Media, LLC 2010

■ MEASUREMENT OF ICP

ICP cannot be reliably estimated from any specific clinical feature or CT finding and must be measured. Different methods of monitoring ICP have been described but two methods are commonly used in clinical practice: intraventricular catheters and intraparenchymal catheter-tip, microtransducer systems. Subarachnoid and epidural devices have much lower accuracy and are currently rarely used. The "gold standard" technique for ICP monitoring is a catheter inserted into the lateral ventricle, usually via a small right frontal burr hole. This can be connected to a standard pressure transducer via a fluid-filled catheter. The reference point for the transducer is the foramen of Munroe, although, in practical terms, the external auditory meatus is often used. Some ventricular catheters have a pressure transducer within their lumen and the ICP waveform is generally of better quality than traditional fluid-filled catheters connected to an external transducer. Ventricular catheters measure global ICP and have the additional advantages of allowing periodic external calibration, therapeutic drainage of CSF, and administration of drugs (e.g., antibiotics). However, placement of the catheter may be difficult if there is ventricular effacement or displacement due to brain swelling or intracranial mass lesions. The use of intraventricular catheters is complicated by infection in up to 11% of cases.

Microtransducer-tipped ICP monitors can be sited in the brain parenchyma or the subdural space, either through a skull bolt, a small burr hole, or during a neurosurgical procedure. They are almost as accurate as ventricular catheters. Fiber-optic strain gauge or pneumatic technologies are used to transduce pressure in modern microtransducer devices.

Transcranial Doppler

Transcranial Doppler is a valuable non-invasive technique which measures systolic flow velocity of the middle cerebral artery. Cerebral blood flow measured with the transcranial Doppler appears to correlate fairly well with more direct measures of flow such as xenon and A–V oxygen content trends.[2] Normal systolic velocity is <120 cm/s. Studies performed at different pCO_2 levels help to determine CO_2 reactivity of cerebral blood flow. Attenuation of the diastolic flow signal may be a sign of intracranial hypertension and diminished effective cerebral perfusion. In addition, the diastolic waveform may indicate early or late signs of elevated ICP as diastolic flow begins to attenuate. A pulsatility index (systolic velocity – diastolic velocity/systolic velocity) >1.6 is a poor prognostic sign.

■ INDICATIONS FOR ICP MONITORING

There are no data from randomized controlled trials that can clarify the role of ICP monitoring in acute coma.[3] Indeed, there are very little data that ICP monitoring improves patient outcome. With the exception of monitoring after TBI, the indications for ICP monitoring are not well established. Despite the absence of evidence demonstrating the benefit of ICP monitoring on outcome after TBI, there is a large body of clinical evidence supporting its use to guide therapeutic interventions, detect intracranial mass lesions early, and assess prognosis. Therefore, ICP monitoring has become an integral part of the management of patients with severe head injuries in virtually all trauma centers in the United States.

The Brain Trauma Foundation recommends ICP monitoring in all patients with a severe TBI (Glasgow Coma Score 3–8) and either an abnormal CT scan or a normal scan and the presence of two or more of the following three risk factors at admission: age >40 years; unilateral or bilateral motor posturing; a systolic BP <90 mmHg.[4] There is around 60% chance of increased ICP in these patients.

The improved outcome of patients with severe head injuries in the United States has been ascribed to intensive management protocols that include ICP monitoring.[4–9] This benefit is based on studies which have used a before–after study design; this study design however has significant limitations. A single concurrent cohort study has been published which failed to demonstrate the benefit of ICP monitoring. Cremer et al.[10] reported a retrospective analysis of severe TBI patients managed at two different trauma centers that differed in the use of ICP monitoring. One center with 122 patients that did not monitor ICP but used ICP lowering treatment (82% sedatives and paralytics, 25% mannitol, 22% hyperventilation, and 2% ventricular drainage) was compared to another center with 211 patients that used ICP monitoring in 67% of severe TBI patients and treated ICP significantly more except for hyperventilation and ventricular drainage which was equally used in both centers. The length of mechanical ventilation was significantly longer in the patients who received ICP monitoring. There was, however, no difference in mortality or 12-month GOS. It therefore appears that true equipoise exists in the role of ICP monitoring in TBI and that a randomized controlled trial is urgently required. It is possible that with such a trial, ICP monitoring will follow the same path as that of the PAC.

■ MANAGEMENT OF RAISED ICP

After the establishment of an airway and a ventilation, the restoration of blood pressure and normal circulating volume is of utmost importance in patients with increased ICP. According to the Brain Trauma Foundation guidelines for the management of severe TBI, a mean arterial pressure of 90 mmHg or greater should be targeted; this was chosen based on attaining cerebral perfusion pressures greater than 70 mmHg. These guidelines use 20 mmHg as the threshold for intracranial hypertension.[4] Patients should be resuscitated with lactated Ringer's solution (see Chapter 8). Norepinephrine should be used to achieve the target MAP once an adequate preload is achieved.

Even though the head-injured patient may be comatose, they require analgesia and sedation as they still respond to painful and noxious stimuli, often with an increase in ICP and blood pressure. Most frequently, narcotics (morphine or fentanyl) should be considered as first-line therapy since they provide both analgesia and depression of airway reflexes, which are required in the intubated patient. Fentanyl has the advantage of having minimal hemodynamic effects.

Other general principles in the management of patients with head injury include lowering the body temperature of patients with fever and prevention of jugular venous outflow obstruction (keeping patient's head midline, avoiding extrinsic compression of the jugular veins by hematomas, masses). While some studies have suggested that CPP is optimal when patients are nursed flat, others have demonstrated that head elevation to 30° lowers ICP without decreasing CPP or cerebral blood flow.[11]

Hyperventilation

Aggressive hyperventilation ($PaCO_2 \leq 25$ mmHg) has traditionally been considered a cornerstone in the management of raised ICP. Hyperventilation reduces ICP by causing cerebral vasoconstriction with a subsequent reduction in CBF. Hyperventilation results in a fall in ICP; however, this is associated with a significant fall in jugular venous O_2 saturation. Skippen and colleagues,[12] using xenon-enhanced computed tomography and cerebral blood flow studies, demonstrated a two-and-a-half-fold increase in the number of regions of brain ischemia in children with TBI who were hyperventilated. In 1991, Muizelaar and colleagues[13] published the results of a prospective randomized clinical study in which they demonstrated that hyperventilation in posthead injury patients was associated with a significantly worse neurological outcome when compared to patients who were kept normocapnic. Based on these data, chronic hyperventilation is no longer recommended.[1,14] Initial target pCO_2 should be 35–40 mmHg.[1,14] Short-term hyperventilation, however, may have a role in reducing ICP in patients who are rapidly deteriorating before other measures can be instituted.[15]

have been shown to lack efficacy and carry the risks of potential side effects (i.e., hyperglycemia, increased risk of infections, myopathy), and their use must be avoided. Indeed, in the CRASH study, high-dose corticosteroids were associated with an increased mortality.[26]

Propofol is the hypnotic agent of choice in patients with an acute neurological insult as it is easily titratable and rapidly reversible once discontinued. Propofol has additional properties that may be beneficial in the head-injured patient including a decrease in cerebral metabolic rate, a decrease in intracranial pressure (ICP), potentiation of GABAminergic inhibition, inhibition of NMDA glutamate receptors and voltage-dependent calcium channels, and prevention of lipid peroxidation.

Prophylactic Hypothermia

Although hypothermia is often induced prophylactically on admission and used for ICP elevation in the ICU in many trauma centers, the scientific literature has failed to consistently support its positive influence on mortality and morbidity. Meta-analyses of hypothermia in patients with TBI have concluded that the evidence was insufficient to support routine use of hypothermia.[27] Ongoing clinical trial should help resolve this important issue.

Mechanical Ventilation

The ventilator settings should be adjusted to maintain the $PaCO_2$ between 35 and 40 mmHg and the PaO_2 above 70 mmHg. While it has been suggested that a high PaO_2 may improve brain tissue oxygenation,[28] this goes against our understanding of human physiology, as tissue oxygen unloading is dependant primarily on the hemoglobin concentration, the P50, and the hemoglobin saturation. The dissolved oxygen fraction makes an insignificant contribution to oxygen transport. A high FiO_2 may, however, promote the formation of reactive oxygen species and increase lipid peroxidation. While it has been suggested that positive end-expiratory pressure (PEEP) and modes of ventilation that increase mean intrathoracic pressure should be avoided in patients with elevated ICP, clinical studies do not support this contention.[29–31] However, in accord with current guidelines, the lowest level of PEEP that maintains adequate oxygenation and prevents end-expiratory alveolar collapse should be used. Continuous pulse oximetry is recommended with the arterial saturation maintained above 94%. Although endotracheal suctioning does cause a transient rise in ICP, it does not produce cerebral ischemia and is required to prevent atelectasis.[32]

Volume Resuscitation

Previous guidelines had advocated moderate to severe dehydration as a treatment modality for cerebral edema. This was based on the assumption that such interventions would decrease brain water content and ICP. This reasoning was seriously flawed as experimental studies demonstrated that cerebral edema was not altered by hydration status and failed to recognize the importance of the cerebral perfusion pressure in preventing secondary brain ischemia.[16] Indeed, acute intracranial disease has been associated with a "cerebral salt-wasting syndrome" characterized by a negative salt balance and a contracted intravascular volume. Fluid restriction therefore exacerbates the underlying volume depletion, leading to an increased risk of cerebral ischemia. Volume resuscitation with isotonic fluids and restoration of a normal intravascular volume are therefore essential in all patients with acute cerebral insults.

Hyperosmotic Agents

If the ICP remains above 20 mmHg, despite adequate sedation and elevation of the head of the bed (to 30°), additional measures are required to lower the ICP. When a ventricular catheter is being used for ICP monitoring, CSF drainage should be used for ICP elevations.[17] If CSF drainage is ineffective, a hyperosmotic agent such as mannitol should be used next. The dose used is 0.25–0.5 g/kg given every 2–6 h to increase the serum osmolarity to 310–320 mOsm/kg H_2O.[18] Mannitol acts acutely by expanding intravascular volume and decreasing blood viscosity, thereby increasing cerebral blood flow.[19] The osmotic movement of fluid out of the cellular compartment is followed by a diuresis which is delayed for 15–30 min, while gradients are established between plasma and cells. The osmotic diuresis following mannitol lasts for between 90 min and 6 h. The prolonged administration of mannitol may lead to intravascular dehydration, hypotension, and prerenal azotemia. The benefit of mannitol in head-injured patients has yet to be determined, and remarkably only one placebo-controlled study has been reported to date.[20] In this study which compared the prehospital administration of mannitol against placebo, mannitol was associated with an increased relative risk for death (1.59; 95% confidence interval 0.44–5.79). Similarly, mannitol has failed to show a benefit in patients with intracerebral hemorrhage.[21,22] Hypertonic saline has been demonstrated to decrease ICP and increase CPP in patients with refractory intracranial hypertension and should be considered an alternative to treatment with mannitol.[23]

Other Interventions

The use of corticosteroids for increased ICP has been efficacious only in cerebral edema associated with tumors.[24,25] In head injuries, steroids

■ REFERENCES

1. Bullock R, Chesnut R, Clifton G, Ghajar J, Marion DW, Narayan RK. *Guidelines for the Management of Severe Head Injury.* New York: Brain Trauma Foundation; 1996.
2. Strauss GI, Moller K, Holm S, et al. Transcranial Doppler sonography and internal jugular bulb saturation during hyperventilation in patients with fulminant hepatic failure. *Liver Transpl.* 2001;7:352–358.
3. Forsyth R, Baxter P, Elliott T, et al. Routine intracranial pressure monitoring in acute coma. *Cochrane Database Syst Rev.* 2001:CD002043.
4. Bratton SL, Chestnut RM, Ghajar J, et al. Guidelines for the management of severe traumatic brain injury. VI. Indications for intracranial pressure monitoring. *J Neurotrauma.* 2007;24(Suppl 1):S37–S44.
5. Colohan AR, Alves WM, Gross CR. Head injury mortality in two centers with different emergency medical services and intensive care. *J Neurosurg.* 1989;71:202–207.
6. Fakhry SM, Trask AL, Waller MA, et al. Management of brain-injured patients by an evidence-based medicine protocol improves outcomes and decreases hospital charges. *J Trauma.* 2004;56:492–499.
7. Palmer S, Bader MK, Qureshi A, et al. The impact on outcomes in a community hospital setting of using the AANS traumatic brain injury guidelines. Americans Associations for Neurologic Surgeons. *J Trauma.* 2001;50:657–664.
8. Bullock MR, Chestnut RM, Clifton GL, et al. Indications for intracranial pressure monitoring. *J Neurotrauma.* 2000;17:479–491.
9. Marshall LF, Gautille T, Klauber MR. The outcome of severe closed head injury. *J Neurosurg.* 1991;75:S28–S36.
10. Cremer OL, van Dijk GW, van Wensen E, et al. Effect of intracranial pressure monitoring and targeted intensive care on functional outcome after severe head injury. *Crit Care Med.* 2005;33:2207–2213.
11. Feldman Z, Kanter MJ, Robertson CS, et al. Effect of head elevation on intracranial pressure, cerebral perfusion pressure, and cerebral blood flow in head-injured patients. *J Neurosurg.* 1992;76:207–211.
12. Skippen P, Seear M, Poskitt K, et al. Effect of hyperventilation on regional cerebral blood flow in head-injured children. *Crit Care Med.* 1997;25:1402–1409.
13. Muizelaar JP, Marmarou A, Ward JD, et al. Adverse effects of prolonged hyperventilation in patients with severe head injury: a randomized clinical trial. *J Neurosurg.* 1991;75:731–739.
14. Bullock RM, Chesnut RM, Clifton GL, et al. Hyperventilation. *J Neurotrauma.* 2000;17:513–520.
15. Qureshi AI, Geocadin RG, Suarez JI, et al. Long-term outcome after medical reversal of transtentorial herniation in patients with supratentorial mass lesions. *Crit Care Med.* 2000;28:1556–1564.

16. Morse ML, Milstein JM, Haas JE, et al. Effect of hydration on experimentally induced cerebral edema. *Crit Care Med.* 1985;13:563–565.
17. Bullock MR, Chestnut RM, Clifton GL, et al. Critical pathway for the treatment of established intracranial hypertension. *J Neurotrauma.* 2000;17:537–547.
18. Marshall LF, Smith RW, Rauscher LA, et al. Mannitol dose requirements in brain-injured patients. *J Neurosurg.* 1978;48:169–172.
19. Rosner MJ, Coley I. Cerebral perfusion pressure: a hemodynamic mechanism of mannitol and the postmannitol hemogram. *Neurosurg.* 1987;21:147–156.
20. Sayre MR, Daily SW, Stern SA, et al. Out-of-hospital administration of mannitol to head-injured patients does not change systolic blood pressure. *Acad Emerg Med.* 1996;3:840–848.
21. Misra UK, Kalita J, Ranjan P, et al. Mannitol in intracerebral hemorrhage: a randomized controlled study. *J Neurol Sci.* 2005;234:41–45.
22. Kalita J, Misra UK, Ranjan P, et al. Effect of mannitol on regional cerebral blood flow in patients with intracerebral hemorrhage. *J Neurol Sci.* 2004;224:19–22.
23. Hartl R, Ghajar J, Hochleuthner H, et al. Hypertonic/hyperoncotic saline reliably reduces ICP in severely head-injured patients with intracranial hypertension. *Acta Neurochir Suppl.* 1997;70:126–129.
24. Gutin PH. Corticosteroid therapy in patients with brain tumors. Natl Cancer Inst Monogr. 1977;46:151–156.
25. Gutin PH. Corticosteroid therapy in patients with cerebral tumors: benefits, mechanisms, problems, practicalities. [Review] [75 refs]. *Sem Oncol.* 1975;2:49–56.
26. Edwards P, Arango M, Balica L, et al. Final results of MRC CRASH, a randomised placebo-controlled trial of intravenous corticosteroids in adult head injury – outcomes at 6 months. *Lancet.* 2005;365:1957–1959.
27. Alderson P, Gadkary C, Signorini DF. Therapeutic hypothermia for head injury. *Cochrane Database Syst Rev.* 2004:CD001048.
28. Menzel M, Doppenberg EMR, Zauneer A, et al. Increased inspired oxygen concentration as a factor in improved brain tissue oxygenation and tissue lactate levels after severe human head injury. *J Neurosurg.* 1999;91:1–10.
29. Clarke JP. The effects of inverse ratio ventilation on intracranial pressure: a preliminary report. *Intensive Care Med.* 1997;23:106–109.
30. Muench E, Bauhuf C, Roth H, et al. Effects of positive end-expiratory pressure on regional cerebral blood flow, intracranial pressure, and brain tissue oxygenation. *Crit Care Med.* 2005;33:2367–2372.
31. McGuire G, Crossley D, Richards J, et al. Effects of varying levels of positive end-expiratory pressure on intracranial pressure and cerebral perfusion pressure. *Crit Care Med.* 1997;25:1059–1062.
32. Kerr ME, Weber BB, Sereika SM, et al. Effect of endotracheal suctioning on cerebral oxygenation in traumatic brain-injured patients. *Crit Care Med.* 1999;27:2776–2781.

50

Subarachnoid Hemorrhage

Subarachnoid hemorrhage (SAH) is a common and devastating condition.[1] Each year approximately 30,000 Americans suffer from a non-traumatic SAH. Patients who have suffered a SAH are best managed in an ICU or a specialized neurological/neurosurgical unit. Despite improved management the outcome following SAH remains poor, with an overall mortality of approximately 25% and significant morbidity amongst the survivors. The most serious complications following the initial bleed are rebleeding and cerebral vasospasm; management of patients with SAH is therefore largely directed to avoiding these complications. The risk of rebleeding (with conservative therapy) is highest in the first month, with a rate of between 20 and 30%. The mortality rate is approximately 70% for patients who rebleed. Angiographic vasospasm probably develops to some degree in most patients who suffer an SAH. However, clinically manifest vasospasm occurs in approximately 40% of patients. Fifteen to twenty percent of these patients will suffer a stroke or die despite aggressive management.

■ DIAGNOSIS AND EVALUATION

CT Scan and Lumbar Puncture

Non-contrast CT scanning is the diagnostic test of choice following a suspected SAH. If the scan is performed within 24 h of the event, clot can be demonstrated in the subarachnoid space in approximately 90% of patients. The diagnostic sensitivity of the CT scan declines after the first

P.E. Marik, *Handbook of Evidence-Based Critical Care*,
DOI 10.1007/978-1-4419-5923-2_50,
© Springer Science+Business Media, LLC 2010

day. A diagnostic lumbar puncture should be performed in a patient with a suspected SAH if the initial CT scan is negative. A normal CT scan and a normal spinal fluid examination exclude a SAH and predict a favorable prognosis in the setting of the sudden onset of a severe headache.

Clinical Classification

The Hunt and Hess classification system is the most commonly used grading system to assess the severity of an SAH. The Hunt and Hess grade has important therapeutic and prognostic implications:

- I – asymptomatic or slight headache
- II – moderate-to-severe headache, nuchal rigidity, no neurological deficit other than cranial nerve palsy
- III – drowsiness, confusion, or mild focal deficit
- IV – stupor, moderate-to-severe hemiparesis
- V – deep coma, decerebrate rigidity

Cerebral Angiography

Selective catheter angiography is currently the standard for diagnosing cerebral aneurysms as the cause of SAH. Approximately 20–25% of cerebral angiograms performed for SAH will not indicate a source of bleeding. It is generally recommended to repeat the angiogram in 2 weeks, because vascular spasm may have obscured the aneurysm. However, only a very small percentage of repeat angiograms will demonstrate an aneurysm. The risk of rebleeding in patients with normal angiograms is low; less than 4% are reported to rebleed when followed for up to 10 years. CT angiography has improved to the point where some centers use it as the primary test to identify an aneurysm.

■ INITIAL MANAGEMENT

General Measures and Measures to Prevent Rebleeding

- Bed rest with elevation of the head to 20–35°.[2]
- Mild sedation/anxiolysis for grade I and II patients.
- Pain management with morphine sulfate or codeine. Meperidine should be avoided as it can precipitate seizures.
- Maintain euvolemia. Careful fluid management is required to avoid hypovolemia, which may reduce the risk of delayed cerebral

ischemia. Despite being widely advocated, data supporting the use of hypervolemia are scant. A prospective randomized trial found no impact of prophylactic hypervolemia on CBF, vasospasm, or outcome.[3]

- Laxatives.
- DVT prophylaxis (stockings/pneumatic boots).
- Nimodipine 60 mg q 4–6 h for prevention of cerebral vasospasm.
- Ventriculostomy for acute obstructive hydrocephalus.
- The routine use of anti-convulsants has been associated with cognitive impairment in patients with SAH and heralded the growing acceptance of reduced use of anti-convulsants.[4,5]
- Corticosteroids have no proven benefit in SAH.

Anti-hypertensive Agents

The role of anti-hypertensive agents in preventing rebleeding is controversial. Rebleeding may be related to variations or changes in blood pressure rather than the absolute blood pressure. However, it is generally advised that the systolic pressure be kept below 150 mmHg. Mild sedation and control of pain may adequately control an elevated blood pressure. If anti-hypertensive agents are used, these should be used with extreme caution. Intravenous agents that can be closely titrated are preferred; an excessive reduction of blood pressure may cause cerebral ischemia. The use of oral or s/l nifedipine is strongly discouraged. Although nitroprusside is a very short-acting, easily titratable anti-hypertensive agent, it has been shown to increase intracerebral pressure. Furthermore, doses in excess of 2 mg/min will lead to cyanide accumulation. Intravenous labetalol is the preferred agent; however, intravenous nicardipine or clevidipine can also be used (see Chapter 25).

Anti-fibrinolytic Therapy

The role of anti-fibrinolytic agent in preventing rebleeding is unclear. While anti-fibrinolytic agents reduce the rate of bleeding, the benefits are offset by a higher incidence of cerebral infarction.[6] Increased use of early aneurysm treatment combined with prophylactic treatment of cerebral vasospasm may reduce the ischemic complications of anti-fibrinolytic agents while maintaining the benefit of reduced preoperative bleeding rates. In a prospective, randomized trial of the anti-fibrinolytic drug tranexamic acid, early rebleeding rates and adverse outcomes were reduced when the drug was administered immediately after the diagnosis of SAH.[2]

■ SURGICAL AND ENDOVASCULAR METHODS OF TREATMENT

In 1991, Guglielmi et al.[7] described the technique of occluding aneurysms from an endovascular approach with electrolytically detachable platinum coils (Guglielmi detachable coils). Guglielmi detachable coils are introduced directly into the aneurysm through a microcatheter and detached from a stainless steel microguidewire by an electric current. The aneurysm is packed with several coils. The coils induce thrombosis, thereby excluding the aneurysm from the circulation. As clinical experience with the technique has increased and technological advances in coil design and adjunctive methods have improved, endovascular treatment has been used with increasing frequency. Improved outcomes have been linked to hospitals that provide endovascular services.

The ISAT trial compared neurosurgical clipping vs. endovascular coiling in 2,143 patients with ruptured aneurysms.[8] In this study which enrolled patients with ruptured intracranial aneurysms suitable for both treatments, endovascular coiling was more likely to result in independent survival at 1 year than did neurosurgical clipping; the survival benefit continued for at least 7 years. The risk of epilepsy was substantially lower in patients allocated to endovascular treatment, but the risk of late rebleeding was higher.

■ MANAGEMENT OF CEREBRAL VASOSPASM

After aneurysmal SAH, angiographic vasospasm is seen in 30–70% of patients, with a typical onset 3–5 days after the hemorrhage, maximal narrowing at 5–14 days, and a gradual resolution over 2–4 weeks. Cerebral vasospasm is associated with reduced CBF. The changes in CBF are coupled to changes in oxygen delivery so that cerebral hypoperfusion leads to inadequate oxygen delivery. In about one half of cases, vasospasm is manifested by the occurrence of a delayed neurological ischemic deficit, which may resolve or progress to cerebral infarction. In contemporary series, 15–20% of such patients suffer stroke or die of vasospasm despite maximal therapy.[1] Often, the development of a new focal deficit, unexplained by hydrocephalus or rebleeding, is the first objective sign of symptomatic vasospasm. In addition, unexplained increases in mean arterial pressure may occur as cerebral arterial autoregulation attempts to improve cerebral circulation to prevent ischemia. Monitoring of vasospasm with transcranial Doppler technology, in addition to clinical observation in the ICU, has been controversial. The literature is inconclusive regarding its sensitivity and specificity.[1]

The goal for the management of cerebral vasospasm is to reduce the threat of ischemic neuronal damage by controlling intracranial pressure, decreasing the metabolic rate of oxygen use, and improving CBF. Since 1976, when Kosnik and Hunt[9] reported on the reversal of neurological deficits by use of induced hypertension and hypervolemia in seven patients who had deteriorated due to vasospasm, the use of "triple-H" therapy in the management of patients with cerebral vasospasm after SAH has been widely accepted. Despite being widely advocated, data supporting the use of triple-H therapy are scant and the relative contribution of each component is debated. A prospective randomized trial found no impact of prophylactic hypervolemia on CBF, vasospasm, or outcome.[3]

It should be noted that hypervolemia is somewhat of a misnomer. In a patient with normal cardiac and renal function, it is not possible to induce a state of hypervolemia; the excess fluid is just "peed out." In patients with cardiac or renal dysfunction and/or alterations in capillary permeability, this approach will lead to pulmonary and tissue (brain) edema (the intravascular and interstitial compartments are in a dynamic equilibrium). Furthermore, it is critical to appreciate that there is no correlation between the CVP/PCWP and the intravascular volume; titrating volume replacement to a predetermined CVP/PCWP is dangerous and is to be strongly discouraged (see Chapter 8).

Cerebral autoregulation is disturbed in patients after SAH, with cerebral perfusion being directly dependent on cerebral perfusion pressure. Vasoactive agents are used to increase the cerebral perfusion pressure. Dopamine and/or norepinephrine may achieve this goal. The systolic blood pressure should be kept between 160 and 200 mmHg (120–150 mmHg for unclipped aneurysms) and titrated to the patients' neurological state. Dopamine should be used cautiously in patients with cardiac disease. Phenylephrine tends to decrease cardiac output (and therefore cerebral blood flow) and should therefore be avoided. The patient should be closely monitored and serial transcranial Dopplers performed to monitor the progress of the patient's condition.

Muench et al.[10] studied the three components of "triple-H" therapy in patients with SAH. Induction of hypertension resulted in a significant increase in regional cerebral blood flow and brain tissue oxygenation at all observation time points. In contrast, hypervolemia/hemodilution induced only a slight increase in regional cerebral blood flow, while brain tissue oxygenation did not improve. Finally, triple-H therapy failed to improve regional cerebral blood flow more than what hypertension did alone and was characterized by the drawback that the hypervolemia/hemodilution components reversed the effect of induced hypertension on brain tissue oxygenation. Using a xenon blood flow tomography-based system, Joseph et al. showed that hypervolemia does not increase CBF. Furthermore, in a clinical series, Ekelund et al.

demonstrated no effect of hypervolemic therapy on rCBF and a pronounced reduction in oxygen delivery capacity. These data suggest that the two "Hs" (hypervolemia + hemodilution) should be dropped from "triple-H" therapy. Transpulmonary thermodilution may be a useful technique to manage fluids and vasopressors in patients with SAH.[11]

In terms of tissue (brain) oxygen delivery, the optimal HCT is probably about 30. However, both hemodilution and blood transfusion to achieve this goal are not recommended (see Chapter 51).

Angioplasty of the implicated vessel, high-dose intravenous nicardipine, and intra-arterial papaverine have been reported in patients with vasospasm. The role of these therapeutic interventions remains to be determined.

■ REFERENCES

1. Bederson JB, Connolly ES, Batjer HH, et al. Guidelines for the management of aneurysmal subarachnoid hemorrhage. A statement for healthcare professionals from a special writing group of the Stroke Council, American Heart Association. *Stroke*. 2009:doi: 10.1161/STROKEAHA.108.191395.
2. Hillman J, Fridriksson S, Nilsson O, et al. Immediate administration of tranexamic acid and reduced incidence of early rebleeding after aneurysmal subarachnoid hemorrhage: a prospective randomized study. *J Neurosurg*. 2002;97:771–778.
3. Lennihan L, Mayer SA, Fink ME, et al. Effect of hypervolemic therapy on cerebral blood flow after subarachnoid hemorrhage: a randomized controlled trial. *Stroke*. 2000;31:383–391.
4. Rosengart AJ, Huo JD, Tolentino J, et al. Outcome in patients with subarachnoid hemorrhage treated with antiepileptic drugs. *J Neurosurg*. 2007;107:253–260.
5. Naidech AM, Kreiter KT, Janjua N, et al. Phenytoin exposure is associated with functional and cognitive disability after subarachnoid hemorrhage. *Stroke*. 2005;36:583–587.
6. Torner JC, Kassell NF, Wallace RB, et al. Preoperative prognostic factors for rebleeding and survival in aneurysm patients receiving antifibrinolytic therapy: report of the Cooperative Aneurysm Study. *Neurosurg*. 1981;9:506–513.
7. Guglielmi G, Vinuela F, Dion J, et al. Electrothrombosis of saccular aneurysms via endovascular approach. Part 2: Preliminary clinical experience. *J Neurosurg*. 1991;75:8–14.
8. Molyneux AJ, Kerr RS, Yu LM, et al. International subarachnoid aneurysm trial (ISAT) of neurosurgical clipping versus endovascular coiling in 2143 patients with ruptured intracranial aneurysms: a

randomised comparison of effects on survival, dependency, seizures, rebleeding, subgroups, and aneurysm occlusion. *Lancet*. 2005;366: 809–817.

9. Kosnik EJ, Hunt WE. Postoperative hypertension in the management of patients with intracranial arterial aneurysms. *J Neurosurg*. 1976;45: 148–154.

10. Muench E, Horn P, Bauhuf C, et al. Effects of hypervolemia and hypertension on regional cerebral blood flow, intracranial pressure, and brain tissue oxygenation after subarachnoid hemorrhage. *Crit Care Med*. 2007;35:1844–1851.

11. Mutoh T, Kazumata K, Ajiki M, et al. Goal-directed fluid management by bedside transpulmonary hemodynamic monitoring after subarachnoid hemorrhage. *Stroke*. 2007;38:3218–3224.

Part VII

Miscellaneous ICU Topics

51

Anemia and RBC Transfusion

Anemia is common in critically ill patients. More than 90% of patients have subnormal hemoglobin by the third day of ICU admission. Despite the fact that blood transfusions have not been shown to improve the outcome of ICU patients (see below) and that the current guidelines recommend blood transfusion only when the hemoglobin falls below 7.0 g/dl, almost half of all patients admitted to an ICU receive a blood transfusion.[1,2] The etiology of anemia of critical illness is multi-factorial and complex. Repeated phlebotomy, gastrointestinal blood loss, and other surgical procedures contribute significantly to the development of anemia. Red cell production in critically ill patients is often abnormal and is involved in the development and maintenance of anemia. The pathophysiology of this anemia includes decreased production of erythropoietin (EPO), impaired bone marrow response to erythropoietin, and reduced red cell survival.

For much of the last century, RBC transfusion has been viewed as having obvious clinical benefit. Blood transfusion was considered as a life-saving strategy and an arbitrary threshold of 10 gm/dl was used as a transfusion trigger. However, over the last 20 years, RBC transfusion practice has come under increased scrutiny. Initially this was driven by concerns over transfusion-related infections, HIV in particular. While the risk of transfusion-transmitted infections has received considerable attention, the risks of this complication with modern blood-banking techniques are now exceedingly remote.[3] On the other hand, it is now becoming clear that there are other important, less-recognized risks of RBC transfusion related to RBC storage effects and to immunomodulating effects of RBC transfusions which occur in almost all recipients.[4]

P.E. Marik, *Handbook of Evidence-Based Critical Care*,
DOI 10.1007/978-1-4419-5923-2_51,
© Springer Science+Business Media, LLC 2010

■ COMPLICATIONS ASSOCIATED WITH BLOOD TRANSFUSION

Infectious

- Human immunodeficiency virus (HIV)
- Hepatitis B, C, D
- Cytomegalovirus
- Parvovirus B19
- Epstein–Barr virus
- Human T-cell leukemia/lymphoma virus
- Human herpes virus 6, 7, and 8
- Toxoplasmosis
- Malaria
- West Nile virus
- TT virus
- Prion disease

Non-infectious

- Immune activation
  - Non-hemolytic febrile reactions
  - Anaphylactoid allergic reactions
  - Acute hemolytic reaction
  - Delayed hemolytic reactions
  - Transfusion-related acute lung injury (TRALI)
  - Delayed TRALI syndrome
  - Transfusion-associated graft vs. host disease
- Immune tolerance
  - Nosocomial/postoperative infections
  - Multi-organ failure
  - Transplant tolerance
  - Cancer recurrence
  - Autoimmune disease

ALERT

Transfused blood contains progenitor stem cells; blood transfusion should be considered to be a mini bone marrow transplant; the immunomodulating effects persist for years; maybe lifelong.[5]

The "toxicity" of blood is related to a number of factors including the following:

- Leukodepleted vs. non-leukodepleted blood
- The length of storage (age of the blood)
- The number of units transfused
- The immune status of the recipient

Furthermore, although blood transfusions increase systemic oxygen delivery, the immediate effectiveness of stored red cell transfusions to augment tissue oxygen consumption in critically ill patients has been questioned in several studies.[6]

We performed a systemic review of the literature to determine the benefits and harm associated with blood transfusion. We included 45 observational studies in our review.[7] In 42 of the 45 studies, the risks of RBC transfusion outweighed the benefits and the risk was neutral in two studies, with the benefits outweighing the risks in a subgroup of a single study (elderly patients with an acute myocardial infarction and a HCT <30%). Seventeen of the eighteen studies demonstrated that RBC transfusions were an independent predictor of death; the pooled OR (12 studies) was 1.7 (95% CI 1.4–1.9). Twenty-two studies examined the association between RBC transfusion and nosocomial infection; in all these studies, blood transfusion was an independent risk factor for infection. The pooled OR (nine studies) for developing an infectious complications was 1.8 (95% CI 1.5–2.2). RBC transfusions similarly increased the risk of developing MODS (three studies) and ARDS (six studies). The pooled OR for developing ARDS was 2.5 (95% CI 1.6–3.3). These data suggest that blood can no longer be regarded as "being safe," that blood transfusions are associated with increased morbidity and mortality, and that the risks and possible benefits of blood transfusion should be evaluated carefully in each patient prior to a transfusion.

Transfusion-related acute lung injury (TRALI) syndrome is an "uncommon" condition characterized by the abrupt onset of respiratory failure within hours of the transfusion of a blood product. It is usually caused by anti-leukocyte antibodies, resolves rapidly, and has a low mortality. A single unit of packed cells or blood component products (FFP and platelets) is usually implicated in initiating this syndrome. It has, however, recently been recognized that the transfusion of blood products in critically ill or injured patients increases the risk for the development of the ALI/acute respiratory distress syndrome (ARDS) 6–72 h after the transfusion. This "delayed TRALI syndrome" is common, occurring in up to 25% of critically ill patients receiving a blood transfusion, and is associated with a mortality rate of up to 40%.[8] While the delayed TRALI syndrome can develop after the transfusion of a single unit, the risk increases as the number of transfused blood products increases. The management of both the classic and delayed TRALI syndromes is essentially supportive.

■ TOLERANCE TO ANEMIA

In health, the amount of oxygen delivered to the whole body exceeds resting oxygen requirements almost fourfold. An isolated decrease in hemoglobin concentration to 10 g/dl with all other parameters remaining constant will result in an oxygen delivery that remains approximately twice that of the resting oxygen consumption. Humans have a remarkable ability to adapt to anemia by increasing cardiac output (in the absence of volume depletion), increasing microcirculatory density, increasing red cell synthesis of 2,3-DPG with a resultant rightward shift of the oxyhemoglobin dissociation curve (aids oxygen unloading), and by increasing oxygen extraction. Healthy volunteers can tolerate isovolemic hemodilution down to a hemoglobin content of 4.5 without apparent harmful effects.[9] However, due to the high extraction ratio of oxygen in the coronary circulation, coronary blood flow appears to be the major factor which limits the tolerance of low hemoglobin concentrations. In experimental animal models of coronary stenosis, depressed cardiac function occurs at hemoglobin concentrations between 7 and 10 g/l.[10,11]

■ WHEN SHOULD PATIENTS BE TRANSFUSED?

Patients without cardiovascular disease may tolerate hemoglobin levels as low as 7 g/dl and possibly lower with minimal sequela. Although physiological reserve decreases with aging, it appears that elderly patients (>65 years) without cardiovascular disease may similarly tolerate hemoglobin concentrations as low as 8 g/dl without untoward effects. The current data clearly demonstrate that blood transfusions increase the risk of infection, ARDS, and death. Evidence-based guidelines would therefore suggest that patients without cardiovascular disease and who are not actively bleeding should be transfused only when the hemoglobin concentration falls below 7 g/dl. Furthermore, it could be argued that even in these patients, a transfusion is indicated only if the patient has symptomatic anemia (i.e., signs of myocardial or tissue ischemia). These recommendations are supported by the landmark Canadian Critical Care Trials Group Study (TRICC) which demonstrated the safety of using a "transfusion trigger" of 7.0 g/dl in critically ill ICU patients.[12] Furthermore, in the subgroup of patients with cardiovascular disease in the TRICC study (none with acute coronary syndromes), the restrictive transfusion strategy was not associated with an increased risk of complications or mortality as compared to the liberal transfusion group.[13]

The traditional 10/30 transfusion trigger can no longer be supported. In the absence of acute bleeding, hemoglobin levels consistent with the TRICC trial (7.0–9.0 g/dl) are well tolerated.[12] The American Association of Blood Banking has recommended titrating transfusion requirements to parameters of severity of illness rather than arbitrarily defined hemoglobin levels.[14] This recommendation is in agreement with the more recent recommendations of the American Society of Anesthesiologists Task Force,[15] as well as the Canadian Guidelines which suggest "there is no single value of hemoglobin concentration that justifies or requires transfusion; an evaluation of the patient's clinical situation should also be a factor in the decision."[16]

The Cardiac Patient

Anemia is well recognized to be a poor prognostic factor in patients with congestive cardiac failure as well as acute coronary syndromes (ACS's).[17,18] Contrary to conventional wisdom, this does not mean that blood transfusion improves outcome. Rao and colleagues[19] examined the potential impact of red blood cell transfusion in 24,111 patients with ACS. Blood transfusion was an independent predictor of myocardial infarction and 30-day all-cause mortality (adjusted hazard ratio 3.94). Furthermore, the 30-day mortality was significantly increased when transfusions were given to patients with hematocrits of 25% or above (compared to those with a hematocrit below 25%). Similarly, Aronson and colleagues[20] demonstrated an increase in mortality and the composite end point of death/recurrent MI/heart failure in patients with acute myocardial infarction who had a hemoglobin >8 g/dl and received a blood transfusion. Similar observations have been made by other authors.[21-23] The increased risk of infarction and death is probably related to the pro-thrombotic and pro-inflammatory properties of stored blood.[24]

The Elective Surgical Patient

Carson and colleagues[25,26] studied patients who underwent surgery and declined blood transfusions for religious reasons. In those patients without cardiovascular disease and who had a baseline hemoglobin of between 6 and 6.9 g/dl, there was no significant increase in perioperative mortality (OR 1.4; 95% CI 0.5–4.2) if the blood loss was less than 2.0 g/dl. However, in patients with cardiovascular disease, preoperative anemia was associated with a significant increase in perioperative mortality. These data confirm that humans can adapt to very low hemoglobin levels, with cardiovascular disease being the major limiting factor. These data suggest that in patients undergoing surgery who have significant coronary artery disease, the hemoglobin should be increased to about 10 g/dl prior to surgery. This is best achieved with the use of EPO and iron, thereby avoiding a blood transfusion. Blood transfusions are independent risk factors for perioperative infections, ARDS, and death (and perhaps tumor recurrence).[7,27]

ALERT

Except for patients with severe acute blood loss, there is no disease state that benefits from *blood transfusion*.
Furthermore, there is no convincing data that blood transfusions acutely increase oxygen uptake in critically ill patients.

Summary of When to Transfuse

- Individualize for each patient
  - Weigh risks vs. benefits
- ACS <8 g/dl
- Significant CAD and surgery <10 g/dl
- All other <6–7 g/dl
  - Tachycardia
  - Lactate
  - MvO_2
  - Mentation

■ CLINICAL PEARLS

- Transfused blood is not the same as the blood in our veins.
- Blood transfusions are associated with significant complications which frequently outweigh any potential benefits.

■ REFERENCES

1. Corwin HL, Gettinger A, Pearl RG, et al. The CRIT Study: Anemia and blood transfusion in the critically ill – current clinical practice in the United States. *Crit Care Med*. 2004;32:39–52.
2. Vincent JL, Baron JF, Reinhart K, et al. Anemia and blood transfusion in critically ill patients. *JAMA*. 2002;288:1499–1507.
3. Busch MP, Kleinman SH, Nemo GJ. Current and emerging infectious risks of blood transfusions. *JAMA*. 2003;289:959–962.
4. Raghavan M, Marik PE. Anemia, allogenic blood transfusion, and immunomodulation in the critically ill. *Chest*. 2005;127:295–307.
5. Beck I, Scott JS, Pepper M, et al. The effect of neonatal exchange and later blood transfusion on lymphocyte cultures. *Am J Reproduct Immunol*. 1981;1:224–225.

6. Marik PE, Sibbald WJ. Effect of stored-blood transfusion on oxygen delivery in patients with sepsis. *JAMA*. 1993;269:3024–3029.
7. Marik PE, Corwin HL. Efficacy of RBC transfusion in the critically ill: a systematic review of the literature. *Crit Care Med*. 2008; 36:2667–2674.
8. Marik PE, Corwin HL. Acute lung injury following blood transfusion: expanding the definition. *Crit Care Med*. 2008;36:3080–3084.
9. Weiskopf RB, Viele MK, Feiner J, et al. Human cardiovascular and metabolic response to acute, severe isovolemic anemia. *JAMA*. 1998;279:217–221.
10. Leung JM, Weiskopf RB, Feiner J, et al. Electrocardiographic ST-segment changes during acute, severe isovolemic hemodilution in humans. *Anesthesiol*. 2000;93:1004–1010.
11. Levy PS, Kim SJ, Eckel PK, et al. Limit to cardiac compensation during acute isovolemic hemodilution: influence of coronary stenosis. *Am J Physiol*. 1993;265:H340–H349.
12. Hebert PC, Wells G, Blajchman MA, et al. A multicenter, randomized, controlled clinical trial of transfusion requirements in critical care. Transfusion Requirements in Critical Care Investigators, Canadian Critical Care Trials Group. *N Engl J Med*. 1999;340:409–417.
13. Hebert PC, Yetisir E, Martin C, et al. Is a low transfusion threshold safe in critically ill patients with cardiovascular diseases? *Crit Care Med*, 2001;29:227–234.
14. Consensus conference. Perioperative red blood cell transfusion. *JAMA*. 1988;260:2700–2703.
15. Practice guidelines for perioperative blood transfusion and adjuvant therapies. An Updated report by the American Society of Anesthesiologists Task Force on Perioperative Blood Transfusion and Adjuvant Therapies. *Anesthesiol*. 2008;105:198–208.
16. Expert Working Group. Guidelines for red blood cell and plasma transfusion for adults and children. *Can Med Assoc J*. 2008;156(11 (suppl.):S1–S24.
17. Nikolsky E, Aymong ED, Halkin A, et al. Impact of anemia in patients with acute myocardial infarction undergoing primary percutaneous coronary intervention: analysis from the Controlled Abciximab and Device Investigation to Lower Late Angioplasty Complications (CADILLAC) Trial. *J Am Coll Cardiol*. 2004;44:547–553.
18. Mozaffarian D, Nye R, Levy WC. Anemia predicts mortality in severe heart failure: the prospective randomized amlodipine survival evaluation (PRAISE). *J Am Coll Cardiol*. 2003;41:1933–1939.
19. Rao SV, Jollis JG, Harrington RA, et al. Relationship of blood transfusion and clinical outcomes in patients with acute coronary syndromes. *JAMA*. 2004;292:1555–1562.
20. Aronson D, Dann EJ, Bonstein L, et al. Impact of red blood cell transfusion on clinical outcomes in patients with acute myocardial infarction. *Am J Cardiol*. 2008;102:115–119.

21. Jani SM, Smith DE, Share D, et al. Blood transfusion and in-hospital outcomes in anemic patients with myocardial infarction undergoing percutaneous coronary intervention. *Clin Cardiol.* 2007;30:II49–II56.
22. Singla I, Zahid M, Good CB, et al. Impact of blood transfusions in patients presenting with anemia and suspected acute coronary syndrome. *Am J Cardiol.* 2007;99:1119–1121.
23. Alexander KP, Chen AY, Wang TY, et al. Transfusion practice and outcomes in non-ST-segment elevation acute coronary syndromes. *Am Heart J.* 2008;155:1047–1053.
24. Twomley KM, Rao SV, Becker RC. Proinflammatory, immunomodulating, and prothrombotic properties of anemia and red blood cell transfusions. *J Thromb Thrombolysis.* 2006;21:167–174.
25. Carson JL, Duff A, Poses RM, et al. Effect of anaemia and cardiovascular disease on surgical mortality and morbidity. *Lancet.* 1996;348:1055–1060.
26. Spence RK, Carson JA, Poses R, et al. Elective surgery without transfusion: influence of preoperative hemoglobin level and blood loss on mortality. *Am J Surg.* 1990;159:320–324.
27. Marik PE. The hazards of blood transfusion. *Br J Hosp Med.* 2009;70:12–15.

52

Coagulopathy and FFP Transfusions

Coagulation disorders are commonly encountered in the ICU. Many conditions including sepsis, malignancy, trauma, vasculitic disorders, and obstetrical accidents may give rise to a coagulopathy. In addition, patients may have medical conditions which predispose them to developing a coagulopathy, e.g., patients with liver disease, renal failure, lupus, leukemia, etc. Sepsis, however, is the single most common factor leading to a coagulopathy and DIC. DIC has been reported in about 10–20% of patients with gram-negative bacteremia and 70% of patients with septic shock. In patients with sepsis, DIC appears to be an important independent predictor of ARDS, multiple organ dysfunction syndrome, and death (see Chapter 10).

A coagulopathy is best defined as the presence of an abnormal coagulation test(s). The Scientific Subcommittee on Disseminated Intravascular Coagulation (DIC) of the International Society on Thrombosis and Haemostasis (ISTH) has suggested that DIC be considered "an acquired syndrome characterized by the intravascular activation of coagulation with loss of localization arising from different causes. It can originate from and cause damage to the microvasculature, which if sufficiently severe, produce organ dysfunction."[1] DIC is characterized by the generation of *fibrin-related products* (soluble fibrin monomer, fibrin degradation products, D-dimer, etc.) and is indicative of an acquired (inflammatory) or a non-inflammatory disorder of the *microvasculature*.

DIC results from the systemic activation of both the clotting and fibrinolytic systems, leading to the consumption of many coagulation factors and platelets. The initial activation of coagulation in sepsis is primarily dependant on activation of the extrinsic (tissue factor-dependant) pathway. DIC is generally considered to be a systemic hemorrhagic

P.E. Marik, *Handbook of Evidence-Based Critical Care*, **543**
DOI 10.1007/978-1-4419-5923-2_52,
© Springer Science+Business Media, LLC 2010

syndrome. However, this is only because hemorrhage is obvious and often impressive. Less commonly appreciated is the formidable microvascular thrombosis that occurs. Fibrin deposition in the microcir-culation is a frequent, if not invariable, finding in patients with DIC. This microvascular thrombosis is closely related to the development of mul-tiple organ dysfunction syndrome and is therefore closely linked to the prognosis of patients with DIC. This microvascular damage is especially pronounced in the lungs and kidneys. In septic patients with DIC, the thrombotic (anti-fibrinolytic) pathways tend to dominate. The DIC that characterizes the early stage of traumatic shock is characteristically hem-orrhagic (fibrinolytic) which then becomes thrombotic by days 2–4; this pattern has important implications with regard to resuscitation with blood and blood products.[2]

A dilutional coagulopathy and DIC frequently occur in cases of mas-sive hemorrhage, regardless of their cause. Coagulation tests can be used to assess the severity of the dilutional coagulopathy and DIC as well as their evolution under the influence of therapeutic interventions. However, coagulation tests fail to predict the risk of bleeding (see below).

The "common" causes of coagulopathy/DIC in the ICU include the following:

- Sepsis with DIC (see Chapter 10)
- Trauma
- Massive hemorrhage
- Organ destruction (e.g., severe pancreatitis)
- Liver disease
  - Chronic liver disease (see Chapter 33)
  - Acute liver failure (see Chapter 35)
- Malignancy
  - Solid tumors
  - Myeloproliferate
- Obstetrical calamities
  - Amniotic fluid embolism
  - Abruptio placentae
- Excessive anti-coagulation
  - Coumadin
  - Heparin
- Vascular abnormalities
  - Kasabach–Merritt Syndrome
  - Large vascular aneurysms
- Toxic or immunological reactions
  - Snake bite
  - Recreational drugs
  - Transfusion reactions
  - Transplant rejection

■ DIAGNOSIS OF DIC

- Laboratory features:
  - Peripheral blood smear will show fragmented red blood cells and thrombocytopenia with large platelets.
  - Prolonged PT and PTT.
  - Thrombocytopenia.
  - Decreased levels of fibrinogen.
  - Decreased levels of Protein C.
  - Decreased levels of anti-thrombin III.
  - Increased levels of fibrin split products and D-dimer.
- Clinical features associated with bleeding:
  - Bleeding from venipuncture sites, mucous membranes, hematuria, GI bleeds, intracerebral bleeds.
  - Petechia, purpura, and subcutaneous hematomas.
- Clinical features of end organ damage due to thrombosis:
  - Acute lung injury.
  - Proteinuria and renal insufficiency.
  - Hepatocellular dysfunction.
  - Mental state changes and neurological deficits.

The ISTH Scoring System for DIC

Step 1. Does the patient have an underlying disorder known to be associated with overt DIC? If yes proceed.[1]

Step 2. Score global coagulation test results:

- Platelet count:
  - >100,000 = 0.
  - <100,000 = 1.
  - <50,000 = 2.
- Elevated FDP:
  - No increase = 0.
  - Moderate increase = 2.
  - Strong increase = 3.
- Prolonged prothrombin time:
  - <3 s = 0.
  - >3 but <6 s = 1.
  - >6 s = 2.
- Fibrinogen level:
  - >100 mg/dl = 0.
  - <100 mg/dl = 1.

Step 3. Calculate score:

- ≥5 compatible with over DIC, repeat score daily.
- <5 suggestive of non-overt DIC.

■ MANAGEMENT

The treatment of DIC remains controversial. This is primarily because there are very few studies which have objectively examined various therapeutic strategies in patients with DIC. The essential therapeutic modality is to treat the triggering disease process. Activated protein C has an important role in the treatment of DIC associated with sepsis (see Chapter 10). FFP and platelet transfusion are indicated only in patients with significant bleeding (see below).

Fresh Frozen Plasma

- Usually derived from whole blood, sometimes apheresis
- Frozen within 8 h of collection
- Volume: 200–250 ml
- Storage: frozen up to 1 year
- Content: "normal" levels of all coagulation factors
- Expiration: 24 h after thawing
- ABO compatibility required, cross matching not required
- FFP is one of the most hazardous individual blood components; the major risks include the following:
  - TRALI
  - Allergic reactions
  - Transmission of infections
  - Fluid overload
  - Increased risk of infections
  - Hemolysis due to anti-A and anti-B

FFP is an important cause of TRALI in ICU patients. Khan et al. demonstrated that ALI was more likely to develop in patients who received FFP transfusions (OR 2.48; 95% CI 1.29–4.74) and platelet transfusions (OR 3.89; 95% CI 1.36–11.52) than in those who received only RBC transfusions (OR 1.39; 95% CI 0.79–2.43).[3] Watson demonstrated that FFP was an independent predictor of MODS and ALI in trauma patients.[4] In addition, similar to blood transfusion, transfusion of FFP has been associated with an increased risk of infection in ICU patients.[5]

Patients with DIC should NOT be given FFP in order to correct abnormal coagulation tests. The administration of FFP should however be considered in patients with DIC who are actively bleeding. Despite the lack of a RCT, it is advisable to transfuse FFP in patients with massive hemorrhage caused by trauma, obstetrical problems, medical problems, or surgery. FFP (10–15 ml/kg, 4–6 units) is recommended to prevent further bleeding.[6] Cryoprecipitate is recommended in patients with a fibrinogen level <100 mg/dl.

FFP Prior to Invasive Bedside Procedures or Surgery

Over 4 million units of FFP are transfused annually in the United States. Approximately one-third of all FFP is used to prepare patients with an elevated INR or PTT for a procedure.[7] Transfusion of FFP prior to an invasive procedure in patients with abnormal coagulation test results rests upon two assumptions[8]

- that abnormal coagulation test results identify patients at increased risk of procedure-related bleeding and
- that transfusion of FFP will reduce that risk.

For patients with mild to moderate abnormalities of coagulation test results, evidence to support these two assumptions is scant to non-existent. A growing body of literature documents that the INR and PTT do not predict which patients will have procedure-related bleeding and should not be used to make decisions about prophylactic preprocedure transfusions.[9]

Several factors account for this lack of predictive value for bleeding. Coagulation tests such as the PT and the PTT were developed primarily to identify specific coagulation deficiencies such as hemophilia. In addition, they are carried out in vitro (in a test tube), at room temperature, and may fail to reflect the efficacy of coagulation pathways in vivo, which are affected by both core temperature and the interaction with circulating cells and substances.

A second assumption of preprocedure FFP transfusion is that the infused product will correct the coagulopathy and reduce the risk of bleeding. For the great majority of patients who are given such transfusions – namely, those with mild to moderate prolongation of the INR – there is very little evidence to support this assumption.[8] In fact, the evidence speaks to the contrary. Holland and Brooks reported the effect of FFP on the INR in 179 patients with a prolonged INR who were given FFP for a variety of indications.[10] For patients with INRs 1.7 or less, infusion of FFP in typical doses used had no effect on the patient's INR. For patients with INR values greater than 2, the correction of INR was modest and incomplete. For example, even for patients with an INR = 4.0, the average correction with FFP transfusion was partial, resulting in an INR = 3.0. Similar findings were reported by Abdel-Wahab et al.,[11] who noted that among 121 adult patients with a pretransfusion INR of 1.6 or less who were given 1–4 units of FFP, the post-transfusion INR corrected to within the normal range in only two patients. The exponential shape of the INR curve implies that increasing the concentration of clotting factors by FFP transfusion will have a substantial correcting effort on the INR when the pretransfusion INR level is markedly prolonged but will have an ever-diminishing impact as the pretransfusion INR approaches the normal physiological range.[8]

These data suggest that as a general rule, FFP should not be transfused prophylactically in patients with an INR <1.8 undergoing an invasive procedure. In patients with an INR ≥1.8 the risk/benefits of preprocedure FFP should be weighed in each patient; should FFP be infused, normalization of the INR should not be attempted. FFP should not be administered prophylactically to patients with normal coagulation tests undergoing high-risk surgery or invasive diagnostic tests in an "attempt to limit bleeding".

Management of Non-therapeutic INRs with or Without Bleeding (Due to Coumadin Therapy)

For most indications, an INR range of 2.0–3.0 is targeted; INR values less than 2.0 are associated with an increased risk for thromboembolism, and INR values greater than 4.0 are associated with an increase in bleeding complications. The risk for bleeding, particularly intracranial bleeding, increases markedly as the INR exceeds 4.5.

The management of patients whose INR is outside the therapeutic range is controversial because many of the various options have not been compared. The interventions include administering vitamin K and/or infusing fresh frozen plasma, prothrombin concentrates, or recombinant factor VIIa. The preferred approach is based largely on the potential risk of bleeding, the presence of active bleeding, and the level of the INR.[12] The response to vitamin K administered subcutaneously is less predictable than that of oral or IV vitamin K. DeZee[13] performed a meta-analysis of trials that used vitamin K to treat patients without major hemorrhage with an INR greater than 4.0. The primary outcome was achievement of the target INR (1.8–4.0) at 24 h after vitamin K administration. This study demonstrated equal efficacy of oral and IV vitamin K (1.0–2.5 mg) in normalizing the INR, whereas subcutaneous vitamin K was no better than placebo.

High doses of vitamin K, though effective, may lower the INR more than is necessary and may lead to warfarin resistance for 1 week or more. Low doses of vitamin K are therefore recommended. A dose of 1.25 is recommended when the INR is between 4.0 and 9.0, but larger doses (i.e., 2.5–5 mg) are required to correct INRs >9.0. Although the ACCP guidelines recommend low-dose vitamin K in patients with an INR between 5 and 10 who are not bleeding,[12] the efficacy of such an approach has recently come into question. Crowther[14] performed an RCT in a cohort of such patients (with an INR 4.5–10) who were randomized to

1.25 mg vitamin K PO or placebo. There was no difference in the number of bleeding events (both minor and major), thromboembolism, or death between groups. While it is possible that the study was not adequately powered to detect a difference in major life-threatening bleeds (and the study recorded all bleeds over a 90-day period), it did demonstrate that this approach was safe and effective in correcting the INR. Based on this study it would still appear to be reasonable to follow the ACCP guidelines (see below).

For life-threatening bleeding, immediate correction of the INR is mandatory. Although fresh frozen plasma can be given in this situation, immediate and full correction can be achieved only by the use of factor concentrates because the amount of FFP required to fully correct the INR is considerable and may take hours to infuse. Prothrombin complex concentrates (PCCs) are recommended in these patients. Profilnine (human prothrombin complex) is currently the only PCC available in the United States. Factor IX complex (Profilnine® SD) is a solvent detergent-treated concentrate of factor IX, factor II, factor X with low levels of factor VIII, which is derived from human plasma.

The following dose is recommended:

- If INR <4
  - Profilnine 25 units/kg by IV push over 2–5 min
- If INR >4
  - Profilnine 50 units/kg by IV push over 2–5 min
- Recheck INR in 4 h
  - Repeat Profilnine if necessary

ACCP Guidelines for Managing Elevated INRs (Due to Coumadin)

- INR more than therapeutic range but <5.0, no significant bleeding[12]:
  - Lower dose or omit dose, monitor INR.
- INR ≥5.0 but <9.0, no significant bleeding:
  - Omit next one or two doses, monitor more frequently, and resume at an appropriately adjusted dose when INR is in therapeutic range. Alternatively, omit dose and give vitamin K (1.25 mg p.o.), particularly if at increased risk of bleeding. If more rapid reversal is required because the patient requires urgent surgery, vitamin K (2.5–5 mg p.o.) can be given with the expectation that a reduction of the INR will occur in 24 h.
- INR ≥9.0, no significant bleeding:
  - Hold warfarin therapy and give higher dose of vitamin K (2.5–5 mg p.o.) with the expectation that the INR will be reduced substantially in 24–48 h (grade 1B). Monitor more frequently and use additional vitamin.

- Serious bleeding at any elevation of INR:
  - Hold warfarin therapy and give vitamin K (10 mg by slow IV infusion), supplemented with PCC depending on the urgency of the situation; vitamin K can be repeated q 12 h.
- Life-threatening bleeding:
  - Hold warfarin therapy and give PCC with vitamin K (10 mg by slow IV infusion). Repeat if necessary, depending on INR.

■ CLINICAL PEARLS

- Patients with an INR of between 1.4 and 1.8 do not routinely require FFP before and after invasive procedure.
- Patients who have a serious bleed while on Coumadin (and have an elevated INR) should receive IV vitamin K (10 mg slow infusion) and a human prothrombin complex.
- Surgical hemostasis is the best method to prevent postprocedure bleeding:
  - A "medical coagulopathy" does not cause bleeding which is localized to the surgical site.

■ REFERENCES

1. Taylor FB Jr, Toh CH, Hoots WK, et al. Towards definition, clinical and laboratory criteria, and a scoring system for disseminated intravascular coagulation. *Thromb Haemost*. 2001;86:1327–1330.
2. Gando S. Acute coagulopathy of trauma shock and coagulopathy of trauma: A Rebuttal. You are now going down the wrong path. *J Trauma*. 2009;67:381–383.
3. Khan H, Belsher J, Yilmaz M, et al. Fresh frozen plasma and platelet transfusions are associated with development of acute lung injury in critically ill medical patients. *Chest*. 2007;131:1308–1314.
4. Watson GA, Sperry JL, Rosengart MR, et al. Fresh frozen plasma is independently associated with a higher risk of multiple organ failure and acute respiratory distress syndrome. *J Trauma*. 2009;67:221–230.
5. Sarani B, Dunkman WJ, Dean L, et al. Transfusion of fresh frozen plasma in critically ill surgical patients is associated with an increased risk of infection. *Crit Care Med*. 2008;36:1114–1118.
6. De Backer D, Vandekerckhove B, Stanworth S, et al. Guidelines for the use of fresh frozen plasma. *Acta Clinica Belgica* 2008;63:381–390.
7. Dzik W, Rao A. Why do physicians request fresh frozen plasma? *Transfusion*. 2004;44:1393–1394.

8. Dzik WH. The James Blundell Award Lecture 2006: transfusion and the treatment of haemorrhage: past, present and future. *Transfus Med.* 2007;17:367–374.

9. Segal JB, Dzik WH. Paucity of studies to support that abnormal coagulation test results predict bleeding in the setting of invasive procedures: an evidence-based review. *Transfusion.* 2005;45:1413–1425.

10. Holland LL, Brooks JP. Toward rational fresh frozen plasma transfusion: the effect of plasma transfusion on coagulation test results. *Am J Clin Path.* 2006;126:133–139.

11. Abdel-Wahab OI, Healy B, Dzik WH. Effect of fresh-frozen plasma transfusion on prothrombin time and bleeding in patients with mild coagulation abnormalities. *Transfusion.* 2006;46:1279–1285.

12. Ansell J, Hirsh J, Hylek E, et al. Pharmacology and management of the vitamin K antagonists: American College of Chest Physicians Evidence-Based Clinical Practice Guidelines (8th Edition). *Chest.* 2008;133:160S–198S.

13. Dezee KJ, Shimeall WT, Douglas KM, et al. Treatment of excessive anticoagulation with phytonadione (vitamin K): a meta-analysis. *Arch Intern Med.* 2006;166:391–397.

14. Crowther MA, Ageno W, Garcia D, et al. Oral vitamin K versus placebo to correct excessive anticoagulation in patients receiving warfarin: a randomized trial. *Ann Intern Med.* 2009;150:293–300.

53

Thrombocytopenia and Platelet Transfusion

■ THROMBOCYTOPENIA IN THE ICU

Thrombocytopenia (defined as a platelet count <100,000/μl) is a common problem in ICU patients and is associated with adverse outcomes. A platelet count of less than 100,000/μl is seen in 20–25% of ICU patients, whereas 12–15% of patients will have a platelet count of <50,000/μl at some point during their ICU admission.[1,2] Typically the ICU patient's platelet count decreases during the first 4 days in the ICU.[3] Regardless of the cause, thrombocytopenia is an independent predictor of ICU mortality in multi-variate analysis with a relative risk of 1.9–4.2 in various studies.[2] In an observational study of 820 patients with severe community-acquired pneumonia admitted to the ICU, Brogly et al.[4] found that thrombocytopenia on admission was an independent predictor of mortality. Moreau reported that a 30% or more decline in platelet count by the fifth ICU day was an independent predictor of death.[5]

The causation of thrombocytopenia in ICU patients is often multifactorial, with sepsis being the most important cause. Thrombocytopenia is an early sign of sepsis and may occur in the absence of other features of DIC. Dilutional thrombocytopenia due to blood and fluid replacement is the second most common cause of thrombocytopenia in the ICU. Other causes include the following:

- Consumptive coagulopathy (DIC) due to liver failure, HELP syndrome, abruptio placentae
- Microangiopathic hemolytic anemia, i.e., thrombotic thrombocytopenic purpura (TTP), hemolytic uremic syndrome (HUS)
- Immune thrombocytopenias

P.E. Marik, *Handbook of Evidence-Based Critical Care*,
DOI 10.1007/978-1-4419-5923-2_53,
© Springer Science+Business Media, LLC 2010

- Idiopathic (ITP)
- Heparin (see below)
- Allo-antibodies
- Collagen vascular diseases
- Malignancy
- Viral
- Drug induced (quinidine)
- Myelosuppressive chemotherapeutic agents
- Drugs are commonly implicated in the etiology of thrombocytopenia. Almost any drug can cause a thrombocytopenia. The commonly implicated drugs include the following:
  - *Anti-microbials*
    - Linezolid
    - Amphotericin
    - Tetracyclines
    - Sulfonamides
    - Penicillins
    - Chloramphenicol
    - Cephalosporins
  - *Anti-convulsants*
    - Phenytoin (Dilantin)
    - Carbamazepine
  - *Diuretics*
    - Furosemide
    - Thiazides
    - Ethacrynic acid
  - *Others*
    - Alcohol
    - Phenylbutazone
    - Aspirin
    - Gold salts
    - Colchicine
    - Chlorpromazine
    - Chlordiazepoxide
    - H2 blockers

A large percentage of thrombocytopenic patients in the ICU receive a platelet transfusion. Many of these transfusions are administered outside of published guidelines.[6] This is important as platelet transfusions are not benign, being associated with many of the same complications as FFP, including TRALI, immune sensitization, etc. The "composition" of pheresed (SDP) as well as single and pooled whole blood-derived platelets (WBDPs) is listed in Table 53-1.

Table 53-1. Platelet product contents.

	Pheresis (SDP)	WBDPs (Single Unit)	WBDP Pool (5 Units)
Platelets Av	$\sim 4.2 \times 10^{11}$	$\sim 7-9 \times 10^{10}$	$\sim 4 \times 10^{11}$
Leukocytes	$10^5 - 10^7$	$\sim 8 \times 10^7$	$\sim 4 \times 10^8$
RBC	Rare	<1 ml	<5 ml
Volume (ml)	200–300	45–60	~ 300
Matching potential	Yes	Yes	No
Shelf life	5 days	5 days	5 days

■ CURRENT GUIDELINES FOR PLATELET TRANSFUSION

- Serious spontaneous hemorrhage due to thrombocytopenia alone is unlikely to occur at platelet counts above $10,000/\mu l$ in non-febrile patients.[6-8] Transfusion to prevent spontaneous bleeding is therefore recommended only below this threshold. In febrile patients, a threshold of $20,000/\mu l$ is suggested.
- Patients with chronic and sustained failure of platelet production, for example, some patients with myelodysplasia or aplastic anemia, may remain free of serious hemorrhage with platelet counts consistently below $10,000/\mu l$ or even $5,000/\mu l$. Prophylactic platelet transfusions may be best avoided in these patients because of the risk of alloimmunization and platelet refractoriness, and other complications of transfusion.[6]
- For epidural anesthesia, gastroscopy and biopsy, transbronchial biopsy, liver biopsy, laparotomy, or similar procedures, the platelet count should be raised to at least $50,000/\mu l$.
- For lumbar puncture, the platelet count should be >$20,000/\mu l$.
- For operations in critical sites such as the brain or eyes, the platelet count should be raised to $100,000/\mu l$.
- The platelet count should not be allowed to fall below $50,000/\mu l$ in patients with acute bleeding.
- It should not be assumed that the platelet count will rise just because platelet transfusions are given, and a preoperative platelet count should be checked to ensure that the above thresholds have been reached.

The platelet count should be measured within an hour of transfusion. Both hemorrhage and the underlying conditions that cause bleeding may increase platelet consumption and appreciably shorten platelet survival. As a general approximation, 1 unit of WBDP/10 kg body weight should increase the platelet count by $30,000/\mu l$. Most ICU patients respond poorly to platelet transfusion. Salman et al.[1] studied 90 ICU patients who received a platelet transfusion; the mean increase in platelet count was 22,600/μl with 64% having a poor response (defined as an increase of <30,000/μl after 6 units of WBDP).

Contraindications to Platelet Transfusion

- Autoimmune idiopathic thrombocytopenic purpura (ITP)
- Thrombotic thrombocytopenic purpura (TTP)
- Heparin-induced thrombocytopenia (HIT)
- Bleeding due to coagulopathy only
- Bleeding due to anatomic defect only

Coagulopathy and Central Venous Catheterization

These "current" guidelines do not address the issue of central venous catheterization in ICU patients with a coagulopathy. This is important as these patients are usually amongst the sickest ICU patients and usually require central venous access for fluid and vasopressor administration. Furthermore, although correction of coagulopathy may be possible, it may not be beneficial and it may be impossible to administer the corrective transfusion factor owing to the lack of venous access, or the condition may not be correctable by transfusion alone. Doerfler[9] described their experience with placement of 104 central lines in 76 coagulopathic medical patients. All insertions were performed by experienced operators; none of the patients received "prophylactic" transfusions of platelets or FFP. There were no serious bleeding complications, with only minor bleeding (skin) in seven (6.5%) patients (who had a mean platelet count of 22,000/μl). Similarly, Mumtaz et al. reviewed their experience in 330 surgical patients with disorders of hemostasis.[10] In 88 of the 330 patients, the underlying coagulopathy was not corrected before catheter placement. In these patients, there were three bleeding complications requiring placement of a purse string suture at the catheter entry site. These authors concluded that "central venous access procedures can be safely performed in patients with underlying disorders of hemostasis. Even patients with low platelet counts have infrequent (3 of 88) bleeding complications, and these problems are easily managed." Fisher and colleagues reported their experience with 658 central venous cannulations in patients with liver disease and a coagulopathy (mean INR 2.4, platelet count 81,000/μl), none of whom received prophylactic transfusions of either FFP or platelets.[11] These authors reported only one major bleeding complication (a hemothorax after accidental subclavian artery cannulation) with minor oozing or local hematoma in 6% of patients. Goldfarb et al. reported their experience with 1,000 cannulations of the internal jugular vein to facilitate obtaining a transvenous liver biopsy.[12] All the patients had coagulopathies (prothrombin time activity less than 50% and/or a platelet count less than 50,000/μl). In 74 patients, the common carotid artery was inadvertently punctured. A clinically detectable hematoma occurred in 10 patients; in one patient, the hematoma compressed the airway; this patient recovered completely after a surgical drainage. In this patient, puncture of the internal jugular vein was difficult because of a goiter, but the carotid artery apparently was not punctured. Similarly, Foster and colleagues reported on their experience with 200 cannulations in patients undergoing liver transplantation who had coagulopathies (that remained uncorrected).[13] These authors reported no cases of bleeding complications.

This data indicates that the risk of bleeding is related to the skill of the operator and not the ability of the blood to clot. In the hands of an experienced operator, the risk of bleeding may be higher in patients with a platelet count less than 20,000/μl; in these patients a platelet transfusion should be considered (if existing venous access allows). In the hands of the inexperienced operator, the femoral site (which is compressible) is recommended (in the coagulopathic patient). However, even in this circumstance, the risks of blood product transfusion likely exceed the benefit.

Paracentesis

According to the position state of the American Association for the Study of Liver Disease (AASLD), "the practice of giving blood products (fresh frozen plasma and/or platelets) routinely before paracentesis in cirrhotic patients with coagulopathy is not data-supported. The risks and costs of prophylactic transfusions exceed the benefit."[14] The guideline states that "since bleeding is sufficiently uncommon, the prophylactic use of fresh frozen plasma or platelets before paracentesis is not recommended."

Thoracentesis and Chest Tube Placement

Hemothorax and pulmonary hemorrhage are very rare complications of thoracentesis; these complications have occurred in patients with normal hemostasis. McVay and Toy[15] reported no bleeding complications in patients with a mild-to-moderate coagulopathy (defined as PT or PTT twice normal or a platelet count of 50,000–99,000/μl) who underwent a thoracentesis. Due to the paucity of data it is difficult to make evidence-based recommendations. Therefore the risks and benefits of the procedure should be evaluated in each patient. However, in keeping with patient undergoing a lumbar puncture, a platelet count above 20,000/μl is suggested in patients undergoing a thoracentesis. As chest tube placement is more "invasive" than thoracentesis, a platelet count >50,000/μl and an INR <2.5–3.0 are suggested (if transfusion of blood products is feasible).

■ HEPARIN-ASSOCIATED THROMBOCYTOPENIA

Recognition of heparin-induced thrombocytopenia (HIT) and HIT with thrombosis (HITT) is of particular importance, given its paradoxical association with thrombosis. HIT/HITT is an immune-mediated disorder that is triggered by exposure to any form of heparin; it is also known as type II HIT to distinguish it from the non-immune-mediated, mild thrombocytopenia associated with heparin termed type I HIT. Type II HIT is caused by the generation of heparin-induced, platelet-activating immunoglobulin G (IgG) antibodies that recognize heparin–platelet factor 4 complexes.[16] The resulting platelet activation and thrombin generation lead to a significant risk of both arterial and venous thrombosis. Depending on the patient population studied, the risk of thrombosis has ranged from 29 to 89%. Even after the cessation of heparin therapy, the threat of thrombosis persists. In one study, the 30-day risk of thrombosis after the diagnosis of HIT was 53%.[17]

The incidence of HIT varies depending on the patient population studied and the type of heparin preparation used. Patients undergoing cardiac or orthopedic surgery are among those at highest risk of developing HIT. HIT is less common in medical patients, with studies suggesting a frequency of 1% or less.[16] Patients receiving unfractionated heparin (UFH) are at increased risk of HIT compared with those given the low molecular weight heparin (LMWH) preparations. Diagnosis of HIT requires consideration of both clinical and serologic findings. Because non-pathogenic heparin–platelet factor 4 antibodies occur commonly in patients treated with heparin, a positive test for HIT antibodies is not sufficient to make the diagnosis. Diagnostic specificity can be increased by the use of a sensitive washed platelet activation assay; a positive platelet activation assay is much more specific for clinical HIT than is a positive platelet factor 4-dependent immunoassay. However, given the risk of thrombosis in patients with HIT, appropriate therapy should not be withheld while awaiting the results of serologic testing. HIT should be suspected in patients who develop thrombocytopenia or experience a relative drop in platelet count of >50%, typically occurring 4–10 days after the initiation of heparin therapy. Thrombocytopenia may occur much more rapidly after exposure to heparin, however, in patients who have received heparin within the previous 100 days. New or recurrent venous or arterial thromboses in patients who are receiving, or have recently received, a heparin product should also raise suspicion for HIT. It should be appreciated that in about 25% of HIT patients, a thrombotic event during heparin treatment precedes the subsequent HIT-associated platelet count fall.[16]

Only a subset of anti-PF4/heparin antibodies activate platelets, which explains the greater diagnostic specificity of the platelet activation assays. There is a correlation between the degree of reactivity in the EIA, expressed in optical density (OD) units, and the presence of PF4/heparin antibodies. Thus, the greater the magnitude of a positive EIA test result, the greater the likelihood that the patient has HIT.

If HIT is suspected, all heparin products must immediately be discontinued. Given the high risk of thrombosis with HIT, it is currently recommended that an alternate, non-heparin anti-coagulant replace heparin in patients strongly suspected of having HIT.[16] In the United States, the direct thrombin inhibitors (DTIs) argatroban and lepirudin are the only agents approved by the FDA for the treatment of HIT. For patients receiving lepirudin, the initial lepirudin infusion rate should be no higher than 0.10 mg/kg/h. The usual starting dose of argatroban is 2.0 μg/kg/min with dosage adjustment according to the PTT. In patients with heart failure, multiple organ system failure, or severe anasarca and in postcardiac surgery patients, an initial infusion at a rate between 0.5 and 1.2 μg/kg/min is recommended.[16]

Coumadin should not be started before the platelet count has increased above 150,000/μl; low-dose Coumadin is recommended (5 mg/day) with the non-heparin anti-coagulant being continued until the platelet count has reached a stable plateau, the INR has reached the intended target range, and after a minimum overlap of at least 5 days between the non-heparin anti-coagulant and Coumadin.

Because thrombocytopenia is common in ICU patients and because these patients are invariably receiving heparin, the possibility of HIT is frequently entertained. It is important to consider HIT in thrombocytopenia patients as the consequences (to the patient and the physician) are devastating should the diagnosis be missed. Consequently, these patients usually undergo an expensive and often frustrating diagnostic workup. This scenario is best avoided by minimizing the use of unfractionated heparin (UH), particularly in high-risk patient groups. Furthermore, it should be noted that UH may not provide adequate DVT prophylaxis for ICU patients (see Chapter 21). As the risk of HIT is lower with LMWH and essentially zero with fondaparinux, these agents are useful alternatives to UH (in patients with normal renal function).

ALERT

Avoid the use of unfractionated heparin in all ICU patients if at all possible.

■ THROMBOTIC THROMBOCYTOPENIC PURPURA

Thrombotic thrombocytopenic purpura (TTP) usually refers to the disorder of thrombocytopenia, hemolysis with schistocytes on blood smears, renal dysfunction, and neurologic abnormalities, such as headache, confusion, focal deficits, seizures, or coma.[18–20] These manifestations are due to widespread microvascular thrombosis involving the capillaries and arterioles of the brain and other organs. Thrombocytopenia results from the consumption of platelets, whereas erythrocyte fragmentation and hemolysis may be due to mechanical injury as the red cells encounter the intravascular thrombi or abnormally high levels of shear stress. Typically, TTP affects previously healthy adolescents or adults and almost invariably follows a rapid course of deterioration and death unless plasma infusion or exchange therapy is instituted immediately. A similar disorder occurs in children, the hemolytic–uremic syndrome (HUS). Childhood HUS, typically preceded by abdominal pain and diarrhea, is recognized as a complication of infection caused by bacteria that produce Shiga toxins, such as *Escherichia coli* O157:H7. Currently, about 90% of children with typical HUS survive with supportive care, without plasma exchange treatment.

ALERT

Thrombocytopenia and acute renal dysfunction or acute CNS abnormalities... THINK...TTP

Common Clinical and Laboratory Features of TTP

- Thrombocytopenia
- Microangiopathic hemolytic anemia
- Neurologic abnormality or complaint
- Renal abnormalities
  - Proteinuria and microscopic hematuria
  - Increased BUN and creatinine
- Temperature >38.3°C
- Microthrombi on tissue biopsy
- Exclusion
  - Evidence of intravascular coagulation
  - Evidence of underlying condition associated with or producing microangiopathic syndrome
  - Positive anti-nuclear antibody or anti-DNA antibody
  - Oliguria or anuria

The pathophysiological hallmarks of acute TTP are von Willebrand factor (VWF)–platelet-rich thrombi occluding the microvasculature. The VWF–platelet thrombi are thought to be the consequence of insufficient processing of newly secreted, extremely adhesive, and ultra large VWF multimers. In a majority of patients, this insufficient processing of ultra large VWF multimers is the result of a severe deficiency of the VWF-cleaving protease, now denoted as ADAMTS13.[18–20] ADAMTS13 activity levels are less than 10% of normal control in patients who have acute TTP. TTP is considered an autoimmune disease, with ADAMTS13-binding IgG detectable in 97–100% of cases.

Platelet transfusion should be avoided because bleeding complications are uncommon in TTP, and marked deterioration in neurological status has been reported in association with platelet transfusions. In acute bouts of acquired TTP, the treatment of choice is daily plasma exchange with replacement of plasma. Plasma exchange should be initiated immediately once a diagnosis of acute TTP is seriously considered or has been established, as deferral in starting treatment is associated with increased numbers of treatment failure and adverse outcome.[21] In case plasma exchange is not available, patients should be treated with plasma infusions until their referral to a center where plasma exchange can be performed. The efficacy of plasma exchange therapy is believed to result from replenishment of the missing ADAMTS13. Although it may also remove the inhibitors, this process is not very effective and by itself is insufficient for therapeutic responses.

Plasma exchange treatment is frequently supplemented with immunosuppressive drugs. Although controlled trials are lacking, the finding that in the majority of patients, idiopathic acquired TTP is an autoimmune disorder with circulating inhibitory anti-ADAMTS13 autoantibodies leading to severe ADAMTS13 deficiency supports the potential efficacy of these drugs. Methylprednisolone is the most commonly used drug. However, the combination of plasma exchange and cyclosporine is an alternative with apparent success.[22] Rituximab, a chimeric monoclonal anti-CD20, has been used with presumed benefits in patients with protracted TTP.

■ REFERENCES

1. Salman SS, Fernandez Perez ER, Stubbs JR, et al. The practice of platelet transfusion in the intensive care unit. *J Intensive Care Med.* 2007;22:105–110.
2. Levi M, Lowenberg EC. Thrombocytopenia in critically ill patients. *Semin Thromb Hemost.* 2008;34:417–424.
3. Akca S, Haji-Michael P, De MA, et al. Time course of platelet counts in critically ill patients. *Crit Care Med.* 2002;30:753–756.

4. Brogly N, Devos P, Boussekey N et al. Impact of thrombocytopenia on outcome of patients admitted to ICU for severe community-acquired pneumonia. *J Infect.* 2007;55:136–140.

5. Moreau D, Timsit JF, Vesin A, et al. Platelet count decline: an early prognostic marker in critically ill patients with prolonged ICU stays. *Chest.* 2007;131:1735–1741.

6. British Society for Haematology. Guidelines for the use of platelet transfusions. Br J Haematol. 2003;122:10–23.

7. Schiffer CA, Anderson KC, Bennett CL, et al. Platelet transfusion for patients with cancer: clinical practice guidelines of the American Society of Clinical Oncology. *J Clin Oncol.* 2001;19:1519–1538.

8. Slichter SJ. Platelet transfusion therapy. *Hematol Oncol Clin North Am.* 2007;21:697–729.

9. Doerfler ME, Kaufman B, Goldenberg AS, et al. Central venous catheter placement in patients with disorders of hemostasis. *Chest.* 1996;110:185–188.

10. Mumtaz H, Williams V, Hauer-Jensen M, et al. Central venous catheter placement in patients with disorders of hemostasis. *Am J Surg.* 2000;180:503–505.

11. Fisher NC, Mutimer DJ. Central venous cannulation in patients with liver disease and coagulopathy – a prospective audit. *Intensive Care Med.* 1999;25:481–485.

12. Goldfarb G, Lebrec D. Percutaneous cannulation of the internal jugular vein in patients with coagulopathies: an experience based on 1,000 attempts. *Anesthesiol.* 1982;56:321–323.

13. Foster PF, Moore LR, Sankary HN, et al. Central venous catheterization in patients with coagulopathy. *Arch Surg.* 1992;127:273–275.

14. Runyon BA. Management of adult patients with ascites due to cirrhosis. *Hepatology.* 2004;39:841–856.

15. McVay PA, Toy PT. Lack of increased bleeding after paracentesis and thoracentesis in patients with mild coagulation abnormalities. *Transfusion.* 1991;31:164–171.

16. Warkentin TE, Greinacher A, Koster A, et al. Treatment and prevention of heparin-induced thrombocytopenia. American College of Chest Physicians evidence-based clinical practice guidelines (8th Edition). *Chest.* 2008;133:340S–380S.

17. Warkentin TE, Kelton JG. A 14-year study of heparin-induced thrombocytopenia. *Am J Med.* 1996;101:502–507.

18. Tsai HM. Thrombotic thrombocytopenic purpura: a thrombotic disorder caused by ADAMTS13 deficiency. *Hematol Oncol Clin North Am.* 2007;21:609–632.

19. George JN. Thrombotic thrombocytopenic purpura. *N Engl J Med.* 2006;354:1927–1935.

20. Kremer Hovinga JA, Meyer SC. Current management of thrombotic thrombocytopenic purpura. *Curr Opin Hematol.* 2008;15:445–450.

21. Pereira A, Mazzara R, Monteagudo J, et al. Thrombotic thrombocy-topenic purpura/hemolytic uremic syndrome: a multivariate analysis of factors predicting the response to plasma exchange. *Ann Hematol.* 1995;70:319–323.
22. Cataland SR, Jin M, Lin S, et al. Cyclosporin and plasma exchange in thrombotic thrombocytopenic purpura: long-term follow-up with serial analysis of ADAMTS13 activity. *Br J Haematol.* 2007;139:486–493.

54

Eclampsia

Hypertension is one of the most common medical disorders affecting pregnancy. It complicates 12% of pregnancies and is responsible for 18% of maternal deaths in the United States.[1] The presentation of a patient with gestational hypertension may range from a mild to a life-threatening disease process. In 2000, the National High Blood Pressure Education Program Working Group on High Blood Pressure in Pregnancy defined four categories of hypertension in pregnancy, namely[2]

- chronic hypertension
- gestational hypertension
- pre-eclampsia
- pre-eclampsia superimposed on chronic hypertension

■ PRE-ECLAMPSIA

Pre-eclampsia is a multi-organ disease process of unknown etiology characterized by the development of hypertension and proteinuria after 20 weeks of gestation. It is characterized by abnormal vascular response to placentation that is associated with increased systematic vascular resistance, enhanced platelet aggregation, activation of the coagulation system, and endothelial dysfunction.[2] Pre-eclampsia is a heterogeneous syndrome with a spectrum of maternal and fetal manifestations with probable multiple causative factors. Clinically pre-eclampsia can manifest as a maternal syndrome with hypertension and proteinuria with/without other multi-system abnormalities and/or a fetal syndrome characterized by fetal growth retardation, reduced amniotic fluid, and abnormal oxygenation. In general, maternal and perinatal outcomes are usually favorable in women with mild pre-eclampsia developing beyond 34 weeks gestation. In contrast, maternal and perinatal morbidities and mortalities are increased in

P.E. Marik, *Handbook of Evidence-Based Critical Care*,
DOI 10.1007/978-1-4419-5923-2_54,
© Springer Science+Business Media, LLC 2010

women who develop the disorder before 33 weeks gestation, in those with pre-existing medical disorders, and in those from developing countries.

Several factors which increase the risk of pre-eclampsia have been identified, including the following:

- Primigravida
- Extremes of age
- Pre-eclampsia in previous pregnancy
- Family history of pre-eclampsia
- Obesity
- Pre-existent thrombophilia
- Chronic hypertension
- Renal disease
- Men who have previously fathered a pre-eclamptic pregnancy

Generally, pre-eclampsia is regarded as a disease of first pregnancy. Eclampsia, the occurrence of seizures superimposed on the syndrome of pre-eclampsia, complicates 1 in 2000 pregnancies in Western nations. In developing countries it is more common, being a common cause of maternal death. It is not clear what percentages of patients with eclampsia have the posterior reversible encephalopathy syndrome (PRES; see Chapter 63).

Diagnosis of Pre-eclampsia

Pre-eclampsia is defined as the presence of hypertension with a blood pressure of at least 140/90 mmHg on at least two occasions 4–6 h apart and proteinuria of 300 mg or more in 24 h. If a 24-h urine sample is not available, proteinuria is defined as a protein concentration of 300 mg/l or more in at least two random samples taken at least 4–6 h apart. However, a quantitative 24-h urine protein should be measured in all patients with suspected pre-eclampsia. The signs and symptoms of pre-eclampsia include the following:

Symptoms

- Severe headache
- Fatigue
- Epigastric/RUQ pain
- Vomiting
- Visual disturbances
- Swelling of hands, face, and feet

Signs

- Hypertension (>140/90 mmHg)
- Proteinuria (>300 mg/day)

- Hyperreflexia
- Oliguria
- Seizures
- Focal neurological signs
- Increased serum creatinine (>0.7 mg/dl)
- Increased serum uric acid (>5.8 mg/dl)
- Intrauterine growth retardation
- Oligohydramnios
- HELLP
    - Reduced platelet count (<100,000/μl)
    - Elevated liver enzymes (AST >70 IU/l)
    - Evidence of microangiopathic hemolytic anemia
        LDH >600 IU/l
        Bilirubin >1.2 mg/dl
        Decreased haptoglobin
        Schizocytes on peripheral smear

Patients with a systolic blood pressure greater than 160 mmhg, a diastolic blood pressure ≥110 mmHg, or severe proteinuria (≥5 g/day) are considered to have severe pre-eclampsia. Furthermore, patients with pulmonary edema, oliguria, severe central nervous system symptoms or the HELLP (hemolysis, elevated liver enzymes, and thrombocytopenia), or posterior reversible encephalopathy (PRES) syndromes are considered to have severe pre-eclampsia. It should be recognized that hypertension or proteinuria may be absent in 10–15% of women who develop the HELLP syndrome and in up to 35% of those who develop eclampsia. Women with systemic lupus erythematosus (SLE) may develop lupus nephritis during pregnancy which may be confused with pre-eclampsia, which is itself more common in women with SLE. An auto-immune workup should be considered in women with severe proteinuria, oliguria, and/or progressive renal dysfunction. As the treatment of these two disorders is quite different, a renal biopsy may be required to confirm the diagnosis.

Complications of Pre-eclampsia

Central Nervous System

- Eclampsia (seizures)
- Cerebral hemorrhage
- Central venous thrombosis
- Hypertensive encephalopathy
- Posterior reversible encephalopathy syndrome (PRES); see Chapter 63
- Seizures/status epilepticus

- Altered mental status
- Cortical blindness

Hepatic

- Jaundice
- Subcapsular/intrahepatic hematoma
- Hepatic rupture

HELLP Syndrome

- Thrombocytopenia
- Hepatic dysfunction
- Microangiopathic hemolytic anemia

Coagulation System

- Disseminated intravascular coagulation
- Microangiopathic hemolysis
- Hematoma
- Hematuria
- Pulmonary embolism

Others

- Acute renal failure
- Cardiogenic/non-cardiogenic pulmonary edema
- Infection/sepsis
- Placenta infarction
- Placenta abruption

Fetal

- Death
- Preterm birth
- Intrauterine growth retardation

HELLP Syndrome

The acronym HELLP describes a variant of severe pre-eclampsia characterized by hemolysis, elevated liver enzymes, right upper quadrant pain, and thrombocytopenia. The development of HELLP syndrome places the pregnant patient at increased risk for morbidity and death. The HELLP syndrome usually develops suddenly during pregnancy (27–37 weeks gestation) or in the immediate puerperium. The HELLP syndrome occurs in up to 20% of pregnancies complicated by severe pre-eclampsia. The clinical presentation of the HELLP syndrome is variable; 12–18% of affected women are normotensive and 13% do not have proteinuria.[3,4] Hepatic injury appears to play a central role in the HELLP syndrome and it has been proposed that placenta-derived proteins damage hepatocytes. Indeed, Strand et al. demonstrated apoptosis in the liver of HELLP patients and cytotoxicity of human hepatocytes exposed to the serum of patients with HELLP.[5] In many respects the HELLP syndrome mimics many of the features of the systemic inflammatory response syndrome (SIRS) which are superimposed on pre-eclampsia.

Posterior Reversible Encephalopathy Syndrome

Posterior reversible encephalopathy syndrome (PRES) is a clinico-neuroradiological entity characterized by headache, vomiting, altered mental status, blurred vision, and seizures with neuroimaging studies demonstrating white–gray matter edema involving predominantly the posterior region of the brain (see Chapter 63).[6] Pre-eclampsia is the commonest cause of PRES. Patients may present with PRES postpartum without the classic pre-eclamptic signs. Furthermore, status epilepticus has been reported to occur in these patients. It is unclear what percentage of patients previously diagnosed with eclampsia or patients with severe eclampsia and neurological signs/symptoms actuality met the diagnostic criteria for PRES. This distinction is important as patients with PRES may require aggressive management of raised intracranial pressure.

Treatment of Pre-eclampsia

Initial therapy of pre-eclampsia includes cautious volume expansion, magnesium sulfate for seizure prophylaxis, and blood pressure control. Delivery is the definitive treatment for pre-eclampsia and eclampsia. The decision to deliver involves balancing the risks of worsening pre-eclampsia against those of prematurity. Delivery is generally not indicated for women with mild pre-eclampsia until 37–38 weeks gestation and should occur by 40 weeks.

Magnesium sulfate prophylaxis reduces the risk of eclampsia and its complications, particularly in women with severe pre-eclampsia.[7,8] In addition, magnesium sulfate reduces the rate of progression of disease in those with mild pre-eclampsia without substantive harmful effects on either mother or child. Magnesium sulfate is clearly the anti-convulsant of choice for treating eclampsia, with substantial reduction in the risk of further seizures compared with diazepam or phenytoin. It is also better at preventing maternal death than is diazepam. Magnesium sulfate is usually given as a loading dose of 4–6 g in 100 ml 5% dextrose–1/4 NS over 15–20 min followed by a constant infusion at a rate of 1–2 g/h.

Magnesium may be given for a total of 24 h or for up to 24 h postpartum. Magnesium is a membrane stabilizer and muscle relaxant. Side effects include flushing, hypotension, muscle weakness, respiratory depression, and confusion. As magnesium is renally excreted, the urine output should be closely monitored and adjustment of the infusion dose is required in patients with impaired renal function.[7] Reduction or loss of tendon reflexes precedes respiratory depression. Tendon reflexes and the respiratory rate should therefore be checked on an hourly basis and the magnesium sulphate infusion adjusted as appropriate to prevent toxicity.[7] While monitoring of magnesium serum levels is not usually required,[7,9] the serum level should be checked in women with suspected toxicity (usual upper limit of therapy is 7.0 mg/dl).

The next step in the management of pre-eclampsia is to reduce the blood pressure to a safe range being diligent to avoid significant hypotension. The objective of treating severe hypertension is to prevent intracerebral hemorrhage and cardiac failure without compromising cerebral perfusion or jeopardizing uteroplacental blood flow which is already reduced in many women with pre-eclampsia.[10] Studies of women with mild pre-eclampsia have shown no benefit with the use of anti-hypertensive therapy (labetalol or calcium channel blockers). Anti-hypertensive therapy is therefore given primarily to prevent complications in the mother. The Working Group Report on High Blood Pressure in Pregnancy recommends initiation of anti-hypertensive therapy for a diastolic blood pressure of 105 mmHg or greater.[2] Furthermore, most authorities and the current guidelines from the American College of Obstetricians and Gynecologists recommend keeping the systolic blood pressure between 140 and 160 mmHg and the DBP between 90 and 105 mmHg.[2,10,11] This recommendation is supported by a recent study which demonstrated that a systolic blood pressure greater than 160 mmHg was the most important factor associated with a cerebrovascular accident in patients with severe pre-eclampsia and eclampsia.[12] This would suggest that a systolic blood pressure between 155 and 160 mmHg should be the primary trigger to initiate anti-hypertensive therapy in a patient with severe pre-eclampsia or eclampsia.[12,13] It should be noted that patients with pre-eclampsia/eclampsia may have a very labile blood pressure; this fact together with the narrow target blood pressure range dictates that these patients be closely monitored in an ICU, preferably with an arterial catheter. Intracerebral hemorrhage is a devastating complication in these patients, which can be avoided by scrupulous attention to blood pressure control.

Anti-hypertensive Agents for the Treatment of Pre-eclampsia

Hydralazine has been recommended as the drug of choice to treat severe pre-eclampsia and eclampsia since the early 1970s.[14] However, hydralazine has a number of properties that make it "unsuitable" for this indication. Its side effects (such as headache, nausea, and vomiting) are common and mimic symptoms of deteriorating pre-eclampsia. Most importantly, however, it has a delayed onset of action, an unpredictable hypotensive effect, and a prolonged duration of action. These properties may result in a precipitous hypotensive overshoot compromising both maternal cerebral blood flow and uteroplacental blood flow. Indeed, in a meta-analysis published by Magee and colleagues,[15] hydralazine was associated with an increased risk of maternal hypotension which was associated with an excess of cesarean sections, placental abruptions, and low Apgar scores. Based on the available data, hydralazine should not be used as first-line treatment of severe hypertension in pregnancy.

Parenteral labetalol is rapidly replacing hydralazine as the most commonly used anti-hypertensive agent in the treatment of severe pre-eclampsia (see Chapter 25). Nicardipine, a dihydropyridine calcium channel blocker, appears to be a safe and effective alternative agent for the control of blood pressure in patients with severe pre-eclampsia. Nitroglycerin, nitroprusside ACE inhibitors, and ARBs are contraindicated in patients with pre-eclampsia.

Corticosteroids and Plasmapheresis as Adjunctive Treatment of HELLP

The development of a SIRS-like condition with increased levels of pro-inflammatory cytokines in patients with HELLP led to the consideration of the use of corticosteroids to treat this disease.[16] A number of retrospective cohort studies have been published which suggest improved maternal and fetal outcome with the use of corticosteroids. In addition, four small randomized controlled studies (RCTs) have been conducted which randomized participants to standard therapy or dexamethasone. A meta-analysis of these RCTs demonstrated no significant difference in maternal mortality or morbidity or fetal outcome; however, hospital stay was significantly shorter in the women allocated to dexamethasone.[17] Furthermore, taken together, most of the studies demonstrate that corticosteroids produce a significant improvement in the hematologic abnormalities associated with the HELLP syndrome together with a more rapid improvement of the clinical features such as mean arterial pressure and urine output. Most of the studies to date used dexamethasone in a dose of 10 mg (equivalent to 200 mg hydrocortisone) every 12 h for 24–36 h. It should be noted that the placenta has a high concentration of the enzyme 11β-hydroxysteroid dehydrogenase (11β–HSD) type 2, which converts cortisol to the inactive metabolite cortisone and prednisolone to prednisone.[18] Inactivation of the synthetic corticosteroid dexamethasone and betamethasone by the placenta is negligible.[19] With our increased understanding of the role of corticosteroids in SIRS, dexamethasone in a dose of 10 mg every 12 h appears appropriate. However, we would recommend treatment for at least 5 days followed by a slow taper (see Chapter 40).

Due to the presence of circulating pro-inflammatory mediators and hepatotoxic factors in the serum of patients with the HELLP syndrome, plasmapheresis would appear to be a logical treatment strategy. Indeed, a number of cases have been reported in which plasmapheresis appeared to be associated with improved patient outcome.[20,21] This treatment modality should be considered in patients with severe HELLP syndrome who have failed traditional treatment measures.

■ CLINICAL PEARLS

- Magnesium sulfate is recommended in all women with preeclampsia.
- Systolic blood pressure should be kept between 140 and 160 mmHg.
- Hydralazine should *not* be used for blood pressure control.
- Labetalol and nicardipine are the drugs of choice for blood pressure control.

■ REFERENCES

1. Koonin LM, MacKay AP, Berg CJ, et al. Pregnancy-related mortality surveillance – United States, 1987–1990. *Morb Mortal Wkly Rep* CDC Surveill Summ. 1997;46:17–36.
2. Gifford RW, August PA, Cunningham G. Report of the national high blood pressure education program working group on high blood pressure in pregnancy. *Am J Obstet Gynecol*. 2000;183:S1–S22.
3. Sibai BM. Diagnosis, controversies, and management of the syndrome of hemolysis, elevated liver enzymes, and low platelet count. *Obstet Gynecol*. 2004;103:981–991.
4. Sibai BM, Ramadan MK, Usta I, et al. Maternal morbidity and mortality in 442 pregnancies with hemolysis, elevated liver enzymes, and low platelets (HELLP syndrome). *Am J Obstet Gynecol*. 1993;169:1000–1006.
5. Strand S, Strand D, Seufert R, et al. Placenta-derived CD95 ligand causes liver damage in hemolysis, elevated liver enzymes, and low platelet count syndrome. *Gastroenterology*. 2004;126:849–858.
6. Hinchey J, Chaves C, Appignani B, et al. A reversible posterior leukoencephalopathy syndrome. *N Engl J Med*. 1996;334:494–500.

7. Altman D, Carroli G, Duley L, et al. Do women with pre-eclampsia, and their babies, benefit from magnesium sulphate? The Magpie trial: a randomised placebo-controlled trial. *Lancet.* 2002;359:1877–1890.

8. Duley L, Gulmezoglu AM, Henderson-Smart DJ. Magnesium sulphate and other anticonvulsants for women with pre-eclampsia. *Cochrane Database of Syst Rev.* 2003;CD000025.

9. Belfort MA, Anthony J, Saade GR, et al. A comparison of magnesium sulfate and nimodipine for the prevention of eclampsia. *N Engl J Med.* 2003;348:304–311.

10. Sibai BM. Diagnosis, prevention, and management of eclampsia. *Obstet Gynecol.* 2005;105:402–410.

11. Diagnosis and management of preeclampsia and eclampsia. ACOG Practice Bulletin No. 33. American College of Obstetricians and Gynecologists. *Obstet Gynecol.* 2002;99:159–167.

12. Martin JN Jr, Thigpen BD, Moore RC, et al. Stroke and severe preeclampsia and eclampsia: a paradigm shift focusing on systolic blood pressure. *Obstet Gynecol.* 2005;105:246–254.

13. Cunningham FG. Severe preeclampsia and eclampsia: systolic hypertension is also important. *Obstet Gynecol.* 2005;105:237–238.

14. Hellman LM, Pritchard JA. *Williams Obstetrics.* 14th ed. New York, NY: Appleton-Century-Crofts; 1971.

15. Magee LA, Cham C, Waterman EJ, et al. Hydralazine for treatment of severe hypertension in pregnancy: meta-analysis. *Br Med J.* 2003;327:955–960.

16. LaMarca BD, Ryan MJ, Gilbert JS, et al. Inflammatory cytokines in the pathophysiology of hypertension during preeclampsia. *Curr Hyperten Rep.* 2007;9:480–485.

17. Matchaba P, Moodley J. Corticosteroids for HELLP syndrome in pregnancy. *Cochrane Database of Syst Rev.* 2004;CD002076.

18. Krozowski Z, MaGuire JA, Stein-Oakley AN, et al. Immunohistochemical localization of the 11 beta-hydroxysteroid dehydrogenase type II enzyme in human kidney and placenta. *J Clin Endocrinol Metab.* 1995;80:2203–2209.

19. Blanford AT, Murphy BE. In vitro metabolism of prednisolone, dexamethasone, betamethasone, and cortisol by the human placenta. *Am J Obstet Gynecol.* 1977;127:264–267.

20. Forster JG, Peltonen S, Kaaja R, et al. Plasma exchange in severe postpartum HELLP syndrome. *Acta Anaesthesiol Scand.* 2002;46:955–958.

21. Del Fante C, Perotti C, Viarengo G, et al. Daily plasma-exchange for life-threatening class I HELLP syndrome with prevalent pulmonary involvement. *Transfus Apheresis Sci.* 2006;34:7–9.

55

Management Issues in the Elderly

People who are greater than 65 years of age are the fastest growing segment of the US population.[1] By 2030 the population older than 65 years will double to approximately 70 million and the fastest growing segment of the population, those >84 years will triple. Age is associated with an increasing prevalence of multiple diseases and disabilities. Age is also associated with a decline in the functional reserve of multiple organ systems and a progressive restriction in personal and social resources. By virtue of have lived longer, increasing numbers of elderly patients (age >65 years) are being admitted to ICUs with diagnoses ranging from exacerbations of chronic illnesses and new onset of catastrophic health problems to trauma caused by home-related incidents and injury-resultant accidents that have occurred outside of the home. Elderly patients currently account for 42–52% of ICU admissions and for almost 60% of all ICU days.[2] A disproportionate number of these ICU days are spent by elderly patients before their death. Forty percent of Medicare descendants are admitted to an ICU during their terminal illness, with descents accounting for one-quarter of all Medicare expenditure.[3] Clearly ICU utilization by the elderly will increase exponentially over the next three decades.

This chapter will review

(i) the physiological changes that occur with aging, particularly as they apply to critically ill patients,

(ii) the outcome of elderly patients admitted to the ICU and prognostic factors which may aid in ICU admission decisions, and

(iii) management issues that pertain particularly to elderly critically ill patients.[4]

P.E. Marik, *Handbook of Evidence-Based Critical Care*,
DOI 10.1007/978-1-4419-5923-2_55,
© Springer Science+Business Media, LLC 2010

■ THE PHYSIOLOGY OF AGING

Aging is a process that converts healthy adults into frail ones, with diminished reserves in most physiological systems and with an exponentially increasing vulnerability to most diseases and to death. At the cellular level, aging can be defined as a progressive deterioration of structure and function that occurs over time.[5] The factors that lead to primary aging are poorly understood; however, the interplay between genetics and oxidant damage is believed to play a major role. The free radical theory of aging postulates that the production of intracellular reactive oxygen species is the major determinant of life span. The changes in cardiopulmonary, renal, and immune function with aging have important implications for the critical care physician and will be briefly reviewed.[4]

Cardiac Function

Cardiovascular performance impacts on critical illness in the elderly in two ways. First, age is a major risk factor for cardiovascular disease, which accounts for over 40% of deaths in those aged 65 years and above.[6] Second, the effect of aging on cardiovascular structure and function has implications for hemodynamic support of the elderly. A substantial lack of cardiac reserve is noted by the age of 70. This lack of reserve may not affect the daily functioning of a "well" older individual, but when this same older person experiences physiological stress such as blood loss, hypoxia, sepsis, or volume depletion, the lack of reserve becomes apparent through cardiac dysfunction.

With aging there is a progressive decrease in the number of myocytes and an increase in myocardial collagen content. Autonomic tissue is replaced by connective tissue and fat, while fibrosis causes conduction abnormalities through intranodal tract and the His bundle. These changes contribute to the high incidence of sick sinus syndrome, atrial arrhythmias, and bundle branch blocks. Arterial distensibility, the major component of afterload, decreases with aging. These changes result in a decrease in left ventricular ejection fraction with compensatory myocyte hypertrophy; consequently, left ventricular mass index increases with aging.[7] Resting cardiac output is maintained despite the increased afterload imposed by the stiffening of the outflow tract. However, maximal heart rate, ejection fraction, and cardiac output decrease with aging. Left ventricular hypertrophy together with increased myocardial collagen results in an overall decline in ventricular compliance. Ventricular relaxation, which is more energy dependent than ventricular contraction and therefore more oxygen dependant, also becomes impaired with aging. Diastolic dysfunction is therefore common in the elderly, particularly in those patients with systemic hypertension.[7-9] Indeed, diastolic dysfunction is responsible for up to 50% of cases of heart failure in patients over the age of 80 years. In critically ill elderly patients, particularly those with coronary artery disease, hypoxemia may compound the pre-existent diastolic dysfunction.

In younger persons, cardiac output is increased predominantly by increasing heart rate in response to β-adrenergic stimulation. With aging there is a relative "hyposympathetic state" in which the heart becomes less responsive to sympathetic stimulation, possible secondary to declining receptor function. The aging heart, therefore, increases cardiac output predominantly by increasing ventricular filling (preload) and stroke volume rather than by increasing heart rate. Because of the dependence of preload, even minor hypovolemia can result in significant cardiac compromise. The dependence on preload to maintain cardiac output is made even more important by the diastolic dysfunction associated with aging. However, due to decreased ventricular compliance, overzealous fluid resuscitation is likely to cause pulmonary edema. These changes dictate scrupulous management of the elderly patients' volume status. The reduction in left ventricular compliance results in a reduction of early diastolic ventricular filling and a compensatory increase in flow due to atrial contraction.[7,9] The contribution of left atrial systole to left ventricular filling increases with age.[9] Atrial fibrillation is therefore poorly handed by elderly patients, particularly those with marked diastolic dysfunction.

The cardiac dysfunction with aging is compounded by the high incidence of cardiac disease, especially coronary artery disease in the elderly. Coronary artery disease may go unrecognized in the elderly, as myocardial ischemia may present with non-specific and atypical symptoms. In the Framingham Heart Study, myocardial infarction was unrecognized or silent in more than 40% of patients over the age of 75 years.[10]

Respiratory Function

Declining respiratory function in the elderly is the result of changes in both the chest wall and the lung. There is a progressive decrease in chest wall compliance caused by structural changes of kyphosis and vertebral collapse. There is a progressive decline in respiratory muscle strength, resulting in a decline in maximal inspiratory and expiratory force by as much as 50%. In the lung there is a loss of elasticity with collapse of the small airways and uneven alveolar ventilation with air trapping. Uneven alveolar ventilation leads to ventilation–perfusion mismatch, which in turn causes a decline in arterial oxygen tension of approximately 0.3 mmHg/year from the age of 30 years. The control of ventilation is also affected by aging. Ventilatory response to hypoxia and hypercapnia falls by 50 and 40%, respectively. Elderly patients have a decreased respiratory reserve and may therefore decompensate quicker than younger patients. Weaning from mechanical ventilation may be more prolonged in these patients. As a consequence of poor nutritional status, decreased cell mediated immune responsiveness, a decline in mucociliary clearance, poor dentition with increased oropharyngeal colonization, and swallow dysfunction, aspiration pneumonia is exceedingly common in elderly patients, particularly those admitted from acute and chronic care facilities.[11]

Renal Function

There is a marked decline in renal function with aging. This decline has important implications for the critically ill patient. Between the ages of 25 and 85 years, approximately 40% of the nephrons become sclerotic. The remaining functional units hypertrophy in a compensatory manner. Sclerosis of the glomeruli is accompanied by atrophy of the afferent and efferent arterioles and a decrease in renal tubular cell number. Renal blood flow falls by approximately 50%. Functionally, there is a decline in glomerular filtration rate of approximately 45% by the age of 80 years. Serum creatinine, however, remains unchanged because there is a concomitant decrease in lean body mass and thus a decrease in creatinine production. Estimates of GFR in the healthy aged can be made from the serum creatinine by using the formula derived by Cockroft and Gault. This formula must be used with caution in critically ill patients as the serum creatinine may be altered by factors other than the GFR including numerous medications and increased muscle breakdown due to sepsis, trauma, protein catabolism, and immobility.

Renal tubular function declines with advancing age. The ability to conserve sodium and excrete hydrogen ions falls, resulting in diminished capacity to regulate fluid and acid–base balance. The aging kidney compensates poorly for non-renal losses of sodium and water. These changes are thought to be due to a decline in the activity of the renin–angiotensin system and decreased end-organ responsiveness to anti-diuretic hormone. Elderly patients are therefore at high risk of becoming dehydrated; this is compounded by the preload dependence of the heart for adequate cardiac output. The decreased GFR with aging has important implications in terms of drug dosing, as most drugs are renally excreted with the fall in renal elimination falling in parallel with the fall in GFR. Therefore, the creatinine clearance (estimated or measured) should be used in dosage calculations for drugs that are renally eliminated.

Energy Expenditure

Body composition and energy expenditure change with aging. There is an increase in body fat and a decrease in lean muscle mass by up to 40% at the age of 80 years. Accompanying this decline in muscle mass is an even greater decline in muscle strength caused by a selective loss of selected muscle fibers. The loss of muscle mass may be compounded by a poor intake of high-quality protein, which is especially common in the elderly. Daily energy expenditure decreases with age. Resting energy expenditure falls by as much as 15%. This decrease is primarily the result of the decrease in lean muscle mass and less physical activity. Following acute illness or injury, the increase in oxygen consumption and energy expenditure in patients over the age of 65 years is approximately 20–25% less than their younger counterparts. These changes in body composition and energy expenditure have important implications with respect to nutritional support. Due to decreased muscle mass in the face of acute illness or even elective surgery, elderly patients may rapidly develop protein–energy malnutrition. Nutritional support should therefore begin within 24 h of admission to the ICU. However, due to their decreased body mass and lower energy expenditure, overfeeding the elderly with the sequelae of "stress hyperglycemia," fatty liver, and excess CO_2 production should be avoided.

Immune System

A progressive decline in the integrity of the immune system occurs with aging.[12] The age-related changes are most evident in the peripheral T-cell pool, which show signs of decreased reactivation to challenge with antigens. The age-related changes in the immune system, together with the increased burden of chronic disease. may explain the increased incidence of sepsis in the elderly. In addition the case–fatality rate of sepsis increases linearly with aging.[13]

Elderly patients are at an increased risk of nosocomial infections. Pneumonia is particularly common in this group of patients; multiple factors contribute to the increased risk of pneumonia including an increased risk for aspiration due to swallow dysfunction, increased oropharyngeal colonization with potentially pathogenic organisms, weak cough, poor ambulation, and altered immune status. Urinary tract infection, decubitus ulcers, and wound infection are also common. In a study of 3,254 trauma patients, 39% of patients older than 65 developed a nosocomial infection as compared to 17% of younger patients.[14] In this study the mortality rate of elderly patients who had nosocomial infection was 28% compared with 5% for younger patients.

■ THE OUTCOME OF ELDERLY PATIENTS ADMITTED TO THE ICU

Severity of illness and age appear to be important factors determining ICU survival.[15] Nicholas et al. analyzed the influence of age on ICU survival from data collected on 792 admissions to eight ICUs in France.[16]

These authors reported that ICU mortality increased progressively with age; over 65 years of age it was more than double that of patients under 45 years (36.8% vs. 14.8%). However, ICU survival may not be the most appropriate end point when evaluating the role of critical care, particularly in the elderly. The goal of critical care medicine is to restore patients to a level of functioning similar to that of their preadmission status and to return patients back into the community from which they came. Therefore, postdischarge disposition and long-term survival (1–3 years) may be more important than hospital survival in evaluating the role of ICU admission.

Somme et al. reported an ICU survival rate of 80, 68, 75, and 69% for those below 75 years, 75–79 years, 80–84 years, and 85 years and older, respectively.[17] However, most deaths occurred during the first 3 months following ICU discharge, with survival rates at 3 months of 54, 56, and 51%, respectively, for those 75–79 , 80–84, and 85 years and older. Rady and Johnson studied the demographics, comorbidities, and outcome of a cohort of 900 octogenarians requiring ICU admission.[18] The octogenarians had a higher hospital mortality (10% vs. 6%, p <0.01) and discharge to a subacute care facility (35% vs. 18%, p <0.01). On follow-up, octogenarian hospital survivors who were discharged to a subacute care facility had a higher mortality than did hospital survivors discharged to home (31% vs. 17%). Preadmission comorbidities and severity of illness were independent predictors of hospital discharge to a subacute care facility. Those comorbidities associated with an increased likelihood of care dependency included degenerative brain disease, cerebrovascular disease, congestive cardiac failure, chronic pulmonary disease, diabetes mellitus, and malnutrition. Kaarlola and colleagues[19] assessed the long-term survival and quality of life of 882 elderly patients (>64 years of age) as compared to 1,827 controls (<65 years of age) admitted to a medical–surgical ICU. The cumulative 3-year mortality rate among the elderly patients was 57% as compared to 40% in the control group (p <0.05). The majority (88%) of the elderly survivors assessed their present health status as good or satisfactory.

An analysis of the available data suggests that functional elderly patients have a favorable long-term outcome following ICU admission. This suggests that age alone should not be used in making ICU triage decisions. The decision to admit an elderly patient to an ICU should be based upon the patient's comorbidities, acuity of illness, and prehospital functional status, which includes "quality of life" and whether the patient was living independently or was admitted from a subacute/chronic healthcare facility. Simultaneously it is imperative to determine the patient's preferences (or surrogates' best estimate of the patient's wishes) with regard to mechanical ventilation and other forms of life-sustaining treatment. For some elderly patients, we should provide the most peaceful and high-quality dying process and avoid admission to the ICU.

■ TRAUMA AND THE ELDERLY PATIENT

Geriatric patients are at high risk of traumatic injuries, particularly those patients with diminished functional status. Falls are the most common mechanism of injury in the elderly population and are responsible for significant morbidity, mortality, and medical costs.[20] Pedestrian–motor vehicle injuries affect the elderly disproportionately and result in a higher mortality as compared with other age groups. Perdue and colleagues reported that trauma patients older than 65 years were 4.6 times likely to die than were younger patients.[21]

A number of factors contribute to the increased mortality of elderly patients after traumatic injuries, most notably their limited physiological reserve together with the presence of comorbid cardiopulmonary disease. Elderly patients compensate poorly following blood loss due to limited chronotropic and inotropic reserve (hypoadrenergic state), diastolic dysfunction, and the inability of the kidney to conserve fluid. Many elderly patients are prescribed β-blockers; these drugs further reduce the ability of the patient to compensate for decreased intravascular volume. In addition, elderly patients are frequently treated with Coumadin and/or antiplatelet drugs which increase the propensity for uncontrolled hemorrhage. Evidence suggests that many injured elderly patients are under-triaged despite the increased risk of death and complications. One possible cause of under-triage is the late presentation of physical findings indicating hypovolemia.

■ SURGERY AND THE ELDERLY

The operative mortality and the incidence of postoperative complications are increased in elderly patients undergoing elective surgery.[22] The operative mortality and the rate of postoperative complication are even higher in elderly patients undergoing emergency surgery. It is not uncommon for elderly patients who appear fit and healthy (physiological age less than chronological age) to do poorly following elective surgery (the "knife" is the great equalizer). The decreased physiological reserve and the increased incidence of comorbidities probably account for this finding. Liu and Leung[23] reported an operative mortality of 4.6% and a postoperative complication rate of 25% in a cohort of octogenarians undergoing non-cardiac surgery. Elderly patients have a high incidence of protracted disabilities following major surgery. Lawrence and coworkers[24] reported a high incidence of functional disabilities at 6 months following major abdominal surgery in a cohort of elderly patients. Postoperative delirium is common following surgery and is associated with increased length of stay, morbidity, and mortality.

> **ALERT**
>
> The "knife" is the great equalizer. Age is associated with a signifi-
> cant decrease in physiological reserve; consequently "healthy" elderly
> patients become old patients after surgery.

Elective surgery must be considered very carefully in the elderly. Most
randomized controlled trials comparing surgical to a more conservative
approach were performed in patients less than 65 years of age. It is probably not appropriate to extrapolate the results of these trials to the elderly
population. Coronary artery bypass surgery is frequently performed in
the elderly with no evidence to support the benefit in this population
of patients. Rady and Johnson[25] compared the outcome from cardiac
surgery in octogenarians to younger patients. The octogenarians had a
significantly higher incidence of postoperative complications and a significantly higher hospital mortality (13.5% vs. 1.3%, p <0.001) than did
the cohort of younger patients. Furthermore, significantly more octogenarians were discharged to a subacute/chronic health-care facility than
were their younger counterparts (39.5% vs. 13%, p <0.001). This study
demonstrated that only 47% of the octogenarians (all who were living at
home and independent prior to surgery) were discharged to home after
surgery and therefore potentially benefitted from undergoing coronary
revascularization.

Over the last few years, geriatricians have developed an approach to
care for the elderly called comprehensive geriatric assessment (CGA).
CGA evaluates the comorbid illnesses, mental status, nutritional status, living circumstances, social support systems, and polypharmacy.[26,27]
The goal of CGA is to provide information to the surgeon, which will
allow more accurate risk assessment for surgery. CGA will also allow
for a pro-active team-based approach to interventions which will limit
complications in those patients who undergo surgery.

■ DELIRIUM IN THE ELDERLY

Postoperative Cognitive Dysfunction (POCD)

Transient POCD is an acute and short-termed disorder of cognition,
memory, and attention (see Chapter 47). An etiologic factor must be
searched for in every patient, since POCD may be the first symptom of a
respiratory (hypoxemia) or cardiac complication, electrolyte disturbance,
infection, or drug interactions. However, in most instances, a specific

cause cannot be identified and may be related to the interaction between anesthesia and the alteration in neurotransmitters involved in the cognitive decline of aging. The prognosis of transient POCD is good in the majority of patients; however, prolonged POCD may occur. Prolonged POCD may last for months to years and is a cause of significant disability. The "long-term postoperative cognitive dysfunction in the elderly study" was a prospective, multi-center study which investigated the incidence and causation of transient and prolonged POCD in elderly patients undergoing major non-cardiac surgery.[28] POCD was present in 26% of patients 1 week after surgery and in 9.9% of patients 3 months after surgery, compared with 3.4 and 2.8% of controls. Increasing age, duration of anesthesia, postoperative infections, and respiratory complications were risk factors for early POCD, but only age was a risk factor for prolonged POCD. POCD is common after cardiac surgery in the elderly, with an incidence of up to 80% at discharge and 50% at 6 weeks.[29,30]

■ DRUG DOSING IN THE ELDERLY

Adverse drug reactions (ADRs) are common causes of complications in hospitalized elderly patients. Age has been shown to be an independent risk factor for ADRs.[31] Aging is associated with decreased renal and hepatic reserve with delayed renal and hepatic clearance of drugs. Due to the myriad of possible drug interactions, the medication list of all elderly patients should be "trimmed" as much as possible.

■ REFERENCES

1. Day JC. Population projections of the United States by age, sex, race and Hispanic origin: 1993–2050, Current Population Reports: US Department of Commerce Bureau of Census. 1993:25–1104.
2. Suresh R, Kupfer YY, Tessler S. The greying of the intensive care unit: demographic changes 1988–1998. *Crit Care Med.* 1999;27(Suppl):A27.
3. Barnato AE, McClellan MB, Kagay CR, et al. Trends in inpatient treatment intensity among Medicare beneficiaries at the end of life. *Health Serv Res.* 2004;39:363–375.
4. Marik PE. Management of the critically Ill geriatric patient. *Crit Care Med.* 2006;34(Suppl):S176–S182.
5. Holloszy JO. The biology of aging. *Mayo Clin Proc.* 2000;75(Suppl): S3–S8.
6. Lakatta EG. Age-associated cardiovascular changes in health: impact on cardiovascular disease in older persons. *Heart Fail Rev.* 2002;7: 29–49.

7. Salmasi AM, Alimo A, Jepson E, et al. Age-associated changes in left ventricular diastolic function are related to increasing left ventricular mass. *Am J Hypertens.* 2003;16:473–477.
8. Gandhi SK, Powers JC, Nomeir AM, et al. The pathogenesis of acute pulmonary edema associated with hypertension. *N Engl J Med.* 2001;344:17–22.
9. Swinne CJ, Shapiro EP, Lima SD, et al. Age-associated changes in left ventricular diastolic performance during isometric exercise in normal subjects. *Am J Cardiol.* 1992;69:823–826.
10. Kannel WB, Dannenberg AL, Abbott RD. Unrecognized myocardial infarction and hypertension: the Framingham Study. *Am Heart J.* 1985;109:581–585.
11. Marik PE. Aspiration pneumonitis and pneumonia: a clinical review. *N Engl J Med.* 2001;344:665–672.
12. Saltzman RL, Peterson PK. Immunodeficiency of the elderly. *Rev Infect Dis.* 1987;9:1127–1139.
13. Martin GS, Mannino DM, Moss M. The effect of age on the development and outcome of adult sepsis. *Crit Care Med.* 2006;34:15–21.
14. Bochicchio GV, Joshi M, Knorr KM, et al. Impact of nosocomial infections in trauma: does age make a difference? *J Trauma.* 2001;50:612–617.
15. Mayer-Oakes SA, Oye RK, Leake B. Predictors of mortality in older patients following medical intensive care: the importance of functional status. *J Am Geriatr Soc.* 1991;39:862–868.
16. Nicolas F, Le GJR, Alperovitch A, et al. Influence of patients' age on survival, level of therapy and length of stay in intensive care units. *Intensive Care Med.* 1987;13:9–13.
17. Somme D, Maillet JM, Gisselbrecht M, et al. Critically ill old and the oldest-old patients in intensive care: short- and long-term outcomes. *Intensive Care Med.* 2003;29:2137–2143.
18. Rady MY, Johnson DJ. Hospital discharge to care facility: a patient-centered outcome for the evaluation of intensive care for octogenarians. *Chest.* 2004;126:1583–1591.
19. Kaarlola A, Tallgren M, Pettila V. Long-term survival, quality of life, and quality-adjusted life-years among critically ill elderly patients. *Crit Care Med.* 2006;34:2120–2126.
20. Mandavia D, Newton K. Geriatric trauma. *Emerg Med Clin North Am.* 1998;16:257–274.
21. Perdue PW, Watts DD, Kaufmann CR, et al. Differences in mortality between elderly and younger adult trauma patients: geriatric status increases risk of delayed death. *J Trauma.* 1998;45:805–810.
22. Barlow AP, Zarifa Z, Shillito RG, et al. Surgery in a geriatric population. *Ann R Coll Surg Engl.* 1989;71:110–114.
23. Liu LL, Leung JM. Predicting adverse postoperative outcomes in patients aged 80 years or older. *J Am Geriatr Soc.* 2000;48:405–412.

24. Lawrence VA, Hazuda HP, Cornell JE, et al. Functional independence after major abdominal surgery in the elderly. *J Am Coll Surg*. 2004;199:762–772.

25. Rady MY, Johnson DJ. Cardiac surgery for octogenarians: is it an informed decision? *Am Heart J*. 2004;147:347–353.

26. Fukuse T, Satoda N, Hijiya K, et al. Importance of a comprehensive geriatric assessment in prediction of complications following thoracic surgery in elderly patients. *Chest*. 2005;127:886–891.

27. Repetto L, Fratino L, Audisio RA, et al. Comprehensive geriatric assessment adds information to Eastern Cooperative Oncology Group performance status in elderly cancer patients: an Italian Group for Geriatric Oncology Study. *J Clin Oncol*. 2002;20:494–502.

28. Moller JT, Cluitmans P, Rasmussen LS, et al. Long-term postoperative cognitive dysfunction in the elderly ISPOCD1 study. ISPOCD investigators. International study of post-operative cognitive dysfunction. *Lancet*. 1998;351:857–861.

29. Santos FS, Velasco IT, Fraguas R Jr. Risk factors for delirium in the elderly after coronary artery bypass graft surgery. *Int Psychogeriatr*. 2004;16:175–193.

30. Newman MF, Kirchner JL, Phillips-Bute B, et al. Longitudinal assessment of neurocognitive function after coronary-artery bypass surgery. *N Engl J Med*. 2001;344:395–402.

31. Onder G, Pedone C, Landi F, et al. Adverse drug reactions as cause of hospital admissions: results from the Italian Group of Pharmacoepidemiology in the Elderly (GIFA). *J Am Geriatr Soc*. 2002;50:1962–1968.

56

Management Issues in the Obese Patient

Obesity is a major health problem worldwide. The number of overweight men and women in the United States has risen steadily since 1960, with a staggering 64.5% of the adult population being overweight in the most recent epidemiological surveys.[1] With the increasing prevalence of obesity in the general population and the association of obesity with many disease states, it is not surprising that a significant proportion of ICU patients are obese. The critically ill obese patient presents the critical care team with many unique problems.

■ EFFECT OF OBESITY ON CRITICAL CARE OUTCOMES

The risk of death from all causes increases throughout the range of moderate and severe overweight for both men and women in all age groups.[2,3] The graphed relationship between body mass index (BMI) and mortality is "J shaped" with increasing death rates with malnutrition and with increasing BMI.[2,4] Obesity is associated with an increased risk of death in hospitalized patients. The association between BMI and mortality is altered in the critically ill. Paradoxically, patients who are overweight (BMI 26–30) and moderately obese (BMI 30–40) have a lower mortality than do patients of normal body weight.[5] The increased production of anti-inflammatory mediators by adipose tissue and the increased energy reserve have been postulated to account for this finding. Morbidly obese patients (BMI >40), however, are at an increased risk of dying. Obesity is however associated with a prolonged duration of mechanical ventilation and increased ICU length of stay.[6]

P.E. Marik, *Handbook of Evidence-Based Critical Care*,
DOI 10.1007/978-1-4419-5923-2_56,
© Springer Science+Business Media, LLC 2010

■ RESPIRATORY EFFECTS OF OBESITY

The effects of obesity on respiratory function are complex and influenced by the degree of obesity, age, and body fat distribution (central or peripheral). The expiratory reserve volume (ERV) is consistently decreased in obese patients, while the FEV1-to-FVC ratio is increased.[7] The vital capacity (VC), the total lung capacity (TLC), and the functional residual volume (FRV) are generally maintained in otherwise normal individuals with mild-to-moderate obesity but are reduced by up to 30% in morbidly obese patients.

Obese patients have an increased work of breathing due to abnormal chest elasticity, increased chest wall resistance, increased airway resistance (R_{aw}), abnormal diaphragmatic position and upper airway resistance, as well as the need to eliminate a higher daily production of carbon dioxide. Patients with morbid obesity are generally hypoxemic, with a widened alveolar–arterial oxygen gradient caused by ventilation–perfusion mismatching. The FRC falls when assuming a supine position, further increasing ventilation–perfusion mismatching Abnormalities in the control of ventilation are common in obese patients with a high percentage of patients having obstructive sleep apnea.

The initial tidal volume should be based on IBW (and not actual weight) and adjusted according to inflation pressures and blood gases (see Chapters 14 and Chapter 19). In patients with chronic CO_2 retention, minute ventilation should be titrated to normalize pH and not pCO_2. The use of positive end-expiratory pressure (PEEP) of 7.5–10 cm H_2O is recommended and may prevent end-expiratory airway closure and atelectasis. Bilevel/APRV may be a particularly useful mode of ventilation in the morbidly obese patient.[8]

ALERT

Lung volumes are determined by height and sex and not by weight. Lung volumes do not increase (grow) with increasing body weight. Tidal volumes *must* therefore be set according to ideal body weight and *not* actual body weight. Using actual body weight will result in severe volutrauma.

Ideal Body Weight

Male: 50 + 0.91 (height in centimeters – 152.4)
Female: 45.5 + 0.91 (height in centimeters – 152.4)

Weaning the obese patient from mechanical ventilation is frequently a difficult and challenging task. Burns and colleagues[9] have demonstrated that in obese patients the reverse Trendelenburg position at 45° resulted in a larger tidal volume and lower respiratory rate than at the 0° or 90° position, and they postulated that this position may facilitate the weaning process.

Obese patients are at particular risk for aspiration pneumonia, especially in the postoperative period. This risk is increased due to several factors, including a higher volume of gastric fluid, a lower than normal pH of gastric fluid in fasting obese patients, increased intra-abdominal pressure, and a higher incidence of gastroesophageal reflux. This is another important reason to nurse the obese patient in the semi-upright position. Obesity is an important risk factor for pulmonary embolism. The high risk of thromboembolic disease in obese ICU patients warrants an aggressive approach to deep venous thrombosis prophylaxis.

Endotracheal intubation can be a challenging experience in the morbidly obese patient. In the Australian Incident Monitoring Study, obesity with limited neck mobility and mouth opening accounted for the majority of cases of difficult intubation.[10] Physicians caring for these patients must be well versed in intubation techniques as well as the use of adjuncts for intubation.

■ CARDIOVASCULAR EFFECTS OF OBESITY

Patients with morbid obesity have an increase in total blood volume and resting cardiac output. Both increase in direct proportion to the amount the patient weighs over the IBW. The cardiac and stroke index are normal in otherwise "healthy" obese patients. Obese patients have an increase in mean oxygen consumption (VO_2) with a normal arteriovenous oxygen difference. Although the resting cardiac output is increased, obese patients have been demonstrated to have an impaired left ventricular contractility and a depressed ejection fraction. The left ventricular filling pressure is elevated in obese patients due to the combination of increased preload and reduced ventricular distensibility. Consequently, fluid loading is poorly tolerated in these patients.

■ DRUG DOSING IN OBESE PATIENTS

Drug distribution, metabolism, protein binding, and clearance are altered by the physiological changes associated with excessive weight. Some of these pharmacokinetic changes may, however, negate the consequences of others and the pharmacokinetic alterations may differ in the morbidly obese compared to the mildly or moderately obese. However, a number of drugs used in the ICU, most notably digoxin, aminoglycosides, and cyclosporin, can cause drug toxicity if obese patients are dosed based on their actual body weight.

In obese patients with renal dysfunction, the creatinine clearance, as calculated using standard formulae, correlates very poorly with the measured creatinine clearance.[11] Therefore, in the obese patient with renal dysfunction, the dosing regimen of renally excreted drugs should be based on the measured creatinine clearance.[12]

■ NUTRITIONAL REQUIREMENTS

Although obese individuals have excess body fat stores and large lean body stores, they are likely to develop protein energy malnutrition in response to metabolic stress, particularly if their nutritional status was poor before injury. Nutrition should not be withheld from the obese patients in the mistaken belief that weight reduction is beneficial during critical illness. Indeed, malnutrition is a recognized risk that is associated with all bariatric surgeries.

In morbidly obese patients, energy expenditure and caloric requirements are best determined by indirect calorimetry.[13] If indirect calorimetry is not available, patients should receive between 20 and 25 kcal/kg of IBW/day (see Chapter 31). Most of the calories should be given as carbohydrates with fats given to prevent essential fatty acid deficiency. It has been suggested that critically ill obese patients receive nutritional support with a hypocaloric high-protein formulation. It has been postulated that if adequate protein is supplied and obligatory glucose requirements are met, endogenous fat stores will be used for energy.[14] Protein requirements in the obese patient may be difficult to determine because of the increased lean body mass. Current consensus recommends a level of 1.5–2.0 g/kg of IBW to achieve nitrogen equilibrium.[14,15]

■ VASCULAR ACCESS IN THE OBESE PATIENT

One of the most challenging features of the morbidly obese patient is venous and arterial access. Poor peripheral venous sites in these patients necessitate more frequent use of central venous access. A short stubby neck, loss of physical landmarks, and a greater skin–blood vessel distance make internal jugular and subclavian vein cannulation technically difficult.

Obese patients have a higher incidence of catheter malpositions and local puncture complications, with catheter-related infections and thromboses. Femoral venous access may not be possible as these patients usually have severe intertrigo and morbid obesity is a major risk factor for catheter-associated bloodstream infection (CRBI) when the femoral site is used.[16] The use of Doppler ultrasound-guided techniques for obtaining central venous access is recommended in these patients. Furthermore, early placement of a PICC should be considered.

■ RADIOLOGICAL PROCEDURES

Bedside radiographs are of very poor quality in the morbidly obese patient, limiting their diagnostic value. Abdominal and pelvic ultrasonographies are limited by extensive abdominal wall and intra-abdominal fat. Percutaneous aspiration and drainage of intraperitoneal and retroperitoneal collections may be hindered by the obese body habitus. Many computed tomography tables have weight restrictions (about 350 lb) that prohibit imaging of morbidly obese patient.

■ CLINICAL PEARLS

- "Prophylactic" PEEP (of 7.5 to 10 cm H20) or APRV should be considered in obese patients who require mechanical ventilation.
- Obese patients are at a high risk of thromboembolic disease, necessitating aggressive DVT prophylaxis.
- Hypocaloric high-protein enteral nutrition is recommended.

■ REFERENCES

1. Flegal KM, Carroll MD, Ogden CL, et al. Prevalence and trends in obesity among US adults, 1999–2000. *JAMA*. 2002;288:1723–1727.
2. Calle EE, Thun MJ, Petrelli JM, et al. Body-mass index and mortality in a prospective cohort of US adults. *N Engl J Med*. 1999;341:1097–1105.
3. Fontaine KR, Redden DT, Wang C, et al. Years of life lost due to obesity. *JAMA*. 2003;289:187–193.
4. Clinical guidelines on the identification, evaluation, and treatment of overweight and obesity in adults. NIH Publication No. 98-4083. 1998. Bethesda, MD: National Institutes of Health.
5. Marik PE. The paradoxical effect of obesity on outcome in critically ill patients. Crit Care Med 2006; 34:1251–53.

6. Akinnusi ME, Pineda LA, El Solh AA. Effect of obesity on intensive care morbidity and mortality: a meta-analysis. *Crit Care Med.* 2008;36: 151–158.

7. Marik PE, Varon J. Management of the critically ill obese patient. *Crit Care Clin.* 2001;17:187–200.

8. Hirani A, Cavallazzi R, Shnister A, et al. Airway pressure release ventilation (APRV) for treatment of severe life-threatening ARDS in a morbidly obese patient. *Crit Care Shock.* 2008;11:132–136.

9. Burns SM, Egloff MB, Ryan B, et al. Effect of body position on spontaneous respiratory rate and tidal volume in patients with obesity, abdominal distension and ascites. *Am J Crit Care.* 1994;3:102–106.

10. Williamson JA, Webb RK, Szekely S, et al. The Australian incident monitoring study. Difficult intubation: an analysis of 2000 incident reports. *Anaesth Intensive Care.* 1993;21:602–607.

11. Snider RD, Kruse JA, Bander JJ, et al. Accuracy of estimated creatinine clearance in obese patients with stable renal function in the intensive care unit. *Pharmacotherapy.* 1995;15:474–453.

12. Erstad BL. Dosing of medications in morbidly obese patients in the intensive care unit setting. *Intensive Care Med.* 2004;30:18–32.

13. Makk LJK, McClave SA, Creech PW. Clinical application of the metabolic cart to the delivery of total parenteral nutrition. *Crit Care Med.* 1990;18:1320–1327.

14. Dickerson RN, Rosato EF, Mullen JL. Net protein anabolism with hypocaloric parenteral nutrition in obese stressed patients. *Am J Clin Nutr.* 1986;44:747–755.

15. Burge JC, Goon A, Choban PS, et al. Efficacy of hypocaloric total parenteral nutrition in hospitalized obese patients: a prospective, double-blind randomized trial. *JPEN.* 1994;18:203–207.

16. Parienti JJ, Thirion M, Megarbane B, et al. Femoral vs. jugular venous catheterization and risk of nosocomial events in adults requiring acute renal replacement: A randomized controlled trial. *JAMA.* 2008;299:2413–2422.

57

Multi-organ Dysfunction Syndrome

With the widespread use of advanced technology for organ support, patients rarely die from their presenting disease but rather from its pathophysiological consequences, namely the sequential dysfunction and failure of several organ systems. This syndrome has been called "multi-system organ failure" (MSOF), "multiple organ system failure" (MOSF), and more recently "multi-organ dysfunction syndrome" (MODS). MODS has an extraordinarily high mortality and, for many patients, the support of this syndrome does not improve survival but rather prolongs the dying process.

MODS is defined as "the presence of altered organ function in an acutely ill patient such that homeostasis cannot be maintained without intervention."[1,2] Earlier terminologies such as MOSF/MSOF should be avoided. These syndromes were defined using physiological parameters to determine either the presence or the absence of a particular organ failure. However, it has become increasing apparent that MODS is not an "all-or-nothing" condition but rather a continuum of dynamically changing organ failure.

In the United States, MODS develops during 15–18% of all ICU admissions.[3] MODS is responsible for up to 80% of all ICU deaths and results in costs of more than US $100,000 per patient or close to half-million dollars per survivor.[3,4] If one examines high-risk populations across the world, the frequency of MODS is remarkably similar and ranges from 7% in victims of multiple trauma to 11% in the general ICU population.[5]

Since 1973, MODS has been increasingly described as the final common pathway (outcome) of critically ill patients in the ICU.[6] However, the first descriptions of this syndrome date back to the early 1940s. During World War II, it was noted that patients with hypovolemic shock due to hemorrhage commonly died 10 days later with renal insufficiency.[7]

P.E. Marik, *Handbook of Evidence-Based Critical Care*,
DOI 10.1007/978-1-4419-5923-2_57,
© Springer Science+Business Media, LLC 2010

Indeed, these observations prompted the use of crystalloid fluids to prevent post-traumatic renal failure during the Korean War. Years later, in the Vietnam conflict, with the use of large volumes of crystalloids, the lungs became the primary organs to deteriorate post-trauma (the so-called shock lung).[8] In the early and mid-1970 s, investigators recognized the association between hemorrhagic shock or infection and multi-organ failure.[9,10] Since then, the failure of multiple organs at the same time or in sequence led some investigators to hypothesize that a common mechanism was responsible.[10]

Sepsis is the most common diagnosis leading to MODS in both non-operative and operative patients. Patients may develop MODS as a consequence of a primary infection or, as is more commonly the case, following nosocomial infections. However, in more than one-third of patients with MODS, no focus of infection can be found on clinical examination or postmortem studies. Other well-recognized risk factors for the development of MODS include severity of disease, age greater than 65 years, persistent deficit in oxygen delivery following resuscitation from circulatory shock, focus of devitalized tissue, severe trauma, major operations, and pre-existing end-stage liver failure.[11]

■ MECHANISMS OF MODS

The pathophysiological process leading to MODS has not been well defined. Tissue injury, whether from infection, blood or volume loss, trauma, or inflammation (such as pancreatitis), induces local and systemic responses. Genetic predisposition has even been cited by some.[12] The systemic responses include shock, reperfusion injuries, and systemic inflammation with organ dysfunction that either becomes progressive and leads to death or from which the patient recovers and enters into a period of prolonged rehabilitation. It is interesting, however, that the progressive dysfunction of organ systems occurs in a predictable manner. During the first 72 h of the original insult, respiratory failure commonly occurs.[13] This is followed by hepatic failure (5–7 days), gastrointestinal bleeding (10–15 days), and finally renal failure (11–17 days), in the typical case. The extent to which an individual organ is likely to be damaged in patients with MODS is variable. There are several hypotheses as to the mechanisms that initiate and perpetuate MODS. Among them, the most commonly cited is the gut hypothesis (the gut is considered the motor of MODS).[14] Splanchnic hypoperfusion is a common finding following multiple trauma, sepsis, shock, or thermal injuries. According to this hypothesis, splanchnic ischemia causes *gut* mucosal injury, which increases mucosal permeability, alters gut immune function, and increases translocation of bacteria.[14–16] Due to hepatic dysfunction, these bacterial toxins escape into the systemic circulation and activate the host's inflammatory response leading to tissue injury and organ dysfunction.

■ DIAGNOSTIC CRITERIA AND SCORING SYSTEMS

At least 20 scoring systems have been described to diagnose and quantify the severity of MODS.[17] These scoring systems differ appreciably, making it extremely difficult to compare the results from different research groups. In 1994, the European Society of Intensive Care Medicine organized a consensus meeting to create the "sepsis-related organ failure assessment (SOFA)" score and to describe and quantitate the degree of organ dysfunction/failure over time in groups of patients and individual patients.[18] The SOFA score was constructed using simple physiological measures of dysfunction in six organ systems. The elements of the SOFA scoring system are depicted in Table 57-1. The SOFA score was not designed to predict outcome but rather to describe and quantitate the sequence of complications in critically ill patients. Using physiological variables similar to those used in the SOFA score, Marshal and colleagues[19] developed the multiple organ dysfunction score.

Table 57-1. The SOFA score.

Sofa Score	1	2	3	4
Respiration PaO_2/FiO_2	<400	<300	<200	<100
Coagulation Platelet ($\times 10^3/\mu l$)	<150	<100	<50	<20
Liver Bilirubin (mg/dl)	1.2–1.9	2.0–5.9	6.0–11.9	>12
CVS Hypotension	MAP <70	Dopamine <5 or dobutamine	Dop >5 Epi ≤0.1 Nor ≤0.1	Dop >15 Epi >0.1 Nor >0.1
CNS GCS	13–14	10–12	6–9	<6
Renal Creatinine or UO	1.2–1.9	2.0–3.4	3.5–4.9 or <500/day	>5.0 or <200

■ CURRENT MANAGEMENT STRATEGIES

The management of the patient with MODS remains a formidable problem. Despite advances in critical care therapeutics, the mortality of multiple organ failure remains unchanged since the syndrome was characterized more than three decades ago. At the present time, there are no modalities that can actively reverse established organ failure; hence, the treatment of these patients consists of metabolic and hemodynamic support until the process reverses itself or death occurs. An increasing emphasis is being placed on the prevention of organ dysfunction, including maintenance of tissue oxygenation, nutrition, and infection control.

Marshall[20] emphasized that one of the keys to managing MODS is to recognize patients at greatest risk. The optimal therapeutic approach should be individualized but the overall goal is to minimize the risk of progression to MODS by

- optimizing supportive management of circulatory and respiratory dysfunction;
- reducing the rate of protein catabolism by prompt surgical debridement, burn wound excision and grafting, and fixation of long bone fractures;
- providing early nutrition support by the enteral route;
- selective, targeted use of antibiotics;
- minimizing blood transfusions.

One of the most common events preceding MODS is circulatory shock, and the risk for developing organ failure can often be predicted by events that occur within the first 24 h of admission. In this regard, inadequate initial resuscitation has been shown to be one of the most important factors increasing the risk of MODS, and optimizing hemodynamic resuscitation is therefore a major therapeutic focus.

■ REFERENCES

1. Society of Critical Care Medicine Consensus Conference Committee. American College of Chest Physicians/Society of Critical Care Medicine Consensus Conference: Definitions for sepsis and organ failure and guidelines for the use of innovative therapies in sepsis. *Crit Care Med.* 1992;20:864–874.
2. Bone RC, Sibbald WJ, Sprung CL. The ACCP-SCCM Consensus Conference on sepsis and organ failure. *Chest.* 1992;101:1481–1483.
3. Tran DD, Groeneveld ABJ, van der Meulen J. Age, chronic disease, sepsis, organ system failure, and mortality in a medical intensive care unit. *Crit Care Med.* 1990;18:474–479.

4. Deitch EA. Multiple organ failure: pathophysiology and potential future therapy. *Ann Surg*. 1992;216:117–134.

5. Deitch EA. Overview of multiple organ failure. In: Prough DS, Traystman RJ, eds. *Critical Care: State of the art*. Anaheim, CA: Society of Critical Care Medicine; 1993: 131–168.

6. Tilney NL, Bailey GL, Morgan AP. Sequential system failure after rupture of abdominal aortic aneurysms: an unsolved problem in post-operative care. *Ann Surg*. 1973;178:117–122.

7. Smith LH, Post RS, Teschan PE. Post-traumatic renal insufficiency in military casualties. II. Management, use of an artificial kidney, prognosis. In: Howard JM, ed. *Battle Casualties in Korea: Studies of the Surgical Research Team*. Washington, DC: Government Printing Office; 1974: 31–50.

8. Petty TL. Adult respiratory distress syndrome: a historical perspective and definition. *Respir Med*. 1981;2:99–103.

9. Eiseman B, Beart R, Norton L. Multiple system organ failure. *Surg Gynecol Obstet*. 1977;144:323–326.

10. Fry DE. Multiple system organ failure. *Surg Clin North Am*. 1988; 68:107–122.

11. Mizock BA. The multiple organ dysfunction syndrome. *Dis Mon*. 2009;55:476–526.

12. Villar J, Maca-Meyer N, Perez-Mendez L, et al. Bench-to-bedside review: understanding genetic predisposition to sepsis. *Crit Care*. 2004;8:180–189.

13. Cerra FB. Multiple organ failure syndrome. *Dis Mon*. 1992;38:843–947.

14. Carrico CJ, Meakins JL, Marshall JC, et al. Multiple-organ-failure syndrome. *Arch Surg*. 1986;121:196–208.

15. Doig CJ, Sutherland LR, Sandham JS, et al. Increased intestinal perme-ability is associated with the development of multiple organ dysfunction syndrome in critically ill ICU patients. *Am J Respir Crit Care Med*. 1998;158:444–451.

16. Deitch EA. Multiple organ failure. *Adv Surg*. 1993;26:333–356.

17. Berrtleff MJOE, Bruining HA. How should multiple organ dysfunction syndrome be assessed? A review of the variations in current scoring systems. *Eur J Surg*. 1997;163:405–409.

18. Vincent JL, Moreno R, Takala J, et al. The SOFA (Sepsis-related Organ Failure Assessment) score to describe organ dysfunction/failure. On behalf of the Working Group on Sepsis-Related Problems of the European Society of Intensive Care Medicine. *Intensive Care Med*. 1996;22:707–710.

19. Marshall JC, Cook DJ, Christou NV, et al. Multiple organ dysfunction score: a reliable descriptor of a complex clinical outcome. *Crit Care Med*. 1995;23:1638–1652.

20. Khadaroo RG, Marshall JC. ARDS and the multiple organ dysfunction syndrome. Common mechanisms of a common systemic process. *Crit Care Clin*. 2002;18:127–141.

58

Therapeutic Hypothermia

In 2002, two landmark studies were published demonstrating that the use of therapeutic hypothermia (TH) after cardiac arrest decreased mortality and improved neurological function.[1,2] Out-of-hospital survivors resuscitated from ventricular fibrillation and ventricular tachycardia were cooled to 32°C–34°C for 12–24 h. Based on these studies, the International Liaison Committee on Resuscitation and the American Heart Association recommended the use of TH after cardiac arrest.[3] Hypothermia has also been used as a treatment for traumatic brain injury, stroke, hepatic encephalopathy, myocardial infarction, and other indications. The mechanisms by which therapeutic hypothermia is neuroprotective are complex and include reduction of cerebral edema and cerebral metabolic rate as well as inhibition of the cascade of cellular events following reperfusion. TH should be strongly considered in comatose survivors of out-of-hospital cardiac arrest. Additional indications include cerebral edema associated with acute liver failure and cerebral edema associated with drug overdose.[4,5] The role of TH in patients with traumatic head injury is controversial.[6] TH is considered to be mild at 32°C–34°C, moderate at 28°C–31.9°C, and deep at 11°C–27.9°C. Arrhythmias become problematic below 30°C. In most therapeutic applications, it is recommended to keep the temperature of patients at 32°C–34°C. The earlier the TH can be instituted, the better the outcome; however, good results have been reported when TH was initiated 24 h after cardiac arrest.[7] However, the optimal duration of induced hypothermia and the optimal degree of hypothermia remain to be determined. A more prolonged period of deep hypothermia may be indicated in patients with severe cerebral edema.[5]

P.E. Marik, *Handbook of Evidence-Based Critical Care*,
DOI 10.1007/978-1-4419-5923-2_58,
© Springer Science+Business Media, LLC 2010

TH can be divided into three distinct phases:

- The induction phase, when the aim is to get the temperature below 34°C and then down to the target temperature as quickly as possible;
- The maintenance phase, when the aim is to tightly control core temperature, with minor or no fluctuations (maximum, 0.2°C–0.5°C);
- The rewarming phase, with slow and controlled warming (target rate, 0.2°C–0.5°C/h).

A number of different techniques have been used to induce therapeutic hypothermia, the most common being surface cooling. Invasive endovascular cooling techniques are more complex; however, they hold promise for the future. Surface cooling is relatively simple to use, but it takes longer to achieve the target body temperature (i.e., average 2–8 h). Surface cooling is best achieved with a microprocessor-controlled total body hyper-hypothermia water therapy system that provides effective patient warming and/or cooling with jackets, blankets, and hoods and that allows for accurate patient temperature control. Surface cooling can also be achieved with ice packs applied to the neck, groin, and axillae, and with rubber cooling blankets. One drawback of external cooling devices is that the shivering response to TH may be increased. However, this can be controlled with pharmacological interventions (see below). The time to achieve the goal temperature is reduced by the infusion of lactated Ringer's solution (4°C) at a dose of 30–40 ml/kg. Accurate, continuous core temperature measurement must guide TH preferably by bladder, rectal, central venous, or esophageal measurement.

TH has a number of side effects including the following:

- Immunosuppression with increased infection risk.
- Cold diuresis.
- Electrolyte disorders:
  - Potassium should be aggressively replaced if <3.8 mEq/dl at the onset of TH and should be reassessed every 3–4 h during the induction phase.
- Insulin resistance.
- Impaired drug clearance.
- Mild coagulopathy.
- Arrhythmias (usually with temperatures below 30°C).

Additional Interventions

- Initial laboratories:
  - ABG.
  - CBC/PT/PTT/INR, fibrinogen.
  - Chem 7, plus iCa/Mg/Phos.
  - Lactate/CPK-MB/CK/troponin.

- Cortisol level.
- Urinalysis.
- Blood cultures and urine cultures.
- Toxicology screen if appropriate.
- Amylase, lipase.
- Beta HCg on all women of child-bearing age.
- Serial laboratories:
  - Lactate q 6 h for 2 days.
  - Repeat CPK-MB/CK/troponin at 6 h.
  - CBC/PT/PTT/INR, Chem 7/Ca/Mg/Phos q 12 h.
  - ABG q 6 h and PRN.
- Central venous access.
- Arterial catheter.
- ECHO (TTE).
- Monitor core temperature.
- Maintain MAP 80–100 mmHg.
- Perform ACTH stimulation test; consider stress doses of corticosteroids.
- Enteral trickle feeding, 20 ml/h, then advance slowly.
- Institute appropriate critical care protocols for sepsis, DVT, and VAP prophylaxis.

Blood gas values are temperature dependent, and if blood samples are warmed to 37°C before analysis (as is common in most laboratories), PO_2 and PCO_2 will be overestimated and pH underestimated in hypothermic patients. The following correction formulas can be used:

- Subtract 5 mmHg PO_2 per 1°C develops (SIRS) that the patient's temperature is <37°C
- Subtract 2 mmHg PCO_2 per 1°C that the patient's temperature is <37°C
- Add 0.012 pH units per 1°C that the patient's temperature is <37°C

During the rewarming phase, hemodynamic instability is common, and as cutaneous vasodilation and an inflammatory postarrest state, clinicians should be prepared to administer intravenous isotonic fluids to maintain adequate preload. Extra care should be taken during rewarming because hyperkalemia may develop during this phase due to the release of potassium sequestered to the intracellular compartment during hypothermia induction. Hyperkalemia can be prevented by slow and controlled rewarming, allowing the kidneys to excrete the excess potassium.

Shivering induces unfavorable effects such as increased oxygen consumption and metabolic rate, excess work of breathing, and increased heart rate with increased myocardial oxygen consumption. Neuromuscular blocking agents (NMBAs) are commonly used during TH to control shivering. NMBAs are however associated with significant complications and are best avoided (see Chapter 9). The failure of a number of clinical trials to demonstrate a benefit of TH may be related to the use of NMBAs. The use of adequate sedation and analgesia and the use of specific anti-shivering agents are usually able to control this problem. Deep sedation with the combination of propofol and fentanyl are recommended. Propofol has the additional benefit of having neuroprotective properties.[8] Additional anti-shivering measures include the following:

- Acetaminophen 650 mg (enteral) every 6 h
- Magnesium sulfate boluses to target a magnesium level of 2.5–3.0 mg/dl
- Meperidine 12.5–25 mg intravenously every 4 h (decrease fentanyl infusion); max. 100 mg/day; contraindicated if renal failure or oliguria present or patient taking an MAO inhibitor, buspirone, or SSRI
- Dexmedetomidine 0.3–1.5 ng/kg/min or clonidine 0.1–0.3 mg (enteral) every 8 h.

■ REFERENCES

1. Bernard SA, Gray TW, Buist MD, et al. Treatment of comatose survivors of out-of-hospital cardiac arrest with induced hypothermia. *N Engl J Med*. 2002;346:557–563.
2. Mild therapeutic hypothermia to improve the neurologic outcome after cardiac arrest. *N Engl J Med*. 2002;346:549–556.
3. Nolan JP, Morley PT, Hoek TL, et al. Therapeutic hypothermia after cardiac arrest. An advisory statement by the Advancement Life support Task Force of the International Liaison committee on Resuscitation. *Resuscitation*. 2003;57:231–235.
4. Raghavan M, Marik PE. Therapy of intracranial hypertension in patients with fulminant hepatic failure. *Neurocrit Care*. 2006;4:179–189.
5. Marik PE, Varon J. Prolonged and profound therapeutic hypothermia for the treatment of "brain death" following a suicidal intoxication. Challenging conventional wisdoms. *Am J Emerg Med*. 2010;28:258. e1–258.e4.
6. Bratton SL, Chestnut RM, Ghajar J, et al. Guidelines for the management of severe traumatic brain injury. III. Prophylactic hypothermia. *J Neurotrauma*. 2007;24(Suppl 1):S21–S25.
7. Varon J, Marik PE. Complete neurological recovery following delayed initiation of hypothermia in a victim of warm water near-drowning. *Resuscitation*. 2006;68:421–423.
8. Marik PE. Propofol: therapeutic indications and side effects. *Curr Pharm Design*. 2004;10:3639–3649.

59

Toxicology

This chapter provides a brief overview on the management of patients following an accidental or a suicidal overdose. The reader is referred to toxicology texts and their local poison center for information on the management of specific intoxications.

■ GENERAL MEASURES

- Stabilization of patient, i.e., airway, breathing, and circulation:
  - Intubate obtunded, comatose and seizing patients.
- Obtain IV access.
- Treat hypotension initially with volume expansion (crystalloids).
- Comatose patients should be given naloxone 0.8 mg IV.
- Flumazenil (a benzodiazepine antagonist) may be indicated in patients who present with obtundation or coma following the ingestion of benzodiazepines. Flumazenil is contraindicated in patients with mixed overdoses (tricyclic anti-depressants and benzo-diazepines) as well as patients with a history of seizures. An initial dose of 0.2 mg intravenously should be given over 30 s. Additional doses of 0.2–0.5 mg can be given up to a total of 3 mg.
- Ipecac is not recommended for ingestions treated in hospital. May be used at home for accidental ingestions in children. Should not be given after ingestion of caustic substances and acids.
- Gastric lavage is indicated in the following circumstances:
  - Recent ingestion (<1 h) of a potentially life-threatening poison;
  - Ingestion of a substance that slows gastric emptying (e.g., anti-cholinergic medications);

P.E. Marik, *Handbook of Evidence-Based Critical Care*,
DOI 10.1007/978-1-4419-5923-2_59,
© Springer Science+Business Media, LLC 2010

- Ingestion of a poison that is slowly absorbed from the gastrointestinal tract;
- Ingestion of a substance that does not bind well to activated charcoal (see below);
- Ingestion of specific life-threatening poisons (e.g., tricyclic antidepressants, theophylline, cyanide);
- Contraindicated in caustic ingestions.

Technique for Performing Gastric Lavage

- Patients who cannot protect their airway *must be intubated* prior to performing gastric lavage.
- Patients are placed in head down lateral position.
- Place large bore lavage tube through mouth.
- Aspirate to empty stomach.
- Lavage with 150–300 ml tepid tap water.

Activated Charcoal

This is the cornerstone of the management of most ingestions. Activated charcoal is administered in a dose of 50–100 g.

- Drugs not well bound to activated charcoal
  - Bromides
  - Caustics
  - Cyanide
  - Ethylene glycol
  - Heavy metals
  - Iron
  - Isopropyl alcohol
  - Lithium
  - Methanol
- Drugs amenable to repeat dose activate charcoal therapy
  - Carbamazepine
  - Diazepam
  - Digitalis
  - Phenobarbital
  - Phenytoin
  - Salicylates
  - Theophylline
  - Tricyclic anti-depressants

Specific antidotes are available for a limited number of intoxications (see Table 59-1).

Table 59-1. Toxic substances with specific antidotes.

Agent	Antidote
Acetaminophen	N-Acetylcysteine
Anti-cholinergic poisoning	Physostigmine
Anti-coagulants	Vitamin K, protamine
Benzodiazepines	Flumazenil
β-Adrenergic antagonists	Glucagon, calcium salts, isoproterenol
Carbon monoxide	Oxygen, hyperbaric oxygen
Cholinergic syndromes	Atropine
Digoxin	Fab antibody, Mg
Ethylene glycol	Fomepizole, thiamine, ethanol
Fluoride	Calcium and Mg salts
Heavy metals	BAL, DMSA, d-penicillamine
Iron	Desferoxime
Isoniazid	GABA antagonists, pyridoxine
Methemoglobinemia	Methylene blue
Opioids	Naloxone

Some drugs are cleared by hemodialysis/hemoperfusion; these techniques should be instituted as clinical circumstances dictate.

- Hemoperfusion
  - Acetaminophen
  - Theophylline
  - Methotrexate
  - Phenylbutazone
  - Procainamide
  - Quinidine
- Hemodialysis
  - Ammonium chloride
  - Amphetamine
  - Atenolol
  - Meprobamate
  - Methyldopa
  - Nadolol
  - Phenobarbital
  - Procainamide
  - Quinidine
  - Sotalol
  - Thallium
  - Ethanol
  - Methanol
  - Ethylene glycol

- Isopropanol
- Aspirin
- Lithium
- Bromide
- Arsenic

In the evaluation of a patient with a possible drug overdose, it is useful to look for symptom complexes or "toxidromes" that may help in identifying the type of drug ingested. The following toxidromes should be identified:

- Depressed level of consciousness
  - Coma, stupor, lethargy, confusion
- Anti-cholinergic signs
  - Mydriasis, increased blood pressure, tachycardia, warm dry skin, erythema, delirium, hallucination, urinary retention
- Cholinergic signs
  - Salivation, lacrimation, urination, defecation (SLUD), miosis, bradycardia, sweating
- Sympathetic signs
  - High blood pressure, tachycardia, hyperthermia, mydriasis
- Serotonin syndrome
  - Confusion, myoclonus, hyperreflexia, diaphoresis, tremor, flushing, diarrhea, fever
- Neurological signs
  - Nystagmus, tremors, hyperreflexia, seizures, extrapyramidal signs, hallucinations

Common agents responsible are the following:

- Depressed level of consciousness
  - Alcohols
  - Anti-cholinergic
  - Anti-convulsants
  - Anti-depressants
  - Anti-histamines
  - Anti-psychotics
  - Barbiturates
  - Benzodiazepines
  - Carbon monoxide
  - Opiates
  - Sulfonylureas
- Seizures
  - Phenytoin
  - β-Blockers
  - Clonidine

- – Theophylline
- – Meperidine
- – Amphetamines
- – Cocaine
- Anti-cholinergic syndrome
  - – Anti-depressants
  - – Anti-histamines
  - – Anti-psychotic
  - – Belladonna alkaloids
  - – Mushrooms
- Cholinergic syndrome
  - – Insecticides
  - – Mushrooms
  - – Nicotine
- Sympathetic syndrome
  - – Cocaine
  - – Amphetamines
  - – Phencyclidine
- Serotonin syndrome
  - – SSRI: fluoxetine, etc.
  - – Isoniazid
  - – Meperidine
  - – Clomipramine
- Extrapyramidal
  - – Anti-psychotic
- Nystagmus
  - – Alcohols
  - – Lithium
  - – Carbamazepine
- Hallucinations
  - – Amphetamines
  - – Cocaine
  - – Phencyclidine
  - – Cannabinoids

■ COMMON INTOXICATIONS

Acetaminophen

Acetaminophen (acetyl-p-aminophenol or APAP) is an active ingredient of several hundred preparations and is the most common drug implicated in both accidental (children) and suicidal overdoses. In 2003, the American Association of Poison Control Centers reported more than 127,000 exposures involving acetaminophen.[1] Of these exposures,

65,000 patients received treatment in a medical facility, and 16,500 received N-acetylcysteine (NAC). There were 214 deaths involving overdose where an analgesic agent was thought to be primarily responsible. In 62 of these cases, APAP was the single agent involved. APAP toxicity is the major cause of fulminant hepatic failure (FHF) and is implicated in as many as 39% of cases presenting to tertiary care hospitals.

Acetaminophen is well absorbed, with peak levels about 4 h after an overdose. After therapeutic doses, approximately 90% of acetaminophen is conjugated by the liver to non-toxic inactive compounds which are renally excreted. About 5% is excreted unchanged in the urine and about 5% is oxidized by the P-450 and mixed function oxidase enzyme to yield highly reactive toxic intermediates which are detoxified by reduced glutathione. After overdosage, the amount of drug metabolized by the P-450 route is increased. The same process occurs in the kidney, and while renal toxicity may occur with acetaminophen overdose, it is far less common than hepatotoxicity. The hepatotoxicity may vary from asymptomatic elevation of liver enzymes to fatal liver failure. Pancreatitis and myocardial necrosis have also been described. It should be noted that stores of reduced glutathione are diminished in alcoholics and malnourished patients, predisposing to hepatic toxicity at therapeutic dosages. Ingestions of greater than 7.5 g in an adult should be considered potentially toxic.

Non-acute ingestions of APAP, frequently referred to as subacute or chronic, are ingestions that take place over a period longer than 4 h. In these cases, the nomogram (Figure 59-1) offers no guidance

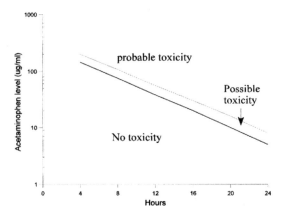

Figure 59-1. Acetaminophen treatment guideline based on serum level Vs. time plot.

in treatment, because it is intended only for use with acute ingestions. Most cases of non-acute ingestion of APAP that results in hepatotoxicity involve persons taking supratherapeutic doses who are at increased risk for APAP-induced hepatotoxicity. However, hepatotoxicity has been reported in patients taking "therapeutic doses" (4 g/day); these patients usually have other risk factors including alcohol abuse, malnutrition, underlying liver disease, or concomitant drugs (including phenytoin).[2,3]

Watkins et al.[4] randomized 147 healthy volunteers to receive acetaminophen (4 g/day), an oral opiate, acetaminophen + an opiate, or placebo. In this study, the daily intake of acetaminophen was associated with normal ALT elevation (>3 times) in up to 44% of patients (risk not influenced by concomitant opiate). The AST levels began to rise on the 5th day and peaked on the 10th day when the drug was stopped. A prospective study of more than 600 patients from 22 US tertiary care centers found that acetaminophen-related liver damage is the leading cause of acute liver failure in the country and that about half of such cases involved unintentional overdose.[5] In the unintentional group, 38% took two or more acetaminophen preparations simultaneously. Based on the risks of hepatotoxicity with the "current dosage" recommendations, the FDA has required a change in the labeling of these products, including reducing the maximum daily dose for both prescription and over-the counter acetaminophen products from 4 g/day to 3,250 mg/day (500 q 4 h or 650 q 6 h), limiting the dose in individual tablets, and adding to the labeling of these products a warning that individuals who chronically use alcohol should use an even lower dose of the drug.[6,7]

Signs and Symptoms

- Stage 1: 12–24 h after ingestion; asymptomatic or mild GI symptoms.
- Stage 2: 24–72 h; right upper quadrant pain, nausea and vomiting, liver enzymes begin to rise.
- Stage 3: 72–96 h; maximal hepatic injury.
- Stage 4: 4 days–2 weeks; patient either improves with normalization of enzymes or progresses to acute hepatic necrosis with liver failure.

Management

Analyzing the serum acetaminophen concentration is essential in all cases of acute overdose (see Figure 59-1). A level prior to 4 h is difficult to interpret. High potential for toxicity exists when serum concentration is >200 µg/ml at 4 h, 50 µg/ml at 12 h, and 7 µg/ml at 24 h after ingestion.

N-Acetylcysteine (NAC) should be administered as soon as possible within the first 24 h of ingestion. However, antidotal therapy is optimal when given within 12 h of acetaminophen ingestion. NAC should be given if the patient has ingested more than 140 mg/kg (or 10 g) acetaminophen, if the serum level is above 140 μg/ml, or if the serum level is in the toxic range. The dose of *N*-acetylcysteine is 140 mg/kg as an initial oral loading dose, followed by 70 mg/kg every 4 h for a total of 17 doses. Nausea and vomiting are reported in 33% of APAP overdoses before NAC and in an estimated 51% during oral NAC therapy. In 2004, *Acetadote* became the first NAC solution approved by the FDA for IV use, allowing the United States to join the rest of the industrialized world, which has been using IV NAC since its introduction in 1977.[8] A 72-h oral, 48-h IV, and 20-h IV protocol have been reported. These protocols have been compared by retrospective study and through meta-analysis.[9] When started within 8 h of ingestion, none of the protocols shows advantage over another. However, the 20-h IV protocol is generally preferred; this is given as a loading dose of 150 mg/kg over 15 min, followed by 50 mg/kg infused over 4 h and 100 mg/kg administered over 16 h as a constant infusion. Although there is general consensus that IV administration is preferable in the face of intractable vomiting, no study shows clear evidence that IV therapy is more or less effective than oral NAC therapy.

It may be useful to measure a second acetaminophen level some time after starting *N*-acetylcysteine in order to determine the half-life of acetaminophen. A half-life greater than 4 h is suggestive of hepatic toxicity. *N*-Acetylcysteine should not be stopped as the level falls to zero, as it is not acetaminophen that is toxic but rather its metabolites.

Salicylates

Signs and Symptoms

Gastric upset, tinnitus, increased depth of breathing, headache, seizures, and coma. Anion gap metabolic acidosis and respiratory alkalosis.

Management

Serum salicylate levels are useful in confirming the diagnosis and assessing the severity of the toxicity but are however not used in directing therapy.

- Supportive measures, GI decontamination, and activated charcoal.
- Forced alkaline diuresis (ion trapping and increased elimination). In cases of severe toxicity, dialysis is useful.
- The decision to dialyze the patient is based on clinical grounds, i.e., seizures, altered level of consciousness.
- Blood level monitoring is useful to monitor drug elimination.

Tricyclic Anti-depressants

The newer cyclic anti-depressants (SSRI agents) are less toxic in over-dose than are the tricyclic drugs. Tricyclic anti-depressants have anti-cholinergic and cardiac effects; however, they can cause seizures, altered mentation and level of consciousness, leading to coma in overdose.

Signs and Symptoms

- *Anti-cholinergic*. mydriasis, blurred vision, dry mouth, tachycardia, hyperpyrexia, urinary retention, decreased GI motility.
- *CNS*. agitation, mental confusion, respiratory depression, seizures, coma.
- *Cardiac*. Quinidine-like action on the heart; widened QRS, PR, and QT intervals, RBBB, torsades de pointes. The best predictor of cardiac arrhythmias and seizures is a QRS complex greater than 0.1 s or a prolonged QTc interval.

Management

- Anti-depressants are highly tissue bound and therefore serum concentrations do not correlate with toxicity and have little clinical value.
- Supportive measures, GI decontamination, and activated charcoal are essential.
- Alkalinization of the serum with bicarbonate to achieve an arterial pH of 7.5–7.55 should be instituted in patients with a prolonged QRS/QTc interval or cardiac arrhythmias. Alkalinization increases plasma protein binding (less free drug) and antagonizes the quinidine-like effects on the His–Purkinje system.
- Seizures are best treated with diazepam/midazolam or intravenous phenobarbital. Phenytoin is ineffective and may be dangerous.

Acute Ethanol Intoxication

Alcohol is the most common poison consumed by Americans; approximately one-third of the population ingests this toxin on a chronic basis. The mechanism of action of alcohol is unclear; no specific ethanol receptors have been identified. It is postulated that ethanol influences multiple ion channels by causing alterations in their tertiary structure due to intercalation of ethanol into the bilipid cell membrane. Ethanol antagonizes the excitatory N-methyl-d-aspartate (NMDA) glutamate receptor and potentiates the inhibitory γ-aminobutyric acid A receptor. These actions may explain the effect of alcohol on the central nervous system; ethanol is a CNS depressant.

Ethanol is readily absorbed from the gastrointestinal tract, with 80% of the absorption occurring in the small intestine. Peak ethanol levels typically occur 30–60 min after ingestion. Metabolism occurs in the liver by first-order kinetics (i.e., at a constant rate unaffected by the serum level), predominantly by alcohol dehydrogenase. The clinical features and associated blood levels of ethanol intoxication are listed in Table 59-2. The blood alcohol level can be estimated by the following formula: EtOH level = osmolar gap × 4.3. Serum ethanol levels decline by about 15–30 mg/dl/h. The treatment of acute alcohol intoxication is largely supportive, with prevention and management of the associated complications. Hemodialysis may be helpful in severe cases. Medical complications associated with acute alcohol ingestion include the following:

Table 59-2. Features of acute alcohol intoxication.

Blood Ethanol Concentration (mg%)	Symptoms and Signs
50–150	Euphoria or dysphoria, uninhibited Impaired concentration and judgment
150–250	Slurred speech, ataxic gait, drowsiness, labile moods, anti-social behavior
250–400	Stupor, incoherent speech, vomiting
400–500	Coma
>500	Death

- Acute myopathy with rhabdomyolysis
- Gastritis
- Esophagitis
- Mallory–Weiss lesion
- Thrombocytopenia
- Pancreatitis
- Alcoholic hepatitis
- Arrhythmias, especially atrial fibrillation
- Decreased myocardial contractility (synergistic with cocaine)
- Peripheral vasodilation and hypotension
- Alcohol withdrawal syndrome and delirium tremens
- Hypoglycemia
- Electrolyte disturbances, including hypokalemia, hyponatremia, hypophosphatemia, hypomagnesemia
- Wernicke's syndrome

Ethylene Glycol and Methanol Poisoning

Ethylene Glycol

Ethylene glycol is found in many deicers, anti-freezes, detergents, polishes, cosmetics, paints, and lacquers. It is colorless and odorless with a slightly sweet taste. Ethylene glycol initially causes an ethanol-like intoxication with little toxicity until it is metabolized in the liver to more harmful metabolites, including several aldehydes, carboxylic acids, and oxalic acid. These intermediates inhibit cellular respiration, protein synthesis, and RNA replication. Ethylene glycol initially undergoes oxidation by hepatic alcohol dehydrogenase to glycolaldehyde, which is then rapidly converted by aldehyde dehydrogenase to glycolic acid. Glycolic acid is converted to glyoxylic acid, whose most toxic metabolite is oxalic acid. Oxalic acid may crystallize as calcium oxalate in many tissues, causing hypocalcemia and tubular obstruction in the kidney. The anion gap acidosis results predominantly from elevated glycolic acid levels.[10]

Classically, ethylene glycol poisoning has been divided into three stages:

- Stage 1 (30 min–12 h) is characterized by CNS effects such as ethanol-like intoxication, stupor, coma and convulsions dominate the clinical picture.
- Stage 2 (12–24 h) is notable for cardiovascular and pulmonary effects such as tachypnea, cyanosis and pulmonary edema, and progressive CNS depression.
- Stage 3 (48–72 h) is characterized by the development of acute renal failure. In addition, during this stage, prolonged generalized seizures may occur.

Methanol

Methanol is found in many cleaning materials, paints and varnishes, antifreeze, duplicating fluids, and gasoline. It is a colorless liquid with a distinct odor. Methanol is about half as potent as ethanol in its ability to cause CNS depression. Like ethylene glycol, it must undergo metabolic transformation before toxicity occurs. Alcohol dehydrogenase catalyzes the formation of formaldehyde, which is converted to formic acid. Formic acid is an inhibitor of mitochondrial cytochrome oxidase, causes histocytotoxic hypoxia, and is responsible for the metabolic acidosis and ocular toxicity seen with methanol. Lactic acidosis may be seen late in the course of methanol toxicity. Neurological, ophthalmologic, and gastrointestinal symptoms dominate the clinical features of methanol toxicity. Features of toxicity include blurred vision, scintillations, loss of sight, unreactive pupils, papilledema, vomiting epigastric pain, convulsions, and coma. An anion gap metabolic acidosis (formate anions) is characteristic.

Management

The serum methanol and ethylene glycol levels should be measured; however they can be estimated from the osmolar gap as follows:

- [Methanol] = 3.2 × osmol gap
- [Ethylene glycol] = 6.2 × osmol gap

Syrup of ipecac should be avoided due to the risk of aspiration. The efficacy of activated charcoal is controversial.

- If pH <7.25, sodium bicarbonate should be given to maintain the pH above 7.25. Large doses of bicarbonate may be required to control severe life-threatening metabolic acidosis. Unlike the metabolites in lactic acidosis and keto-acidosis, the metabolites of ethylene glycol cannot be converted back to bicarbonate.
- *Ethanol*. Ethanol slows down the metabolism of both methanol and ethylene glycol reducing their toxicity. Ethanol should be given to patients with ocular symptoms, acidosis, or patients with a serum methanol or ethylene glycol level greater than 20 mg/dl:
  - Loading dose: 600 mg/kg IV.
  - Maintenance dose: 100–150 mg/h. The infusion should be titrated to maintain a serum ethanol level of 100–150 mg/dl.
- *Fomepizole*. Fomepizole is a potent inhibitor of alcohol dehydrogenase and is used as an alternative to ethanol. Fomepizole has been used successfully to treat methanol, ethylene glycol, and diethylene glycol poisoning in humans. The indications for fomepizole are the same as those for ethanol. The currently approved dose consists of a loading dose of 15 mg/kg IV over 30 min, followed by 10 mg/kg every 12 h for four doses, then 5 mg/kg every 12 h thereafter.[11]
- *Hemodialysis*. Hemodialysis facilitates the removal of methanol, ethylene glycol, and their metabolites. Hemodialysis should be instituted in all patients with a serum level above 50 mg/dl, patients with ocular symptoms (methanol), and in patients with a significant metabolic acidosis. The ethanol infusion rate should be increased during dialysis as it is also removed during dialysis.
- In methanol poisoning, folic/folinic acid (50–100 mg q 4 h) may mitigate the toxic effects of formate. Pyridoxine (100 mg) and thiamine (100 mg) should be given daily in ethylene glycol poisoning.

Isopropyl Alcohol

In general, isopropyl alcohol is less toxic than either methanol or ethylene glycol. It is metabolized to acetone. Neither a metabolic acidosis nor an ion gap characteristically occurs.

Signs and Symptoms

- Dizziness, confusion, slurred speech, headache, ataxia, stupor, and coma
- Nausea, vomiting, abdominal pain, hemorrhagic gastritis, diarrhea
- Hypotension, bradycardia, rhabdomyolysis, hemolysis

Management

Treatment is essentially supportive. Hemodialysis is recommended in severe poisoning, especially when accompanied by hypotension.

Digitalis

Signs and Symptoms

Nausea, vomiting, diarrhea, fatigue, malaise, headache, confusion, delusions, hallucinations, blurred vision, disorder of green–yellow color perception, visualization of halos around objects, and cardiac arrhythmias, including paroxysmal atrial tachycardia (PAT) with 2 to 1 block, junctional tachycardia, varying degrees of heart block, ventricular ectopy, ventricular tachycardia, ventricular fibrillation.

Management

- Due to high degree of tissue binding, serum drug levels do not accurately reflect tissue levels. Diagnosis of toxicity is a clinical diagnosis. The majority of patients who show signs of toxicity have a serum level above 2 ng/ml; however, some patients may exhibit toxicity below this level. Similarly patients may have a level above 2 ng/ml with no signs of toxicity.
- Gastric lavage and activated charcoal (acute ingestion).
- Continuous ECG monitoring, evaluating old ECGs.
- Correction of electrolytes. *Beware*: K+ may increase acutely with digoxin overdose.
- Atropine for conduction disturbances.
- Phenytoin or lidocaine for arrhythmias of impulse formation.

- Temporary pacemaker for arrhythmias that are resistant to atropine.
- Digoxin-specific antibodies (digoxin Fab fragment antibodies) for serious arrhythmias and severe toxicity. Digoxin Fab (Digibond) dosing:
  - Extreme caution if patient in renal failure.
  - Serum levels not useful once FAB given.
  - Dose dependent on body load; each vial contains 40 mg FAB and binds 0.6 mg digoxin.
  - Body load of digoxin = (serum digoxin concentration $\times$ 5.6 $\times$ weight in kilograms)/1,000. Dose (vials) = body load/0.6.

Phenytoin

Signs and Symptoms

Nystagmus, ataxia, slurred speech, confusion, seizures

Management

Phenytoin is highly protein bound; therefore serum levels do not correlate well with toxicity. Free levels are a better indicator of toxicity (>2 μg/ml). Treatment includes gastric lavage and repeated activated charcoal.

Lithium

Signs and Symptoms

Mild-to-moderate toxicity occurs when the serum concentration is between 1.5 and 2.5 mEq/l and severe toxicity occurs when the levels are between 2.5 and 3.5 mEq/l. Levels above 3.5 mEq/l are life threatening. Symptoms however do not necessarily correlate with lithium levels and symptoms of toxicity may occur at therapeutic levels. Neurological symptoms dominate the clinical picture of lithium toxicity. Symptoms include nausea, vomiting, diarrhea, polyuria, blurred vision, muscular weakness, confusion, vertigo, increased deep tendon reflexes, myoclonus, choreoathetoid movements, urinary and fecal incontinence, stupor, coma, seizures, cardiac arrhythmia, cardiovascular collapse, and death.

Predisposing Factors to Lithium Toxicity

- Infections
- Volume depletion
- Gastroenteritis
- Renal insufficiency

- Congestive cardiac failure
- Non-steroidal anti-inflammatory drugs
- Diuretics
- Tetracycline

Management

Management includes gastric lavage and supportive therapy. Activated charcoal is not effective in removing lithium. Dehydrated patients should be actively rehydrated; however, forced saline diuresis is not recommended. Hemodialysis is indicated in patients with levels above 4 mEq/l or in patients with signs of serious toxicity and levels above 2 mEq/l. The duration of dialysis should be guided by the serum levels. It is important to bear in mind that serum levels may rebound up following dialysis and require repeat dialysis.

Opiates

Signs and Symptoms

Constricted pupils, bradycardia, hypotension, hypothermia, pulmonary edema, respiratory depression, and coma.

Management

Management of opiate toxicity includes supportive therapy and the administration of the opiate antagonist naloxone (Narcan). Naloxone should be given as an initial intravenous bolus of 0.4 mg. A bolus of between 0.4 mg and 2 mg can be repeated every 3–5 min up to a total dose of 10 mg. Naloxone has a duration of action of about 45–60 min, which is considerably shorter than that of all the opiate agonists. Therefore, should the patient respond to the boluses of naloxone, a continuous infusion should be started by placing 8 mg into 1,000 ml of 5% D/W and infusing at a rate of 0.4–0.8 mg/h.

Cocaine

Cocaine is a naturally occurring substance found in the leaves of the rythroxylum coca plant. The plant is endogenous to South America, Mexico, Indonesia, and the West Indies. Cocaine hydrochloride is a water-soluble powder which can be absorbed through the nasal mucosa or injected intravenously. Cocaine hydrochloride has a high melting point and decomposes when burnt; this form of cocaine is therefore not suitable for smoking. Cocaine can be effectively smoked when it has been transformed into an alkaloid form, either "freebase" or "crack." Freebase and crack are the same chemical form of cocaine but are made using different techniques.

Cocaine abuse and dependence is epidemic in the United States. More than 50 million Americans have used cocaine, and more than 6 million Americans of all ages use it on a regular basis. The national prevalence of cocaine use is highest among 18- to 25-year olds but is becoming quite popular in the teenage group. In New York City between 1990 and 1992, 26.7% of fatal injury victims had cocaine metabolites in their urine or blood.[12] Death after cocaine use is one of the five leading causes of death in the 15- to 44-year-old age group. Cocaine is the most frequent drug-related cause of emergency department (ED) visits in the United States. In 2006, hospitals in the United States provided a total of 113 million ED visits; the Drug Abuse Warning Network (DAWN) estimates that 958,164 of these visits involved an illicit drug, with cocaine being involved in 548,608 cases (both cocaine and alcohol in 101,588 cases).[13]

Analysis of street samples of cocaine has found an average purity rate of 40%.[14] Therefore, adulterants represent more than half of the composition of all cocaine sold. Local anesthetics are among the most frequent contaminants of cocaine. Local anesthetics have psychoactive and reinforcing properties similar to cocaine and can thus potentiate these effects when combined along with cocaine. Other additives include sugars, talc, and cornstarch.

Cocaine acts by promoting the release and blocking the reuptake of neurotransmitters (norepinephrine, dopamine, and serotonin) at synaptic junctions, resulting in increased neurotransmitter concentrations. This results in sympathic and central nervous stimulation. Cocaine like other amide local anesthetic agents blocks initiation and conduction of nerve impulses by deceasing axonal membrane permeability to sodium ions. At high doses, cocaine has Class 1 anti-arrhythmic effects.

Cocaine can be smoked, nasally insufflated, or injected intravenously. Smoking "crack" cocaine is a popular and potentially dangerous route of administration. Due to the large absorptive surface area of the lung, very high serum levels can be achieved within seconds. Nasal insufflation produces euphoria in about 3–5 min, with peak cocaine levels being achieved in 30–60 min. The biological half-life in the blood is about 1 h. Cocaine is metabolized to benzoylecgonine and ecgonine, which are excreted in the urine. Less than 5% of cocaine is excrete unchanged in the urine. Most urinary excretion occurs within 24 h of administration. Most assays for detecting cocaine measure urinary benzoylecgonine levels. This assay will be positive for up to 6 days after a single use and as long as 21 days with high-dose long-term use.

Alcohol enhances the euphoric effects of cocaine. Each year, approximately 12 million Americans use this drug combination. Cocaethylene is produced by the liver from the combination of cocaine and ethanol. Cocaethylene produces intense dopaminergic stimulation in the brain and the myocardium. The risk of sudden death is 25 times greater in persons who abuse both alcohol and cocaine than in those who use only cocaine.

Chest pain is the most frequent cocaine-related symptom and accounts for up to 40% of cocaine-related ED visits. In the COCaine Associated CHest PAin (COCHPA) study, cocaine-associated MI occurred in 6% of patients who presented to the ED with chest pain after cocaine use.[15] Cocaine-associated chest pain may be caused by not only MI but also by aortic dissection, and this must be considered in the differential diagnosis. In the COCHPA study, the sensitivity of an ECG revealing ischemia or MI to predict a true MI was only 36%. The specificity, positive predictive value, and negative predictive value of the ECG were 89.9, 17.9, and 95.8%, respectively. High-risk patients with ST-segment elevation or depression >1 mm, elevated serum cardiac markers, recurrent chest pain, or hemodynamic instability should be admitted to the ICU/CCU.

Complications Associated with the Use of Cocaine

- Sudden death, due to arrhythmias, intracerebral bleeds, respiratory arrest, seizures, hyperthermia, and myocardial infarction.
- Psychiatric: Cocaine use is associated with altered behavior, psychological, personality, and psychomotor alterations. Patients may have an underlying depression or personality disorder.
- Cardiovascular:
  - Myocardial ischemia and infarction: The coronary arteries are usually normal; cocaine increases myocardial oxygen demand, induces coronary spasm, and increases platelet aggregation and has a procoagulant effect by depleting protein C and antithrombin III.
  - Myocarditis and cardiomyopathy.
  - Severe hypertension.
  - Dissecting aortic aneurysm (often fatal).
  - Arrhythmias ,including supraventricular tachycardia, ventricular tachycardia, and fibrillation.
- Pulmonary:
  - Asthma.
  - Thermal airway injury.
  - Non-cardiogenic pulmonary edema.
  - Pulmonary hemorrhage.
  - COP (cryptogenic organizing pneumonia).
  - Pneumothorax and pneumomediastinum.
  - Interstitial pneumonitis.

- Neurological:
  - Seizures.
  - Hemorrhagic strokes.
  - Cerebral infarctions.
  - Ruptured aneurysms.
- Renal:
  - Rhabdomyolysis and acute renal failure.
- Other:
  - Intestinal ischemia.
  - Gastroduodenal perforations.
  - DIC.
  - Placental abruption.
  - Hyperthermia.

The Management of Cocaine Toxicity

- CBC, Chem 7, troponins and CPKs, PT, PTT, ECG, CXR as well as a toxicology screen should be performed in all patients with suspected cocaine toxicity.
- Agitation is best treated with benzodiazepines.
- *Seizures.* Solitary seizures usually do not require therapy. Status epilepticus, however, requires aggressive treatment with intravenous benzodiazepines followed by a loading dose of phenytoin.
- Hyperthermia must be treated immediately with cool-water washes and/or with cooling blankets.
- *Hypertension.* This is usually self-limiting. However, severe or sustained hypertension should be treated. β-Blockers (including labetalol) may cause paradoxical worsening of hypertension as a result of unopposed alpha stimulation. Severe hypertension is best treated with a combination of benzodiazepines and calcium channel blockers (verapamil or nicardipine).
- Myocardial ischemia/infarction:
  - In cases of myocardial ischemia or impending infarction, calcium channel blockers (verapamil or diltiazem), aspirin, and nitroglycerin are recommended. Nitroglycerin and verapamil reverse cocaine-induced hypertension and coronary arterial vasoconstriction; therefore, they are the agents of choice in treating patients with cocaine-associated chest pain.
  - Timely percutaneous coronary intervention by experienced operators in high-volume centers is preferred over fibrinolytics in ST-segment elevation MI and is even more desirable in the setting of cocaine use.[16]
  - Thrombolytics should be avoided in patients with cocaine-related infarction because of the increased risk of bleeding in these

patients as well as the unreliable electrocardiographic criteria to identify myocardial infarction.[16]

- β-Adrenergic blocking agents (including labetalol) may exacerbate cocaine-induced coronary arterial vasoconstriction, thereby increasing the magnitude of myocardial ischemia.
- Nifedipine should not be used as this agent may potentiate seizures and death.

Carbon Monoxide Poisoning

Carbon monoxide (CO) intoxication is the leading cause of death due to poisoning in the United States. Epidemics of CO poisoning commonly occur during winter months and sources include smoke from fires, fumes from heating systems, burning fuels, and exhaust fumes from motor vehicles. CO combines preferentially with hemoglobin to produce carboxyhemoglobin (COHb), displacing oxygen and reducing systemic arterial oxygen (O_2) content. CO binds reversibly to hemoglobin with an affinity 200–230 times that of oxygen. Consequently, relatively minute concentrations of the gas in the environment can result in toxic concentrations in human blood. The history of exposure and carboxyhemoglobin levels should alert the physician to this diagnosis. In the absence of exposure history, CO poisoning should be considered when two or more patients are simultaneously sick with similar non-specific symptoms.

Many victims of CO poisoning die or suffer permanent, severe neurological injury despite treatment. In addition, as many as 50% of those who recover consciousness and survive may experience varying degrees of more subtle but disabling neuropsychiatric sequelae. The features of acute CO poisoning are more dramatic than those resulting from chronic exposure. At low COHb levels, chronic cardiopulmonary problems, such as angina and chronic obstructive pulmonary disease, may be exacerbated, since cardiac myoglobin binds with great affinity and rapidly reduces myocardial O_2 reserve. Chest pain due to myocardial ischemia may occur, as can cardiac arrhythmias. Subacute or chronic CO poisoning presents with less severe symptoms (e.g., nausea, vomiting, headache) and patients may initially be misdiagnosed as having other illnesses.

The clinical presentation of acute CO poisoning is variable, but in general, the severity of observed symptoms correlates roughly with the observed level of COHb. However, in terms of diagnostic value, the non-specificity of these presenting symptoms makes definitive diagnosis difficult. In addition, there have been several reports of levels near zero with patients showing neurological deficits ranging from partial paralysis to coma. With levels less than 10%, the patient is usually asymptomatic. As COHb increases above 20%, the patient may develop headache, dizziness, confusion, and nausea. Coma and seizures due to cerebral edema are common with levels greater than 40%, and death is likely above 60%. In reality, these symptom-level guidelines tend to be unreliable because of prehospital delays and early oxygen therapy and with concomitant poisoning from cyanide.

The mainstay of therapy for CO poisoning is supplemental O_2, ventilatory support, and monitoring for cardiac arrhythmias. There is general agreement that 100% oxygen should be administered prior to laboratory confirmation when CO poisoning is suspected. The goal of oxygen therapy is to improve the O_2 content of the blood by maximizing the fraction dissolved in plasma (PaO_2).Once treatment begins, O_2 therapy and observation must continue long enough to prevent delayed sequelae as carboxymyoglobin unloads. Unfortunately, there are no useful guidelines as to the length of the observation period.

The role of hyperbaric oxygen in the management of carbon monoxide poisoning is controversial, although both physiological data and some randomized trial data suggest a potential benefit. Hyperbaric-oxygen therapy elevates arterial and tissue oxygen tensions, promoting carbon monoxide elimination, and also increases adenosine triphosphate production and reduces oxidative stress and inflammation.[17] A single-center, prospective trial showed that the incidence of cognitive sequelae was lower among patients who underwent three hyperbaric-oxygen sessions (an initial session of 150 min, followed by two sessions of 120 min each, separated by an interval of 6–12 h) within 24 h after acute carbon monoxide poisoning than among patients treated with normobaric oxygen (25% vs. 46%, $p = 0.007$ and 0.03 after adjustment for cerebellar dysfunction and stratification variables). However, a Cochrane review of six trials, including two published only in abstract form, did not support the use of hyperbaric oxygen for patients with carbon monoxide poisoning.[18] The Undersea and Hyperbaric Medical Society recommends hyperbaric-oxygen therapy for patients with serious carbon monoxide poisoning – as manifested by transient or prolonged unconsciousness, abnormal neurological signs, cardiovascular dysfunction, or severe acidosis – or patients who are 36 years of age or older, were exposed for 24 h or more (including intermittent exposures), or have a carboxyhemoglobin level of 25% or more.[19]

■ REFERENCES

1. Watson WA, Litovitz TL, Klein-Schwartz W, et al. 2003 Annual report of the American Association of poison control centers toxic exposure surveillance system. *Am J Emerg Med.* 2004;22:335–404.

2. Pearce B, Grant IS. Acute liver failure following therapeutic paracetamol administration in patients with muscular dystrophies. *Anaesthesia.* 2008;63:89–91.

3. Suchin SM, Wolf DC, Lee Y, et al. Potentiation of acetaminophen hepatotoxicity by phenytoin, leading to liver transplantation. *Dig Dis Sci.* 2005;50:1836–1838.
4. Watkins PB, Kaplowitz N, Slattery JT, et al. Aminotransferase elevations in healthy adults receiving 4 grams of acetaminophen daily: a randomized controlled trial. *JAMA.* 2006;296:87–93.
5. Larson AM, Polson J, Fontana RJ, et al. Acetaminophen-induced acute liver failure: results of a United States multicenter, prospective study. *Hepatology.* 2005;42:1364–1372.
6. Kuehn BM. FDA focuses on drugs and liver damage: labeling and other changes for acetaminophen. *JAMA.* 2009;302:369–371.
7. Borman, MS. Organ-specific warnings; Internal Analgesic, Antipyretic, and Antirheumatic Drug Products for over the counter human use; Final Monograph. Available at: http://edocket.access.gpo.gov/2009/pdf/E9-9684.pdf FDA-1977-N-0013. 2009. Department of Health and Human Services, Food and Drug administration. Accessed August 26, 2009.
8. Prescott LF, Illingworth RN, Critchley JA, et al. Intravenous N-acetylcysteine: the treatment of choice for paracetamol poisoning. *Br Med J.* 1979;2:1097–1100.
9. Buckley NA, Whyte IM, O'Connell DL, et al. Oral or intravenous N-acetylcysteine: which is the treatment of choice for acetaminophen (paracetamol) poisoning? *J Toxicol Clin Toxicol.* 1999;37:759–767.
10. Brent J. Current management of ethylene glycol poisoning. *Drugs.* 2001;61:979–988.
11. Brent J, McMartin K, Phillips S, et al. Fomepizole for the treatment of ethylene glycol poisoning. *N Engl J Med.* 1999;340:832–838.
12. Marzuk PM, Tardiff K, Leon AC, et al. Fatal injuries after cocaine use as a leading cause of death among young adults in New York City. *N Engl J Med.* 1995;332:1753–1757.
13. Drug Abuse Warning Network, 2006: National Estimates of Drug-Related emergency Department Visits. Available at: https://dawninfo.samhsa.gov/files/ED2006/DAWN2k6ED.pdf. US Department of Health and Human Services. Substance Abuse and Mental Health Services Administration. Accessed August 8, 2009.
14. Shannon M. Clinical toxicity of cocaine adulterants. *Ann Emerg Med.* 1988;17:1243–1247.
15. Hollander JE, Hoffman RS, Gennis P, et al. Prospective multicenter evaluation of cocaine-associated chest pain. Cocaine Associated Chest Pain (COCHPA) Study Group. *Acad Emerg Med.* 1994;1:330–339.
16. McCord J, Jneid H, Hollander JE, et al. Management of cocaine-associated chest pain and myocardial infarction. A scientific statement from the American Heart Association acute cardiac care committee of the Council on Clinical Cardiology. *Circulation.* 2008;117:1897–1907.
17. Weaver LK. Clinical practice. Carbon monoxide poisoning. *N Engl J Med.* 2009;360:1217–1225.

18. Juurlink DN, Buckley N, Stanbrook MB, et al. Hyperbaric oxygen for carbon monoxide poisoning. Cochrane Database Syst Rev. 2005;CD002041.
19. Hyperbaric oxygen 2009; indications and results: The Hyperbaric Oxygen Therapy Committee report. Gesell, L. B. 2008. Durham, NC: Undersea and Hyperbaric Medical Society.

60

Alcohol Withdrawal Syndromes

Approximately 11–15 million people report heavy alcohol use or alcohol abuse and dependence in the United States; not surprisingly, alcohol-related medical problems are commonly encountered in critically ill and injured patients. Alcohol withdrawal syndrome (AWS) consists of symptoms and signs arising in alcohol-dependent individuals, typically within 24–48 h of consumption of their last drink. Delirium tremens (DTs), a severe and potentially fatal form of AWS, typically occurs 48–96 h after withdrawal of alcohol. AWS is usually mild and self–limiting; however, approximately 5% of patients develop DTs with a mortality approaching 15%. Older age, underlying disease, and comorbid liver disease are associated with an increased mortality risk. Although AWS occurs intentionally in those seeking abstinence, it may arise unexpectedly in an alcohol-dependent patients after admission to hospital. This disorder usually manifests itself on hospital days 3–5 and usually lasts less than 1 week although prolonged DTs has been described.

Alcohol affects many of the regulatory systems in the body including an increase in the release of endogenous opiates, activation of the γ-aminobutyric acid type A receptor (GABA-A), inhibition of the N-methyl-D-aspartate (NMDA) receptor, and interactions with both serotonin and dopamine receptors. Chronic exposure to the inhibitory GABA-A and excitatory NMDA receptors is thought to be involved in the pathogenesis of alcohol withdrawal.

The key clinical findings in AWS include the following:

- Anxiety
- Tremor
- Headache

P.E. Marik, *Handbook of Evidence-Based Critical Care*,
DOI 10.1007/978-1-4419-5923-2_60,
© Springer Science+Business Media, LLC 2010

- Disorientation
- Agitation
- Delirium
- Hallucinations
- Insomnia
- Anorexia, nausea, vomiting
- Diaphoresis
- Hyperreflexia
- Tachycardia
- Hypertension
- Seizures
- Low-grade fever
- Hyperventilation

Although AWS is usually mild and does not require treatment, if severe, it may be complicated by alcohol withdrawal seizures and delirium tremens, which is characterized by the following:

- A severe hyperadrenergic state
- Disorientation
- Impaired attention and consciousness
- Visual and auditory hallucinations

By definition, in order to make the diagnosis of AWS, the patient must have two or more of the following after cessation or reduction of alcohol use that has been heavy or prolonged:

- Autonomic hyperactivity
  - Sweating
  - Tachycardia
- Increased hand tremor
- Insomnia
- Nausea or vomiting
- Transient hallucinations or illusions
- Psychomotor agitation
- Anxiety
- Tonic–clonic seizures

AWS can be classified as follows:

- Mild – tremors and minimal sympathetic symptoms
- Moderate – hallucinations and sympathetic symptoms
- Severe – seizure activity, fever, change in mental status, and significant alteration in vital signs. Severe AWS is also known as delirium tremens (DTs).

■ THE CLINICAL INSTITUTE WITHDRAWAL ASSESSMENT SCALE FOR ALCOHOL (CIWA-AR)

The CIWA-Ar is a useful assessment tool to quantitate the severity of the AWS and to guide therapy.[1]

The elements of the CIWA-Ar include the following:

- Nausea and vomiting
- Tremor
- Paroxysmal sweats
- Anxiety
- Agitation
- Tactile disturbances
- Auditory disturbances
- Visual disturbances
- Headache/fullness in head
- Orientation and clouding of sensorium

■ DIFFERENTIAL DIAGNOSIS

In hospitalized medical and surgical patients who become confused or delirious, it is *essential* to exclude organic, pharmacological, or metabolic causes of altered mental state. This is particularly so in elderly patients who "have a few drinks at night." To complicate matters, AWS may coexist with many of these disorders.

The differential diagnosis includes but is not limited to the following:

- Hypoxia
- Sepsis
- Subdural hematoma
- Stroke
- Hypertensive encephalopathy/PRESS
- Metabolic/septic encephalopathy
- Epilepsy (alcohol reduces the seizure threshold)
- Electrolyte disturbances, particularly
  - Hyponatremia (common in chronic alcoholics)
  - Hypophosphatemia
  - Hypocalcemia
- Endocrine and metabolic disturbances
  - Hypothyroidism
  - Adrenal insufficiency
  - Uremia
  - Liver failure
  - Wernicke's syndrome (delirium, amnesia, ataxia, and ophthalmoplegia)

- Pharmacological
  - Serotonin syndrome
  - Benzodiazepine withdrawal
  - Drug-induced psychosis/drug reactions

■ TREATMENT

- Benzodiazepines form the cornerstone of therapy for AWS.[2,3] Benzodiazepines are used primarily to control agitation:
  - All the benzodiazepines have similar modes of action (bind to benzodiazepine receptors on the GABA receptor) and all are metabolized by the liver. They differ, however, in their pharmacokinetic profile and the presence of active metabolites.
  - Symptom-triggered bolus dosing of benzodiazepines as compared to a fixed-dose approach is associated with less complications and a shorter period of treatment.[4,5]
  - A continuous infusion (titrated to control agitation) should however be considered in intubated patients requiring high dosages of benzodiazepine.
  - Lorazepam is the drug of choice for the treatment of AWS in the ICU. The dosage depends on the severity of the withdrawal syndrome, some patients requiring in excess of 20 mg/h.
  - Lorazepam is the drug of choice in patients with alcohol withdrawal seizures. Lorazepam has been shown to reduce the risk of recurrent seizures.
- β-Blockers, clonidine, and haloperidol have been shown to be useful as adjunctive therapy:
  - A β-blocker (atenolol or metoprolol) and/or clonidine should be added in patients showing marked autonomic instability, i.e., tachycardia and hypertension.[6]
  - Haloperidol is the drug of choice for control of delirium and hallucinations.
- A number of case reports have described the successful use of dexmedetomidine in patients with DTs (see Chapter 9).[7,8] This drug may prove to be a very useful agent in the treatment of AWS, particularly when used as an adjunct with benzodiazepines.
- In cases of AWS refractory to standard therapy, propofol is very effective.[9] It is recommended that propofol be added to lorazepam once the dose of lorazepam exceeds 20–30 mg/h (in intubated patients).[9] Propofol's mechanism of action is thought to be similar to the action of alcohol on the central nervous system. Propofol directly activates the GABA-A receptor–chloride ionophore complex increasing chloride conductance. In addition, propofol inhibits the NMDA subtype of glutamate receptor. In addition,

propofol is associated with less cross tolerance than are benzodiazepines, is easily titratable, and has a rapid metabolic clearance.

- Phenytoin has no role in the management of withdrawal seizures. Placebo-controlled trials have demonstrated phenytoin to be ineffective in the secondary prevention of alcohol withdrawal seizures.[10,11]
- Chlorpromazine should be avoided as it is epileptogenic.
- Valproic acid and divalproex sodium (Depakote) may be a safe and efficacious alternative/adjunctive agent to benzodiazepines for the treatment of AWS.

Other Treatment Considerations

- Hypomagnesemia, hypokalemia, and hypophosphatemia are particularly common in chronic alcoholic patients; these electrolyte disorders may become life threatening after the initiation of nutrition (refeeding syndrome). These electrolytes should be routinely supplemented and closely monitored.
- Alcoholic ketoacidosis may be seen in malnourished, non-diabetic alcoholic patients. Restoration of normal fluid balance with glucose-containing saline solution (with added thiamine) usually reverses this syndrome.
- Hypoglycemia may occur in the withdrawing alcoholic, since malnutrition and liver disease impair the storage of glycogen. This mandates monitoring the serum glucose in the withdrawing alcoholic.
- Patients who abuse alcohol are at risk of developing acute pancreatitis, erosive gastritis, and acute alcoholic hepatitis. Hence, a serum amylase/lipase and liver function tests should be performed in all acutely ill alcoholic patients.
- Due to the increase in sympathetic activity, patients with coronary artery disease are at an increased risk of myocardial ischemia.

Prevention of Postoperative DTs

- The best way to prevent postoperative AWS and its complications is to screen for high-risk patients preoperatively.
- A scheduled low-dose benzodiazepine regimen supplemented by symptom-triggered dosing is recommended in high-risk patients.
- Intravenous ethanol has no role in the prevention of AWS.[12]

■ CLINICAL PEARLS

- Lorazepam is the drug of choice for AWS in the ICU.
- Symptom-triggered dosing of benzodiazepines is recommended.

- β-Blockers should be considered in patients with excessive tachycardia.
- Haloperidol is the drug of choice for delirium.
- Dexmedetomidine may be a useful adjunctive agent in patients with severe AWS.

■ REFERENCES

1. Sullivan JT, Sykora K, Schneiderman J, et al. Assessment of alcohol withdrawal: the revised clinical institute withdrawal assessment for alcohol scale (CIWA-Ar). *Br J Addict.* 1989;84:1353–1357.
2. Ntais C, Pakos E, Kyzas P, et al. Benzodiazepines for alcohol withdrawal. *Cochrane Database Syst Rev.* 2005;CD005063.
3. Mayo-Smith MF. Pharmacological management of alcohol withdrawal. A meta-analysis and evidence-based practice guideline. American Society of Addiction Medicine Working Group on Pharmacological Management of Alcohol Withdrawal. *JAMA.* 1997;278:144–151.
4. Esteban A, Frutos F, Tobin MJ, et al. A comparison of four methods of weaning patients from mechanical ventilation. Spanish lung failure collaborative group. *N Engl J Med.* 1995;332:345–350.
5. Spies CD, Otter HE, Huske B, et al. Alcohol withdrawal severity is decreased by symptom-orientated adjusted bolus therapy in the ICU. *Intensive Care Med.* 2003;29:2230–2238.
6. Kraus ML, Gottlieb LD, Horwitz RI, et al. Randomized clinical trial of atenolol in patients with alcohol withdrawal. *N Engl J Med.* 1985;313:905–909.
7. Baddigam K, Russo P, Russo J, et al. Dexmedetomidine in the treatment of withdrawal syndromes in cardiothoracic surgery patients. *J Intensive Care Med.* 2005; 20:118–123.
8. Darrouj J, Puri N, Prince E, et al. Dexmedetomidine infusion as adjunctive therapy to benzodiazepines for acute alcohol withdrawal. *Ann Pharmacother.* 2008;42:1703–1705.
9. McCowan C, Marik P. Refractory delirium tremens treated with propofol: a case series. *Crit Care Med.* 2000;28:1781–1784.
10. Hillbom M, Pieninkeroinen I, Leone M. Seizures in alcohol-dependent patients: epidemiology, pathophysiology and management. *CNS Drugs.* 2003;17:1013–1030.
11. Polycarpou A, Papanikolaou P, Ioannidis JP, et al. Anticonvulsants for alcohol withdrawal. *Cochrane Database Syst Rev.* 2005;CD005064.
12. Weinberg JA, Magnotti LJ, Fischer PE, et al. Comparison of intravenous ethanol versus diazepam for alcohol withdrawal prophylaxis in the trauma ICU: results of a randomized trial. *J Trauma.* 2008;64:99–104.

61

Serotonin Syndrome

Serotonin syndrome is characterized by the triad of neuromuscular hyperactivity, autonomic hyperactivity, and change in mental status.[1,2] It is not an idiosyncratic drug reaction but is a predictable response to serotonin excess in the central nervous system (CNS). It can occur from an overdose, a drug interaction, or an adverse drug effect involving serotonergic agents. Most severe cases result from a drug combination, especially the combination of selective serotonin reuptake inhibitors (SSRIs) and monoamine oxidase inhibitors (MAOIs). It occurs in approximately 15% of patients with SSRI overdose. The death of an 18-year-old patient named Libby Zion in New York City more than 20 years ago, which resulted from the coadministration of meperidine and phenelzine, remains the most widely recognized and dramatic example of this preventable condition.[3]

Serotonin syndrome may result from a large number of drugs and drug combinations:

- Selective serotonin reuptake inhibitors
  - Fluoxetine, paroxetine, sertraline, citalopram, and escitalopram
- Anti-depressants
  - Venlafaxine, trazodone, nefazodone, clomipramine, and St. John's wort
- Monoamine oxidase inhibitors
  - Phenelzine, moclobemide, tranylcypromine, clorgyline, and isocarboxazid
- Antibiotics
  - Linezolid (a monoamine oxidase inhibitor) and ritonavir (acts through inhibition of cytochrome P450 $3A_4$)

P.E. Marik, *Handbook of Evidence-Based Critical Care*,
DOI 10.1007/978-1-4419-5923-2_61,
© Springer Science+Business Media, LLC 2010

- Serotonin-releasing agents
  - Fenfluramine, methylenedioxymethamphetamine (MDMA or ecstasy), and amphetamine
- Analgesics
  - Meperidine, fentanyl, and tramadol
- Anti-emetics
  - Ondansetron, granisetron, and metoclopramide
- Others
  - Lithium, tryptophan, and sumatriptan

■ PATHOPHYSIOLOGY

Serotonin (5-hydroxytryptamine or 5-HT) is produced by decarboxylation and hydroxylation of L-tryptophan[1,2]. Serotonin syndrome results from an excess of serotonin in the central nervous system that may result from the following:

- Inhibition of serotonin metabolism (MAOI)
- Inhibition of serotonin reuptake in nerve terminals (SSRI)
- Increase in serotonin precursor (tryptophan) or serotonin release (serotonin-releasing agents)

The excess serotonin in the CNS stimulates the serotonin receptors found primarily in midline raphe nuclei, located in the brain stem. There are seven subtypes of serotonin receptors ($5\text{-}HT_1$ to $5\text{-}HT_7$); the $5\text{-}HT_{2A}$ receptors are mostly involved in the pathophysiology of serotonin toxicity.

■ DIAGNOSIS

A history of exposure to drugs known to cause the serotonin syndrome is key to considering the diagnosis, together with the clinical triad of neuromuscular hyperactivity, autonomic hyperactivity, and change in mental status:

- Neuromuscular hyperactivity
  - Shivering, tremor, hypertonia, and rigidity
- Autonomic hyperactivity
  - Hyperthermia, flushing, diaphoresis, and diarrhea
- Mental status changes
  - Confusion, anxiety, agitation, and hypomania

There are two recognized sets of criteria that are used to confirm the diagnosis of serotonin syndrome.

Sternbach's Criteria

- Recent addition or increase in a known serotonergic agent[4]
- Absence of other possible etiologies (infection, substance abuse, or drug withdrawal)
- No recent addition or increase of a neuroleptic agent
- At least three of the following symptoms
  - Mental status changes (confusion and hypomania)
  - Agitation
  - Myoclonus
  - Hyperreflexia
  - Diaphoresis
  - Shivering
  - Tremor
  - Diarrhea
  - Incoordination
  - Fever

Hunter Serotonin Toxicity Criteria

- A history of exposure to serotonergic agents and the presence of any one of the following is diagnostic of serotonin toxicity[5]:
  - Spontaneous clonus
  - Inducible clonus or ocular clonus with agitation or diaphoresis
  - Tremor and hyperreflexia
  - Hypertonia and hyperthermia (temperature >38°C) with inducible clonus or ocular clonus

Most of the laboratory abnormalities are a consequence of poorly treated hyperthermia:

- Elevated serum creatinine and aminotransferase
- Metabolic acidosis
- Elevated serum creatinine kinase

■ DIFFERENTIAL DIAGNOSIS

- Malignant hyperthermia
  - Inhalation anesthesia

- Neuroleptic malignant syndrome
  - Dopamine antagonist
- Anti-cholinergic delirium
- Heat stroke
- CNS infection (meningitis/encephalitis)
- Sympathomimetic toxicity
- Acute baclofen withdrawal

■ CLINICAL PRESENTATION

Serotonin toxicity can classified as follows:

- Mild
  - Serotonergic symptoms that may or may not concern the patient
- Moderate
  - Toxicity causing significant distress but not life threatening
- Severe
  - Life-threatening toxicity causing severe hyperthermia, muscle rigidity, and multi-organ failure

Hyperthermia develops in approximately half of cases and results from increased muscle activity due to agitation and tremor. A core temperature as high as 40°C is common in moderate-to-severe cases. Tachycardia, hypertension, mydriasis, hyperactive bowel sounds, myoclonus, and ocular clonus are common; however, not all of these symptoms are present in every patient.

Hyperreflexia, clonus, and hypertonicity are greater in lower extremities than in upper extremities. Sustained clonus is usually found at the ankles.

■ TREATMENT

- The most important step is the removal of the offending drug.
- Mild cases (e.g., tremors and hyperreflexia) are managed with supportive care and treatment with benzodiazepines. Control of agitation with benzodiazepine is an essential step in the management.
- 5-HT$_{2A}$ antagonists (cyproheptadine and chlorpromazine) have been used in moderate-to-severe cases. There are no randomized clinical trials demonstrating the effectiveness of 5-HT$_{2A}$ antagonists:
  - Cyproheptadine is available only in oral form; the initial dose is 12 mg followed by 2 mg every 2 h until symptoms improve, and patients may require up to 12–32 mg of the drug in 24-h period.

- Sublingual olanzapine (an atypical anti-psychotic drug with 5-HT$_{2A}$ antagonist activity) has also been used.
- Chlorpromazine is the only 5-HT$_{2A}$ antagonist available in parenteral form; 50–100 mg of intramuscular chlorpromazine may be administered.

Supportive Care

- Focus on stabilization of airway, breathing, and circulation.
- Supportive care includes passive and active cooling of the patient, sedation, and intubation.
- Physical restraints are discouraged because they can increase hyperthermia, rhabdomyolysis, and lactic acidosis.
- Aggressive volume resuscitation is required because patients have volume loss due to hyperthermia.

Patients should be aware about the possibility of recurrence of the symptoms, especially after re-exposure to serotonergic drugs.

Complications

- Rhabdomyolysis
- Renal failure
- Venous thromboembolism
- Decubitus ulcers
- Disseminated intravascular coagulation
- Seizures

■ REFERENCES

1. Boyer EW, Shannon M. The serotonin syndrome. *N Engl J Med.* 2005;352:1112–1120.
2. Isbister GK, Buckley NA, Whyte IM. Serotonin toxicity: a practical approach to diagnosis and treatment. *Med J Aust.* 2007;187:361–365.
3. Asch DA, Parker RM. The Libby Zion case. One step forward or two steps backward? *N Engl J Med.* 1988;318:771–775.
4. Sternbach H. The serotonin syndrome. *Am J Psychiatry.* 1991;148: 705–713.
5. Dunkley EJ, Isbister GK, Sibbritt D, et al. The hunter serotonin toxicity criteria: simple and accurate diagnostic decision rules for serotonin toxicity. *QJM.* 2003;96:635–642.

62

Radiology

■ THE CHEST RADIOGRAPH

Interpretation of the bedside (anteroposterior, supine) chest radiograph (CXR) is fraught with numerous pitfalls. These include the following:

- On the AP view, the heart and the mediastinum appear about 15% wider than are on an upright PA chest radiograph (false impression of cardiomegaly and mediastinal widening).
- Portable chest radiographs may be difficult to interpret due to poor positioning.
- Pleural effusions and pneumothoraces are frequently "missed" because the patient is in the supine position.
- The pulmonary vasculature is distorted on supine radiographs because blood no longer flows preferentially to the lower lobes.
- Because lateral chest films cannot be obtained, abnormalities in the posterior costophrenic angles (retrocardiac), within the mediastinum and adjacent to the spine, can easily be missed.

It should be appreciated that the CXR is a two-dimensional image of a complex three-dimensional structure and that even on the "best" bedside CXR, significant pulmonary pathology may be missed, e.g., pneumothorax, airspace consolidation, abscesses, and interstitial lung disease.[1] The "astute" clinician should therefore have a low threshold for performing a chest CT scan; however, the risks of moving a patient to the radiology suite must be weighed against the possible benefits (see Chapter 66). CT scanning performed in the ICU must be in our future.[2]

Despite these limitations, a careful review of the bedside AP CXR is an invaluable tool in the management of patients with respiratory failure. In previous years, the standard practice was to obtain daily CXRs in

P.E. Marik, *Handbook of Evidence-Based Critical Care*,
DOI 10.1007/978-1-4419-5923-2_62,
© Springer Science+Business Media, LLC 2010

all ICU patients. Recently, however, a number of well-conducted studies indicate that this is not a cost-effective practice and that CXRs should be performed only on "demand," i.e., as clinical circumstances dictate.[3,4] These studies have demonstrated that it is rare that such an approach leads to findings that would have been missed had daily CXR been performed. However, all patients require a CXR on admission to the ICU, after endotracheal intubation and after insertion of a subclavian or an internal jugular central venous catheter.

The chest radiograph should be studied systematically; first, the position of all the tubes and catheters should be evaluated, followed by an evaluation of the lung parenchyma, the pleura, the mediastinum, and the diaphragm followed by a search for signs of extraalveolar air.

Position of Tubes and Catheters

- *Endotracheal tube.* With the head in a neutral position the tip of the tube should be 4–6 cm from the carina. It should be noted that with movement of the head, from a flexed to an extended position, the tube can move by as much as 4 cm. A useful landmark for the tip of the ET tube is the superior border of the aortic notch (Marik's sign) or the upper border of T4 (see Figure 62-1):
  - The aortic arch is the "center of an imaginary sphere"; so even if the CXR is rotated, Marik's sign can still be used to determine the position of the ET tube.
- *Central venous catheters.* The tip of the catheter should be located beyond the venous valves of the subclavian or the internal jugular vein but proximal to the right atrium (i.e., above the superior vena cava–right atrial junction). Placement in the right atrium may result in atrial perforation. Two useful radiographic landmarks for the position of the tip of the catheter are as follows(see Figure 62-1):
  - The first costochondral junction.
  - A point 2 cm inferior to a line joining inferior margins of the clavicular heads.
- The position of other tubes and catheters, such as the nasogastric tube, the feeding tube, chest tubes, the intra-aortic balloon catheter, and pacing wires, should be noted.

Lung Parenchyma, Pleura, and Mediastinum

The presence of pulmonary infiltrates should be noted. It should be noted whether the infiltrate is interstitial or alveolar (or both), unilateral or bilateral, and patchy or diffuse. An infiltrate may be caused by water (cardiogenic or non-cardiogenic pulmonary edema), cells (infection), and/or

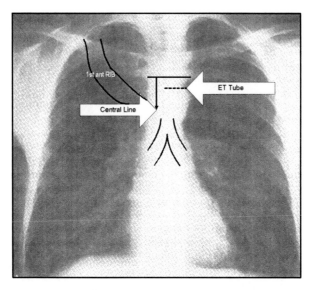

Figure 62-1. Idealized CXR demonstrating the position of the central line and the endotracheal tube.

blood (pulmonary hematoma, intra-alveolar bleed). It should be appreciated that it may not be possible to distinguish between these entities by examination of the chest film alone. The following radiographic findings may help distinguish cardiac and non-cardiac pulmonary edema:

- Non-cardiac pulmonary edema (acute lung injury)
  - Normal heart shape
  - Absence of septal lines
  - No peribronchial cuffing
  - Frequent air bronchograms
  - Patchy increased lung density
  - Peripheral increased lung density
- Cardiogenic pulmonary edema
  - Base-to-apex blood flow inversion
  - Even distribution of increased lung density
  - Septal lines
  - Peribronchial cuffing

In the supine position, fluid tracks posteriorly, resulting in a diffuse haziness of the lung fields. It is therefore very easy to miss a significant pleural collection. Fluid collections can be confirmed by ultrasonography.

The width of the mediastinum (normal; <10 cm) as well as the presence of mediastinal nodes or masses should be noted.

The traditional apicolateral collection of air may not be present on portable supine films of patients with pneumothoraces. Free air will often be located in the anterior costophrenic sulcus as this is the most superior portion of the pleural space in the supine patient. Other radiographic signs of a pneumothorax in the supine position include a relative hyperlucency over the upper abdominal quadrants and a deep costophrenic angle (the deep sulcus sign).

The portable chest radiograph is not ideal for evaluating the hilum and the lung parenchyma. Conventional and high-resolution computed tomography (HRCT) may be useful for the evaluation of aortic dissection, pleural disease, the lung parenchyma (especially in immunocompromised patients with pulmonary infiltrates), characterization of diffuse infiltrative pulmonary disease, and evaluation of suspected masses in the mediastinum or the hilum. Routine CT evaluation of the chest can be done with or without intravenous administration of contrast media. Contrast is reserved for those cases in which mediastinal or hilar pathology is suspected.

HRCT differs from conventional CT not only in the use of a thinner X-ray beam (e.g., 1.5 mm vs. 1 cm) but also in the use of digitized X-ray construction which allows for better spatial resolution and for more detailed images of the lung parenchyma. HRCT is therefore useful in the evaluation of patients with diffuse infiltrative lung diseases. Spiral CT differs from conventional CT primarily in that it allows continuous scanning of the patients. In spiral CT, the X-ray tube makes continuous 360° revolutions without interruption. The patient is moved through the circulating beam at a predetermined speed, and imaging information is then obtained as a solid cylinder, instead of one slice at a time. Spiral CT is most helpful in evaluating lesions at or near the diaphragm (less motion artifact), vascular structures (main pulmonary arteries in suspected pulmonary embolism), and small pulmonary nodules.

■ PLAIN ABDOMINAL RADIOGRAPHY

Plain abdominal radiographs are commonly requested for patients with non-specific abdominal symptoms and signs, yet this test has limited diagnostic and clinical utility.[5,6] This is particularly true in ICU patients in whom plain abdominal radiographs rarely impact management decisions. This diagnostic test should therefore be obtained only in specific clinical circumstances. The most useful diagnostic findings include free air under the diaphragm (indicative of bowel perforation) and features suggestive of bowel obstruction such as dilated loops of bowel, lack of rectal gas, and fecal impaction. Plain films may also be useful in the evaluation of suspected bowel ischemia because certain findings (e.g., pneumatosis intestinalis and portal venous gas) are pathognomonic for this condition. In addition, plain abdominal films (or a half/half film) are required to confirm the position of NG and feeding tubes. Beyond these clinical indications, plain abdominal radiographs have limited diagnostic utility. Andrews and colleagues[7] evaluated the role of plain abdominal films in patients admitted to the ICU with GI bleeding. In this study, abdominal radiography failed to reveal a single abnormality that changed management or outcome. It has been suggested that a normal or a negative study is implicitly valuable because of the reassurance provided to the requesting physician. However, the sensitivity of this test is too low to exclude significant abdominal pathology with any degree of certainty and "abnormal" findings lack diagnostic specificity.

■ COMPUTED TOMOGRAPHY (CT)

While portable computed tomographic (CT) scanners are becoming available,[2,8] in most hospitals, ICU patients are transported to the radiology department. Transporting patients out of the ICU carriers a risk of serious physiological changes and life-threatening complications (see Chapter 66). Therefore, only those patients whose treatment is likely to be changed should undergo CT scanning. With advances in portable CT technology, it is likely that portable scanners will become ubiquitous. Additional concerns with CT scanning include radiocontrast agent-induced renal dysfunction (see Chapter 44), allergic reactions, and radiation exposure (especially with repeated tests).

Ahvenjarvi et al.[9] evaluated the role of abdominal and thoracic CT scanning in 64 ICU patients who underwent 82 CT examinations. Seventy-one percent of the examinations (58/82) were made to identify a possible focus of infection. Fifty of the 82 (61%) examinations resulted in a new treatment intervention directly or after additional examinations. Similarly, Barkhausen and colleagues[10] demonstrated the utility of thoracic and abdominal CT scans in the evaluation of patients with fever or sepsis without a known source. In this study, a septic focus was detected by CT in 19% of the patients, which directly altered patient management with changes in the antibiotic regimen, percutaneous drainage, and/or surgery. These studies demonstrate the utility of "body CT scanning" in patients with sepsis and an unclear focus of infection. In addition, CT scans have specific indications in patients with suspected pulmonary embolism, pulmonary infiltrates of unclear cause, suspected sinusitis, as well as patients with severe pancreatitis, mesenteric ischemia, and colitis, to name but a few.

Neurological dysfunction is common in patients admitted to the ICU. Clinically these patients present with a spectrum of neurological findings including depressed consciousness, delirium, seizures as well as focal neurological signs. The use of sedative drugs (especially benzodiazepines and opiates), the systemic inflammatory response as well as metabolic and endocrine disturbances may lead to reversible neurological syndromes (depressed consciousness, confusion, and delirium). However, due to hemodynamic instability and coagulation abnormities, this group of patients is at high risk for cerebrovascular accidents which have important therapeutic and prognostic implications. Salerno et al. reviewed the utility of head CT scans performed in 123 MICU patients.[11] A new finding was present in 26 (21.1%) patients. In the patients with a new CT finding, there was a change in diagnosis in 11 patients and a change in treatment in 6 patients. The presence of an acute brain abnormality detected by head CT scanning could not be reliably predicted by patient characteristics or other clinical variables. Rafanan and colleagues[12] reviewed the medical records of 230 MICU patients who underwent head CT scanning. These authors reported that 31% of their patients had new findings on their CT scans, with ischemic stokes (49%) being the commonest lesion. While a focal neurological deficit was more common in the patients with a positive scan, the patients' clinical characteristics were poorly predictive of new CT findings. These studies suggest that all patients with unexplained acute neurological findings should undergo CT scanning. Head imaging is not usually considered in the diagnostic workup of ICU patients who develop confusion/delirium (see Chapter 47).[13–15] However, it is likely that with widespread head CT scanning, many of these patients may be determined to have ischemic strokes. The identification of new findings on head imaging has important prognostic and therapeutic implications.

■ REFERENCES

1. Romano L, Pinto A, Merola S, et al. Intensive-care unit lung infections: the role of imaging with special emphasis on multi-detector row computed tomography. *Eur J Radiol.* 2008;65:333–339.
2. Masaryk T, Kolonick R, Painter T, et al. The economic and clinical benefits of portable head/neck CT imaging in the intensive care unit. *Radiol Manage.* 2008;30:50–54.
3. Clec'h C, Simon P, Hamdi A, et al. Are daily routine chest radiographs useful in critically ill, mechanically ventilated patients? A randomized study. *Intensive Care Med.* 2008;34:262–270.
4. Graat ME, Kroner A, Spronk PE, et al. Examination of daily routine chest radiographs in a mixed medical–surgical intensive care unit. *Intensive Care Med.* 2007;33:639–644.

5. Feyler S, Williamson V, King D. Plain abdominal radiographs in acute medical emergencies: an abused investigation? *Postgrad Med J.* 2002;78:94–96.
6. Flak B, Rowley VA. Acute abdomen: plain film utilization and analysis. *Can Assoc Radiol J.* 1993;44:423–428.
7. Andrews AH, Lake JM, Shorr AF. Ineffectiveness of routine abdominal radiography in patients with gastrointestinal hemorrhage admitted to an intensive care unit. *J Clin Gastroenterol.* 2005;39:228–231.
8. Gunnarsson T, Theodorsson A, Karlsson P, et al. Mobile computerized tomography scanning in the neurosurgery intensive care unit: increase in patient safety and reduction of staff workload. *J Neurosurg.* 2000;93:432–436.
9. Ahvenjarvi LK, Laurila JJ, Jartti A, et al. Multi-detector computed tomography in critically ill patients. *Acta Anaesthesiol Scand.* 2008;52:547–552.
10. Barkhausen J, Stoblen F, Dominguez-Fernandez E, et al. Impact of CT in patients with sepsis of unknown origin. *Acta Radiologica.* 1999;40:552–555.
11. Salerno D, Marik PE, Daskalakis C, et al. The role of head computer tomographic scans on the management of MICU patients with neurological dysfunction. *J Intensive Care Med.* 2009;24:372–375.
12. Rafanan AL, Kakulavar P, Perl J, et al. Head computed tomography in medical intensive care unit patients: clinical indications. *Crit Care Med.* 2000;28:1306–1309.
13. Ely EW, Shintani A, Truman B, et al. Delirium as a predictor of mortality in mechanically ventilated patients in the intensive care unit. *JAMA.* 2004;291:1753–1762.
14. Girard TD, Pandharipande PP, Ely EW. Delirium in the intensive care unit. *Crit Care.* 2008;12(Suppl 3):S3.
15. Devlin JW, Fong JJ, Fraser GL, et al. Delirium assessment in the critically ill. *Intensive Care Med.* 2007;33:929–940.

63

PRES

Posterior reversible encephalopathy syndrome (PRES), first described by Hinchey and colleagues in 1996, is a *clinico-neuro-radiological entity* characterized by headache, vomiting, altered mental status, blurred vision, and seizures with neuroimaging studies, demonstrating white–gray matter edema involving predominantly the posterior region of the brain.[1] PRES is most commonly associated with pre-eclampsia, hypertensive encephalopathy, and immunosuppressive/cytotoxic drugs.[2–4] One of the distinctive characteristics of PRES is the reversibility of the clinical and radiological abnormalities once treatment is instituted. Most patients usually make a complete recovery within few weeks. A delay in the recognition and treatment of the syndrome may result in permanent neurological sequela.

■ ETIOLOGY AND PATHOGENESIS

Hypertension, Hypertensive Crises, and Their Role in PRES

The exact pathogenesis of PRES remains incompletely understood but is probably related to the failure of cerebral autoregulation and endothelial damage. The favored pathogenetic theory suggests autoregulatory disturbance with hyperperfusion, resulting in blood–brain barrier breakdown with reversible edema, without infarction.[2] In particular, in conditions accompanied by high blood pressure (e.g., hypertensive encephalopathy), it has been suggested that the increased systemic pressure exceeds the autoregulatory mechanisms of the cerebral vasculature, sufficient to overcome the blood–brain barrier, hence allowing extravasation of fluid and blood into the brain parenchyma. It is not well known why the posterior circulation is preferentially affected. A possible explanation is the

P.E. Marik, *Handbook of Evidence-Based Critical Care*,
DOI 10.1007/978-1-4419-5923-2_63,
© Springer Science+Business Media, LLC 2010

lower sympathetic innervation of posterior cerebral arterial circulation than in the internal carotid artery territory, with a consequent reduced autoregulation of already impaired cerebral areas. Not all patients who develop PRES are hypertensive, suggesting that endothelial damage may play a role in the pathogenesis of this disorder.[5] Best studied in pre-eclampsia/eclampsia, laboratory evidence of endothelial injury is often present with platelet consumption (thrombocytopenia) and evidence of red cell fragmentation [schistocyte formation and increase in lactate dehydrogenase (LDH)].

Pregnancy-Induced PRES

Pre-eclampsia is the commonest cause of PRES. Patients may present with PRES postpartum without the classic pre-eclamptic signs.[2,6] Furthermore, status epilepticus has been reported to occur in these patients.

Drugs Associated with PRES

A number of drugs have been implicated in the causation of PRES, including the following:[2]

- Cyclosporin
- Tacrolimus
- Sirolimus
- Oxaliplatin
- Bevacizumab (a recombinant humanized monoclonal antibody)
- Sunitinib (a tyrosine kinase inhibitor)
- Gemcitabine (a pyrimidine nucleoside analogue)

Miscellaneous Conditions Associated with PRES

- Sepsis and septic shock[5]
- Porphyria[7]
- Liver failure (chronic)[8]
- SLE[9]
- Thrombotic thrombocytopenic purpura/hemolytic uremic syndrome
- Acute renal failure
- High-dose corticosteroids
- Bone marrow transplant

■ CLINICAL FEATURES

The clinical spectrum of PRES includes the following:

- Headache
- Altered level of consciousness
  - Lethargy
  - Stupor
  - Somnolence
  - Coma
- Visual disturbances
  - Blurred vision
  - Cortical blindness
  - Visual field defects
- Seizures and status epilepticus
- Hemiparesis, dystonia, etc. (rare)

■ DIAGNOSTIC STUDIES

Cerebrospinal Fluid (CSF) Analysis

Invasive diagnostic methods such as lumbar puncture (LP) to evaluate CSF are not needed; however, in the setting of SLE or acquired immunodeficiency syndrome in which other causes of the neurological picture have to be ruled out, the CSF analysis serves as an important differential diagnostic tool.

Imaging Studies

Computed tomography (CT) scan findings are negative in almost all cases of PRES and when positive, it is difficult to distinguish between PRES and acute stroke. Therefore, the image study of choice is magnetic resonance imaging (MRI).[3,10,11]

The most common MRI findings are those of bilateral edema in the white matter of posterior portions of the brain, particularly occipital and parietal areas. Other area may also be involved including the postfrontal cortical, the subcortical white matter, the cortex, the brainstem, the basal ganglia, and the cerebellum. Covarrubias et al.[12] reported that the occipitoparietal areas were involved in 100% of the cases with involvement of anterior structures (i.e., temporal and frontal lobes) in more than 80% of cases.

■ MANAGEMENT

It is important to treat patients with PRES as soon as the condition is
recognized to avoid the risk of irreversible brain injury. The treatment of
PRES includes the following:

- Removal/significant reduction in the causative factors/medications.
- Maintenance of hydration (intravenous crystalloid fluids), adequate
  arterial oxygenation, and correction of electrolyte disturbances.
- Monitoring of airways and ventilation.
- Delivery or cesarean section in pregnant women.
- Lowering of blood pressure:
  - MAP of 105–125 mmHg, with not more than 10–15% reduction
    within the first hour (see Chapter 25).
- Treatment of status epilepticus:
  - Lorazepam 0.1 mg/kg over 2–5 min (see Chapter 48).
  - Pregnant women: magnesium sulfate (see Chapter 54).
  - Refractory status epilepticus: propofol or midazolam.
  - Continuous electroencephalographic monitoring.
- Nitroglycerin should be *avoided*; it has been reported to aggra-
  vate edema in these patients, probably by further enhancing brain
  vasodilatation.[13]

■ REFERENCES

1. Hinchey J, Chaves C, Appignani B, et al. A reversible posterior leukoencephalopathy syndrome. *N Engl J Med.* 1996;334:494–500.
2. Servillo G, Bifulco F, De Robertis E, et al. Posterior reversible
   encephalopathy syndrome in intensive care medicine. *Intensive Care
   Med.* 2007;33:230–236.
3. Bartynski WS. Posterior reversible encephalopathy syndrome, part 1:
   fundamental imaging and clinical features. *AJNR.* 2008;29:1036–1042.
4. Gocmen R, Ozgen B, Oguz KK. Widening the spectrum of PRES: series
   from a tertiary care center. *Eur J Radiol.* 2007;62:454–459.
5. Bartynski WS, Boardman JF, Zeigler ZR, et al. Posterior reversible
   encephalopathy syndrome in infection, sepsis, and shock. *AJNR.*
   2006;27:2179–2190.
6. Servillo G, Striano P, Striano S, et al. Posterior reversible encephalopathy
   syndrome (PRES) in critically ill obstetric patients. *Intensive Care Med.*
   2003;29:2323–2326.
7. Celik M, Forta H, Dalkilic T, et al. MRI reveals reversible lesions resembling posterior reversible encephalopathy in porphyria. *Neuroradiology.*
   2002;44:839–841.

8. Chawla R, Smith D, Marik PE. Near fatal posterior reversible encephalopathy syndrome complicating chronic liver failure treated by induced hypothermia and dialysis: a case report. *J Med Case Rep.* 2009;3:6623.
9. Baizabal-Carvallo JF, Barragan-Campos HM, Padilla-Aranda HJ, et al. Posterior reversible encephalopathy syndrome as a complication of acute lupus activity. *Clin Neurol Neurosurg.* 2009;111:359–363.
10. McKinney AM, Short J, Truwit CL, et al. Posterior reversible encephalopathy syndrome: incidence of atypical regions of involvement and imaging findings. *AJR.* 2007;189:904–912.
11. Casey SO, Sampaio RC, Michel E, et al. Posterior reversible encephalopathy syndrome: utility of fluid-attenuated inversion recovery MR imaging in the detection of cortical and subcortical lesions. *AJNR Am J Neuroradiol.* 2000;21:1199–1206.
12. Covarrubias DJ, Luetmer PH, Campeau NG. Posterior reversible encephalopathy syndrome: prognostic utility of quantitative diffusion-weighted MR images. *AJNR.* 2002;23:1038–1048.
13. Finsterer J, Schlager T, Kopsa W, et al. Nitroglycerin-aggravated pre-eclamptic posterior reversible encephalopathy syndrome (PRES). *Neurology.* 2003;61:715–716.

64

End-of-Life Issues

The prime goal of the intensive care unit is to provide temporary physiological support for patients with potentially reversible organ failure and to prevent additional complications while allowing their acute illness to resolve enabling them to return to their previous level of functioning. The care provided in an ICU may, however, be detrimental to patients by providing overly aggressive treatments which may result in increased pain and complications. Ideally, patients should be admitted to an ICU if they are likely to benefit from admission with a decreased risk of death. However, with increasing frequency, patients with end-stage and terminal illnesses are being admitted to the ICU. Angus et al.[1] have demonstrated that 60% of all hospital deaths in the United States occur after admission to the ICU, with patients spending on average 8 days in the ICU before their death. Rady and Johnson[2] reviewed all hospital deaths over a 2-year period at a teaching hospital in Phoenix, AZ. Of the 252 patients who died in hospital, 196 (78%) were treated and subsequently 165 (65%) died in the ICU.

Admission of a dying patient with irreversible disease to the ICU serves only to transform death into a prolonged and painful experience. It should be appreciated that death is the only certainty of life and that the ICU is not a halfway station between life on earth and the hereafter. The function of the ICU should not be to prolong death. In terminal or incurable illnesses, our aim should not be to preserve biological life but to make the life that remains as comfortable and as meaningful as possible. The culture of our current health-care system is highly invested in "aggressive" treatment of terminal disease with the notion that death represents medical failure. However, public interest in decisions regarding the use of medical technologies and pain control near the end of life is strong and growing. In addition, policy statements of national organizations recognize the right of competent patients to forgo treatment,

P.E. Marik, *Handbook of Evidence-Based Critical Care*,
DOI 10.1007/978-1-4419-5923-2_64,
© Springer Science+Business Media, LLC 2010

even if refusal may lead to death.[3-5] Withholding and withdrawing life-supportive measures, a practice which was once considered controversial, is now widely accepted. As a general principle, when the goals of cure cannot be achieved with aggressive life-sustaining treatments such as mechanical ventilation, it is appropriate to withdraw these treatments and to allow death to occur.[4-7]

Because most critically ill patients are unable to participate in end-of-life treatment decisions, family members are generally asked to speak for the patients and to varying degrees to participle in decision making. Yet shared decision making about end-of-life treatment choices is often incomplete, with families having a poor understanding of the ultimate decisions that are made.[8] Patients and relatives faced with end-of-life issues identify poor communication with the treating physicians as the greatest source of frustration and anxiety.[9,10] Azoulay and colleagues[11] interviewed family members of ICU patients after meeting with a treating physician. In 54% of cases the family representative failed to understand the diagnosis, prognosis, or treatment plan of the patient.

■ PALLIATIVE CARE

Palliative care originated as end-of-life care in the 1960s. Since then the scope of practice of palliative care has expanded far beyond its roots. The goal of palliative care is to maintain and improve the quality of life of all patients and their families during any stage of illness, whether acute, chronic, or terminal.[5]

According to the World Health Organization (WHO), palliative care aims to prevent and relieve suffering by early identification, assessment, and treatment of pain and other types of physical, psychological, emotional, and spiritual distress.[12] Ideally, all patients should receive palliative care concurrently, the elements and intensity of which are individualized to meet the patient's and family's needs and preferences.

The primary goal of palliative care is to achieve the best possible quality of life for patients as long as they are alive and to support the patient's family while the patient is alive and after death. Clearly, palliative care should be available near the end of life. However, it should also be available at any point during the course of a progressive or chronic disease or critical illness when the patient becomes symptomatic. An important concept is that, in general, palliative care should be available when curative/restorative care begins, while curative/restorative care continues, after life-prolonging treatments are withheld or withdrawn, and, for the patient's family, after the patient's death.

"Principles" of Palliative Care

- Palliative care is foremost centered on the patient and the patient's family (with the patient defining his/her family constellation).[5] It recognizes the right of competent adult patients to determine their goals of care both before and after they face disabling symptoms and approach their end of life.
- Palliative care includes identification of, and respect for, the preferences of patients and families. This should be done through careful assessment of their values, goals, and priorities, as well as their cultural context and spiritual needs.
- Palliative care encourages and supports family involvement in planning and providing care to the extent desired by the patient.
- Palliative care should begin at ICU admission and then be adjusted, analogous to curative/restorative care, to meet the needs of the patient and the family in accordance with their preferences.
- All patients with symptomatic or life-threatening diseases, particularly those with chronic or advanced diseases or critical illnesses, regardless of age or social circumstances, should have access to palliative care.
- Health-care providers should strive to develop a comprehensive, interdisciplinary approach that provides palliative care sensitive to the patient's and family's needs and respectful of their cultural and spiritual values.
- Bereavement care for families is an integral part of palliative care.
- Health-care providers should have an appropriate level of competence in palliative care. Their training and educational experiences should help them to acquire the core competencies necessary to provide compassionate and individualized palliative care. They should appreciate the limits of their knowledge and skills and know when to seek consultation from palliative care experts.

There is evidence that palliative care programs in the ICU play a key role in improving communication with patients' families regarding diagnosis, prognosis, goals of care, management of pain and anxiety and provision of spiritual and emotional support.[13-15] Palliative care programs that include structured family meetings to discuss patient-specific goals and advance care planning and which address the emotional and spiritual well-being of patients and families have led to improvement in quality of care, effective use of resources, and enhanced staff satisfaction.[16] A study done by Nelson and colleagues suggest that an ICU "palliative care bundle" improves patient comfort, family communication, and end-of-life decision making.[17] This bundle of palliative care measures includes

- the identification of a medical decision maker
- advance directives

- resuscitation status
- pain assessment and optimal pain management
- spiritual support
- multi-disciplinary family meetings

Family meetings are considered to have a central role in providing families with information concerning their loved one's diagnosis, prognosis, and treatment options. Such meetings allow families to make decisions based on the patient's wishes and current prognosis. Not only do these meetings address the patient's medical condition and quality of life, but they also provide emotional and spiritual support for the patient and the family at the time of significant stress.[16] Lautrette and colleagues[10] randomized family members of 126 patients dying in the ICU to a pro-active communication strategy or to a customary end-of-life conference. In this study, the family members who participated in the pro-active communication meetings suffered less anxiety, depression, and post-traumatic stress after the death of the patient.

While we specifically encourage dialogue between each patient's family and the ICU treating team on a daily basis, we recommend a "pro-active" multi-disciplinary family meetings in patients who are at imminent risk of death and patients who have required 5 or more days of mechanical ventilation. While the prognosis of patients on admission to the ICU is often uncertain, studies suggest that after 5 days of supportive care, the outcome is easier to predict.[18] The family meeting should follow a structured format to ensure that all the elements of the "palliative care bundle" are addressed. Family meetings should include the key physicians involved in the patient's care (including subspecialties), the patient's bedside nurse, and representatives from pastoral and palliative care with participation by all the patient's close relatives. The meetings should be held in a quiet room outside of the ICU, with adequate and comfortable seating and appropriate furnishings. Furthermore, the meeting should be planned at a time that allows for uninterrupted discussions with ample time for the family to voice their feelings and concerns and have all their questions answered.

Adequate preparation is a key component to the success of a family meeting. This includes ensuring participation by key family members and subspecialists involved in the patients care. Clinicians should review the patient's medical history as well as what is known about the patient's disease, including treatment options and likely outcomes. Any disagreements among health-care providers must be resolved prior to meeting with the family. Staff–staff conflict will only increase the family's anxiety and lead to mistrust. The premeeting for clinicians is a good strategy to resolve any conflict and clarify goals of the family meeting. The premeeting can be brief but is an important step in preparation for a successful family meeting. A knowledge of family dynamics and their religious background and beliefs aids in the preparation of the meeting.

■ MY LIVING WILL

I, Paul Marik, being of sound mind and body, do not wish to be resuscitated should my heart cease beating and even if it does not. I do not want a feeding tube inserted into me, unless the tube is big enough to carry a pizza. I want to have pizza regularly – and by "regularly," I mean at least three times a day. I do not wish to be kept alive indefinitely by artificial means; if a reasonable amount of time passes and I fail to ask for at least one of the following, chocolate, ice cream, steak, sex, French fries, potato chips, chocolate, coffee, or hamburger, it should be presumed that I won't ever get better. When such a determination is reached, I hereby instruct my appointed person and attending physicians to pull the plug, reel in the tubes, and call it a day! I would be remiss if I didn't mention organ donation. I want all my organs donated: my eyes to a blind person, my legs to a ballerina, and my brain ... well never mind.

■ REFERENCES

1. Angus DC, Barnato AE, Linde-Zwirble W, et al. Use of intensive care at the end of life in the United States: an epidemiologic study. *Crit Care Med.* 2004;32:638–643.
2. Rady MY, Johnson DJ. Admission to intensive care unit at the end-of-life: is it an informed decision? *Palliat Med.* 2004;18:705–711.
3. Snyder L, Leffler C. Ethics manual: fifth edition. *Ann Intern Med.* 2005;142:560–582.
4. Truog RD, Campbell ML, Curtis JR, et al. Recommendations for end-of-life care in the intensive care unit: a consensus statement by the American College of Critical Care Medicine. *Crit Care Med.* 2008;36:953–963.
5. Lanken PN, Terry PB, Delisser HM, et al. An official American Thoracic Society clinical policy statement: palliative care for patients with respiratory diseases and critical illnesses. *Am J Respir Crit Care Med.* 2008;177:912–927.
6. Rubenfeld GD. Principles and practice of withdrawing life-sustaining treatments. *Crit Care Clin.* 2004;20:435–451.
7. Cook D, Rocker G, Giacomini M, et al. Understanding and changing attitudes towards withdrawal and withholding of life support in the intensive care unit. *Crit Care Med.* 2006;34(Suppl):S317–S323.

8. White DB, Braddock CH, III, Bereknyei S, et al. Toward shared decision making at the end of life in intensive care units: opportunities for improvement. *Arch Intern Med.* 2007;167:461–467.

9. Nelson JE, Angus DC, Weissfeld LA, et al. End-of-life care for the critically ill: a national intensive care unit survey. *Crit Care Med.* 2006;34:2547–2553.

10. Lautrette A, Darmon M, Megarbane B, et al. A communication strategy and brochure for relatives of patients dying in the ICU. *N Engl J Med.* 2007;356:469–478.

11. Azoulay E, Chevret S, Leleu G, et al. Half the families of intensive care unit patients experience inadequate communication with physicians. *Crit Care Med.* 2000;28:3044–3049.

12. World Health Organization. WHO definitions of palliative care – 2005. Available at: http://www.who.int/cancer/palliative/definition/en/,2005, WHO. Accessed September 21, 2009.

13. Billings JA, Keeley A, Bauman J, et al. Merging cultures: palliative care specialists in the medical intensive care unit. *Crit Care Med.* 2006;34:S388–S393.

14. Curtis JR, Engelberg RA. Measuring success of interventions to improve the quality of end-of-life care in the intensive care unit. *Crit Care Med.* 2006;34:S341–S347.

15. Mularski RA, Curtis JR, Billings JA, et al. Proposed quality measures for palliative care in the critically ill: a consensus from the Robert Wood Johnson Foundation Critical Care Workgroup. *Crit Care Med.* 2006;34:S404–S411.

16. Lautrette A, Ciroldi M, Ksibi H, et al. End-of-life family conferences: rooted in the evidence. *Crit Care Med.* 2006;34:S364–S372.

17. Nelson JE, Mulkerin CM, Adams LL, et al. Improving comfort and communication in the ICU: a practical new tool for palliative care performance measurement and feedback. *Qual Saf Health Care.* 2006;15:264–271.

18. Lecuyer L, Chevret S, Thiery G, et al. The ICU trial: a new admission policy for cancer patients requiring mechanical ventilation. *Crit Care Med.* 2007;35:808–814.

65

What Defines an Intensive Care Unit? Implications for Organizational Structure

Critical care medicine combines physicians, nurses, and allied health professional in the coordinated and collaborative management of patients with life-threatening single- or multiple-organ failures, including stabilization after surgical interventions.[1] Critical care medicine requires the continuous (i.e., 24 h) monitoring and support of failing or threatened organ systems while at the same time treating the patients' underlying disease process. The common goals of the intensive care unit (ICU) are to restore and maintain the function of vital organs, to enhance the patient's chance of survival, and to achieve an acceptable clinical outcome.

■ THE HISTORY OF CRITICAL CARE MEDICINE

George Edward Fell (1849–1918), chair of Physiology at the Medical Department of Niagara University in New York, is believed to be the first physician to apply intermittent positive pressure to a human and is widely regarded as the first "intensivist."[2,3] On July 23, 1887, Fell performed a tracheotomy and applied "forced respiration" with a household bellow to a patient who had overdosed on morphine (later estimated to be 1,296 mg) and was at the "near-final stage of asphyxia."[4] Remarkably, the patient made a full recovery. Fell applied this technique to over 100

P.E. Marik, *Handbook of Evidence-Based Critical Care*,
DOI 10.1007/978-1-4419-5923-2_65,
© Springer Science+Business Media, LLC 2010

other patients. He was, however, severely criticized for his work and was treated with contempt on presenting his pioneering case at the 9th International Medical Conference held in Washington, DC.[3] Fell made a number of critical observations which took over 100 years for the scientific community to confirm, including the concept that "overinflation of the lungs" could be harmful. Fell took on cases at any hour of the day or night, stayed with his patients until too exhausted to continue, and developed teams to share the burden of his work (the foundations on which the specialty of critical care medicine are based). In 1929, Dr. Cecil Drinker, a Harvard professor of Physiology, developed the negative-pressure tank ventilator, which became known as the "iron lung."[5] However, it would not be until the late 1940s as polio ravaged Europe and North America that the Drinker tank ventilator would first be used to provide ventilator support to a child at Boston City Hospital who had been stricken with respiratory paralysis caused by polio. During the Copenhagen polio epidemic of 1952, tracheotomy and continuous manual ventilation by intermittent positive ventilation replaced the iron lung. The successful application of positive-pressure ventilation led to the design of a large number of volume-cycled and time-cycled ventilators in Scandinavia, Germany, and the United Kingdom and established intermittent positive ventilation as a standard ventilation practice. One of the first widely available American ventilators was the Jefferson ventilator developed at Jefferson Medical College in Philadelphia.[5] Others, including the Bennet and Bird "Mark 4," soon became available.

What appears to be the world's first ICU was established at the Municipal Hospital of Copenhagen in December 1953 by the Danish anesthesiologist Bjorn Ibsen during the polio epidemic of 1952–1953.[6] The first patient admitted to the unit was a 43-year-old man who had unsuccessfully attempted to hang himself. The patient had a tracheotomy performed and received manual positive-pressure ventilation with 60% oxygen in N_2O. A review of the patient's chart illustrates many aspects of critical care medicine as we know it today, namely the continuous recording of the function of vital organs, immediate interventions when changes in the patient's condition mandated it, and monitoring of the effects of the intervention.[6] The unit was initially called the "Anesthesiologic Observation Unit" but changed to the "Intensive Therapy Unit" (ITU) in 1966. What appears to be the first ICU in the United States was a three-bed unit for postoperative neurosurgical patients opened by W.E Dandy at John Hopkins Hospital in Baltimore in the early 1950s.[7] The first physician-staffed ICUs in the United States were developed in 1958 by Max Harry Weil and Herbert Shubin at the Los Angeles County General Hospital and by Peter Safar in Baltimore.[8,9] Both these units were staffed by a multi-disciplinary team representing both medical and surgical specialties with a 24-h/day, 7-day/week physician commitment.

■ ICU DEFINITION

An ICU is best defined as a geographically distinct area of a hospital where critically ill and injured patients undergo continuous monitoring of multiple physiological and clinical parameters and where multiple interventions are made on an iterative basis based on the dynamic changes in those parameters. A defining feature of an ICU is a low nurse-to-patient ratio (1:1 or 1:2) and the frequent presence of clinicians at the patients' bedside.

ICU clinical care builds on a foundation of relevant and timely physiological monitoring of clinically relevant variables that are readily measured at the bedside. Effective monitoring technologies should measure a physiologic variable that can be acted upon to improve patient outcome. Ideally, they should detect an incipient problem before it causes significant morbidity or requires intensive intervention. Such monitoring technologies should be accurate, precise, and reproducible; they should be easy to implement without disrupting routine care processes, easy to consistently apply and interpret, and they should not increase risk to the patient. Finally, such technologies should be cost effective. The "five vital signs" (heart rate, blood pressure, respiratory rate, temperature, and arterial saturation) remain the core variables upon which most ICU monitoring is based. Increasingly, however, additional measures have been added to our "monitoring armamentarium" including those derived from the mechanical ventilator, non-invasive hemodynamic monitors, and scales for the assessment of sedation, delirium, pain, and neurological status.

Prior to the 1960s, clinicians were unable to detect hypoxemia until clinical cyanosis developed. Arterial blood gas analysis introduced in the late 1960s became the definitive technology of the ICU and remains an essential monitoring tool today.[10–12] The introduction of the pulmonary artery catheter (PAC) in the early 1970s defined critical care medicine for the next two decades.[13,14] However, by 1996, the safety and effectiveness of the PAC came under increasing scrutiny.[15] Studies demonstrated that the PAC provided "physiological variables" (PCWP and CVP) whose highly variable interpretation could lead to inappropriate therapeutic interventions and that the routine use of the PAC did not improve patient outcomes.[16–18] The PAC has now fallen by the wayside. Currently, pulse oximetry, electrocardiography, and bedside echocardiography stand alone with blood gas analysis as monitoring tools with a favorable risk–benefit profile that likely improve patient outcome.[19–21] The clinical benefits of "emerging" technologies such as transpulmonary thermodilution, lithium dilution, pulse contour analysis, and intra-abdominal and esophageal pressure monitoring remain to be determined.[22–25]

■ DATA MANAGEMENT AND PROCESSING IN THE ICU

Data overload is no more apparent than in the ICU, where intensivists are confronted with over 1,000 pieces of information on each of their patients each day.[26] This situation is compounded by a paper-based ICU record system. While a large volume of complex data can be handled by an integrated electronic medical record and order entry system, there are safety risks and adverse events associated with and perpetuated by electronic systems.[27,28] However, clinical information systems in the ICU have the potential to improve access to clinical data, to increase the quality and coherence of the patient care process, to automate guidelines and care pathways, and to achieve better processes and outcomes. Computer decision support systems that make use of intelligent monitoring algorithms and allow early intervention for physiological derangements may become standard and essential components of the emerging ICU.

■ ICU ORGANIZATIONAL STRUCTURE

While technology appears to be a necessary feature of the modern ICU, it is by no means sufficient without health care professionals collaborating to form an effective team. Critical care as first practiced by Fell and later by Bjorn Ibsen, Max-Hary Weil, and Peter Safar required the near-continuous presence of physicians (intensivists) at the patient's bedside supported by a multi-disciplinary team of health-care professionals engaged in continuous physiological monitoring and support of failing organ systems. The first guideline published (in 1972) by the Society of Critical Care Medicine states that "24-h in-house physician staffing and the assignment of physicians full time to a unit distinguish the facility capable of rendering critical care medicine from a facility that is merely a special nursing unit."[29] Furthermore, it states that "it is essential that final responsibility for patient care resides with the physician who provides continuous patient observation and has the most experience in critical care medicine." Both the founding and subsequent guidelines of the Society of Critical Care Medicine endorse the concept that critically ill patients are best managed by an intensivist-led team of health-care professionals which includes ICU nurses, respiratory therapists, clinical pharmacist, dietician, and palliative care practitioners.[29-32] The role of the intensivist is to oversee all aspects of patient care and to assume final responsibility for the management of the patient. This is known as a "closed" ICU model.

The organizational structure of ICUs is usually classified according to two types of models, namely a low- or high-intensity model and an open- or closed ICU model.[31,33] In a low-intensity ICU, patients are managed by non-intensivists; however an intensivist may be consulted on some cases (open model), whereas in a high-intensity model, intensivists are consulted on all patients (open model) or the intensivist assumes responsibility for the patient and directs all aspects of the care (closed model). The admission and discharge practices differ between open and closed units. Closed units are those in which the intensivist screens all admissions and discharges, and assumes full responsibility for all aspects of the patient care. Open units are those in which admission of patients to the ICU is uncontrolled and management of the patients is at the discretion of each attending physician. Admissions are based on a first-come, first-served basis.

In a systematic review evaluating the association between ICU physician staffing and patient outcomes, Pronovost and colleagues[33] analyzed data from 26 studies, which compared a high- with a low-intensity staffing model. All the studies were observational, and 19 studies used historical control with a before-and-after design. High-intensity staffing was associated with a lower risk of death (OR 0.71; 95% CI 0.62–0.82). A more recent study using a cohort rather than a before–after study design demonstrated that patients with acute lung injury cared for in closed ICUs had reduced hospital mortality (OR 0.68; 95% CI 0.53–0.89). However, in this study a consultation by a pulmonologist/intensivist was not associated with improved outcome.[34] Similarly, Hawari and colleagues[35] demonstrated a significant reduction in 28-, 60-, and 90-day mortality, as well as ICU efficiency and bed utilization, when their oncology ICU transitioned from an open ICU managed largely by oncologists to a Leapfrog-compliant closed ICU staffed by intensivists. These data suggest that closed ICUs are associated with a 30–40% reduction in the risk of death when compared to an open ICU staffing model. Contrary to the extensive and consistent data supporting that high-intensity ICU staffing improves outcome, a report by Levy and colleagues has shown opposite results.[36] This report, however, has a number of methodological issues which cast doubt as to the validity of the findings.[37]

Optimal ICU Organizational Structure

The care of the critically ill patients requires knowledge of multiple-organ pathological alterations and their interactions, appropriate analysis and understanding of numerous data, timely initiation of effective therapy, and a good grasp of ethical issues. An intensivist-led multi-disciplinary team functioning in a closed ICU is the model which provides the optimal care of critically ill and injured patients and maximizes the likelihood of a good outcome, limits complications, and is associated with a reduced length of stay. There is ample evidence supporting the superiority of a closed ICU model over an open/low-intensity staffing model in improving patient outcome. The Society of Critical Care Medicine's recommendations for critical care delivery in the ICU indicate that "a multidisciplinary ICU team should be led by a full-time critical care-trained physician available in a timely fashion to the ICU 24 h/day."[31] The intensivist should be continuously available at the bedside (during the day) and perform rounds twice daily: multi-disciplinary/teaching rounds in the morning and business/sign-out rounds in the afternoon. The intensivist or his designee should be solely responsible for writing orders. This model does not exclude the patients' primary care physician, the oncologist, or the surgeon from the patients' care; they remain an important part of the multi-disciplinary team and should remain actively involved in the care of their patient and interact collaboratively with the intensivist.

The preponderance of evidence supports the concept that critically ill patients are best managed in a closed ICU by dedicated critical care physicians who have undergone specialized multi-disciplinary training which provides them with the necessary knowledge, skills, and attitudes to achieve the best outcomes for critically ill patients. In critical care, it is the intensive attention at the bedside by dedicated physicians and nurses working together in a compassionate and caring environment that will achieve the best outcome for our patients.[37]

■ REFERENCES

1. De Lange S, Van AH, Burchardi H. European Society of Intensive Care Medicine statement: intensive care medicine in Europe – structure, organisation and training guidelines of the Multidisciplinary Joint Committee of Intensive Care Medicine (MJCICM) of the European Union of Medical Specialists (UEMS). *Intensive Care Med.* 2002;28:1505–1511.

2. Garrrison GF. *History of Medicine.* 1st ed. Philadelphia, PA: WB Saunders; 1913.

3. Trubuhovich RV. 19th century pioneers of intensive therapy in North America. Part 1: George Edward Fell. *Crit Care Resus.* 2007;9: 377–393.

4. Fell GE. Forced respiration in opium poisoning- its possibilities, and the apparatus best adapted to produce it. *Bufffalo Med Surg J.* 1887;28: 145–157.

5. Grenvik A, Eross B, Powner D. Historical survey of mechanical ventilation. *Int Anesthesiol Clin.* 1980;18:1–10.

6. Berthelsen PG, Cronqvist M. The first intensive care unit in the world: Copenhagen 1953. *Acta Anaesthesiol Scand.* 2003;47:1190–1195.

7. Long DM. A century of change in neurosurgery at Johns Hopkins: 1889–1989. *J Neurosurg.* 1989;71:635–638.

8. Weil MH, Shoemaker WC. Pioneering contributions of Peter Safar to intensive care and the founding of the Society of Critical Care Medicine. *Crit Care Med.* 2004;32:S8–S10.
9. Safar P, Dekornfeld TJ, Pearson JW, et al. The intensive care unit. A three year experience at Baltimore city hospitals. *Anaesthesia* 1961;16: 275–284.
10. Severinghaus JW, Bradley AF. Electrodes for blood pO_2 and pCO_2 determination. *J Appl Physiol.* 1958;13:515–520.
11. Clark LC. Monitor and control of blood and tissue O2 tensions. *Trans Am Soc Artif Intern Organs.* 1956;2:41–48.
12. Stow RW, Baer RF, Randall B. Rapid measurement of the tension of carbon dioxide in the blood. *Arch Phys Med Rehabil.* 1957;38: 646–650.
13. Ganz W, Donosco R, Marcus HS, et al. A new technique for measurement of cardiac output by thermodilution in man. *Am J Cardiol.* 1971;27:392–396.
14. Swan HJ, Ganz W, Forrester J, et al. Catheterization of the heart in man with use of a flow-directed balloon-tipped catheter. *N Engl J Med.* 1970;283:447–451.
15. Connors AF, Speroff T, Dawson NV, et al. The effectiveness of right heart catheterization in the initial care of critically ill patients. *JAMA.* 1996;276:889–897.
16. Marik PE, Baram M, Vahid B. Does the central venous pressure predict fluid responsiveness? A systematic review of the literature and the tale of seven mares. *Chest.* 2008;134:172–178.
17. Harvey S, Harrison DA, Singer M, et al. Assessment of the clinical effectiveness of pulmonary artery catheters in management of patients in intensive care (PAC-Man): a randomised controlled trial. *Lancet.* 2005;366:472–477.
18. Sandham JD, Hull RD, Brant RF, et al. A randomized, controlled trial of the use of pulmonary-artery catheters in high-risk surgical patients. *N Engl J Med.* 2003;348:5–14.
19. Beaulieu Y, Marik PE. Bedside ultrasonography in the ICU, Part 1. *Chest.* 2005;128:881–895.
20. Moller JT, Johannessen NW, Espersen K, et al. Randomized evaluation of pulse oximetry in 20,802 patients: II. Perioperative events and postoperative complications. *Anesthesiol.* 1993;78:445–453.
21. Neff TA. Routine oximetry. A fifth vital sign? *Chest.* 1988;94:227.
22. Marik PE, Cavallazzi R, Vasu T, et al. Dynamic changes in arterial waveform derived variables and fluid responsiveness in mechanically ventilated patients. A systematic review of the literature. *Crit Care Med.* 2009;37:2642–2647.
23. Cheatham ML. Intraabdominal pressure monitoring during fluid resuscitation. *Curr Opin Crit Care.* 2008;14:327–333.

24. Talmor D, Sarge T, Malhotra A, et al. Mechanical ventilation guided by esophageal pressure in acute lung injury. *N Engl J Med.* 2008;359: 2095–2104.

25. Pittman J, Bar-Yosef S, SumPing J, et al. Continuous cardiac output monitoring with pulse contour analysis: a comparison with lithium indicator dilution cardiac output measurement. *Crit Care Med.* 2005;33: 2015–2021.

26. Morris AH. Developing and implementing computerized protocols for standardization of clinical decisions. *Ann Intern Med.* 2000;132: 373–383.

27. Kuehn BM. IT vulnerabilities highlighted by errors, malfunctions at veterans' medical centers. *JAMA.* 2009;301:919–920.

28. Koppel R, Metlay JP, Cohen A, et al. Role of computerized physician order entry systems in facilitating medication errors. *JAMA.* 2005;293:1197–1203.

29. Downes JJ Jr, Del Guercio L, Grace WJ, et al. Guidelines for organization of critical care units. *JAMA.* 1972;222:1532–1535.

30. Durbin CG Jr. Team model: advocating for the optimal method of care delivery in the intensive care unit. *Crit Care Med.* 2006;34:S12–S17.

31. Brilli RJ, Spevetz A, Branson RD, et al. Critical care delivery in the intensive care unit: defining clinical roles and the best practice model. *Crit Care Med.* 2001;29:2007–2019.

32. Guidelines for categorization of services for the critically ill patient. Task Force on Guidelines; Society of Critical Care Medicine. *Crit Care Med.* 1991;19:279–285.

33. Pronovost PJ, Angus DC, Dorman T, et al. Physician staffing patterns and clinical outcomes in critically ill patients: a systematic review. *JAMA.* 2002;288:2151–2162.

34. Treggiari MM, Martin DP, Yanez ND, et al. Effect of intensive care unit organizational model and structure on outcomes in patients with acute lung injury. *Am J Respir Crit Care Med.* 2007;176:685–690.

35. Hawari FI, Al Najjar TI, Zarru L, et al. The effect of implementing high-intensity intensive care unit staffing model on outcome of critically ill oncology patients. *Crit Care Med.* 2009;37:1967–1971.

36. Levy MM, Rapoport J, Lemeshow S, et al. Association between critical care physician management and patient mortality in the Intensive Care Unit. *Ann Intern Med.* 2008;148:801–809.

37. Marik PE, Myburgh J, Annane D, et al. Association between critical care physician management and patient mortality. *Ann Intern Med.* 2009;149:770–771.

66

Intrahospital Transport

The safest place for the critically ill patient is stationary in the ICU, connected to a sophisticated ventilator with all infusion pumps running smoothly, complete monitoring installed, and with a nurse present to care for the patient. However, with increasing technological advancements, it is almost routine for critically ill patients to be transported out of the ICU for a variety of tests and procedures. Data suggest that between 25 and 50% of patients undergo intrahospital transports during their ICU stay, with many patients having multiple transports. The commonest reason for an intrahospital "road trip" is transport to the radiology suite for a CT scan.[1,2] Hurst et al.[2] reported that the average duration of an intrahospital critical care transport was 74 min. In general, transported patients have significantly higher severity of illness scores, greater use of vasopressors and mechanical ventilation, and longer ICU and hospital length of stay and higher hospital mortality than do non-transported patients.[1] These patient factors significantly increase the risks of transport.

Adverse events occur in up to 70% of intrahospital transports.[2–6] There are two general categories of adverse events. The first is based on mishaps that occur during the intensive care monitoring (e.g., lead disconnections, loss of intravenous access, depleted oxygen supply, equipment failure). The second category is the physiological deterioration of the patient related to the critical illness (e.g., hypotension, arrhythmias, hypoxia, increased intracranial pressure). Beckmann and colleagues[4] report on their analysis of incidents and adverse events affecting patients during intrahospital transfer, obtained from the database of the Australian Incident Monitoring Study in Intensive Care. Between 1993 and 1999, 176 reports were submitted describing 191 incidents. Seventy-five reports (39%) identified equipment problems, relating prominently to battery/power supply, transport ventilator and monitor function, and

P.E. Marik, *Handbook of Evidence-Based Critical Care*,
DOI 10.1007/978-1-4419-5923-2_66,
© Springer Science+Business Media, LLC 2010

access to patient elevators and intubation equipment. One hundred and sixteen reports (61%) identified patient/staff management issues including poor communication, inadequate monitoring, incorrect setup of equipment, artificial airway malpositioning, and incorrect positioning of patients. Serious adverse outcomes occurred in 55 reports (31%) including major physiological derangement in 27 (15%). Of 900 contributing factors identified, 46% were system based and 54% human based. Communication problems, inadequate protocols, in-servicing/training, and faulty equipment were prominent causes of equipment-related incidents. Errors of problem recognition and judgment, failure to follow protocols, inadequate patient preparation, haste, and inattention were common management-related incidents.

Airway mishaps are common in intubated patients during a transport and may lead to a fatal outcome.[3,4] These mishaps include endotracheal tube migration (with overventilation and barotrauma), tube dislodgment, tube kinking and tube disconnection. These events frequently occur in the confined space of an elevator making their detection difficult and the performance of cardiopulmonary resuscitation nearly impossible. Additional problems include hypoxemia due to inadequate "bagging" or problems with the supply of oxygen. Furthermore, intrahospital transport appears to be a significant risk factor for the development of ventilator-associated pneumonia (possibly due to an increased risk of aspiration).[7] These data suggest that practitioners competent in managing the airway (i.e., respiratory therapists) should accompany all intubated patients during an intrahospital transport.

The risk of an intrahospital transport can be minimized and the outcomes improved with careful planning, the use of appropriately qualified personnel, and the availability of appropriate equipment. During transport, there should be no hiatus in the monitoring or the maintenance of a patient's vital functions. All critical care transports (both inter- and intrahospital) should be performed by specially trained individuals. Furthermore, the decision to transport a critically ill patient, either within a hospital or to another facility, should be based on an assessment of the potential benefits of transport weighed against the potential risks. If a diagnostic test or a procedural intervention under consideration is unlikely to alter the management or the outcome of that patient, then the need for transport must be questioned. When feasible, diagnostic testing or simple procedures in unstable or potentially unstable patients are best performed at the bedside.

The American College of Critical Care Medicine (ACCM) in collaboration with the American Association of Critical Care Nurses (AACN) has developed guidelines for the transport of critically ill patients.[5] These guidelines recommend that all critical care transports be performed by a dedicated, specially trained transport team. Stearley et al.[6] demonstrated that critically ill patients that are transported by a specialized transport team have an overall complication rate of 15.5%, compared with the national complication rate which may be as high as 75%.

Because the transport of critically ill patients to procedures or tests outside the ICU is potentially hazardous, the transport process must be organized and efficient. To facilitate a safe transport, the ACCM guidelines suggest that the following four issues be addressed.[5]

■ PRETRANSPORT COORDINATION AND COMMUNICATION

When an alternate team at a receiving location will assume management responsibility for the patient after arrival, continuity of patient care will be ensured by physician-to-physician and/or nurse-to-nurse communication to review the patient's condition and the treatment plan in operation. This communication should occur each time patient care responsibility is transferred. Before transport, the receiving location should confirm that it is ready to receive the patient for the procedure or the test. Other members of the transport team (e.g., respiratory therapy, hospital security) should then be notified as to the timing of the transport and the equipment support that will be needed. The responsible physician(s) should be made aware of the transport. Documentation in the medical record includes the indications for the transport and patient's status throughout the time away from the unit of origin.

■ PERSONNEL

It is strongly recommended that a minimum of two people accompany the critically ill patient during a transport. One of the accompanying personnel should be a critical care nurse who is "transport certified"[5,6]. Additional personnel may include a respiratory therapist, a registered nurse, or a critical care technician as needed. It is strongly recommended that a physician with training in airway management, advanced cardiac life support, and critical care/emergency medicine accompany unstable patients.

■ EQUIPMENT

- Cardiac monitor/defibrillator.
- Airway management equipment and resuscitation bag of proper size and fit for the patient.
- Oxygen source of ample volume to provide the patient's needs for the projected time out of the ICU with an additional 30 min reserve.

- Standard resuscitation drugs (e.g., epinephrine, lidocaine, atropine, sodium bicarbonate).
- Blood pressure cuff.
- Ample supply of the intravenous fluids and continuous drip medications (regulated by battery-operated infusion pumps) being administered to the patient.
- Additional medications to provide the patient's scheduled intermittent medication doses and to meet anticipated needs (e.g., sedation) with appropriate orders to allow their administration if a physician is not present.
- For patients receiving mechanical support of ventilation, a device capable of delivering the same minute ventilation, pressure, FiO_2, and PEEP that the patient is receiving in the ICU. For practical reasons, in adults, an FiO_2 of 1.0 is most feasible during transport because this eliminates the need for an air tank and an air–oxygen blender.
- A resuscitation cart and a suction equipment need not accompany each patient being transported, but such equipments shall be stationed in areas used by critically ill patients and be readily available (within 4 min) by a predetermined mechanism for emergencies that might occur on route.

For practical reasons, bag-valve ventilation is most commonly employed during intrahospital transports. Portable mechanical ventilators are, however, preferred as they more reliably administer the prescribed minute ventilation, PEEP, and desired oxygen concentrations. It should be appreciated that prolonged bag-valve ventilation may be dangerous in patients with severe respiratory failure. The receiving location should have a ventilatory equipment capable of delivering ventilatory support equivalent to that being delivered at the patient's origin. The endotracheal tube position should be noted and secured before transport and the adequacy of oxygenation and ventilation reconfirmed. When a transport ventilator is employed, it must have alarms to indicate disconnection and excessively high airway pressures and must have a backup battery power supply.

■ MONITORING

All critically ill patients undergoing transport should receive the same level of basic physiological monitoring during transport as they had in the intensive care unit. This includes, at a minimum, continuous electrocardiographic monitoring, continuous pulse oximetry, and periodic measurement of blood pressure, pulse rate, and respiratory rate.

■ INTERHOSPITAL TRANSPORT

Patient outcomes depend to a large degree on the technology and expertise of personnel available within each health-care facility. When services are needed that exceed available resources, a patient ideally should be transferred to a facility that has the required resources. Interhospital transportation poses many of the same risks that are associated with intrahospital transport. Interhospital patient transfers should therefore occur only when the benefits to the patient exceed the risks of the transfer (dead or near-dead patients should not be transferred to another facility). The decision to transfer a patient is the responsibility of the attending physician at the referring institution. Once this decision has been made, the transfer should be effected as soon as possible. Resuscitation and stabilization should begin before the transfer (this does not mean a 22 g IV), realizing that complete stabilization may be possible only at the receiving facility. In the United States, it is essential for practitioners to be aware of federal and state laws regarding interhospital patient transfers. In general, under COBRA/EMTALA, financially motivated transfers are illegal and put both the referring institution and the individual practitioner at risk for serious penalty. Current regulations and good medical practice require that a competent patient, guardian, or the legally authorized representative of an incompetent patient give informed consent before interhospital transfer. The informed consent process includes a discussion of the risks and benefits of transfer. These discussions should be documented in the medical record before transfer.

■ CLINICAL PEARLS

- The safest place for the critically ill patient is stationary in the ICU.
- The risk and benefits must be evaluated before the transport of every ICU patient.
- Both intra- and interhospital transports require careful planning, the use of appropriately qualified personnel, and the availability of appropriate equipment.

■ REFERENCES

1. Voigt LP, Pastores SM, Raoof ND, et al. Review of a large clinical series: intrahospital transport of critically ill patients: outcomes, timing, and patterns. *J Intensive Care Med*. 2009;24:108–115.
2. Hurst JM, Davis K Jr, Johnson DJ, et al. Cost and complications during in-hospital transport of critically ill patients: a prospective cohort study. *J Trauma*. 1992;33:582–585.

3. Waydhas C. Intrahospital transport of critically ill patients. *Crit Care*. 1999;3:R83–R89.
4. Beckmann U, Gillies DM, Berenholtz SM, et al. Incidents relating to the intra-hospital transfer of critically ill patients. An analysis of the reports submitted to the Australian Incident Monitoring Study in Intensive Care. *Intensive Care Med*. 2004;30:1579–1585.
5. Warren J, Fromm RE Jr, Orr RA, et al. Guidelines for the inter- and intrahospital transport of critically ill patients. *Crit Care Med*. 2004;32: 256–262.
6. Stearley HE. Patients' outcomes: intrahospital transportation and monitoring of critically ill patients by a specially trained ICU nursing staff. *Am J Crit Care*. 1998;7:282–287.
7. Bercault N, Wolf M, Runge I, et al. Intrahospital transport of critically ill ventilated patients: a risk factor for ventilator-associated pneumonia – a matched cohort study. *Crit Care Med*. 2005;33:2471–2478.

67

Limiting Errors and Avoiding Litigation

Shit happens

– Old Chinese Proverb

- "Suits for malpractice are so frequent that many doctors have abandoned the practice of surgery, leaving it to those who, with less skill and experience, have less reputation and property to lose" – *NY Medical Journal*, 1856.
- In 1986, a Philadelphia jury awarded $1 million to a "spiritual advisor" who claimed in a medical malpractice case to have lost her psychic powers as a result of a negligently administered CT scan.
- "Florida hospital surgeons mistakenly amputate wrong leg of patient" – March 1995.
- "Doctors let patient bleed to death in operating room" (C-section performed with heparin infusion running and PTT >120 s) – NJ, 2006.

These statements/cases highlight the complexity and enormous problems associated with medical malpractice in the United States. This is a rather unfortunate topic for a text on *Evidence-Based Critical Care Medicine*, as the practice of evidence-based medicine should protect the intensivist against litigation. However, medical malpractice is a reality of American medicine and intensivists (and their delegates) are not immune from litigation. The purpose of this chapter is to provide an overview of medical malpractice litigation in the United States and to provide the reader with proactive steps he/she can take to reduce the risk of litigation.

P.E. Marik, *Handbook of Evidence-Based Critical Care*,
DOI 10.1007/978-1-4419-5923-2_67,
© Springer Science+Business Media, LLC 2010

Regardless of the merits of a case, litigation is best avoided (at all costs) as the personal, financial, and professional toll can be overwhelming.

■ THE FACTS

Causes of Death in the United States (Cases/Year)

- Cardiovascular – 710,760[1]
- Cancer – 553,091
- Medical errors/adverse events – 225,400
- Stroke – 166,661
- Chronic respiratory disease – 122,009
- Accidents – 97,900

Errors in the ICU

- Due to the complexity of ICU patients, the complexity of care, and the delegation of tasks to many individuals (often with minimal understanding of the issues), "errors" in the ICU are common.
- Studies suggest that between 20 and 30% of patients suffer from an iatrogenic injury in the ICU, with many of these events being life threatening.[2,3]
- Donchin and colleagues[4] reported that 1.7 errors occur per patient per day in the ICU.
- The Multinational Sentinel Events Evaluation (SEE) study reported 38.8 sentinel events per 100 ICU patient days.[5] Medication errors, vascular access, airway complications and equipment failure were responsible for the majority of these events.
- Medication errors are the commonest type of errors in the ICU[2,6,7]:
  - Wrong drug.
  - Wrong dose.
  - Wrong route.
  - Drug interaction overlooked.
- Autopsy studies find missed diagnoses that would have changed therapy and improved outcome in >30% of deceased ICU patients.[8,9]

Limiting Errors

- Do the right thing; *do not cut corners* (see   Chapter 68):
  - You may get away with it "most" of the time, but eventually you will fall in the "big hole."

- Communicate directly with the ICU nurse so that he/she understands the treatment plan. Inform him/her of new orders or changes in existing orders.
- Be diligent and systematic.
- Avoid arrogance and dogmatisms.
- Limit fragmentation of care:
  - Need a "captain of the ship," i.e., a full-time dedicated intensivist who assumes responsibility for the patients' overall care (i.e., must have a plan).
- Improve communication with your colleagues:
  - Speak with them directly; the chart is a poor medium for communication. While originally conceived as a method to document a patients' progress in the hospital, the "chart" has become the domain of the billing clerk, risk managers (and lawyers), and JACHO, and currently serves very little useful purpose!
  - The cell phone is a remarkable invention that allows people to speak to each other.[10]
- Improve hand offs.
- One house officer should not cover more than 6 ICU patients during the day and 12 patients at night:
  - Preventing intern fatigue (work hour reduction) reduces errors in the ICU.[11]
- Establish a clear chain of command.
- A clinical pharmacist should be involved in multi-disciplinary ICU rounds and should review ICU medication/orders.

Litigation and Errors: The Facts

- Studies have shown that about 1% of all hospitalized patients suffer a permanent injury (or death) as a result of medical negligence.[12-15]
- These same studies demonstrate that only between 3 and 10% of patients who actually suffer from medical negligence file a suit.
- About 40,000 claims are filed annually in the United States.
- Of all the suits filed, an error in care (medical malpractice) is reported to occur in about 65% of cases (i.e., 35% of cases may be frivolous).[16]
- Approximately 17,000 malpractice payments are made annually.[17]
- The National Practitioner Data Bank (NPDB) has recorded 235,942 physician malpractice reports (1990–2006), with a total of 164,819 physicians being listed with 1.87 reports per physician[17]:
  - About 0.9% were residents at the time of the report.
- The most frequent types of claims against internal medicine specialists include the following:[18]

- Errors in diagnosis (24%).
- Improper performance of a procedure (14%).
- Failure to supervise care (12%).
- Medication error (12%).
- Common errors in diagnosis/treatment:
  - The failure to diagnose and/or the timely treatment of an infection/sepsis.
  - Missed pulmonary embolism.
  - Failure of prophylaxis against DVT/PE.
  - Missed HIT.
  - Failure to follow-up on an abnormal test (pulmonary nodule, abnormal lab test).
  - Failure to be "aware" of an abnormal test result, e.g., potassium, troponin, ECG, etc.
  - Failure to recognize/treat hypoxemia and/or intubate in a timely manner.
  - Failure to move patient to a higher level of care (i.e., ICU).
- "Standard of care" refers to the quality of care that would be expected of an ordinary or a reasonable (prudent) physician in the same specialty in a similar circumstance.[18]
- Standard of care for residents:
  - The general view of the law today is that resident physicians must conform at least to the standard of care expected of a general practitioner in that field, i.e., they are held accountable to the "standard" of their attendings and *not* their peers.[19]
  - The implications for attendings is that they are responsible for the conduct and supervision of their residents.
  - The implications for residents is that they *must* seek the help, advice, and counsel of their attendings.

Avoiding Litigation

- Develop a good relationship with your patient and/or their relatives[20]:
  - Be respectful.
  - Be courteous.
  - Be honest.
  - Listen to what they have to say.
  - Tell them the truth (as it relates to the diagnosis and prognosis).
- Never "piss off" your patient and/or their family, no matter how obnoxious they are.
- Keep up-to-date.
- Acknowledge your mistake(s):
  - And learn from your mistakes.

- The dictum "if it's not documented, it was not done" holds true (unfortunately):
  - Document whatever you do and say (to the patient or the family) to cover your ass.
  - *Every* entry into the chart (orders as well as progress notes/consults) *must* be dated, timed, and signed.
  - Your notes/orders *must* be legible.
  - If you make a mistake, draw a line through the note, write "Error" next to the line, and then date, time, and sign. *Do not* try and "blackout" the note; this is an invitation for trouble.
- Informed consent:
  - All procedures and surgeries in the ICU/operating room require informed consent; exceptions include NG/OG tubes, feeding tubes, peripheral venous access, and *emergent* procedures.
  - Informed consent must be truly "informed" and involves much more than just obtaining a signature.
  - You *must* not get consent for another operator (else you will both be in trouble).
  - Must explain the nature of the procedure.
  - The most common risks as well as the risk of death (if this may occur) must be discussed.
  - Alternative treatments and associated risks must be discussed.
  - All these *must* be documented in the chart.
  - Be cautious when obtaining consent from a patient that does not understand English (or your native tongue). Do not use a family member to translate; a hospital translator is imperative and the details should be well documented.

■ REFERENCES

1. Starfield B. Is US health really the best in the World? *JAMA.* 2000;284:483–485.
2. Rothschild JM, Landrigan CP, Cronin JW, et al. The critical care safety study: The incidence and nature of adverse events and serious medical errors in intensive care. *Crit Care Med.* 2005;33:1694–1700.
3. Giraud T, Dhainaut JF, Vaxelaire JF, et al. Iatrogenic complications in adult intensive care units: a prospective two-center study. *Crit Care Med.* 1993;21:40–51.
4. Donchin Y, Gopher D, Olin M, et al. A look into the nature and causes of human errors in the intensive care unit. *Crit Care Med.* 1995;23:294–300.
5. Valentin A, Capuzzo M, Guidet B, et al. Patient safety in intensive care: results from the multinational Sentinel Events Evaluation (SEE) study. *Intensive Care Med.* 2006;32:1591–1598.

6. Valentin A, Capuzzo M, Guidet B, et al. Errors in administration of parenteral drugs in intensive care units: multinational prospective study. *BMJ*. 2009;338:b814.

7. van den Bemt PM, Fijn R, van der Voort PH, et al. Frequency and determinants of drug administration errors in the intensive care unit. *Crit Care Med*. 2002;30:846–850.

8. Perkins GD, McAuley DF, Davies S, et al. Discrepancies between clinical and postmortem diagnoses in critically ill patients: an observational study. *Crit Care*. 2003; 7:R129–R132.

9. Combes A, Mokhtari M, Couvelard A, et al. Clinical and autopsy diagnoses in the intensive care unit: a prospective study. *Arch Intern Med*. 2004;164:389–392.

10. Soto RG, Chu LF, Goldman JM, et al. Communication in critical care environments: mobile telephones improve patient care. *Anesth Analg*. 2006;102:535–541.

11. Landrigan CP, Rothschild JM, Cronin JW, et al. Effect of reducing interns' work hours on serious medical errors in intensive care units. *N Engl J Med*. 2004;351:1838–1848.

12. Localio AR, Lawthers AG, Brennan, TA et al. Relation between malpractice claims and adverse events due to negligence. Results of the Harvard Medical Practice Study III. *N Engl J Med*. 1991;325:245–251.

13. Studdert DM, Thomas EJ, Burstin HR, et al. Negligent care and malpractice claiming behavior in Utah and Colorado. *Med Care*. 2000;38: 250–260.

14. Cohen TH, Hughes KA. Medical Malpractice Insurance Claims in Seven States, 2000–2004 (NCJ-216339). Available at: http://www.ojp.usdoj.gov/bjs/pub/pdf/mmicss04.pdf. 2007. Department of Justice, Washington, DC.

15. California Medical Association. *Medical Insurance Feasibility Study*. San Francisco, CA: Sutter Publication; 1977.

16. Studdert DM, Mello MM, Gawande AA, et al. Claims, errors, and compensation payments in medical malpractice litigation. *N Engl J Med*. 2006;354:2024–2033.

17. National Practitioner Data Bank. 2006 Annual Report. 2007. Washington, DC, US Department of Health and Human Services.

18. Luce JM. Medical malpractice and the chest physician. *Chest*. 2008;134:1044–1050.

19. Kachalia A, Studdert DM. Professional liability issues in graduate medical education. *JAMA*. 2004;292:1051–1056.

20. Hoffman PJ, Plump JD, Courtney MA. The defense counsel's perspective. *Clin Orthop Rel Res*. 2005;15–25.

68

Avoiding Therapeutic Misadventures in the ICU

- Do not give a β-blocker to a patient with sinus tachycardia:
  - The patient usually has a tachycardia for a reason (low stroke volume/cardiac output, fever, etc). A β-blocker is a very effective method of "knocking off" a septic, hypovolemic patient with a severe tachycardia.
  - Exceptions to this rule include patients with acute coronary syndromes, delirium tremens, and thyrotoxicosis.
- Do not give a non-intubated COPD patient a benzodiazepine; this will cause them to stop breathing (which is usually a bad thing).
- Do not use an intravenous anti-hypertensive agent (e.g., hydralazine) in a patient unless the patient has a true hypertensive emergency.
- *Never* prescribe sublingual nifedipine.
- Never remove a central line with the patient sitting up, unless you wish to cause an air embolism. This should be done with the patient lying flat and during a valsalva maneuver.
- Never ignore an abnormal lab value; if it seems "wrong," repeat it "stat."
- Hyperkalemia, hypokalemia, and hypophosphatemia should always be treated emergently.
- Oliguria (and intravascular volume depletion) should never be treated with Lasix (furosemide).
- Delirium (agitation) should be treated with haloperidol/dexmedetomidine and not a benzodiazepine.

P.E. Marik, *Handbook of Evidence-Based Critical Care*,
DOI 10.1007/978-1-4419-5923-2_68,
© Springer Science+Business Media, LLC 2010

- Pain should be treated with an analgesic (usually an opiate) and not a benzodiazepine or with propofol.
- Do not "paralyze" an agitated patient or one with ventilator dyssynchrony (this is torture):
  - Treat the underlying problem.
- Do not use NIPPV in an uncooperative/somnolent patient.
- Suture your central line/arterial line, else it will "fall out."
- Secure the ET tube, else it will "fall out."
- Patients on high FiO$_2$ (>80%) and high PEEP (>12 cm H$_2$O) should not travel outside the ICU unless absolutely necessary.
- Check the dosages of the following drugs carefully:
  - Heparin.
  - Insulin.
  - Morphine.
- Oral hypoglycemic drugs should not be prescribed in the ICU:
  - Hypoglycemia kills.
- Limit the use of Coumadin in the ICU (it is rat poison and cannot be good for humans),

69

The "Devil's" Medicine Bag

The following "drugs" especially in the "wrong hands" are likely to cause more harm than to be of any benefit:

- Nitroprusside
- IV hydralazine
- Nifedipine (short acting)
- TPN
- Lasix®
- Blood mixed with some FFP

Remember, Coumadin is "rat poison"; it was designed to kill rats!

P.E. Marik, *Handbook of Evidence-Based Critical Care*,
DOI 10.1007/978-1-4419-5923-2_69,
© Springer Science+Business Media, LLC 2010

70

Words of Wisdom

- Always be honest.[1]
- Failure is success if you learn from it.
- It is a privilege to practice medicine; do not abuse that privilege.[2]
- Common sense occurs uncommonly.[3]
- Common things occur commonly[3]:
  - If it looks like a horse, whines like a horse and smells like a horse, do not expect a zebra to appear.
- The less a procedure is indicated, the more likely that it will be accompanied by a complication.[3]
- If a patient is reluctant to undergo a procedure, do not force the issue; that is the patient who will have a complication.
- When doing a procedure, remember that nature always sides with the hidden flaw.
- Never open a can of worms unless you plan to go fishing.
- No individual has a monopoly on the truth.[2]
- A physicians error is often the result of overconfidence.[2]
- We only see what we know (or look for).
- When you do not know what to do, do nothing:
  - *Corollary*: Doing something harmful is not better than doing nothing.
- Do not assume the obvious and do not make assumptions.
- The Law of Sub-specialization:
  - If you are a hammer, the world looks like a nail.
- An acute surgical abdomen is when a good surgeon says it is an acute surgical abdomen. There is no test for it.
- Before ordering a test, decide what you will do if it is (a) positive or (b) negative. If both answers are the same, do not do the test.
- There is no manifestation that cannot be caused by a given drug.
- If a drug is not working, stop it.

P.E. Marik, *Handbook of Evidence-Based Critical Care*,
DOI 10.1007/978-1-4419-5923-2_70,
© Springer Science+Business Media, LLC 2010

- If it cannot be read, do not write it.
- Any order that can be misunderstood will be misunderstood.
- Respect your fellow health-care workers; they are your most important clinical asset.[2]
- Never ignore an ICU nurse's observation.
- Be kind to nurses, and they will be kind to you. Be unkind to nurses and they will make your life miserable.
- It is the highest form of self-respect to admit our errors and mistakes and make amends for them. To make a mistake is only an error in judgment, but to adhere to it when it is discovered shows infirmity of character – Dale E. Turner.

"Banned Word(s)" in the ICU

- Pan culture
- CVP
- Culture of sputum
- IV hydralazine
- "Vec" for vent synchrony
- TPN
- Coumadin
- Lantus

■ REFERENCES

1. Pausch R. *The Last Lecture*. New York, NY: Hyperion; 2008.
2. Alpert JS. "Common sense is not so common" (What we all need to remember) – Part Two. *Am J Med*. 2009;122:789–790.
3. Alpert JS. "Commom sense is not so common" (What we all need to remember) – Part One. *Am J Med*. 2009;122:700–701.

Subject Index

Note: The letters 'f' and 't' following the locators refer to figures and tables respectively.

A

AACN, *see* American Association of Critical Care Nurses (AACN)

Abdominal compartment syndrome, 66–67

Abdominal perfusion pressure (APP), 55, 65–67

"AbNormal Saline," 68–69

Acalculous cholecystitis, 141, 143–144

Accelerated idioventricular rhythm, 318

ACCESS, *see* Acute Candesartan Cilexetil Evaluation in Stroke Survivors (ACCESS)

ACCM, *see* American College of Critical Care Medicine (ACCM)

ACE inhibitors (ACEI), 291

Acetyl-*p*-aminophenol (APAP), 607

Acid–base disturbances, 453–460
  acid–base disorders, 454t
  an approach to arterial blood gas analysis, 453–456
  compensation for, 455t
  metabolic acidosis, 456–459
    bicarbonate and ketoacidosis, 458

diagnostic algorithm, 457

D-lactic acidosis, 458–459

indications for bicarbonate therapy, 458

use of bicarbonate, 456

metabolic alkalosis (MA), 459
  adverse effects, 459
  therapeutic maneuver, 459

normal acid–base values, 454t

osmolal gap and lethal intoxications, 456t

traditional acid–base definitions, 454t

Acidosis, 267, 448, 454t, 456, 465, 467, 475, 622

acute respiratory acidosis, 179

anion gap (AG) acidosis, 68, 100, 613

"dilutional acidosis," 70

D-lactic acidosis, 458–459

extracellular acidosis, 223

gastric intramucosal acidosis, 184

hypercapnic respiratory acidosis, 155, 222–223

hyperchloremic acidosis, 457f, 458

intracellular acidosis, 223, 458

P.E. Marik, *Handbook of Evidence-Based Critical Care*,
DOI 10.1007/978-1-4419-5923-2,
© Springer Science+Business Media, LLC 2010

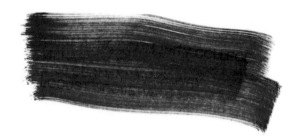

Breinigsville, PA USA
13 October 2010
247250BV00012B/2/P